WITHDRAWN
WRIGHT STATE UNIVERSITY LIBRARIES

MEDICAL THERAPY OF ISCHEMIC HEART DISEASE
NITRATES, BETA BLOCKERS, AND CALCIUM ANTAGONISTS

MEDICAL THERAPY OF ISCHEMIC HEART DISEASE

NITRATES, BETA BLOCKERS, AND CALCIUM ANTAGONISTS

EDITED BY

JONATHAN ABRAMS, M.D.
Professor of Medicine, University of
New Mexico School of Medicine, Albuquerque

CARL J. PEPINE, M.D.
Professor of Medicine, University of Florida
College of Medicine; Associate Director,
Division of Cardiology, Shands Hospital, Gainesville

UDHO THADANI, M.B.B.S.
Professor of Medicine, University of Oklahoma College of Medicine;
Director of Clinical Cardiology, and Vice Chief, Cardiovascular Section,
University of Oklahoma Health Sciences Center, Oklahoma City

LITTLE, BROWN AND COMPANY
BOSTON/TORONTO/LONDON

Copyright © 1992 by Jonathan Abrams, Carl J. Pepine, and Udho Thadani

First Edition

All rights reserved. No part of this book may be reproduced in any form or by any electronic or mechanical means, including information storage and retrieval systems, without permission in writing from the publisher, except by a reviewer who may quote brief passages in a review.

Library of Congress Catalog Card No. 91-62510

ISBN 0-316-00471-5

Printed in the United States of America

RRD-VA

CONTENTS

Preface *vii*
Contributing Authors *ix*

1. Pathophysiology of Myocardial Ischemia: Major Clinical Syndromes   1
   Udho Thadani, Edwin G. Olson, and Stephen F. Hamilton

2. Approach to Therapy of Ischemic Heart Disease   37
   Lyle J. Swenson

3. Mechanism of Actions of Nitrates   79
   Jonathan Abrams

4. Mechanism of Actions of Beta Blockers   97
   Edwin G. Olson, Stephen F. Hamilton, and Udho Thadani

5. Mechanism of Actions of Calcium Antagonists   137
   Charles R. Lambert and Carl J. Pepine

6. Pharmacology and Pharmacokinetics of Nitrates   151
   Elizabeth Kowaluk and Ho-Leung Fung

7. Pharmacology and Pharmacokinetics of Beta Blockers   177
   Stephen F. Hamilton, Beth H. Resman-Targoff, Edwin G. Olson, and Udho Thadani

8. Pharmacology and Pharmacokinetics of Calcium Antagonists—Individualized Dosing Regimens and Drug Interactions   207
   Larry M. Lopez and Carl J. Pepine

9. Nitrates in Transient Ischemic Syndromes   233
   Jonathan Abrams

10. Beta Blockers in Transient Ischemic Syndromes   259
    Udho Thadani, Vasu D. Goli, Edwin G. Olson, and Stephen F. Hamilton

11. Calcium Antagonists in Transient Myocardial Ischemic Syndromes and Systemic Hypertension 287
    Deborah A. Jalowiec and Carl J. Pepine

12. The Role of Nitrates in Acute Myocardial Infarction and Post-Infarction 309
    John T. Flaherty

13. The Role of Beta Blockers in Acute Myocardial Infarction and Post-Infarction 329
    Vasu D. Goli, Edwin G. Olson, Stephen F. Hamilton, and Udho Thadani

14. The Role of Calcium Antagonists in Acute Myocardial Infarction and Post-Infarction 355
    Charles R. Lambert and Carl J. Pepine

15. Problems with Nitroglycerin and Nitrates, Including Nitrate Tolerance 369
    Jonathan Abrams

16. Problems with Beta Blocker Therapy 395
    Stephen F. Hamilton, Beth H. Resman-Targoff, Edwin G. Olson, and Udho Thadani

17. Problems with Calcium Antagonist Therapy 427
    Charles R. Lambert and Carl J. Pepine

18. An Approach to Antianginal Drug Therapy 441
    David Hoekenga and Jonathan Abrams

19. When to Use Angioplasty or Bypass Surgery 463
    Barry F. Rose and Carl J. Pepine

    Index 503

PREFACE

Medical Therapy of Ischemic Heart Disease provides a comprehensive overview of the three major classes of antianginal or anti-ischemic drugs: the organic nitrates, the beta-adrenergic blockers, and the calcium channel antagonists. Although revascularization procedures are widely utilized and provide important clinical improvement to many patients with severe coronary disease, the majority of individuals with coronary atherosclerosis do not have coronary bypass surgery or percutaneous coronary angioplasty. In addition, patients who have undergone a revascularization procedure are often required to continue their antianginal medications for a variety of reasons. After coronary revascularization, many patients have a recurrence of angina or other manifestations of ischemia in the months to years following the procedure, and thus require therapy with antianginal drugs. This book provides an updated assessment of the three groups of drugs. A coherent approach to each pharmacologic class has been used; this book should provide a useful comparative analysis for the reader.

In the initial chapters, the *mechanism of actions* and the pertinent clinical *pharmacology* and *pharmacokinetics* of each group of drugs provide an important background for their use in various ischemic syndromes, which is discussed in subsequent chapters. Both *stable* and *unstable angina pectoris* are discussed; it is of interest that all three groups of drugs are used in both types of angina with considerable success. There are interesting and important differences in the results of administering the various anti-ischemic drugs during an *acute myocardial infarction*. Importantly, each of these drug classes may have a role in specific conditions of postinfarct patients. *Adverse effects* as well as nitrate tolerance may limit or preclude the use of one or another drug class for a given disorder. These issues are carefully reviewed.

In the present era, it would be inappropriate to ignore the importance of revascularization for the ischemic syndromes, and this approach to patients is reviewed in the final chapter. However, this discussion is not meant to comprehensively cover the indications for the revascularization techniques or the detailed results of coronary bypass surgery or coronary angioplasty.

Several chapters are designed to provide an overview of the various syndromes of myocardial ischemia and an appropriate overall approach to therapy (Chapters 1, 2, 18, and 19). This information should be useful in placing each of the three drug groups in a clinical perspective when considering coronary revascularization.

We have had considerable experience with clinical research and bedside administration of antianginal drugs. The contributed chapters have been written by a variety of experts who also provide considerable expertise and insight.

J. A.
C. J. P.
U. T.

CONTRIBUTING AUTHORS

JONATHAN ABRAMS, M.D.
Professor of Medicine, University of New Mexico School of Medicine, Albuquerque

JOHN T. FLAHERTY, M.D.
Associate Professor of Medicine, Johns Hopkins University School of Medicine; Attending Physician, Cardiology Division, Johns Hopkins Hospital, Baltimore

HO-LEUNG FUNG, PH.D.
Chairman, Department of Pharmaceutics, State University of New York at Buffalo, Buffalo

VASU D. GOLI, M.D.
Assistant Professor of Medicine, University of Oklahoma College of Medicine; Director of Echocardiography, Cardiology Section, Oklahoma Medical Center, Oklahoma City

STEPHEN F. HAMILTON, PHARM.D.
Associate Professor of Pharmacy Practice, and Adjunct Associate Professor of Medicine, University of Oklahoma College of Pharmacy; Clinical Pharmacist, Oklahoma Medical Center, Oklahoma City

DAVID HOEKENGA, M.D.
Former Professor of Medicine, University of New Mexico School of Medicine, Albuquerque; Private Practice in Cardiology, Las Cruces

DEBORAH A. JALOWIEC, M.D.
Instructor, Department of Medicine, University of Florida College of Medicine; Attending Physician, Division of Cardiology, Shands Hospital, Gainesville

ELIZABETH KOWALUK, PH.D.
Research Associate, Department of Pharmaceutics, State University of New York at Buffalo, Buffalo

CHARLES R. LAMBERT, M.D., PH.D.
Abraham Mitchell Chair in Invasive Cardiology, University of South Alabama College of Medicine, Mobile

LARRY M. LOPEZ, PHARM.D.
Associate Professor of Pharmacy and Medicine, University of Florida; Clinical Pharmacist, Division of Cardiology, Veterans Administration Medical Center, Gainesville

EDWIN G. OLSON, M.D.
Associate Professor of Medicine, University of Oklahoma College of Medicine; Director of Cardiac Center, Cardiology Section, Oklahoma Medical Center, Oklahoma City

CARL J. PEPINE, M.D.
Professor of Medicine, University of Florida College of Medicine; Associate Director, Division of Cardiology, Shands Hospital, Gainesville

BETH H. RESMAN-TARGOFF, PHARM.D.
Clinical Assistant Professor of Pharmacy Practice, University of Oklahoma College of Pharmacy; Clinical Pharmacist, Oklahoma Medical Center, Oklahoma City

BARRY F. ROSE, M.D.
Clinical Assistant Professor, Department of Medicine, Memorial University of Newfoundland Faculty of Medicine, St. John's, Newfoundland

LYLE J. SWENSON, M.D.
Assistant Professor of Medicine, University of Minnesota School of Medicine, Minneapolis; Attending Physician, St. Paul-Ramsey Medical Center, St. Paul

UDHO THADANI, M.B.B.S.
Professor of Medicine, University of Oklahoma College of Medicine; Director of Clinical Cardiology, and Vice Chief, Cardiovascular Section, University of Oklahoma Health Sciences Center, Oklahoma City

MEDICAL THERAPY OF ISCHEMIC HEART DISEASE
NITRATES, BETA BLOCKERS, AND CALCIUM ANTAGONISTS

Notice
The indications and dosages of all drugs in this book have been recommended in the medical literature and conform to the practices of the general medical community. The medications described do not necessarily have specific approval by the Food and Drug Administration for use in the diseases and dosages for which they are recommended. The package insert for each drug should be consulted for use and dosage as approved by the FDA. Because standards for usage change, it is advisable to keep abreast of revised recommendations, particularly those concerning new drugs.

CHAPTER 1

PATHOPHYSIOLOGY OF MYOCARDIAL ISCHEMIA: MAJOR CLINICAL SYNDROMES

UDHO THADANI
EDWIN G. OLSON
STEPHEN F. HAMILTON

A normally functioning heart is able to increase its output and, hence, coronary blood flow in response to its metabolic requirements. Inadequate coronary blood flow to a region of the heart in relation to the regional myocardial oxygen and metabolic requirements reduces oxygen delivery to the mitochondria and results in myocardial ischemia. The latter differs from myocardial hypoxia in that, in addition to oxygen deprivation, there is accumulation of toxic metabolites due to impaired blood flow only during myocardial ischemia.

The most common predisposing underlying factor responsible for myocardial ischemia is narrowing of the coronary arteries due to atherosclerosis. The atherosclerotic plaque may rupture or fissure. This may lead to aggregation of platelets, thrombus formation, and spasm, with resultant cessation or reduction of blood flow in the involved vessel. Myocardial ischemia may occasionally occur in the presence of normal coronary arteries either due to a marked increase in myocardial oxygen demand or a reduction in blood flow secondary to the spasm of epicardial coronary arteries, thrombosis, increased blood viscosity, hypercoagulable state, small vessel disease, or coronary artery embolization.

Ischemic heart disease, due to all etiologies but especially due to underlying atherosclerosis, is the leading cause of morbidity and mortality in the Western world. In the United States, it accounts for an annual mortality of more than 600,000 and much morbidity in the form of stable and unstable angina, myocardial infarction, ischemic cardiomyopathy, and heart failure.

This chapter discusses the regulation of coronary blood flow, factors that determine myocardial oxygen requirement, pathogenesis of myocardial ischemia in general and in various clinical ischemic syndromes, and therapy guidelines for different clinical syndromes.

MYOCARDIAL OXYGEN CONSUMPTION (UPTAKE)

The heart is an aerobic organ that needs oxygen in order to oxidize substances and produce energy for contraction and other functions. Heart work, comprised of pressure work and kinetic work, is not analogous to myocardial oxygen consumption. Only a certain fraction of oxygen consumption and ATP production is translated into mechanical work [55]. A great deal is spent on heat production, which keeps the temperature of the body above environmental values. Under normal circumstances, pressure work, which approximates peak systolic pressure and cardiac output [70], is the major component of the work performed by the heart, while kinetic work, which depends on the cardiac output, blood viscosity, cross-sectional area of the major resistance site (aortic valve), and ejection time, contributes little to total work. In aortic stenosis and hypertrophic obstructive cardiomyopathy,

TABLE 1-1. *Determinants of Myocardial Oxygen Demand*

Major
  Heart rate
  Contractility
  Intraventricular pressure in systole
  Ventricular dimension
  Ventricular wall thickness
Minor
  Electrical excitation
  Depolarization
  Maintenance of active state

---

both pressure and kinetic work increase due to an increase in intraventricular pressure and reduction in cross-sectional area of aortic valve or left ventricular outflow tract.

In the resting (basal) state, the oxygen consumption of the beating heart ranges from 8 to 15 ml/minute per 100 grams of tissue and this decreases markedly when contractile function of the heart ceases [90]. Oxygen cost of electrical depolarization is trivial in relation to the cost of contractile activity [77]. The various determinants of myocardial oxygen consumption are shown in Table 1-1. Of these, the most important are heart rate, wall stress (tension), and contractility [15, 117, 122, 132]. Each cardiac cycle requires certain amounts of oxygen. More oxygen will be required as the heart beats faster. The rapid heart rate also increases the force of myocardial contraction (treppe phenomenon or Bowditch staircase phenomenon), which increases myocardial oxygen consumption [10]. Thus, tachycardia from any cause increases myocardial oxygen needs. Wall stress is a more appropriate term than tension, although the terms are used interchangeably. According to Laplace's law, wall stress is directly related to intraventricular pressure and radius and inversely to wall thickness.

$$\text{wall stress} = \frac{\text{pressure} \times \text{radius}}{2 \times \text{wall thickness}}$$

In a spherical or ellipsoidal model (human heart), wall stress is more accurately expressed by the formula:

$$\text{wall stress} = \frac{P \times R_1}{2h (1 + h/2 R_1)}$$

where P = pressure, R_1 = internal radius, and h = wall thickness.

Sarnoff utilized time in the equation and used the term tension time index, that is, the area under the ventricular pressure curve, as the major determinant of oxygen consumption of the contracting heart (Fig. 1-1) [122]. Without knowledge of radius or chamber size and wall thickness, however, the term pressure time index is more accurate than

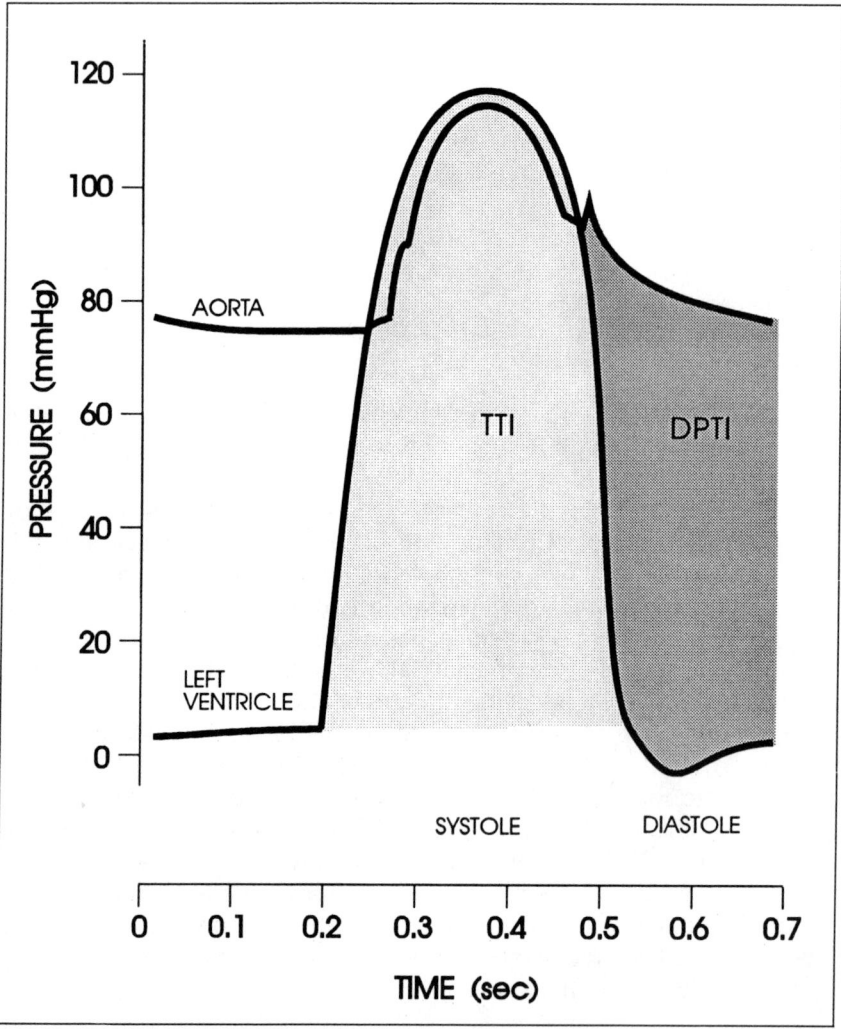

FIG. 1-1. Diagrammatic representation of tension time index (TTI) and diastolic pressure time index (DPTI). TTI in reality is pressure time and is determined by intraventricular systolic pressure and duration of systole which, in turn, is determined by heart rate. Coronary blood flow occurs in diastole and is determined by diastolic arterial pressure and duration of diastole. The ratio of TTI and DPTI is termed *endocardial viability ratio*. (From Ref. 122, with permission.)

tension time index. In clinical situations, it is often difficult to measure the radius and wall thickness of the ventricle and, therefore, one often utilizes pressure time index as the determinant factor for myocardial oxygen uptake. Further, wall stress does not take into account the effect of myocardial contractility, which under increased inotropic stimulation such as physical or mental stress, may be the major determinant of myocardial oxygen demand [132].

Although heart rate, wall stress, and contractility are the primary determinants of myocardial oxygen consumption, in certain pathologic circumstances there may be metabolic oxygen wastage, that is, when fuel supplied to the heart is primarily free fatty acids, which have been shown to increase myocardial oxygen consumption considerably [93].

Variations in tension development, heart rate, and contractility are constantly occurring and regulate mechanical work of the heart. Thus, myocardial oxygen requirements vary widely depending on the physical state of the individual. The variation in mechanical work of the heart is most obvious during physical activity, which enhances sympathetic tone and leads to an increase in heart rate, contractility, and blood pressure. These changes augment myocardial performance at the cost of increased myocardial oxygen uptake, which in normal individuals is balanced by a parallel increase in coronary blood flow and, hence, myocardial oxygen supply. However, in pathological states such as coronary artery stenosis, the increased demand may outstrip the supply, with detrimental consequences.

CORONARY BLOOD FLOW (OXYGEN SUPPLY)

The most important determinant of coronary blood flow is myocardial oxygen demand [5]. This autoregulation of flow helps to maintain variable blood supply and, hence, oxygen supply to the myocardium. Under basal conditions, coronary blood flow varies between 60 to 90 ml/minute per 100 grams of myocadium but can decrease by 50 percent when metabolic requirements decrease, as during total body hypothermia or cardiac arrest.

Under basal conditions, myocardial oxygen extraction is near maximum as indicated by very low coronary sinus blood oxygen saturation. Therefore, an increase in myocardial oxygen supply can be achieved primarily by an increase in coronary blood flow. It has been proposed that the myocardium communicates its oxygen requirements to the coronary arteries by the rate of production of adenosine [7]. The breakdown of high-energy phosphate compounds during increased myocardial oxygen demand produces enough adenosine, which in turn produces coronary vasodilation and, hence, increase in coronary blood flow [47]. The other proposed mechanisms of coronary dilation

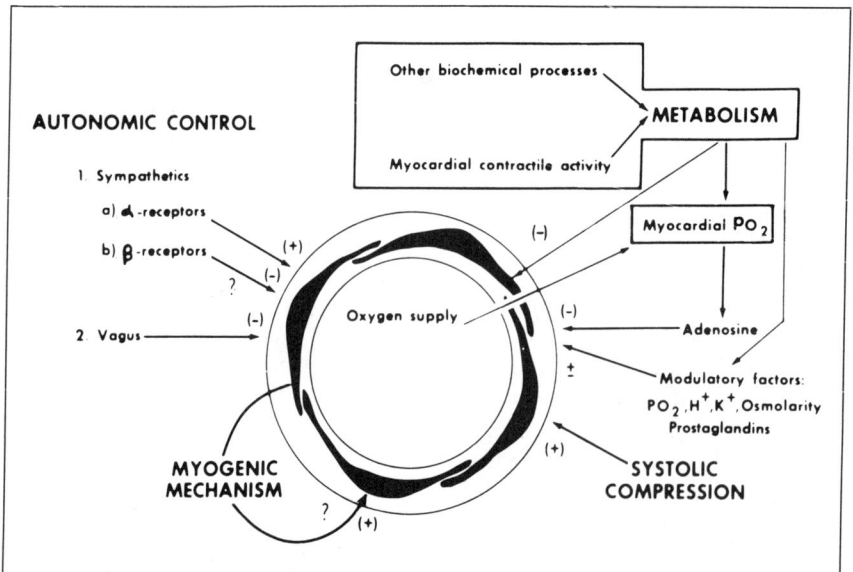

FIG. 1-2. Positive and negative influences of autonomic and metabolic factors on coronary blood flow. Positive factors reduce the arterial lumen, while negative factors increase the arterial lumen. (From Ref. 7, with permission.)

are prostaglandins, protons, and other vasoactive compounds such as potassium and lactate. However, none are as potent as adenosine [16].

In humans, the myocardium is supplied by two coronary arteries, the right and the left. The left coronary artery usually supplies the left ventricle while the right coronary artery supplies the right ventricle, and its posterior descending branch present in 85 percent of subjects supplies the posterior part of the interventricular septum. The main coronary arteries traverse first in the epicardium and have branches that penetrate the myocardium and then branch into smaller arteries and, finally, arterioles and capillaries. The regulation of coronary blood flow occurs at the level of arterioles and precapillary sphincters. The resistance in these vessels is affected by metabolic, neurogenic, myogenic, and hormonal factors (Fig. 1-2) that determine the net myocardial blood flow and, hence, oxygen supply to the myocardium [16]. In addition to the metabolic factors, coronary arteries contain both alpha- and beta-adrenergic receptors; the stimulation of the former produces constriction while stimulation of the latter produces coronary vasodilation [95, 143]. Parasympathetic nerves also control coronary flow and their stimulation usually leads to vasodilation and augmentation in coronary blood flow [48]; a 25 percent increase in blood flow has been documented in animals following pharmacologic blockade [48].

In the normal heart, there are over 2000 capillaries per cubic millimeter; only 60 to 80 percent function normally [153]. When myocardial oxygen tension falls, more capillaries are recruited. This capillary recruitment is important in meeting the increased myocardial oxygen requirements.

In the left ventricle, the throttling effect of the myocardium during systole on the penetrating coronary vessels severely impairs coronary blood flow [13]. The epicardial blood flow is less impaired than the subendocardial flow as the intramyocardial pressure is maximal in the subendocardial region. Therefore, blood flow occurs in the left coronary artery predominantly in diastole (Fig. 1-3) and to a small extent in systole (15 percent) [6]. In contrast, in the right coronary artery, because the right ventricular intramyocardial pressure is low, blood flow occurs both in systole and diastole [6] except in the pathological condition of severe pulmonary hypertension when diastolic blood flow in the right coronary artery becomes predominant. Very low coronary blood flow in systole in the left ventricle induces vasodilation in the subendocardial vessels and augments blood flow in diastole and, thus, the 1:1 endocardial to epicardial flow is maintained [59]. Subendocardial blood flow in the left ventricle is also influenced by the end-diastolic pressure in the left ventricle, which if high can impede blood flow to the subendocardial regions. The net coronary flow in diastole is determined by the perfusion pressure, which, in the case of the left coronary artery, is the difference between the diastolic coronary arterial pressure (or aortic diastolic pressure in the absence of coronary stenosis) and the coronary sinus pressure, which, in turn, is influenced by the right atrial pressure. In the case of the right coronary artery, the perfusion pressure is the difference between the systolic or diastolic blood pressure in the right coronary artery and the right ventricular systolic or end-diastolic pressures, respectively. In the left ventricle, coronary blood flow is determined by the diastolic pressure time index (DPTI), which is the area under the aortic pressure curve during diastole (Fig. 1-1).

In the normal heart, changes in perfusion pressure vary coronary blood flow only transiently and, thus, autoregulation of coronary arteries plays a dominant role in maintaining coronary flow at various perfusion pressures. This autoregulation is brought about by changes in resistance at the level of precapillary sphincters and arterioles and by capillary recruitment or capillary shutoff. When perfusion pressure decreases, arterioles dilate and resistance falls, with resultant increase in flow. An opposite situation arises when perfusion pressure increases.

Since the coronary blood flow occurs predominantly in diastole, the duration of diastole assumes great importance; the longer the diastole, the greater the flow. Thus, tachycardia not only increases myocardial oxygen requirement but also can decrease coronary blood flow during each cardiac cycle.

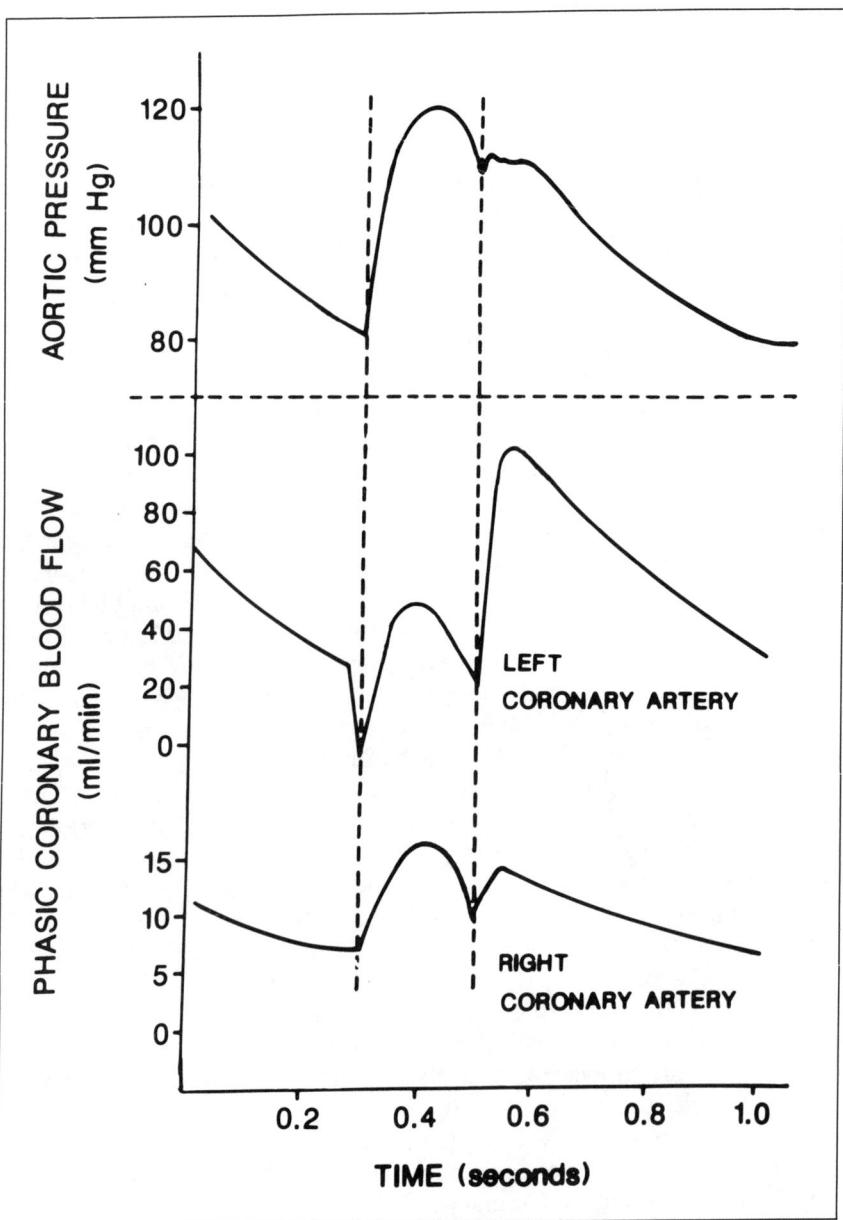

FIG. 1-3. Right and left coronary artery blood flow in relation to aortic blood pressure. (From Berne, R. M. and Levy, M. B., *Cardiovascular Physiology*, 22nd Ed., St. Louis: CV Mosby Co., 1972, with permission.)

MYOCARDIAL ISCHEMIA

An imbalance between myocardial oxygen requirement and myocardial oxygen supply leads to myocardial ischemia (Fig. 1-4). The consequences are produced by the lack of oxygen and the accumulation of metabolites due to a relative or absolute lack of blood flow. Although myocardial ischemia can occur in the presence of normal coronary arteries, the most common underlying mechanism is coronary atherosclerosis, which produces narrowing of the coronary arteries. The latter increases resistance to blood flow across the stenosis. The resistance increases by a power of four as the radius decreases (Poiseuillie's law), so that reducing the internal diameter by 70 to 80 or 90 percent dramatically elevates the resistance (Fig. 1-5) [78]. Basal coronary flow falls when the luminal area is reduced by 90 percent or more [58]. With a reduction in coronary blood flow, there is a compensatory vasodilation in the ischemic bed. However, the maximal vasodilatory reserve is impaired in the presence of coronary stenosis producing a 50 percent reduction in luminal area, or greater [78].

The length of stenosis also plays an important role in determining coronary blood flow. Stenosis of more than 5 mm and multiple stenosis in the same coronary artery have more profound deleterious effects on coronary flow than single stenosis of less than 5 mm [49]. When atherosclerosis is eccentric, normal portions of the coronary artery can undergo dynamic changes in tone, which, if augmented, can produce critical stenosis (Fig. 1-6). When stenosis is severe, poststenotic perfusion pressure may decrease beyond the critical level of 50 mmHg with loss of autoregulation by failure of compensatory vasodilation [78]. This further robs the blood flow in an already ischemic myocardium with resultant severe subendocardial or even transmural ischemia.

The net coronary flow in the presence of coronary stenosis is not only determined by the net perfusion pressure but also by the presence or absence of collaterals to the ischemic region [65].

Severe myocardial ischemia also leads to contractile failure of the myocardium with resultant increase in left ventricular diastolic pressure and increase in resistance to the blood flow in the subendocardial tissue.

An alternate mechanism of reduction in coronary artery flow is coronary artery spasm, which occurs primarily at the site of epicardial vessels that may be normal or involved with atherosclerosis [87]. Spasm, when extreme, may cause complete cessation of flow with transmural ischemia, but gradation of spasm can occur with variable effects.

Within 30 seconds of coronary occlusion, there is loss of contractility coincident with a decline in myocardial oxygen tension; the marginal zone contracts weakly, whereas the nonischemic myocardium exhibits a compensatory increase in its force of contraction [73]. However, cessation of coronary blood flow for less than 15 minutes produces only

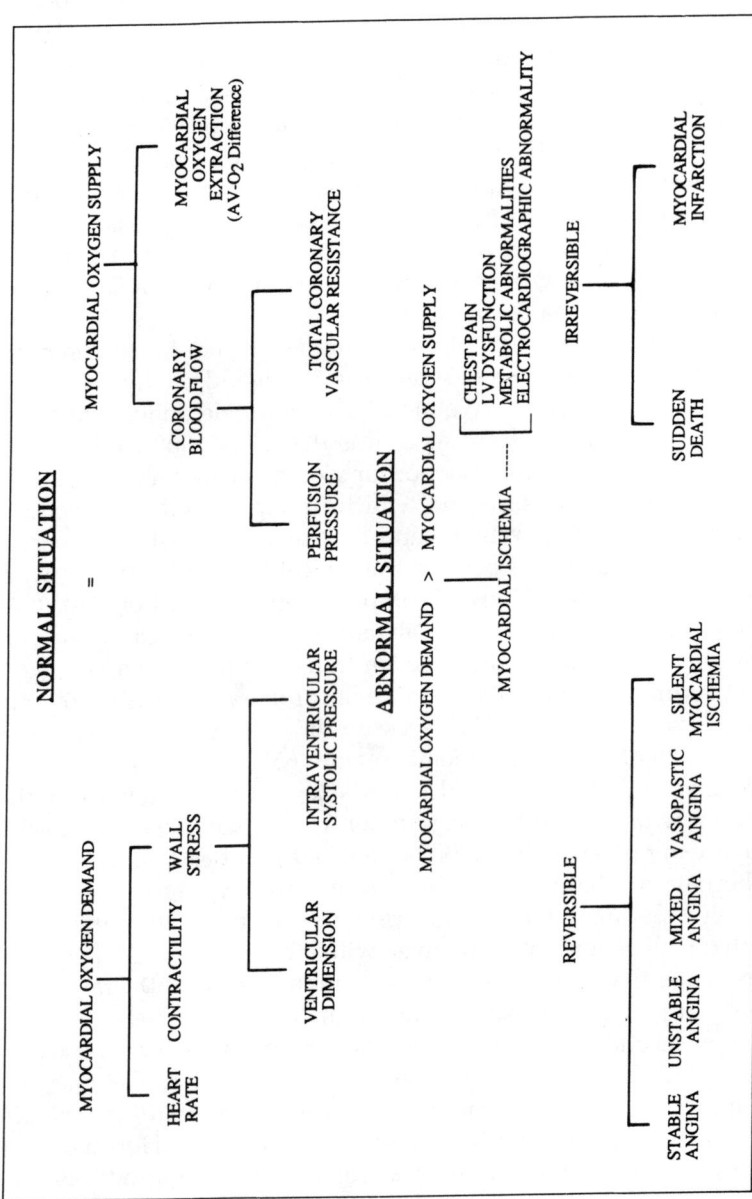

FIG. 1-4. Myocardial oxygen demand and supply under normal and abnormal situations. Relative increase in myocardial oxygen demand (MVO_2) due to either an increase in MVO_2 or actual reduction in coronary blood flow produces myocardial ischemia.

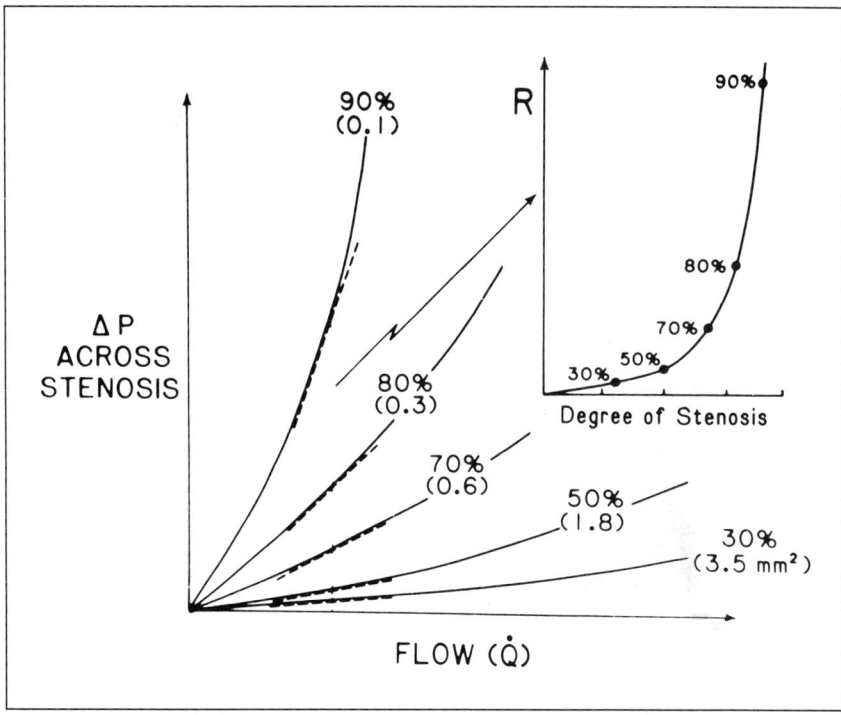

FIG. 1-5. The effect of the severity of coronary stenosis (internal diameter) and flow on vascular resistance (R). (From Ref. 25, with permission.)

reversible ischemia, but when flow is interrupted for more than 15 minutes, irreversible changes occur and the extent of damage is dependent on the duration of interruption of blood flow and the presence or absence of collateral blood flow to the ischemic region [68].

The results of myocardial ischemia in humans are determined by the territory supplied by the stenotic or blocked coronary artery and the extent of collateral vessels. Since collateral vessels are not always visible and there is an overlap of flow by two adjacent branches of coronary arteries, the ischemic area produced by coronary obstruction is always less than the area supplied by the obstructed vessel. Because subendocardial regions are more vulnerable, ischemia initially starts in the subendocardial region and advances eventually to the subepicardial region (an advancing wave front phenomenon) (Fig. 1-7) [113]. With branch arterial narrowing, subendocardial flow falls at about 25 percent occlusion with metabolic changes developing at about 60 percent occlusion and contractility and ECG changes at 75 percent occlusion [58]. With major artery occlusion, such events occur at about 25 to 40 percent flow reduction [58].

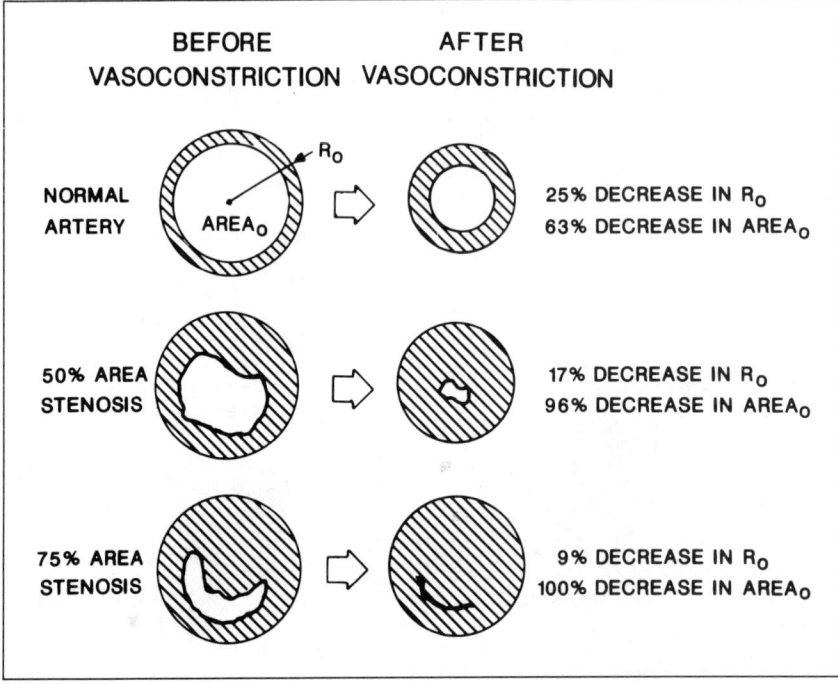

FIG. 1-6. Effect of changes in vasomotor tone on radius and area. In a diseased vessel, minor changes in external diameter can produce critical stenosis of normal and diseased coronary artery. (From Ref. 82, with permission.)

PATHOGENESIS OF ISCHEMIC HEART DISEASE IN HUMANS

In humans, atherosclerosis, thrombus, spasm, and embolism alone or in combination play a major role in the pathogenesis of ischemic heart disease. Various clinical syndromes are produced depending on the chronicity or suddenness of the coronary occlusive lesions.

Atherosclerosis is the major disease affecting the coronary arteries. The lesions may vary from fatty streaks to complicated plaques [154]. Fatty streaks are focal accumulation of lipid-laden smooth muscle cells that are believed by some to be the earliest lesions of atherosclerosis. How these fatty streaks progress to complicated plaques is not known. Fibrous plaque is a more advanced lesion and is composed of lipid-laden myointimal cells and collagen fibers. These may produce luminal narrowing. The most advanced lesion is the complicated plaque, which is both a proliferative and degenerative lesion. It is composed of fibrous tissue, fibrin, necrotic debris, intra- and extracellular lipid and focal calcification. It is an amorphous material with raised surface that occludes the arterial lumen to a variable degree. Complicated plaques are

1. PATHOPHYSIOLOGY OF MYOCARDIAL ISCHEMIA

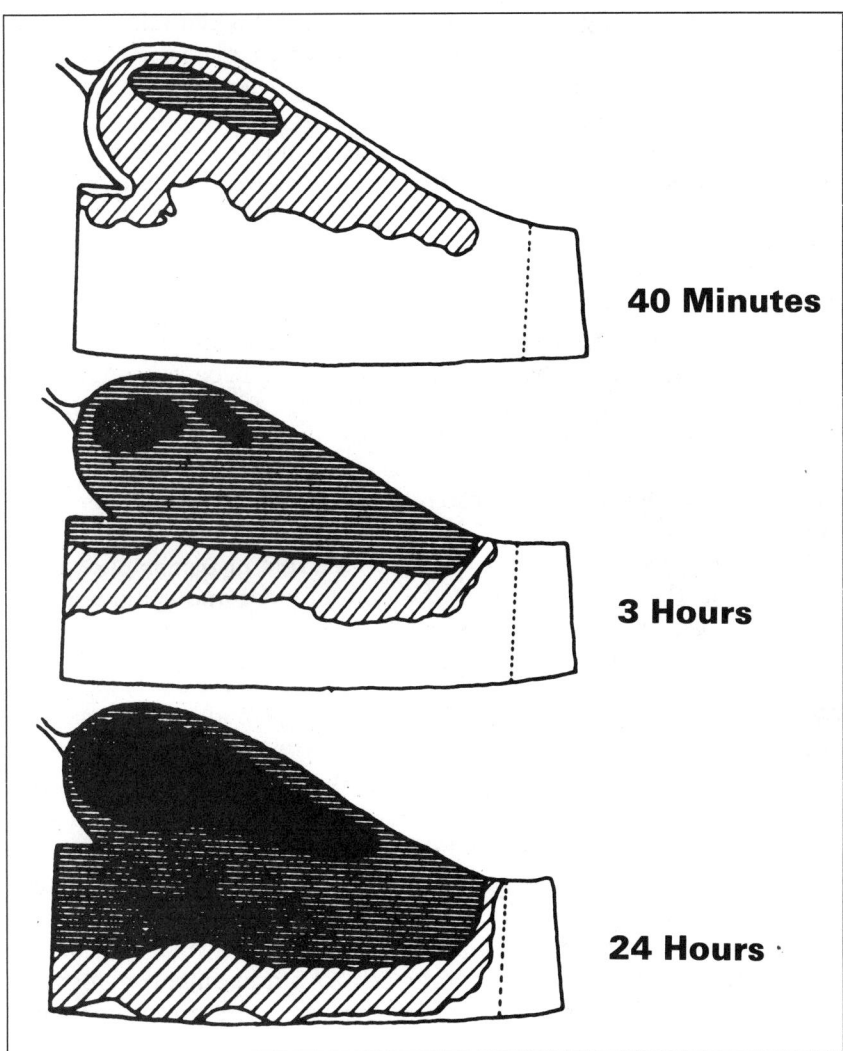

FIG. 1-7. Progression of the wavefront of ischemic cell death with respect to duration of coronary occlusion. Necrosis (*all shaded areas*) progresses from subendocardial to subepicardial regions with time. (From Ref. 113, with permission.)

invariably covered by a fibrous cap that overlies a central, frequently degenerated liquified core. It is the complicated plaque that is most often associated with plaque rupture, fissuring, hemorrhage, endothelial damage, and mural thrombosis [115].

The pathogenesis of the atherosclerotic plaque still remains controversial. Mechanical injury, internal hemorrhage, lipid accumulation, thrombosis, and encrustation have all been implicated. Myocyte migration to the intima also plays a major role in the pathogenesis of atherosclerosis. Lipogenic theory has been proposed on the basis of production of lesions in experimental animals fed high-lipid diets [133]. But the lesions produced are more akin to lipid storage disease rather than complicated lesions of atherosclerosis. The only analogous condition in humans to the experimental lesions perhaps is atherosclerotic disease seen in familial hypercholesterolemia where deficiency of LDL receptors in the liver and elsewhere leads to excessively high cholesterol levels [18]. But how the raised cholesterol level produces atherosclerosis is not fully established.

The thrombogenic theory emphasizes the role of platelet and fibrin thrombi and the endothelium in the development and progression of atherosclerosis plaques [96]. Previous and recent evidence suggests that this mechanism may be more important than realized.

Nonatherosclerotic Ischemic Heart Disease

Coronary artery embolism may occur with previously normal or diseased coronary arteries. Emboli usually arise from within the heart from a transmural thrombus, platelet thrombi on the valves or the left atrium as in atrial fibrillation, or valvular heart disease. However, distal platelet emboli in the coronary arteries arise often from the proximal complicated atherosclerotic plaque [35].

Coronary artery dissection is a rare entity but spontaneous or traumatic dissection may abruptly occlude the artery and produce myocardial ischemia [21].

Coronary artery spasm is a more common etiology of myocardial ischemia than previously recognized [87]. The site of spasm is usually the epicardial portion of the coronary arteries, which may or may not be involved with the atherosclerotic process. Spasm is usually transient but often recurrent and produces reversible myocardial ischemia. Rarely spasm is prolonged and may lead to myocardial infarction [101]. Spasm of small coronary vessels has been reported in scleroderma heart disease [20].

The mechanism by which coronary artery spasm is produced still remains a subject of great debate and speculation. Platelet aggregation is known to release substances that trigger potent endothelial-dependent inhibitory responses of the smooth muscle in the media. Thromboxane A_2, released by the platelets, increases coronary smooth muscle contraction, which is not endothelial-dependent and may explain spasm in both the normal and atherosclerotic coronary arteries [141]. However, cyclo-oxygenase inhibitors do not alter response of coronaries to aggregating platelets [141]. Serotonin, released by platelets, may produce coronary artery contraction, but serotonin blocker katenserin does not prevent coronary artery spasm [141]. Other substances that have been implicated are adenosine nucleolide ADP, ATP, and platelet activating factor [141]. In the absence of endothelium or damaged vessel, platelet aggregation and thrombin produce local contraction and decrease of coronary artery lumen [72]. Excessive alpha-adrenergic stimulation or increase in parasympathetic tone has also been implicated but remains speculative in the pathogenesis of spasm [155].

Current evidence suggests that arterial spasm is multifactorial in origin and can invariably be induced by intravenous ergonovine and reversed by intravenous or intracoronary nitrates and calcium channel blocking agents. It has been suggested that there exists a local coronary supersensitivity to diverse vasoconstriction stimuli that accounts for spasm in the epicardial arteries [141].

Coronary Thrombosis
Recent studies have clearly documented that coronary thrombosis plays an important role in the causation of both reversible and irreversible ischemic myocardial syndromes [27, 41, 53]. In the presence of atherosclerotic coronary artery disease, fissuring or rupture of a complicated plaque exposes the raw arterial intima and media to platelets and blood constitutes; platelets aggregate and thrombi and fibrin are deposited at the raw surface. The thrombus so formed may lyse spontaneously or may progress with complete occlusion of the vessel. The result would be reversible ischemia if clot lysis occurs spontaneously, but permanent damage will result if thrombus does not lyse. In the pathogenesis of thrombosis, factor VII, thrombi, and fibrinogen all play a major role both in the presence and absence of atherosclerotic coronary artery disease [91].

Diminished Coronary Vascular Flow Reserve
In the presence of normal coronary arteries, myocardial ischemia may still occur due to an abnormally high resistance at the level of small coronary arteries or arterioles with a reduction in maximum coronary vascular flow reserve. In this situation, the increase in myocardial oxygen demand during stress cannot be matched by an increase in supply. In some patients with hypertension, aortic stenosis, or hypertrophic cardiomyopathy, this mechanism has been shown to account for myocardial ischemia in the presence of normal coronary arteries [45, 108]. Similar mechanism has been shown to operate in some patients who do not have thick ventricles but experience classical angina pectoris in

the presence of normal coronary arteries [103]. This syndrome has been called syndrome X by some workers [71].

Intermittent Platelet Aggregation

In the presence of coronary obstruction, intermittent reductions in flow may occur due to platelet aggregates at the site of stenosis. Phasic flow reductions have been well documented in animal experiments where coronary stenosis has been produced by external compression [50], and there is evidence of a similar phenomenon in humans [36]. Washout of platelet plug may cause distil embolization and myocardial damage [35].

Platelet aggregation at the atherosclerotic or damaged vessel site releases vasoactive substances that may produce coronary artery spasm and further reduction of blood flow to the ischemic regions [141].

MANIFESTATIONS OF MYOCARDIAL ISCHEMIA

Depending on the severity, duration, and extent of ischemic period, there may be reversible or irreversible myocardial damage with resultant biochemical, mechanical, electrocardiographic, and clinical consequences. Thus, myocardial ischemia may be transient (reversible) or permanent (irreversible).

Reversible Myocardial Ischemia

Reversible myocardial ischemia is manifested by reduction in regional contractility secondary to a reduction in ATP levels [62]. Subsequently, there is impairment in diastolic relaxation [144], and leakage of K^+ from the myocardium cells is responsible for changes of action potential and ST segment shifts [148]. Anaerobic metabolism is responsible for accumulation of lactate and H^+ ions, which further impair systolic function [32]. Subendocardial ischemia produces ST segment depression while transmural ischemia causes ST segment elevation; reversal of ischemia leads to normalization of processes but myocardial stunning with depressed function or biochemical abnormalities may persist for minutes or hours [14].

In animals, complete occlusion of a vessel for up to 15 minutes leads to depletion of ATP stores and accumulation of metabolites [68]. These changes produce depression of contractile and diastolic function of the ventricle but no tissue necrosis occurs when flow is restored, although ATP stores may remain depleted for several minutes and systolic dysfunction may persist for a long time.

In humans, the clinical examples of transient reversible ischemia are: (1) stable angina pectoris, (2) unstable angina, (3) variant angina, (4) mixed angina, and (5) silent myocardial ischemia. Although these clinical syndromes are the end result of reversible myocardial ischemia, the pathogenesis for these syndromes varies widely.

Stable Angina Pectoris

The term *angina pectoris* was first used by Heberden in 1772 to describe a strangling feeling localized in the retrosternal and substernal regions [63]. The pain was usually intermittent and often precipitated by activity. Now we use the term stable angina pectoris to describe ischemic myocardial pain that is substernal, retrosternal, or transternal in location and may radiate to the neck or left arm and sometimes to the right arm or back. The pain is usually precipitated by activity or emotional upset and is relieved after discontinuation of activity or ingestion of a sublingual nitroglycerin. By definition, the frequency of angina episodes has been stable without deterioration for at least a period of 3 to 6 months. A good history will document this fact.

Pathophysiology of Stable Angina

The underlying cause of stable angina is invariably atherosclerotic coronary artery disease. Because of coronary artery narrowing, coronary blood flow is restricted and cannot increase in proportion to increase in myocardial oxygen demand. In a majority of the patients, angina can be reproduced by exercise at identical workloads and rate pressure product [116]. However, in some patients angina threshold may vary from day to day [46]. As the severity of disease worsens, effort tolerance decreases progressively and it may be difficult to avoid angina even with minimal effort like brushing the teeth or toweling. Thus, the major pathogenetic factor for stable angina is an increase in myocardial oxygen demand in the presence of relatively fixed coronary blood supply (Fig. 1-8). In some patients, an increase in coronary tone during exercise may bring out a reduction in blood flow and aggravate ischemia [54].

The mechanism by which pain is produced is not known but may be related to stretching of the ischemic myocardium or stimulation of the nerve endings due to accumulation of metabolites or a change in the pH.

During an episode of angina pectoris, there is often evidence of subendocardial ischemia manifested by ST segment depression and when the territory of ischemia is large, one may observe changes in systolic and diastolic function. Depending on the extent of ischemia, global ejection fraction may or may not decrease but regional function often shows some abnormality.

The overall prognosis of patients with stable angina pectoris is relatively good, with an annual mortality of 1.6 to 3.3 percent [94]. High-risk groups can usually be identified by exercise testing, assessment of

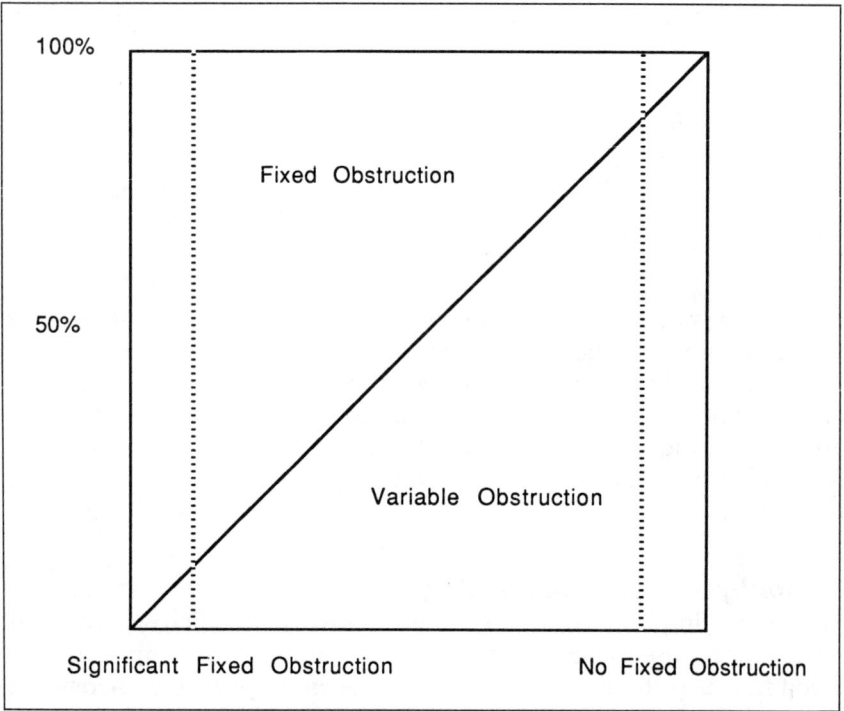

FIG. 1-8. Relationship between fixed and variable (dynamic) coronary obstruction in the production of myocardial ischemia in patients with stable, unstable, and variant angina. In patients with stable angina, fixed obstruction plays a major role, while in patients with unstable angina, variable obstruction due to intermittent platelet or thrombotic occlusion plays a major role. In patients with variant angina, spasm plays a dominant role in production of ischemia.

left ventricular function at rest and during exercise, and coronary anatomy [11, 22, 28, 127].

Treatment Strategy for Stable Angina

The treatment strategy for patients with stable angina pectoris is to lower myocardial oxygen demand and/or to increase coronary blood flow to the ischemic region. Nitrates, by reducing ventricular dimension, reduce wall stress. By dilating the eccentrically stenotic artery and collateral vessels, nitrates may improve coronary blood flow to the ischemic areas [17, 56, 89, 136]. Beta adrenoceptor blocking drugs reduce myocardial oxygen demand by reducing heart rate and contractility [110, 131]. These agents also attenuate the rise in systolic blood pressure during exercise [137]. Calcium channel blocking agents work primarily by reducing afterload and contractility but may also dilate stenotic arteries and improve coronary blood flow [12].

In patients who remain symptomatic despite pharmacologic therapy, it is necessary to consider other alternatives such as coronary angioplasty [67] or coronary bypass surgery, procedures that usually increase coronary blood flow [127].

Some patients with classical exertional angina do not have underlying coronary artery disease. In these patients, recent evidence suggests that there is impairment in maximum coronary flow reserve due to an abnormally high tone in the arterioles or precapillary sphincters [45, 71, 103, 108]. Some of these patients also have small vessel disease that cannot be visualized by conventional angiography. These patients have been shown to have diminished coronary flow reserve during pharmacologic vasodilation induced by agents like dyprimadole or papaverine [45, 108]. In this group of patients, calcium channel antagonists and nitrates may be effective for symptomatic relief. The long-term prognosis is usually excellent in the absence of any obstructive coronary artery disease. In patients with hypertrophic cardiomyopathy with diminished coronary flow reserve and diastolic dysfunction who have angina pectoris, beta blockers and/or verapamil are more effective [118], while vasodilators may aggravate the outflow tract obstruction by reflexly increasing the contractility.

In a minority of patients with stable angina and severe obstructive coronary artery disease, a superimposed coronary artery spasm may compromise flow; this has been recently documented during exercise [54]. Whether this represents a spasm or collapse of an artery due to alterations in perfusion pressure distal to the stenosis in response to diminishing myocardial oxygen requirements in an ischemic segment remains unknown at the present time [76]. If spasm is suggested, nitrates and calcium channel antagonists are often the drugs of choice.

Some patients with severe aortic regurgitation and normal coronary arteries may experience angina. This can be explained on the basis of raised left ventricular end-diastolic pressure and reduced flow in diastole in the coronary arteries due to aortic regurgitation. The treatment in such patients is usually aortic valve replacement.

Unstable Angina Pectoris

The clinical syndrome of unstable angina is secondary to reversible myocardial ischemia. Unstable angina has been used to describe four entities [24, 126]: (1) progressive or crescendo angina in a patient with a previous history of stable angina; (2) angina of recent onset precipitated by minimal exertion; (3) angina at rest during which pain lasts more than 15 minutes and may or may not be relieved by sublingual nitroglycerin; this form has also been called preinfarction angina or intermediate syndrome; and (4) angina occurring within 4 weeks of acute myocardial infarction (postinfarction angina). Although it is desirable to document ST-T wave changes during an episode of pain,

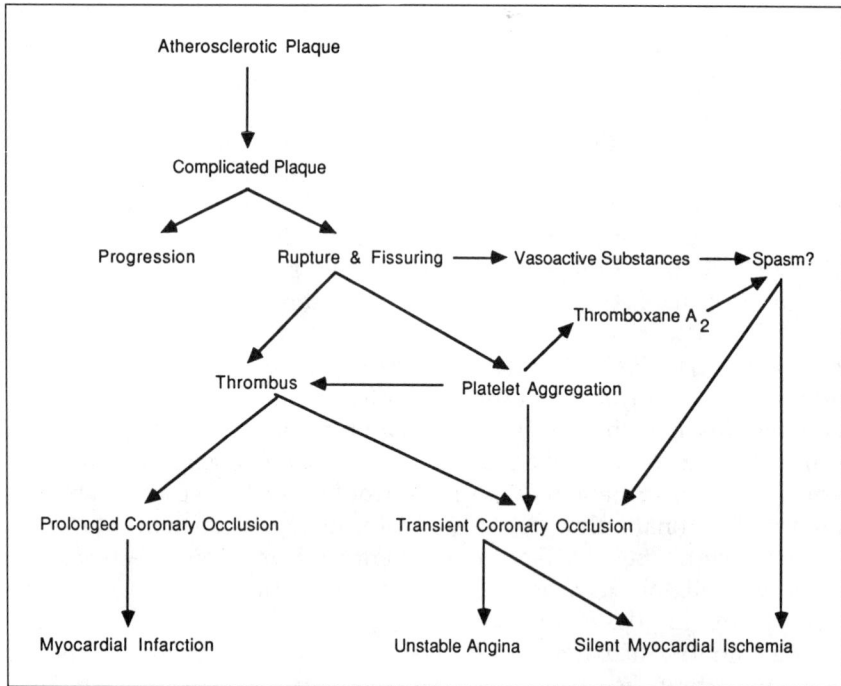

FIG. 1-9. Role of plaque progression, rupture or fissuring, platelets, and thrombus in myocardial ischemic syndromes, unstable angina, and myocardial infarction.

some patients with unstable angina may experience pain without electrocardiographic changes.

Pathophysiology of Unstable Angina Pectoris

There is convincing evidence that primary reduction in myocardial oxygen supply due to a reduction in coronary blood flow plays a major role in the majority of patients with unstable angina and especially in those with rest angina [27, 53, 129]. The reduction in coronary blood flow is brought about by a complex interaction between the platelet aggregation or thrombus formation at the complicated atherosclerotic plaque site and alterations in coronary vasomotor tone (Fig. 1-9).

Recent data suggests that increased platelet aggregation and thrombus formation at the site of atherosclerotic plaque that has undergone recent fissuring or progression plays the predominant role in producing the syndrome of unstable angina [2, 129, 152]. The waxing and waning nature of thrombus accounts for variable prognosis in this group of patients. Although coronary artery spasm has been claimed to play a major role [84], several observations suggest otherwise: (1) a recent report of higher mortality after nifedipine therapy, a drug known to relieve coronary artery spasm in comparison to either placebo therapy or a combination of beta blocker–nitrate therapy in patients with unstable angina [114]; (2) high incidence of subsequent myocardial infarction and death despite aggressive medical treatment with calcium channel antagonists [97]; and (3) reduction in mortality and morbidity with antiplatelet and antithrombotic agents [81].

In some patients with unstable angina, especially in those with progressive or recent onset angina, increase in myocardial oxygen demand rather than a decrease in coronary blood flow via the increase in heart rate, blood pressure, or myocardial contractility may precipitate ischemic episodes [112, 120].

The incidence of severity of coronary artery disease in unstable angina is similar to that of stable angina, with the exception that a 10 to 12 percent incidence of left main coronary artery disease and a 10 to 13 percent incidence of normal coronary arteries has been reported [109]. The remaining patients have one-, two-, or three-vessel disease.

Treatment Strategy in Unstable Angina

Based on current data, the initial treatment strategy for all patients with unstable angina should be the use of aspirin or intravenous heparin, provided there are no contraindications. Symptomatic treatment with nitrates to reduce myocardial oxygen demand and wall stress, and beta blockers and calcium channel antagonists to reduce myocardial oxygen demand is also justified. Nitrates and calcium channel antagonists reduce vascular tone and coronary artery spasm and thus may benefit patients who experience myocardial ischemia due to phasic alterations in coronary tone.

The final treatment plan should be made on the basis of underlying coronary anatomy and pathophysiology of unstable angina pectoris. However, current evidence would favor use of aspirin [25, 81] or anticoagulants [135] for the short and intermediate management of these patients until the condition stabilizes. Trials with thrombolytic agents in a small number of patients have produced conflicting reports. Routine coronary bypass surgery is not warranted in view of similar medical and surgical mortality and myocardial infarction rates over a 10-year period in patients with unstable angina [121]. High-risk groups can usually be detected either by exercise testing or by coronary angiography. In those with critical proximal stenosis and poor left ventricular function or left main disease, coronary bypass surgery may be warranted. In selected patients, coronary angioplasty may be indicated but it is preferable to delay this procedure as reocclusion and complication rate during urgent angioplasty is high [39].

Variant (Vasospastic) Angina Pectoris
This syndrome was first described by Prinzmetal [111] and is also referred to as vasospastic angina. It is characterized by pain at rest with associated ST elevation due to transmural myocardial ischemia but at times there is only ST segment depression [30, 87]. The pain is usually episodic and occurs at night and may wake the patient from sleep. Pain may last several minutes. In some patients pain may be brought on by exertion, but in a majority of the patients exercise performance is usually normal. Painful episodes may recur for several weeks or months and then may disappear spontaneously [128, 147]. In 85 percent of patients, there is evidence of underlying atherosclerosis while the rest may have normal-looking arteries, although one cannot with certainty exclude minor degrees of atherosclerosis.

Pathophysiology of Variant Angina
There is good evidence to suggest that the syndrome is produced by focal spasm of epicardial coronary artery or arteries [141]. However, the mechanism that triggers spasm still remains speculative. A local hypersensitivity of a segment of a coronary artery to various stimuli of a nonspecific nature is responsible for spasm [141].

Treatment Strategy for Variant Angina
In the absence of specific etiology, the treatment for this syndrome is prevention or abolition of spasm with drugs such as nitrates or calcium channel antagonists. In patients who are refractory to pharmacologic therapy and have severe proximal coronary artery disease, coronary bypass surgery or angioplasty may be warranted. In the absence of obstructive coronary artery disease, it is rare for these patients to have a myocardial infarction [141], although occasional cases have been reported [101, 141]. Sudden release of spasm, which occurs invariably after an episode of spasm, makes these patients especially prone to reperfusion ventricular arrhythmias.

Mixed Angina Pectoris
Some patients with angina pectoris do not fit into any of the categories described earlier. They may have classical exertional angina, but in addition may also experience resting chest pain or their exercise tolerance may vary on the same day or on different days [86].

Pathophysiology of Mixed Angina
The fact that coronary artery atherosclerosis is often eccentric allows one to speculate that the normal segment of the coronary artery may undergo episodic changes in tone or undergo spasm. This dynamic nature of coronary arteries can reduce the noncritical stenosis to a critical stenosis (Fig. 1-6) with resultant myocardial ischemia even at rest or low levels of exercise. It is now recognized that this syndrome is more

common than originally thought [86]. However, one cannot be absolutely sure if the variation in angina threshold is due to an increase in coronary artery tone or spasm, intermittent platelet aggregation, or thrombosis at the atherosclerotic plaque site.

Treatment Strategy for Mixed Angina
Treatment with agents that reduce myocardial oxygen demand and drugs that decrease coronary artery tone is usually effective. In patients who do not respond, addition of aspirin is desirable. If patients still remain symptomatic, a more aggressive approach is indicated.

Silent Myocardial Ischemia
Originally, silent myocardial ischemia was used for electrocardiographic ST segment depression or elevation during ambulatory monitoring in the absence of symptoms [134]. The definition has been broadened to include ST changes, a fall in ejection fraction, or an abnormal thallium myocardial uptake during exercise in asymptomatic patients. Recent studies have shown that silent myocradial ischemia occurs more frequently than episodes associated with symptoms [38, 130]; an incidence as high as 80 percent has been reported in patients with stable angina pectoris [38].

Pathophysiology of Silent Myocardial Ischemia
Some of the episodes of silent ischemia on a 24-hour Holter monitor are due to an increase in myocardial oxygen demand as evidenced by an increase in heart rate and/or blood pressure; many episodes are, however, recorded in the absence of an increase in heart rate or blood pressure [38, 107]. A reduction in coronary blood flow secondary to a reduction in coronary artery lumen due to increased coronary vascular tone, frank spasm, or platelet aggregation is probably responsible for a majority of these episodes.

Why patients with silent ischemia do not experience pain is not known. Pain threshold is elevated in patients with silent ischemia in comparison to those who experience symptoms [83]. Stating that elevated endorphin levels explain silent ischemia remains controversial at the present time [85]. It has been suggested that the extent of ischemic territory is smaller in the painless ischemic group than in those who experience painful ischemia [29].

At present, the long-term prognosis of silent ischemia in patients who are completely asymptomatic is not well defined. Preliminary data suggests that in patients with unstable angina frequent episodes of painless ischemia are of prognostic importance [57, 130]. Treatment is usually aimed at altering the underlying pathophysiologic mechanism.

Irreversible Myocardial Ischemia

Prolonged periods of myocardial ischemia eventually lead to myocardial cell damage and myocardial infarction. However, myocardial damage is dependent on: (1) site and duration of obstruction to flow, (2) presence or absence of collaterals, and (3) the area of the myocardium supplied by the obstructed vessel.

Consequences of Irreversible Myocardial Ischemia

At first, there is depletion of ATP, which leads to impaired contractility and eventually systolic bulging of the infarcted area [80]. Inhibition of a sodium pump leads to edema formation and K^+ leakage from the cell [34]. Intracellular acidosis impairs left ventricular function further. In addition, lysozymes and free oxygen radicals may play an important role in aggravating necrosis [149]. When spontaneous reperfusion occurs, calcium enters the cells and may account for reperfusion injury characterized by band necrosis and arrhythmias [98]. Presence of dead cells in the infarcted region and viable cells in the peri-infarct zone account for many of the arrhythmias seen in these patients.

Pathophysiology of Irreversible Myocardial Injury

Recent evidence suggests that: (1) complete occlusion of a coronary artery supplying the infarcted region (Q wave infarct) is found in approximately 85 percent of patients when the angiogram is performed within 4 hours of symptoms [41]; (2) plaque fissuring is probably the initial factor that eventually leads to formation of a thrombus due to adhesion of platelets, liberation of vasoactive substances, and probably an increase in coronary vasomotor tone [36]; (3) thrombotic process may progress, red thrombus may propagate; (4) myocardial salvage may be possible for several hours depending on collateral flow to the infarcted region [9, 100]; (5) catecholamines can aggravate ischemia and produce an increase in infarct zone; 6) spontaneous reperfusion may occur in 20 to 40 percent of patients but may cause reperfusion necrosis and arrhythmias due to calcium influx [74, 98]; (7) presence of dead cells in the infarcted region and viable cells in the peri-infarct zone account for many of the arrhythmias [44]; and (8) arrhythmias following myocardial infarction are either secondary to the reentry mechanism due to the peri-infarction block, increased automaticity, or late triggered activity [43, 44].

ACUTE MYOCARDIAL INFARCTION

An abrupt cessation of coronary blood flow is the cause of acute myocardial infarction. Clinical and pathologic studies have shown that in patients with acute myocardial infarction the occluded artery is narrowed by a preexisting atherosclerotic lesion and other arteries may be involved with the same process. Half the patients have triple-vessel disease and more than 80 percent have at least double-vessel disease. Thrombotic occlusion is present in patients with transmural infarction [41]. In patients with nontransmural infarction, thrombotic occlusion may be present in 40 percent of patients; the possible explanation of low incidence is spontaneous recanalization of the thrombus [42]. The reocclusion and recurrence of infarction is very high in patients with subendocardial and nontransmural infarction. Although clinical separation of Q wave and non-Q wave infarction is useful, many of the patients without Q waves may have a transmural infarction and vice versa. The differences in subendocardial and transmural necrosis may be explained on the basis of duration of ischemia and the presence or absence of collaterals. In animal models, necrosis is invariably subendocardial after 40 minutes of occlusion; after 24-hour occlusion, most infarcts extend into the epicardium [113]. A wave front of ischemic cell death progresses from endocardium to epicardium over a period of time (Fig. 1-7).

The irreversible damage to the myocardium is often accompanied by chest pain and characteristic electrocardiographic changes. Some patients (15 to 20 percent) may experience myocardial infarction without pain—silent myocardial infarction [69].

The extent of myocardial damage is dependent on the territory supplied by the blocked artery and collateral flow to the ischemic region either via bridge collaterals or overlap of blood supply from adjacent arteries. Spontaneous reperfusion will permit some antegrade flow and reduce the amount of damage. Both the antegrade flow and retrograde flow via the collaterals vary from patient to patient. This makes exact determination of infarct size difficult if not impossible. In the absence of collaterals and spontaneous resolution of thrombosis, the infarct size is invariably transmural and large.

Determinants of Outcome After Acute Myocardial Infarction

Three important variables that determine early outcome are: (1) infarct size, (2) infarct site, and (3) coexisting coronary artery disease.

Patients dying of cardiogenic shock usually have 40 percent or more damaged myocardium [1, 105]. This can be assessed on clinical characteristics developed by Killip and Kimball [75], signs of presence of left ventricular dysfunction, or alternatively by objective assessment of global left ventricular function by nuclear ventriculography or echocardiography.

In patients with uncomplicated infarcts, hospital mortality is in the range of 5 percent; patients with primary ventricular fibrillation or those with signs of mild to moderate congestive heart failure have a mortality of 10 to 15 percent. Patients with pulmonary edema have a mortality of 30 to 40 percent, and those with cardiogenic shock have a mortality of more than 90 percent [138, 145, 151].

Anterior myocardial infarction, especially secondary to the occlusion of the left anterior descending artery, causes more dysfunction and carries a worse prognosis than an inferior infarct or a lateral infarction [138]. Anterior infarcts are also apt to infarct expansion, aneurysmal formation, and mural thrombi and rupture [3, 51, 92].

Occlusion of a circumflex coronary artery usually results in an anterolateral infarct, although in some 15 percent of patients in whom the circumflex artery supplies the posterior descending artery, circumflex occlusion may cause posteroinferior infarction.

Occlusion of the right coronary artery usually causes an inferior or posteroinferior infarction and because of the infarction of the posterior papillary muscle may cause acute papillary muscle rupture and fulminant acute mitral regurgitation. Cardiogenic shock and pulmonary edema may exist in this setting of a relatively small infarct.

Right ventricular infarction rarely occurs in isolation but is found in 10 to 15 percent of patients with an inferior myocardial infarction [146]. It leads to an elevation of jugular venous pressure and low output state. Due to impaired venous return to the left ventricle, hypovolemic shock may ensue. However, this is potentially reversible by volume replacement [33]. Right ventricular and inferior infarction cause a higher incidence of atrioventricular block, nausea, and symptoms due to increased vagal tone [19].

Whether the infarction is transmural or not has a major implication [26]. Aneurysms develop only in the presence of a transmural infarction. On the other hand, patients with a subendocardial infarction are more prone to extend the infarct.

Previous myocardial infarction in a patient with a recent infarction also carries a grave prognosis. Patients with coexistent disease in other arteries are more at risk of developing further ischemia, and postinfarction angina may occur either due to ischemia in an area distant from the occluded artery or ischemia in the area supplied by occluded artery that has undergone partial resolution. Patients with ischemia at a distance have been reported to have a higher mortality than those with ischemia in the infarct region [126].

Infarct expansion, rupture, and aneurysm formation are all complications of a transmural infarction and are not seen in patients with subendocardial or nontransmural infarction [19]. Left ventricular aneurysm often develops at the apex or lateral wall; about half of the cases are complicated by intramural thrombus, which may predispose the patient to systemic embolization [3, 51]. Patients in whom aneurysms are lined by shiny fibroelastic layer are more prone to ventricular arrhythmias [64].

Treatment Strategy

The goal of therapy in patients with an acute myocardial infarction is to limit the infarct size and prevent subsequent complications. This can be achieved to some extent by restoration of coronary blood flow before complete and irreversible damage has occurred and reduction of myocardial oxygen demand. Thrombolytic agents, streptokinase, and recombinant tissue-type plasminogen (rtPA) restore flow in the occluded artery when given within 6 hours after onset of chest pain in 50 to 76 percent of patients [60, 119, 139, 140, 142, 150]. Successful recanalization is higher with intracoronary infusion than via intravenous route, but the former is impractical for the majority of the patients. However, even after recanalization, reocclusion may occur in 20 to 30 percent of patients [124]. Residual stenosis in the infarct-related artery after successful thrombolytic therapy has persuaded many to perform urgent angioplasty [119, 140], but reocclusion rate and complications are high in comparison to elective angioplasty performed at a later date [140]. Well-designed double-blind studies are urgently needed to evaluate the effectiveness of this treatment modality.

With any intervention, the salvage of myocardium is dependent on the rapidity with which intervention is applied following the onset of symptoms [88]. Some myocardium may be salvaged for up to 6 hours. Urgent coronary bypass surgery may be indicated in some patients and in a small series has been shown to reduce mortality [40].

Another strategy to reduce infarct size is to reduce myocardial oxygen demand by pharmacological means. In this setting, the role of beta blockers is well established [8, 61, 99] and the role of nitrates and calcium channel antagonists is being intensely investigated.

Patients who develop postinfarct angina may require invasive studies and revascularization if they fail to respond to medical therapy. Acute mitral regurgitation due to ruptured papillary muscle or acute ventricular septal defect require surgical intervention. In patients who develop left ventricular aneurysms and have a mural thrombus, anticoagulation therapy for 3 to 6 months prevents systemic embolization. Patients who develop cardiac failure secondary to a ventricular aneurysm may benefit from aneurysmal resection.

Early reinfarction and death within the first few months to 1 year of infarction remains a major issue. High-risk patients with global ejection fraction less than 50 percent need the most attention and can be identified by clinical features and noninvasive workup [4, 104]. In unselected group of patients, long-term beta blocker therapy reduces the rate of sudden death and reinfarction [8].

Sudden Cardiac Death

Sudden death syndrome is a common presentation of ischemic heart disease. Ventricular fibrillation is the most common cause of death within 1 hour of an acute myocardial infarction [31, 106]. Survivors of sudden death and myocardial infarction are also at a risk of sudden death in subsequent years [31].

Pathophysiology of Sudden Cardiac Death

Earlier studies suggested that coronary thrombosis accounted for a minority of patients with sudden death. Recent careful pathologic studies have, however, shown that intraluminal thrombi occur in 74 percent of those in whom sudden cardiac ischemic death occurred compared with none of those dying suddenly from other causes [36]. This study also showed evidence of plaque fissuring in 86 of the 90 patients (90.5 percent) dying suddenly. Platelet aggregates have been found in small intramyocardial vessels in 30 percent of patients [35]. Platelet aggregates are often confined to the segment of the myocardium downstream of a major epicardial coronary artery containing an atherosclerotic plaque that had undergone fissuring and on which mural thrombus had developed [35, 36, 37]. Thus, recent data supports the view that platelet aggregation in the small coronary arteries represents an embolic phenomenon. The association of myocardial ischemia with such emboli could precipitate sudden death and ventricular fibrillation. This early pathogenesis of sudden death is different than subsequent sudden death in the hospital survivors of sudden death or myocardial infarction [23]. In this group of patients, there is usually a preceding episode of ventricular tachycardia, which may degenerate into ventricular fibrillation [23]. The mechanism of arrhythmias in this group of patients probably is reentrant excitation of relatively discrete circuits that form during the healing of acute infarction.

Treatment Strategy

The treatment focus should be the prevention of plaque fissuring and subsequent platelet aggregation and thrombus formation. However, in survivors of sudden death, prevention of recurrence of ventricular arrhythmia is warranted. This can be achieved by identifying a drug that will abolish reentrant excitation or, in the absence of a suitable drug, resection of the area responsible for the reentry mechanism, or implantation of a permanent defibrillator [23].

ISCHEMIC CARDIOMYOPATHY

Dilated cardiomyopathy secondary to severe underlying coronary artery disease is a relatively uncommon presentation of ischemic heart disease [125]. Usually there is evidence of multiple sites of injury rather than extensive myocardial infarction. It has been suggested that this is due to repeated bouts of ischemia in multiple regions that lead to cardiac dilation. This has been termed hibernating myocardium due to persistent ischemic injury and may be potentially reversible by successful revascularization [14].

REFERENCES

1. Alonso, D. R., Scheidt, S., Post, M., and Killip, T. Pathophysiology of cardiogenic shock: Quantification of myocardial necrosis, clinical, pathologic and electrocardiographic correlations. *Circulation* 48:588, 1973.
2. Ambrose, J. A., Winters, S. L., Stern, A., et al. Angiographic morphology and the pathogenesis of unstable angina. *J. Am. Coll. Cardiol.* 5:609, 1985.
3. Asinger, R. W., Mikell, F. L., Elsperger, J., and Hodges, M. Incidence of left-ventricular thrombosis after acute transmural myocardial infarction: Serial evaluation of two-dimensional electrocardiography. *N. Engl. J. Med.* 305:297, 1981.
4. Beller, G. A., and Gibson, R. S. Risk stratification after myocardial infarction. *Mod. Concepts Cardiovasc. Dis.* 55:5, 1986.
5. Berne, R. M. Regulation of coronary blood flow. *Physiol. Rev.* 44:1, 1964.
6. Berne, R. M., and Levy, M. N. *Cardiovascular Physiology* (5th ed.). St Louis: C. V. Mosby Co., 1986.
7. Berne, R. M., and Rubio, R. Coronary circulation. In R. M. Berne, N. Sperelakis, and S. R. Geiger (eds.), *Handbook of Physiology: A critical, comprehensive presentation of physiological knowledge and concepts.* Section 2. The Cardiovascular System. Bethesda: American Physiological Society, 1979:873.
8. Beta-blocker Heart Attack Trial Research Group. A randomized trial of propranolol in patients with acute myocardial infarction. I. Mortality results. *JAMA* 247:1707, 1982.
9. Blumgart, H. L., Schlesinger, M. J., and Davis, D. Studies on the relation of the clinical manifestations of angina pectoris, coronary thrombosis, and myocardial infarction to the pathologic findings. *Am. Heart J.* 19:1, 1940.
10. Boerth, R. C., Covell, J. W., Pool, P. E., and Ross, J., Jr. Increased myocardial oxygen consumption and contractile state associated with increased heart rate in dogs. *Circ. Res.* 24:725, 1969.
11. Bonow, R. O., Bacharach, S. L., Green, M. V., et al. Prognostic implications of symptomatic versus asymptomatic (silent) myocardial ischemia induced by exercise in mildly symptomatic and in asymptomatic patients with angiographically documented coronary artery disease. *Am. J. Cardiol.* 60:778, 1987.
12. Braunwald, E. Mechanisms of action of calcium-channel-blocking agents. *N. Engl. J. Med.* 307:1618, 1982.
13. Braunwald, E., Ross, J., Jr., and Sonnenblick, E. H. Regulation of coronary blood flow. In E. Braunwald, J. Ross, Jr., and E. H. Sonnenblick (eds.), *Mechanisms of Contraction of the Normal and Failing Heart.* Boston: Little, Brown, 1976. P. 200.
14. Braunwald, E., and Rutherford, J. B. Reversible ischemic left ventricular dysfunction: Evidence for the "hybernating myocardium." *J. Am. Coll. Cardiol.* 8:1467, 1986.
15. Braunwald, E., Sarnoff, S. J., Case, R. B., et al. Hemodynamic determinants of coronary flow: Effect of changes in aortic pressure and cardiac output on the relationship between myocardial oxygen consumption and coronary flow. *Am. J. Physiol.* 192:157, 1958.
16. Braunwald, E., and Sobel, B. E. Coronary blood flow and myocardial ischemia. In E. Braunwald (ed.), *Heart Disease: A textbook of cardiovascular medicine.* Philadelphia: Saunders, 1984. P. 1235.

17. Brown, G., Bolson, E., Pedersen, R. B., et al. The mechanisms of nitroglycerin action: Stenosis vasodilatation as a major component of drug response. *Circulation* 64:1089, 1981.
18. Brown, M. S., and Goldstein, J. L. Familial hypercholesterolemia: A genetic defect in the low-density lipoprotein receptor. *N. Engl. J. Med.* 294:1386, 1976.
19. Bulkley, B. H. Site and sequelae of myocardial infarction. *N. Engl. J. Med.* 305:337, 1981.
20. Bulkley, B. H., Klacsmann, P. G., and Hutchins, G. M. Angina pectoris, myocardial infarction and sudden cardiac death with normal coronary arteries: A clinicopathologic study of 9 patients with progressive systemic sclerosis. *Am. Heart J.* 95:563, 1978.
21. Bulkley, B. H., and Roberts, W. C. Dissecting aneurysm (hematoma) limited to coronary artery: A clinicopathologic study of six patients. *Am. J. Med.* 55:747, 1973.
22. Burggraf, G. W., and Parker, J. O. Prognosis in coronary artery disease: Angiographic, hemodynamic, and clinical factors. *Circulation* 51:146, 1975.
23. Buxton, A. E. Sudden cardiac death—1986. *Ann. Intern. Med.* 104:716, 1986.
24. Cairns, J. A. Unstable angina: 1985 update. *Can. Med. Assoc. J.* 134: 741, 1986.
25. Cairns, J. A., Gent, M., Singer, J., et al. Aspirin, sulfinpyrazone, or both in unstable angina. Results of a Canadian multicenter trial. *N. Engl. J. Med.* 313:1369, 1985.
26. Cannom, D. S., Levy, W., and Cohen, L. S. The short- and long-term prognosis of patients with transmural and nontransmural myocardial infarction. *Am. J. Med.* 61:452, 1976.
27. Capone, G., Wolf, N. M., Meyer, B., and Meister, S. G. Frequency of intracoronary filling defects by angiography in angina pectoris at rest. *Am. J. Cardiol.* 56:403, 1985.
28. Chaitman, B. R., Bourassa, M. G., Wagniart, P., Corbara, F., and Ferguson, R. J. Improved efficiency of treadmill exercise testing using a multiple lead ECG system and basic hemodynamic exercise response. *Circulation* 57:71, 1978.
29. Chierchia, S., Lazzari, M., Freedman, B., et al. Impairment of myocardial perfusion and function during painless myocardial ischemia. *J. Am. Coll. Cardiol.* 1:924, 1983.
30. Chierchia, S., Marchesi, C., and Maseri, A. Evidence of angina not caused by increased myocardial metabolic demand and patterns of electrocardiographic and hemodynamic alterations during "primary" angina. In A. Maseri, G. A. Klassen, and M. Lesch (eds.), *Primary and Secondary Angina Pectoris*.New York: Grune & Stratton, 1976. P. 145.
31. Cobb, L. A., Baum, R. S., Alvarez, H., III, and Schaffer, W. A. Resuscitation from out-of-hospital ventricular fibrillation: 4 years follow-up. *Circulation* 52 (Suppl III):III-223, 1975.
32. Cobbe, S. M., and Poole-Wilson, P. A. The time of onset and severity of acidosis in myocardial ischaemia. *J. Mol. Cell Cardiol.* 12:745, 1980.
33. Cohn, J. N. Right ventricular infarction revisited. *Am. J. Cardiol.* 43:666, 1979.
34. Dalby, A. J., Bricknell, O. L., and Opie, L. H. Effect of glucose-insulin-potassium infusions on epicardial ECG changes and on myocardial metabolic changes after coronary artery ligation in dogs. *Cardiovasc. Res.* 15:588, 1981.
35. Davies, M. J., Path, F. R. C., Thomas, A. C., et al. Intramyocardial platelet aggregation in patients with unstable angina suffering sudden ischemic cardiac death. *Circulation* 73:418, 1986.

36. Davies, M. J., and Thomas, A. C. Thrombosis and acute coronary-artery lesions in sudden cardiac ischemic death. *N. Engl. J. Med.* 310:1137, 1984.
37. Davies, M. J., and Thomas, A. C. Plaque fissuring—the cause of acute myocardial infarction, sudden ischaemic death, and crescendo angina. *Br. Heart J.* 53:363, 1985.
38. Deanfield, J. E., Selwyn, A. P., Chierchia, S., et al. Myocardial ischaemia during daily life in patients with unstable angina: Its relation to symptoms and heart rate changes. *Lancet* 2:753, 1983.
39. De Feyter, P. J., Serruys, P. W., Soward, A., et al. Coronary angioplasty for early post infarction unstable angina. *Circulation* 74:1365, 1986.
40. DeWood, M. A., Spores, J., Berg, R., Jr., et al. Acute myocardial infarction: A decade of experience with surgical reperfusion in 701 patients. *Circulation* 68(Suppl II):II-8, 1983.
41. DeWood, M. A., Spores, J., Notske, R., et al. Prevalence of total coronary occlusion during the early hours of transmural myocardial infarction. *N. Engl. J. Med.* 303:897, 1980.
42. DeWood, M. A., Stifter, W. F., Simpson, C. S., et al. Coronary arteriographic findings soon after non-Q-wave myocardial infarction. *N. Engl. J. Med.* 315:417, 1986.
43. El-Sherif, N., Hope, R. R., Scherlag, B. J., and Lazzara, R. Re-entrant ventricular arrhythmias in the late myocardial infarction period. II. Patterns of initiation and termination of re-entry. *Circulation* 55:702, 1977.
44. El-Sherif, N., Scherlag, B. J., and Lazzara, R. Electrode catheter recordings during malignant ventricular arrhythmia following experimental acute myocardial ischemia: Evidence for re-entry due to conduction delay and block in ischemic myocardium. *Circulation* 51:1003, 1975.
45. Epstein, S. E., and Cannon, R. O., III. Site of increased resistance to coronary flow in patients with angina pectoris and normal epicardial coronary arteries. *J. Am. Coll. Cardiol.* 8:459, 1986.
46. Epstein, S. E., and Talbot, T. L. Dynamic coronary tone in precipitation, exacerbation and relief of angina pectoris. *Am. J. Cardiol.* 48:797, 1981.
47. Feigl, E. O. Coronary physiology. *Physiol. Rev.* 63:1, 1983.
48. Feigl, E. O., Buffington, C. W., and Nathan, H. J. Adrenergic coronary vasoconstriction during myocardial underperfusion. *Circulation* 75(Suppl I):I-5, 1987.
49. Feldman, R. L., Nichols, W. W., Pepine, C. J., and Conti, C. R. Hemodynamic significance of the length of a coronary arterial narrowing. *Am. J. Cardiol.* 41:865, 1978.
50. Folts, J. D., Gallagher, K., and Rowe, G. G. Blood flow reductions in stenosed canine coronary arteries: Vasospasm or platelet aggregation? *Circulation* 65:248, 1982.
51. Forman, M. B., Collins, W., Kopelman, H. A., et al. Determinants of left ventricular aneurysm formation after anterior myocardial infarction: A clinical and angiographic study. *J. Am. Coll. Cardiol.* 8:1256, 1986.
52. Friedman, P. L., Stewart, J. R., and Wit, A. L. Spontaneous and induced cardiac arrhythmias in subendocardial purkinje fibers surviving extensive myocardial infarction in dogs. *Circ. Res.* 33:612, 1973.
53. Fuster, V., and Chesebro, J. H. Mechanisms of unstable angina. *N. Engl. J. Med.* 315:1023, 1986.
54. Gage, J. E., Hess, O. M., Murakami, T., et al. Vasoconstriction of stenotic coronary arteries during dynamic exercise in patients with classic angina pectoris: Reversibility by nitroglycerin. *Circulation* 73:865, 1986.
55. Gibbs, C. L. Cardiac energetics. In G. A. Langer and A. J. Brady (eds.), *The Mammalian Myocardium*. New York: Wiley, 1974. P. 105.
56. Gorlin, R., Brachfeld, N., MacLeod, C., and Bopp, P. Effect of nitroglycerin

on coronary circulation in patients with coronary artery disease or increased left ventricular work. *Circulation* 19:705, 1959.
57. Gottlieb, S. O., Weisfeldt, M. L., Ouyang, P., et al. Silent ischemia as a marker for early unfavorable outcomes in patients with unstable angina. *N. Engl. J. Med.* 314:1214, 1986.
58. Gregg, D. E., and Bedyneck, J. L., Jr. Compensatory changes in the heart during progressive coronary artery stenosis. In A. Maseri, G. A. Klassen, and M. Lesch (eds.), *Primary and Secondary Angina Pectoris*. New York: Grune & Stratton, 1976. P. 3.
59. Gregg, D. E., Khouri, E. M., and Rayford, C. R. Systemic and coronary energetics in the resting unanesthetized dog. *Circ. Res.* 16:102, 1965.
60. Gruppo Italiano per Lo Studio Della Streptochinasi Nell'Infarto Miocardico (GISSI). Effectiveness of intravenous thrombolytic treatment in acute myocardial infarction. *Lancet* 1:397, 1986.
61. Hammerman, H., Kloner, R. A., Briggs, L. L., and Braunwald, E. Enhancement of salvage of reperfused myocardium by early beta-adrenergic blockade (timolol). *J. Am. Coll. Cardiol.* 3:1438, 1984.
62. Hearse, D. J., Crome, R., Yellon, D. M., and Wyse, R. Metabolic and flow correlates of myocardial ischaemia. *Cardiovasc. Res.* 17:452, 1983.
63. Heberden, W. Some account of a disorder of the breast. *Med. Trans. Roy. Coll. Phys.* 2:59, 1772.
64. Hochman, J. S., Platia, E. V., and Bulkley, B. H. Differences in LV aneurysms by endocardial pathology: Relationship to ventricular tachycardia in a surgical population. *J. Am. Coll. Cardiol.* 1:733, 1983.
65. Hoffman, J. I. E. A critical view of coronary reserve. *Circulation* 75(Suppl I):I-6, 1987.
66. Hoffman, J. I. E. Determinants and prediction of transmural myocardial perfusion. *Circulation* 58:381, 1978.
67. Holmes, D. R., Jr., and Vlietstra, R. E. Percutaneous transluminal coronary angioplasty: Current status and future trends. *Mayo Clin. Proc.* 61:865, 1986.
68. Jennings, R. B., and Ganote, C. E. Mitochondrial structure and function in acute myocardial ischemic injury. *Circ. Res.* 38(Suppl I):I-80, 1976.
69. Kannel, W. B., and Abbott, R. D. Incidence and prognosis of unrecognized myocardial infarction: An update on the Framingham Study. *N. Engl. J. Med.* 311:1144, 1984.
70. Kannengiesser, G. J., Opie, L. H., and Van Der Werff, T. J. Impaired cardiac work and oxygen uptake after reperfusion of regionally ischaemic myocardium. *J. Mol. Cell Cardiol.* 11:197, 1979.
71. Kaski, J. C., Crea, F., Nihoyannopoulos, P., et al. Transient myocardial ischemia during daily life in patients with syndrome X. *Am. J. Cardiol.* 58:1242, 1986.
72. Kaski, J. C., Crea, F., Meran, D., et al. Local coronary supersensitivity to diverse vasoconstriction stimuli in patients with variant angina. *Circulation* 74:1255, 1986.
73. Katz, A. M. Effects of ischemia on the contractile processes of heart muscle. *Am. J. Cardiol.* 32:456, 1973.
74. Kennedy, J. W., Ritchie, J. L., Davis, K. B., and Fritz, J. K. Western Washington randomized trial of intracoronary streptokinase in acute myocardial infarction. *N. Engl. J. Med.* 309:1477, 1983.
75. Killip, T., III, and Kimball, J. T. Treatment of myocardial infarction in a coronary care unit: A two-year experience with 250 patients. *Am. J. Cardiol.* 20:457, 1967.
76. Klein, L. W., Segal, B. L., and Helfant, R. H. Dynamic coronary stenosis behavior in classic angina pectoris: Active process or passive response? *J. Am. Coll. Cardiol.* 10:311, 1987.

77. Klocke, F. J., Braunwald, E., and Ross, J., Jr. Oxygen cost of electrical activation of the heart. *Circ. Res.* 18:357, 1966.
78. Klocke, F. J. Measurements of coronary blood flow and degree of stenosis: Current clinical implications and continuing uncertainties. *J. Am. Coll. Cardiol.* 1:31, 1983.
79. Klocke, F. J. Coronary blood flow in man. *Progr. Cardiovasc. Dis.* 19:117, 1977.
80. Kubler, W., and Katz, A. M. Mechanism of early "pump" failure of the ischemic heart: Possible role of adenosine triphosphate depletion and inorganic phosphate accumulation. *Am. J. Cardiol.* 40:467, 1977.
81. Lewis, H. D., Jr., Davis, J. W., Archibald, D. G., et al. Protective effects of aspirin against acute myocardial infarction and death in men with unstable angina: Results of a Veterans Administration Cooperation Study. *N. Engl. J. Med.* 309:396, 1983.
82. MacAlpin, R. N. Contribution of dynamic vascular wall thickening to luminal narrowing during coronary arterial constriction. *Circulation* 61:296, 1980.
83. Malliani, A. The elusive link between transient myocardial ischemia and pain. *Circulation* 73:201, 1986.
84. Maseri, A., L'Abbate, A., Baroldi, G., et al. Coronary vasospasm as a possible cause of myocardial infarction: A conclusion derived from the study of "preinfarction" angina. *N. Engl. J. Med.* 299:1271, 1978.
85. Maseri, A., Chierchia, S., Davies, G., and Glazier, J. Mechanisms of ischemic cardiac pain and of silent myocardial ischemia. *Am. J. Med.* 79(Suppl IIIA):III-7, 1985.
86. Maseri, A., Chierchia, S., and Kaski, J. C. Mixed angina pectoris. *Am. J. Cardiol.* 56:30E, 1985.
87. Maseri, A., Mimmo, R., Chierchia, S., et al. Coronary artery spasm as a cause of acute myocardial ischemia in man. *Chest* 68:625, 1975.
88. Mathey, D. G., Sheehan, F. H., Schofer, J., and Dodge, H. T. Time from onset of symptoms to thrombolytic therapy: A major determinant of myocardial salvage in patients with acute myocardial infarction. *J. Am. Coll. Cardiol.* 6:518, 1985.
89. McGregor, M. Pathogenesis of angina pectoris and role of nitrates in relief of myocardial ischemia. *Am. J. Med.* 74:21, 1983.
90. McKeever, W. P., Gregg, D. E., and Canney, P. C. Oxygen uptake of the nonworking left ventricle. *Circ. Res.* 6:612, 1958.
91. Meade, T. W. Thrombosis and ischaemic heart disease. *Br. Heart J.* 53:473, 1985.
92. Meizlish, J. L., Berger, H. J., Plankey, M., et al. Functional left ventricular aneurysm formation after acute anterior transmural myocardial infarction: Incidence, natural history, and prognostic implications. *N. Engl. J. Med.* 311:1001, 1984.
93. Mjos, O. D. Effect of free fatty acids in myocardial function and oxygen consumption in intact dogs. *J. Clin. Invest.* 50:1386, 1971.
94. Mock, M. B., Ringqvist, I., Fisher, L. D., et al. Survival of medically treated patients in the coronary artery surgery study (CASS) registry. *Circulation* 66:562, 1982.
95. Mohrman, D. E., and Feigl, E. O. Competition between sympathetic vasoconstriction and metabolic vasodilation in the canine coronary circulation. *Circ. Res.* 42:79, 1978.
96. Moore, S. Thrombosis and atherogenesis—The chicken and the egg: Contribution of platelets in atherogenesis. *Ann. N.Y. Acad. Sci.* 454:146, 1985.
97. Muller, J. E., Turi, Z. G., Pearle, D. L., et al. Nifedipine and conventional

therapy for unstable angina pectoris: A randomized, double-blind comparison. *Circulation* 69:728, 1984.
98. Nayler, W. G., and Elz, J. S. Reperfusion injury: Laboratory artifact or clinical dilemma? *Circulation* 74:215, 1986.
99. Norris, R. M., Brown, M. A., Clarke, E. D., et al. Prevention of ventricular fibrillation during acute myocardial infarction by intravenous propranolol. *Lancet* 2:883, 1984.
100. O'Brien, C. M., Carroll, M., O'Rourke, P. T., et al. The reversibility of acute ischemic injury to the myocardium by restoration of coronary flow. *J. Thorac. Cardiovasc. Surg.* 64:840, 1972.
101. Oliva, P. B., and Breckinridge, J. C. Arteriographic evidence of coronary arterial spasm in acute myocardial infarction. *Circulation* 56:366, 1977.
102. Oliveros, R. A., Boucher, C. A., Haycraft, G. L., and Beckmann, C. H. Myocardial oxygen supply-demand ratio: A validation of peripherally vs. centrally determined values. *Chest* 75:693, 1979.
103. Opherk, D., Mall, G., Zebe, H., et al. Reduction of coronary reserve: A mechanism for angina pectoris in patients with arterial hypertension and normal coronary arteries. *Circulation* 69:1, 1984.
104. O'Rourke, R. A. Clinical decisions for postmyocardial infarction patients. *Mod. Concepts Cardiovasc. Dis.* 55:55, 1986.
105. Page, D. L., Caulfield, J. B., De Sanctis, R. W., Kastor, J. A., and Sanders, C. A. Myocardial changes associated with cardiogenic shock. *N. Engl. J. Med.* 285:133, 1971.
106. Pantridge, J. F., and Geddes, J. S. A mobile intensive-care unit in the management of myocardial infarction. *Lancet* 2:271, 1967.
107. Pepine, C. J. Clinical aspects of silent myocardial ischemia in patients with angina and other forms of coronary heart disease. *Am. J. Med.* 80:25, 1986.
108. Picano, E., Simonetti, I., Masini, M., et al. Transient myocardial dysfunction during pharmacologic vasodilation as an index of reduced coronary reserve: A coronary hemodynamic and echocardiographic study. *J. Am. Coll. Cardiol.* 8:84, 1986.
109. Plotnick, G. D., and Conti, C. R. Unstable angina: angiography, short- and long-term morbidity, mortality and symptomatic status of medically treated patients. *Am. J. Med.* 63:870, 1977.
110. Prichard, B. N. C. Beta-adrenergic receptor blocking drugs in angina pectoris. *Drugs* 7:55, 1974.
111. Prinzmetal, M., Kennamer, R., Merliss, R., et al. Angina pectoris. I. A variant form of angina pectoris. *Am. J. Med.* 27:375, 1959.
112. Quyyumi, A. A., Efthimiou, J., Quyyumi, A., et al. Nocturnal angina: Precipitating factors in patients with coronary artery disease and those with variant angina. *Br. Heart J.* 56:346, 1986.
113. Reimer, K. A., Lowe, J. E., Rasmussen, M. M., and Jennings, R. B. The wavefront phenomenon of ischemic cell death. I. Myocardial infarct size vs. duration of coronary occlusion in dogs. *Circulation* 56:786, 1977.
114. Report of the Holland Interuniversity Nifedipine/Metoprolol Trial (HINT) Research Group. Early treatments of unstable angina in the coronary care unit: A randomised, double blind, placebo controlled comparison of recurrent ischaemia in patients treated with nifedipine or metoprolol or both. *Br. Heart J.* 56:400, 1986.
115. Roberts, W. C. The coronary arteries in coronary heart disease: Morphologic observations. In H. L. Ioachim (ed.), *Pathobiology Annual*. New York: Appleton-Century-Crofts, 1975, P. 249.
116. Robinson, B. F. Relation of heart rate and systolic blood pressure to the onset of pain in angina pectoris. *Circulation* 35:1073, 1967.
117. Rodbard, S., Williams, C. B., Rodbard, D., and Berglund, E. Myocardial tension and oxygen uptake. *Circ. Res.* 14:139, 1964.

118. Rosing, D. R., Kent, K. M., Maron, B. J., and Epstein, S. E. Verapamil therapy: A new approach to the pharmacologic treatment of hypertrophic cardiomyopathy. II. Effects on exercise capacity and symptomatic status. *Circulation* 60:1208, 1979.
119. Rothbaum, D. A., Linnemeier, T. J., Landin, R. J., et al. Emergency percutaneous transluminal coronary angioplasty in acute myocardial infarction: A 3 year experience. *J. Am. Coll. Cardiol.* 10:264, 1987.
120. Roughgarden, J. W. Circulatory changes associated with spontaneous angina pectoris. *Am. J. Med.* 41:947, 1966.
121. Russel, R. O., Rackley, C. E., and Kouchoukos, N. T. Unstable angina pectoris: Management based on available information. *Circulation* 65(Suppl II):II-72, 1982.
122. Sarnoff, S. J., Braunwald, E., Welch, G. H., Jr., et al. Hemodynamic determinants of oxygen consumption of the heart with special reference to the tension-time index. *Am. J. Physiol.* 192:148, 1958.
123. Scanlon, P. J., Nemickas, R., Moran, J. F., et al. Accelerated angina pectoris clinical, hemodynamic, arteriographic, and therapeutic experience in 85 patients. *Circulation* 47:19, 1973.
124. Schaer, D. H., Ross, A. M., and Wasserman, A. G. Reinfarction, recurrent angina, and reocclusion after thrombolytic therapy. *Circulation* 76(Suppl II):II-57, 1987.
125. Schuster, E. H., and Bulkley, B. H. Ischemic cardiomyopathy: A clinicopathologic study of fourteen patients. *Am. Heart J.* 100:506, 1980.
126. Schuster, E. H., and Bulkley, B. H. Early post-infarction angina: Ischemia at a distance and ischemia in the infarct zone. *N. Engl. J. Med.* 305:1101, 1981.
127. Second Interim Report by the European Coronary Surgery Study Group. Prospective randomised study of coronary artery bypass surgery in stable angina pectoris. *Lancet* 2:491, 1980.
128. Severi, S., Davies, G., Maseri, A., et al. Long-term prognosis of "variant" angina with medical treatment. *Am. J. Cardiol.* 46:226, 1980.
129. Sherman, C. T., Litvack, F., Grundfest, W., et al. Coronary angioscopy in patients with unstable angina pectoris. *N. Engl. J. Med.* 315:913, 1986.
130. Singh, B. N., and Nademanee, K. Prevalence and prognostic significance of silent myocardial ischemia in patients with unstable angina. *Circulation* 75(Suppl II):II-40, 1987.
131. Sonnenblick, E. H., Braunwald, E., Williams, J. F., and Glick, G. Effects of exercise on myocardial force-velocity relations in intact unanesthetized man: Relative roles of changes in heart rate, sympathetic activity, and ventricular dimensions. *J. Clin. Invest.* 44:2051, 1965.
132. Sonnenblick, E. H., Ross, J., Jr., Covell, J. W., et al. Velocity of contraction as a determinant of myocardial oxygen consumption. *Am. J. Physiol.* 209:919, 1965.
133. Stehbens, W. E. Vascular complications in experimental atherosclerosis. *Progr. Cardiovasc. Dis.* 29:221, 1986.
134. Stern, S., and Tzivoni, D. Early detection of silent ischaemic heart disease by 24-hour electrocardiographic monitoring of active subjects. *Br. Heart J.* 36:481, 1974.
135. Telford, A. M., and Wilson, C. Trial of heparin versus atenolol in prevention of myocardial infarction in intermediate coronary syndrome. *Lancet* 1:1225, 1985.
136. Thadani, U. Current status of nitrates in angina pectoris. *Mod. Concepts of Cardiovasc. Dis.* 56:49, 1987.
137. Thadani, U., Sharma, B., Meeran, M. K., et al. Comparison of adrenergic beta-receptor antagonists in angina pectoris. *Br. Med. J.* 1:138, 1973.

138. The Multicenter Postinfarction Research Group. Risk stratification and survival after myocardial infarction. *N. Engl. J. Med.* 309:331, 1983.
139. The TIMI Study Group. The thrombolysis in myocardial infarction (TIMI) trial. Phase I findings. *N. Engl. J. Med.* 312:932, 1985.
140. Topol, E. J., Califf, R. M., George, B. S., et al. A randomized trial of immediate versus delayed elective angioplasty after intravenous tissue plasminogen activator in acute myocardial infarction. *N. Engl. J. Med.* 317:581, 1987.
141. Vanhoutte, P. M., and Houston, D. S. Platelets, endothelium, and vasospasm. *Circulation* 72:728, 1985.
142. Verstraete, M., Bory, M., Collen, D., et al. Randomised trial of intravenous recombinant tissue-type plasminogen activator versus intravenous streptokinase in acute myocardial infarction. Report from the European Cooperative Study Group for Recombinant Tissue-type Plasminogen Activator. *Lancet* 1:842, 1985.
143. Vlahakes, G. J., Baer, R. W., Uhlig, P. N., et al. Adrenergic influence in the coronary circulation of conscious dogs during maximal vasodilation with adenosine. *Circ. Res.* 51:371, 1982.
144. Vogel, W. M., Apstein, C. S., Briggs, L. L., et al. Acute alterations in left ventricular diastolic chamber stiffness. Role of the "erectile" effect of coronary arterial pressure and flow in normal and damaged hearts *Circ. Res.* 51:465, 1982.
145. Volpi, A., Maggioni, A., Franzosi, M. G., et al. In-hospital prognosis of patients with acute myocardial infarction complicated by primary ventricular fibrillation. *N. Engl. J. Med.* 317:257, 1987.
146. Wackers, F. J. T., Lie, K. I., Sokole, E. B., et al. Prevalence of right ventricular involvement in inferior wall infarction assessed with myocardial imaging with thallium-201 and technetium-99m pyrophosphate. *Am. J. Cardiol.* 42:358, 1978.
147. Walling, A., Waters, D., Miller, D. D., et al. Long-term prognosis of patients with variant angina. *Circulation* 76:990, 1987.
148. Weiss, J., and Shine, K. I. Extracellular potassium accumulation during myocardial ischemia: Implications for arrhythmogenesis. *J. Mol. Cell Cardiol.* 13:699, 1981.
149. Werns, S. W., Shea, M. J., and Lucchesi, B. R. Free radicals and myocardial injury: Pharmacologic implications. *Circulation* 74:1, 1986.
150. White, H. D., Norris, R. M., Brown, M. A., et al. Effect of intravenous streptokinase on left ventricular function and early survival after acute myocardial infarction. *N. Engl. J. Med.* 317:850, 1987.
151. Wiener, R. S., Moses, H. W., Richeson, J. F., and Gatewood, R. P., Jr. Hospital and long-term survival of patients with acute pulmonary edema associated with coronary artery disease. *Am. J. Cardiol.* 60:33, 1987.
152. Wilson, R. F., Holida, M. D., and White, C. W. Quantitative angiographic morphology of coronary stenoses leading to myocardial infarction of unstable angina. *Circulation* 73:286, 1986.
153. Winbury, M. M., Howe, B. B., and Hefner, M. A. Effect of nitrates and other coronary dilators on large and small coronary vessels: An hypothesis for the mechanism of action of nitrates. *J. Pharmacol. Exp. Ther.* 168:70, 1969.
154. Wissler, R. W. Principles of the pathogenesis of atherosclerosis. In E. Braunwald (ed.), *Heart Disease: A Textbook of Cardiovascular Medicine.* Philadelphia: Saunders, 1984. P. 1183.
155. Yasue, H., Horio, Y., Nakamura, N., et al. Induction of coronary artery spasm by acetylcholine in patients with variant angina: Possible role of the parasympathetic nervous system in the pathogenesis of coronary artery spasm. *Circulation* 74:955, 1974.

CHAPTER 2

APPROACH TO THERAPY OF ISCHEMIC HEART DISEASE

LYLE J. SWENSON

Ischemic heart disease is the leading cause of death in the United States, accounting for more than one-third of all deaths. It is estimated that approximately five million people suffer from ischemic heart disease in the United States and that there are 1.5 million myocardial infarctions each year, over 35 percent of these resulting in death [122]. Over half of the deaths due to myocardial infarction occur outside the hospital, most often within 2 hours after the onset of symptoms.

Despite these staggering statistics, there may be some cause for optimism since the mortality from ischemic heart disease is declining and has been since 1968. The reasons for this decline are not well understood but probably involve many different changes in the development and treatment of ischemic heart disease. It is likely that improvements in the detection and control of hypertension, decreased use of cigarettes, decreased consumption of saturated fats, and increased health awareness and health education have contributed to this decline. Nevertheless, ischemic heart disease continues to be one of the most, if not the most, important public health problem in the developed countries of the world.

Angina pectoris is the most common chronic manifestation of ischemic heart disease. It is typically induced by exercise and is an important cause of disability. The approach to the management of chronic angina pectoris has relied upon three classes of antianginal agents in attempts to prevent or at least limit the frequency and severity of angina: long-acting nitrates of various forms, a wide range of beta blockers, and the calcium channel antagonists. Newer agents and newer formulations of older agents have been introduced recently with advantages and disadvantages requiring tailoring of therapy to the individual patient. The particular presentation of the patient influences tremendously the approach to therapy, depending on whether the patient has typical exercise-induced angina, mixed angina, or variant angina due to coronary artery spasm. For those patients whose symptoms are not controlled with medical therapy, coronary artery bypass graft (CABG) has proven an effective form of therapy for the relief of angina. More recently percutaneous transluminal coronary angioplasty (PTCA) has become an appealing alternative to CABG for the therapy of patients with ischemic heart disease.

Unstable angina has gone by many different names in the past and continues to be redefined based on our growing understanding of the pathophysiology of this disorder. Unstable angina currently includes three sometimes related but different presentations of ischemic heart disease: (1) angina of recent onset, (2) crescendo angina superimposed on a stable pattern, and (3) angina at rest. These entities are generally thought to be intermediate syndromes between chronic stable angina and acute myocardial infarction and clearly represent a wide spectrum of ischemic heart disease. Another presentation of angina, that of recurrent ischemic chest pain following myocardial infarction, is sometimes included in the category of unstable angina.

The approach to the patient with unstable angina involves not only myocardial oxygen supply-demand issues but also consideration of the thrombosis, vasospasm, and platelet aggregation that contribute to the development of this disorder. Most patients with unstable angina can be stabilized with medical therapy, which includes anticoagulation as well as antianginal therapy. The use of thrombolytic agents is being actively investigated. Even though the medical therapy of unstable angina continues to improve, many of these patients will require early intervention with coronary angiography and revascularization with either PTCA or CABG because of refractory symptoms.

Acute myocardial infarction is a common presentation of ischemic heart disease and caused 513,700 deaths in 1987 [122]. Most of these deaths occurred outside of hospitals. For those patients with myocardial infarction that are admitted to the hospital, therapy will be influenced by how early in the course of the infarction they present and by the technological capabilities and responsiveness of the institution where they are initially cared for. Advances in our understanding of the pathophysiology of acute myocardial infarction have led to the use of reperfusion therapy involving thrombolytic therapy as well as percutaneous transluminal coronary angioplasty and coronary artery bypass graft surgery. These approaches have all been found to be successful in reperfusing acutely occluded coronary vessels, with encouraging results in terms of improvement of left ventricular function. Intravenous thrombolytic therapy, the only reperfusion therapy that currently has widespread applicability, has clearly been shown to result in improved survival.

In the past few years there has been a growing interest in the evaluation, therapy, and clinical significance of asymptomatic, or silent, ischemic episodes in patients with coronary artery disease. Our understanding of the influence of silent ischemia on the course of ischemic heart disease continues to grow.

Other manifestations of ischemic heart disease, not the least of which are sudden cardiac death and chronic congestive heart failure, may complicate the therapy of the patient with angina and are sometimes the primary or earliest manifestations of ischemic heart disease. In these more complex patients, evaluation and management may require use or consideration of the entire range of our diagnostic and therapeutic armamentariums.

EVALUATION OF THE PATIENT WITH ISCHEMIC HEART DISEASE

The evaluation of patients with suspected or established ischemic heart disease often begins with the evaluation of chest pain. Use of the term angina pectoris to describe the chest pain of ischemic heart disease was originated by Dr. William Heberden in 1772 [82]. His classic description identified the qualities we now use to define typical angina pectoris: substernal or retrosternal chest discomfort that is precipitated by exertion and relieved by rest. The major clinical syndromes of ischemic heart disease (chronic stable angina, unstable angina, and myocardial infarction, as well as variant angina), all have angina pectoris as the most prominent symptom. Other presentations such as ventricular arrhythmias, congestive heart failure, and ischemic cardiomyopathy may have chest pain as part of the presentation and only the recently described entity of totally asymptomatic or silent myocardial ischemia does not have angina as part of the syndrome. Angina may also be present in other cardiac disorders, such as aortic stenosis and hypertrophic cardiomyopathy, to name two common examples, but it is often difficult to know whether coronary obstruction is not also present. The chest pain of some cardiac disorders may, at times, be difficult to differentiate from angina pectoris, but clarification of the etiology most often will not require invasive diagnostic techniques.

A number of features of ischemic heart disease make the evaluation of this common disorder a complicated feat. As previously alluded to, the manifestations of ischemic heart disease are protean and range from the patient with minimal atherosclerosis and no symptoms to the patient with severe stenosis of all major coronary vessels and left ventricular dysfunction who may present with severe symptoms. This broad range of presentations with markedly different outcomes compels the physician to modify the approach to evaluation and management of the patient dependent on the severity and urgency of the presentation.

An important part of the evaluation of patients with ischemic heart disease is the determination of high-risk subsets, such as left main coronary artery stenosis and important stenosis of all three major epicardial coronary vessels with left ventricular dysfunction. Unfortunately, the history, physical examination, and noninvasive testing do not have the sensitivity to identify reliably all these high-risk patients. Cardiac catheterization accurately identifies these subsets but involves some risk to the patient, although generally that risk is very low.

Further confounding the rational attempts of clinicians to evaluate their patients with ischemic heart disease is the changing prognosis of this disease. With improved medical and surgical therapy, there has been a trend toward improved prognosis of ischemic heart disease [51, 115, 117, 130]; this will affect the need and justification for diagnostic testing and therapeutic intervention. In addition, as advances are made in diagnostic and therapeutic techniques, these may be incorporated into medical practice at a pace that is sometimes faster than can be efficiently accommodated. At times, technological advances precede our ability to utilize them to their fullest potential.

TABLE 2-1. *Evaluation of Patient with Ischemic Heart Disease*

History
  Elucidation of basic descriptors of chest pain
  Elucidation of other cardiovascular symptoms
  Past medical history
  Family history
Physical examination
  Diagnostic information
  Functional assessment
Laboratory investigation
  Electrocardiogram
  Ambulatory electrocardiography
  Exercise testing
    Thallium-201 scintigraphy
    Equilibrium radionuclide angiocardiography
    Echocardiography
  Myocardial imaging
    Positron-emission tomography
    Single photon-emission computed tomography
Cardiac catheterization
  Hemodynamic evaluation
  Coronary angiography
  Left ventriculography
  Assessment of coronary flow reserve

History

Despite the vast array of sophisticated diagnostic and therapeutic modalities available to us, the patient history is the first, and sometimes most important, step in the evaluation of the patient with chest pain and suspected ischemic heart disease [30, 56, 135] (Table 2-1). As with symptoms of any disease state, the clinician must elucidate the basic properties of chest pain to determine its etiology: location, quality, severity, chronology, setting in which it occurs, aggravating or alleviating factors, and associated symptoms. The earliest report of angina pectoris, by Heberden, described the chest discomfort as a sense of "strangling and anxiety" [82]. Additional descriptions in use today include the terms crushing, heavy, squeezing, pressure-like, and constricting. The location is usually substernal or retrosternal, with radiation of the pain to the left shoulder and arm, throat, neck, jaw, and teeth being relatively common. Typical angina pectoris is precipitated by exertion or emotion and relieved by rest.

Other symptoms may occur during myocardial ischemia such as dyspnea, nausea, fatigue, and faintness and have been termed anginal equivalents. Symptoms of congestive heart failure such as fatigue, dyspnea on exertion, orthopnea and edema, and of arrhythmias, such as palpitations and syncope, must also be elucidated. The past medical history, family history, and risk factor assessment are also particularly important parts of the clinical history when evaluating the patient with ischemic heart disease.

Although the clinical history is tremendously helpful diagnostically and can give some indication of the extent of atherosclerotic involvement of the coronary arteries [31], it is clear that the distribution of chest pain, the precipitating factors of angina, and the duration of angina have no good correlation with prognosis or the anatomic extent of coronary disease seen angiographically [8, 58, 131, 170].

There are some subsets of patients with ischemic heart disease in whom the history is generally less helpful. Some patients, for reasons as yet unclear, do not have angina pectoris or other ischemic symptoms despite objective documentation of ischemia, a clinical entity currently labeled silent myocardial ischemia [106]. On the other hand, some patients with coronary artery disease, notably women under 50 years of age, tend to have chest pain syndromes with atypical features [173].

Physical Examination

The physical examination can provide important clues to the presence of coronary disease, even though not diagnostic. The findings of hypertension, peripheral vascular disease, signs of hypercholesterolemia such as xanthomas and xantholasmas, and arcus senilis raise the possibility of coronary artery disease. The cardiac examination is of obvious importance in the evaluation of any cardiac disorder and may also aid in the diagnosis and assessment of severity of involvement in the patient with suspected or documented ischemic heart disease. Abnormalities of cardiac rhythm, abnormal precordial impulses, decreased intensity of the first heart sound, abnormal splitting of the second heart sound, ventricular and atrial gallop sounds, the murmur of mitral regurgitation in the absence of mitral valve disease, elevation of jugular venous pressure, pulmonary rales, peripheral edema, and, rarely, the presence of a diastolic murmur from coronary artery stenosis all give important diagnostic and functional information [27].

Electrocardiogram

The laboratory evaluation of the patient with suspected or documented ischemic heart disease begins with the electrocardiogram (ECG). The resting ECG will frequently be normal in patients with angina pectoris when performed in the absence of chest pain. Abnormalities that may be found include nonspecific ST-T abnormalities, evidence of prior myocardial infarction, and, possibly, conduction abnormalities. Unfortunately, only Q waves indicative of myocardial infarction have specificity for coronary artery disease.

The electrocardiogram performed during chest pain, however, provides valuable information whether normal or abnormal. The resting

ECG in patients with unstable angina is characterized by ST segment depression or elevation in the vast majority, and the remainder will generally show T-wave inversion [120]. Patients with variant angina, or coronary artery spasm, typically develop ST segment elevation on the electrocardiogram during chest pain [28]. Ambulatory electrocardiographic monitoring is another useful tool in evaluating both symptomatic and asymptomatic ischemia [29, 38].

Exercise Testing

Exercise testing is indicated in patients with symptoms or signs suggestive of coronary artery disease or with known coronary artery disease to establish the diagnosis, assess functional capacity, and assess prognosis [30, 56, 135, 77]. When used to aid in the diagnosis of coronary artery disease the results of exercise stress testing must be interpreted in light of the prevalence of disease in the population being tested (Bayes theorem of conditional probability) [44]. Males with typical angina pectoris have a 90 percent likelihood of having coronary artery disease on angiography, and exercise testing would most often only confirm the initial impression [172]. Females with typical angina, however, have a prevalence of 60 to 70 percent [172]. Females also have a higher rate of false positive ST segment response with exercise testing, and therefore a positive test does not greatly improve the predictive accuracy of the history alone [77]. Exercise testing can be helpful diagnostically in males with atypical chest pain, but because of the problem with false positives, it is of limited value in women with atypical symptoms [77]. In asymptomatic men, exercise testing has a sensitivity of 50 percent and specificity of 90 percent [77]. The addition of Thallium-201 scintigraphy to exercise testing improves sensitivity and specificity, although interpretation is also dependent on the prevalence of disease in the population being tested [123]. The use of equilibrium radionuclide angiocardiography (gated blood pool imaging) in conjunction with exercise testing to diagnose coronary artery disease was initially said to have very high sensitivity and specificity [123]. Highly selected populations were used, however, and subsequent studies have shown lower sensitivity and specificity, with specificity as low as 31 percent [142]. Combining echocardiography with exercise testing results in improved sensitivity and specificity compared with exercise electrocardiography alone and in experienced hands is comparable to planar thallium imaging [7]. Pharmacologic stress testing, utilizing agents such as dipyridamole and dobutamine, can be used to diagnose ischemic heart disease in patients who cannot exercise.

Another important indication for exercise testing, in addition to aiding in diagnosis, is to determine prognosis and identify patients with coronary artery disease who are at high risk because of extensive disease or left ventricular dysfunction. Certain outcomes have been found to

TABLE 2-2. *Exercise Test Parameters Associated with Poor Prognosis and/or Increased Severity of CAD*

Duration of symptom-limiting exercise
  Failure to complete stage II of Bruce protocol or equivalent workload (≤ 6.5 METS*) with other protocols
Exercise heart rate (HR) at onset of limiting symptoms
  Failure to attain HR ≥ 120/min (off beta blockers)
Time of onset, magnitude, morphology, and postexercise duration of abnormal horizontal or downsloping ST segment depression
  Onset of HR < 120/min or ≤ 6.5 METS
  Magnitude ≥ 2.0 mm
  Postexercise duration ≥ 6 min
  Depression in multiple leads
Systolic BP response during or following progressive exercise
  Sustained decrease of > 10 mm Hg or flat BP response (≤ 130 mm Hg) during progressive exercise)
Other potentially important determinants
  Exercise-induced ST segment elevation in leads other than aVR
  Angina pectoris during exercise
  Exercise-induced U wave inversion
  Exercise-induced ventricular tachycardia

*Energy expenditure at rest, equivalent to an oxygen uptake of approximately 3.5 ml O_2 per kilogram body weight per minute.
Source: From R. C. Schlant, et al., Guidelines for Exercise Testing. A Report of the American College of Cardiology/American Heart Association Task Force on Assessment of Cardiovascular Procedures. (Subcommittee on exercise testing.) *J. Am. Coll. Cardiol.* 8:725–38, 1986.

be associated with a poor prognosis [77] (Table 2-2). On the other end of the spectrum, patients who can exercise for 9 minutes or more of a Bruce protocol exercise test and have less than 1 mm of ST segment depression have a good prognosis and will seldom have advanced coronary disease [172]. Thallium-201 scintigraphy again improves the usefulness of exercise testing in establishing prognosis. In one study, the number of myocardial segments with transient thallium defects was the only significant predictor of future cardiac events when compared with clinical, angiographic, and exercise test information [16]. Exercise testing is also indicated and helpful in the evaluation of patients following revascularization and in the assessment of functional capacity [77].

Myocardial Imaging

Recent advances in the field of radionuclide cardiac imaging have made it possible to detect the presence of ischemia, determine regional and global left ventricular systolic function, and quantitate regional myocardial necrosis, all with one imaging technique [156]. Both positron-emission tomography (PET) and single photon-emission computed tomography (SPECT) have these capabilities. It is hoped that these methodologies will be able to detect areas of ischemic but still viable myocardium, something our currently available technology cannot adequately predict.

Cardiac Catheterization

Coronary angiography and left ventriculography remain the standard for establishing the diagnosis of coronary artery disease. These techniques also furnish important information used to assess prognosis [147] and direct patient management. Coronary angiography does not provide physiologic information, however, and has been demonstrated to be inaccurate in the assessment of the physiologic significance of coronary stenosis if only the percent diameter stenosis is used [174]. Other techniques used in conjunction with coronary angiography, such as the assessment of coronary flow reserve assessed either by digital radiography [10] or by a Doppler tipped catheter [181], are being actively investigated to quantitate accurately the physiologic importance of coronary stenoses.

GOALS OF THERAPY

It is imperative that goals of therapy be established and kept in mind in the management of the patient with ischemic heart disease. In most patients, *relief of symptoms and improvement in quality of life* is the most important goal. This is the objective in the day-to-day care of patients receiving medical therapy and one that can be achieved in a large proportion of patients undergoing revascularization. It should also be considered in the setting of acute ischemic events, both short term and long term, as may be influenced by potential salvage of jeopardized myocardium. A second important goal is to *prevent cardiac events*, such as episodes of unstable angina, myocardial infarction, and life-threatening arrhythmias. Another major goal of therapy, which is closely linked to the prevention of cardiac events, is *improvement in survival*. These are sometimes difficult goals to achieve, but with identification of high-risk subsets, specific medical and surgical interventions have been clearly shown to be of benefit in these respects. A less well publicized but extremely important goal is *patient education*. Patients with ischemic heart disease will accept their situation and be more compliant and willing to participate in the achievement of other therapeutic goals if they have a good understanding of their disease, its natural history, and its treatment. This is a continuing educational process. The final goal is to *halt the progression of ischemic heart disease*. This can be achieved in some patients by recognition and modification of risk factors. In the age of interventional cardiology, this goal is too often forgotten or neglected. Reduction of serum cholesterol [107], control of hypertension [87], and cessation of smoking [54, 83, 92] have all been shown to reduce the risk of coronary artery disease. The national decline in mortality from ischemic heart disease may be due in part to improvements in these and other risk factors; preventive efforts continue to be justified.

APPROACH TO THERAPY

The therapy of ischemic heart disease continues to evolve and change rapidly. Since the introduction of nitroglycerin for the relief of angina pectoris over 100 years ago [17], medical therapy has changed tremendously, most notably in the past decade, with the addition of beta blockers and calcium channel antagonists, as well as a wide range of long-acting nitroglycerin preparations. One of the most important advances in the therapy of patients with ischemic heart disease has been the surgical technique of coronary artery bypass grafting (CABG), which was developed in the mid-1960s [39, 52]. Surgical revascularization results in relief of symptoms in most patients with angina pectoris, although angina may recur due to continued progression of disease. Certain anatomic subsets have improved survival after undergoing CABG. This procedure continues to be refined, and results have improved with newer techniques such as the use of cold cardioplegia for myocardial protection and the use of the internal mammary artery graft. The use of percutaneous transluminal coronary angioplasty (PTCA) has undergone remarkable growth since it was first performed by Grüntzig in 1977 [73]. Early evaluation of PTCA focused on the successful dilation of coronary artery stenoses. PTCA is now beginning to be evaluated in terms of its efficacy in relieving symptoms, salvage of myocardium in acute ischemic syndromes [124], economic comparisons with other forms of therapy [94], and its effect on survival.

In addition to PTCA, other interventional techniques are being developed to treat ischemic heart disease. Laser angioplasty is being evaluated clinically [146] and other mechanical means of improving coronary flow have been investigated [93].

During the same period of time that PTCA was rapidly becoming a part of the therapy of ischemic heart disease, an older medical therapy was being resurrected. Thrombolytic therapy has been extensively investigated over the past 20 years with mixed results [49, 102, 151]. With the advent of aggressive coronary angiography in the setting of acute myocardial infarction, it became clear that thrombosis at the site of a severe coronary stenosis, resulting in coronary artery occlusion, is the cause of approximately 90 percent of all transmural myocardial infarctions [42]. This confirmation of a theory proposed many years earlier led to a rebirth of thrombolytic therapy for acute myocardial infarction. Many studies of thrombolytic therapy during the early phase of this rebirth used intracoronary administration of streptokinase relatively late after the onset of symptoms. These studies when considered together conferred no benefit in survival [57]. Studies using streptokinase early in the course of acute myocardial infarction, however, have shown dramatic salvage of jeopardized myocardium whether given intravenously [100] or by the intracoronary route [35]. More recent evaluations of intravenous administration of thrombolytic agents for acute myocardial infarction have clearly demonstrated improved survival with the use of streptokinase [75, 90], tissue plasminogen activator [175], and anisoylated plasminogen streptokinase activator complex (APSAC) [3].

The major syndromes of ischemic heart disease are chronic stable angina, unstable angina, and acute myocardial infarction. Although the distinctions between these entities sometimes become unclear and some patients don't fit well into any of these categories, it is useful to develop an approach to the therapy of ischemic heart disease using these major syndromes as starting points. Guidelines for the management of stable angina, unstable angina, and myocardial infarction will be pertinent to the management of mixed angina, variant angina, and silent ischemia, although these syndromes have unique characteristics that require special consideration.

CHRONIC STABLE ANGINA

Chronic angina with a stable clinical course is typically a manifestation of fixed obstruction in the epicardial coronary arteries secondary to atherosclerosis. The development of angina in this syndrome can be thought of as an imbalance in the myocardial oxygen supply-demand ratio [171]. In the presence of severe coronary stenosis, supply to the coronary circulation distal to the stenosis may not be able to increase to meet increased demand, resulting in ischemia, which typically manifests itself clinically as angina pectoris. The approach to the patient with chronic stable angina must therefore include consideration of the major determinants of myocardial oxygen supply and demand. Myocardial oxygen supply depends mainly on adequate oxygenation and adequate coronary blood flow, which is dependent on, and related intimately to, perfusion pressure. The major determinants of myocardial oxygen demand are left ventricular systolic pressure, left ventricular size, contractility, and heart rate. Efforts to limit myocardial oxygen demand, and thus to prevent ischemia, include prevention of systolic hypertension, reduction of ventricular size, reduction of the inotropic state of the heart or contractility, and control of heart rate. Increases in coronary vasomotor tone, or vasospasm, may play a role in limiting coronary blood flow and may be responsible for the development of angina at different levels of myocardial oxygen demand or when demand is unchanged.

Medical Therapy
Nitroglycerin preparations, beta blockers, and calcium channel antagonists all have beneficial effects on the major determinants of myocardial

oxygen demand and have proven benefit in the management of chronic stable angina. If the evaluation of stable angina reveals no indication of high risk, medical therapy will frequently control ischemic symptoms, thus accomplishing one of the major goals of therapy. In early studies of the natural history of coronary artery disease, the annual mortality was 2 to 3 percent, 7 to 8 percent, and 11 percent for one-, two-, and three-vessel disease, respectively [18, 136]. More recent studies of medically treated patients show better survival in comparison. The Veterans Administration multicenter trial's annual mortality for medically treated patients was 4 percent [117]. Patients with mild symptoms of angina in the Coronary Artery Surgery Study (CASS) who were treated medically had annual mortality rates of approximately 2 percent, 4 percent, and 8 percent for one-, two-, and three-vessel disease, respectively [115]. Even though the patients in the CASS study had less symptomatic coronary artery disease, these trends toward improved survival probably reflect improved medical therapy. Prognosis can be estimated not only by the location and number of stenotic major epicardial coronary arteries but also by the global left ventricular ejection fraction. Following myocardial infarction, survival is directly related to the ejection fraction (Fig. 2-1).

For those patients with disabling angina on medical therapy, assessment with coronary angiography and consideration of revascularization is indicated. Patients identified as being at high risk for cardiac events or early mortality by noninvasive testing are also candidates for angiographic assessment and revascularization.

Coronary Artery Bypass Graft Surgery

Coronary artery bypass graft surgery (CABG) emerged in the 1960s as the preferred surgical procedure for myocardial revascularization [39, 52]. This procedure utilizes the patient's saphenous vein to bypass obstructed coronary arteries. Use of the internal mammary artery after being dissected free from the chest wall has been employed more frequently in recent years, and its use is supported by studies showing improved graft patency with this technique [20, 159]. The in-hospital mortality for elective CABG performed by experienced surgical teams is probably 1 to 2 percent [95], although the large randomized trials of CABG versus medical therapy show a higher operative mortality of 4 to 5.6 percent [133]. The incidence of perioperative myocardial infarction is approximately 5 percent for elective CABG [95, 101]. It is clear that perioperative infarction adversely affects survival [119]. The use of cold cardioplegia for myocardial protection during surgery has reduced the incidence of perioperative myocardial infarction, and recent results may be improved [133]. Using saphenous veins, graft patency is 85 to 93 percent postoperatively, 75 to 90 percent at 1 year, and thereafter the vein graft occlusion rate is approximately 2 percent per year [13, 21].

The ability of myocardial revascularization with CABG to abolish or

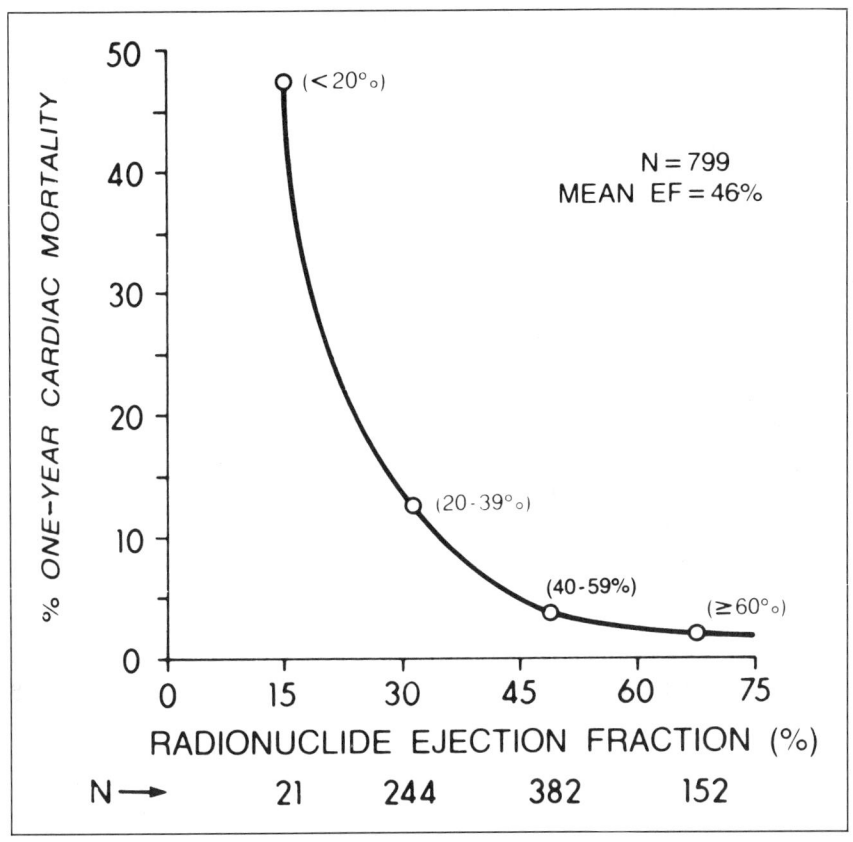

FIG. 2-1. Cardiac mortality rate in four categories of radionuclide Ejection Fraction (EF) determined before discharge. N denotes the number of patients in the total evaluation and in each category. Of 811 patients in whom the ejection fraction was recorded, 12 were lost to follow-up during the first year after hospitalization. (From The Multicenter Postinfarction Research Group: Risk stratification and survival after myocardial infarction. *N. Engl. J. Med.* 309:331–36, 1983, with permission.)

improve anginal symptoms in the majority of patients, and do so more effectively than medical therapy, is well established [126, 140]. Objective improvement in exercise performance has also been documented [103]. Surgical revascularization is not a cure, however, and angina commonly recurs in a number of years [22] and is related to graft patency. None of the large randomized trials of CABG for chronic angina has shown a difference in the incidence of myocardial infarction, and this is accounted for by the perioperative infarction rate in the surgically treated patients [133].

Although debate continues, survival is improved in certain anatomic subsets, as determined by cardiac catheterization, in patients undergoing CABG. In those patients with significant stenosis of the left main coronary artery, especially those identified as being high risk on the basis of a history of infarction, hypertension, functional class III or IV, or resting ECG abnormalities, survival is improved with surgery compared to medical therapy [51, 157, 158]. Proximal disease of both the left anterior descending and circumflex coronary arteries does not have the same prognosis as left main coronary artery stenosis and cannot be considered as a left main equivalent [133]. Patients with significant stenosis of all three major epicardial coronary arteries (three-vessel disease) and the same high-risk characteristics had improved survival with surgery in the VA Cooperative Trial [117]. The European Coronary Surgery Study of patients with coronary disease and good left ventricular function showed there was improved 6-year survival in the surgically treated patients with three-vessel disease (CABG 94 percent vs. medical 80.4 percent) [50]. There was no significant difference in 5-year survival for those patients with three-vessel disease in the CASS study who were either asymptomatic or had mild angina (CABG 93 percent vs. medical 89 percent) [23]. There was improved survival, however, in the patients with three-vessel disease and reduced ejection fraction (50 percent). The medically treated patients in the CASS study had surprisingly good survival, which is probably a reflection of their mild symptoms, in comparison to patients in the other large randomized trials of CABG in chronic angina.

In patients with two-vessel disease, prognosis varies dependent on whether the left anterior descending coronary artery (LAD) is involved [50]. Those with LAD involvement have poorer survival, although surgery does not clearly improve survival in these patients. There are still some uncertainties regarding the effect of CABG on survival, and reanalysis of the available studies continues as improved medical and surgical therapies are instituted [78]. However, some important guidelines can be established from the information produced by the large randomized trials of medical and surgical therapy of coronary artery disease.

1. Coronary artery bypass graft surgery confers a survival advantage in patients with hemodynamically significant left main coronary artery disease.
2. Coronary artery bypass graft surgery also confers a survival advantage to those patients with three-vessel disease and impaired ventricular function or who are otherwise identified to be high risk on the basis of functional classification, prior myocardial infarction, hypertension, or resting ECG abnormalities.
3. Coronary artery bypass graft surgery does not prevent myocardial infarction compared to medical therapy.
4. Patients with coronary artery disease whose symptoms are adequately treated with medical therapy may be continued on medical

therapy until surgery is indicated on the basis of high-risk anatomic features as described in statements 1 and 2 above or their symptoms become unresponsive to medical therapy.

Percutaneous Transluminal Coronary Angioplasty

Percutaneous transluminal coronary angioplasty (PTCA) was initially recommended for a narrowly defined subset of patients with chronic stable angina: those with single-vessel atherosclerotic stenosis that is severe, discrete, proximal, noncalcified, and concentric, with normal left ventricular function, and refractory symptoms [118]. With increased experience and rapid technical advances, indications for PTCA have broadened considerably and currently include multivessel disease, prior CABG, acute myocardial infarction, and unstable angina, as well as patients with advanced age and poor left ventricular function [80]. Primary success in achieving an improvement in coronary stenosis has improved from approximately 63 percent as reported by the National Heart, Lung and Blood Institute (NHLBI) Registry in 1983 [96] to as high as 91 percent at institutions with many years of experience that perform a high volume of procedures and use recent technological advances. The primary success rate for single-vessel PTCA by experienced operators is expected to be 85 to 90 percent [12]. Reported primary success rates for two-vessel disease are 85 percent [112] and for multi-vessel PTCA 87 percent [167]. Completely occluded vessels may be opened in approximately half of all cases if the occlusion has been relatively recent in onset [98].

The NHLBI PTCA Registry reported an overall complication rate of 21 percent in the first 3 ½ years of PTCA, with a major complication rate of 9.2 percent (myocardial infarction, emergency CABG, or death). Emergency surgery was required in 6 to 8 percent, and the mortality rate was 1.1 percent. These results included the learning curve of institutions, institutions with a low volume of procedures, and a fixed guidewire system.

Complication rates have improved with experience, better patient selection, and improved angioplasty systems. Results from experienced institutions have Q wave infarction rates and requirements for emergency surgery as low as 1.1 percent and 3.1 percent, respectively [72]. For most institutions, the emergency surgery rate is 2.5 percent, the myocardial infarction rate is 2.3 percent, and the mortality rate is approximately 1 percent [74]. Restenosis rates vary considerably but are probably in the range of 15 to 30 percent in native vessels [12], and often higher. The restenosis rate of dilated bypass grafts is as high as 50 percent [46]. Successful PTCA is associated with improvement in symptoms in approximately 80 percent [96] as well as improvement in left ventricular function and hemodynamics [97, 178]. Information on the influence of PTCA on survival is not available.

TABLE 2-3. *Comparison of PTCA and CABG for Therapy of Ischemic Heart Disease*

	PTCA	CABG
Advantages	Lower cost	Applicable to most patients
	Short hospitalization	Associated cardiac abnormalities can be treated
	Less morbidity	Improved survival in certain anatomical subsets
	Decreased duration of disability	Cardiopulmonary bypass allows treatment of complications
Disadvantages	Significant incidence of restenosis	More costly
	Not applicable to many patients	Longer hospital stay
	Complications may require emergency CABG	Increased morbidity
	Long-term consequences largely unknown	Increased duration of disability
		Gradual attrition of saphenous vein bypass grafts

PTCA has been developed into a safe and clinically effective technique of myocardial revascularization and has become a proven alternative to CABG in selected patients (Table 2-3). As this technique continues to improve, the indications for PTCA will most probably continue to broaden. In comparison to CABG, PTCA is less expensive [94], requires less hospitalization, and is associated with less morbidity [85, 91].

The disadvantages of PTCA include failure to achieve a primary success in all patients, restenosis in a significant number of patients, anatomy unsuitable for the procedure in many patients, and the need for emergency surgery in 2 to 5 percent of procedures. PTCA is also a specialized procedure that does not address other potentially correctable cardiac disorders. The ability to relieve symptoms of ischemia is similar for PTCA and CABG.

Symptomatic patients with a single discrete proximal coronary artery stenosis are still the most appropriate candidates for PTCA. For most patients with multivessel disease, especially three-vessel disease, and those with totally occluded vessels for more than a few months, coronary artery bypass surgery remains the logical choice of therapy. The best form of therapy for patients with two- and three-vessel coronary disease is still being investigated.

In the future, newer forms of percutaneous revascularization may prove beneficial. These procedures may involve laser angioplasty, modified forms of angioplasty balloons, and atherectomy.

UNSTABLE ANGINA

Patients with unstable angina almost invariably have severe atherosclerotic coronary artery disease. In addition, approximately 75 percent of these patients can be shown to have progression of their disease angiographically [116]. In the past, the mechanism of unstable angina was thought to be the same as stable angina. It was also believed that anginal episodes were primarily precipitated by increased myocardial oxygen demand in the presence of a fixed oxygen supply due to severe fixed atherosclerotic obstruction. There is a growing body of evidence, however, indicating that thrombosis plays an important role in the development of unstable angina [65, 109, 160, 161, 169, 181] and that the pathophysiology may be similar to acute myocardial infarction [4]. Coronary angiography performed in the setting of unstable angina frequently demonstrates complex atherosclerotic obstruction suggesting rupture of atherosclerotic plaques, partially occlusive thrombi, or both [5]. Coronary angioscopic studies of patients with unstable angina show that increases in the frequency and severity of angina are associated with ulceration of atherosclerotic plaques and suggest that the subsequent development of thrombus may cause unstable rest angina [150]. Coronary vasospasm has been shown to be involved in the pathogenesis of this disorder [111]. It is also thought that platelet aggregation participates in the development of unstable angina since platelet aggregates can form and obstruct flow in an experimentally narrowed canine coronary artery [55] and because antiplatelet therapy has a convincing beneficial effect on the outcome of patients with this syndrome [19, 105].

As the pathophysiology of unstable angina becomes more completely understood, the approach to therapy has shifted. In the past, most interventions in unstable angina were aimed at decreasing myocardial oxygen demands. The therapy of this disorder now includes efforts to improve myocardial oxygen supply as well and to reverse the thrombosis, spasm, and platelet aggregation that may precipitate the development of unstable angina.

The prognosis of unstable angina varies with the type of presentation. Recent onset angina has a more favorable prognosis than crescendo angina or angina at rest, with less chance of myocardial infarction or death and a greater chance of becoming asymptomatic [11, 47, 129]. Patients with crescendo angina have infarction and death rates similar to recent onset angina but are less likely to improve symptomatically.

Angina at rest has a poorer outcome generally, with high rates of myocardial infarction and death [34, 60, 113].

Medical Therapy

Most patients with ischemic chest pain at rest associated with electrocardiographic changes of ischemia can be controlled with medical therapy including, at least, beta blockers and nitroglycerin preparations [144]. This includes patients with transient ST elevation during pain [145].

There has been some controversy over the use of beta blockers in patients with angina at rest, especially those with ST segment elevation, because of the theoretic risk of enhanced coronary vasoconstriction due to unopposed alpha-adrenergic tone [141]. Beta blockers, however, when used in conjunction with vasodilators, have been shown to reduce both symptomatic and silent episodes of ischemia without producing clinical deterioration [69].

Nitroglycerin preparations should be employed; they have a beneficial effect on ischemia by decreasing myocardial oxygen demand through a reduction in left ventricular size and systemic resistance [2]. Intravenous nitroglycerin infusions have the advantage of being rapidly titrated to the desired effect [34]. Hypotension is the most worrisome side effect of nitrate therapy and must be avoided.

The addition of calcium channel antagonists to nitrate and beta blocker therapy in unstable angina has been shown to have a beneficial effect in terms of the incidence of sudden death, myocardial infarction, and persistent angina [61, 121, 125]. In patients with angina at rest due to coronary artery spasm, calcium channel antagonists reduce the frequency of anginal episodes both acutely and chronically [6].

A number of treatment strategies have been employed to address thrombosis and platelet aggregation, which are thought to play an important role in the development of unstable angina. Intravenous infusion of heparin reduces the incidence of refractory angina and myocardial infarction in patients with unstable angina [160, 161]. Two large, randomized trials of aspirin therapy in unstable angina both revealed a reduced incidence of myocardial infarction and subsequent death in the aspirin-treated group [19, 105]. The combination of intravenous heparin and oral aspirin appears to not have any therapeutic advantage over intravenous heparin alone and is associated with a slightly higher complication rate [161].

Thrombolytic Therapy

Thrombolytic therapy using streptokinase administered by the intracoronary route has been evaluated in small studies of unstable angina and these have shown improvement in symptoms in the treated patients [109, 169]. The use of intravenous tissue plasminogen activator for unstable angina has been associated with rapid improvement of symptoms and marked reduction in the prevalence of intracoronary thrombus demonstrated angiographically [65], but the overall treatment effect is mild and not clearly more beneficial than the combination of heparin and aspirin [180].

Medical Versus Surgical Therapy

Randomized trials comparing medical and surgical therapy of unstable angina have shown no overall improvement in survival with surgery [108, 132, 144, 149]. The trial sponsored by the National Heart, Lung and Blood Institute [144] showed low in-hospital mortality for both surgically and medically treated patients, as well as similar late mortality. Myocardial infarction rates were not significantly different between treatment groups, although they were somewhat higher in the surgically treated group. This trial was conducted prior to the widespread use of cold cardioplegia for myocardial protection, however, and it is likely that perioperative infarction rates are now lower [86]. It is interesting and important to note that during the follow-up period of 30 months, over a third of the medically treated patients (36 percent) required surgical intervention for recurrent angina refractory to medical therapy. This study and others support the concept that unstable angina can be controlled effectively in most patients with aggressive medical management and that coronary angiography and revascularization can be performed electively.

The largest and most recent comparison of medical and surgical therapy for unstable angina, the Veterans Administration Cooperative Study [108], has confirmed the findings of the earlier trials but also demonstrated that the subset of patients with depressed left ventricular ejection fraction (0.30 to 0.59) who underwent surgery had improved survival compared with those who were treated medically. All the trials comparing medical and surgical therapy of unstable angina, however, have been performed prior to the widespread use of anticoagulant therapy and calcium channel antagonists and also do not address the role PTCA may have in the therapy of patients with unstable angina.

Percutaneous Transluminal Coronary Angioplasty

PTCA is an alternative to CABG in selected patients with unstable angina. In those patients with unstable angina and single-vessel disease, PTCA can be performed safely and with a high success rate [53, 179]. Mortality and morbidity in this subset of patients is similar to CABG. Both procedures provide marked symptomatic improvement, although PTCA may be more successful in this regard [53]. Highly selected patients with multivessel disease and refractory unstable angina who have normal or near normal left ventricular function may also undergo PTCA safely and with a high success rate [40]. The role of PTCA in patients with multivessel disease remains controversial, however. Randomized trials comparing PTCA to other therapies in unstable angina are needed to clarify further the benefits of PTCA in patients with multivessel disease who present with this disorder.

The application of PTCA to the syndrome of unstable angina is limited by unsuitable coronary anatomy in approximately half of all patients with this disorder [68]. Another major limitation is the incidence of restenosis in the dilated segment, which is probably similar to the restenosis rate in stable angina [40]. Despite these limitations, PTCA will probably be used more commonly for patients with unstable angina in the future.

Treatment Strategy of Unstable Angina

Even though the outlook for patients with unstable angina has improved with the advent of newer medical therapies and revascularization strategies, this syndrome still requires immediate attention by highly trained medical personnel. Hospitalization in an intensive care setting with electrocardiographic monitoring is indicated in these patients. Precipitating problems such as anemia, hypoxia, hypertension, congestive heart failure, valvular heart disease, and thyroid disorders must be investigated and treated appropriately. A trial of sublingual nitroglycerin should be given to patients with ongoing ischemic chest pain and no hypotension or signs of hypovolemia. Antianginal therapy, including nitrates, beta blockers, and calcium channel antagonists should also be instituted if no contraindications exist (Fig. 2-2). Anticoagulation with intravenous heparin infusion and/or oral aspirin is justified. Thrombolytic therapy may, in the future, be indicated, and its role in unstable angina is being actively investigated.

Coronary angiography is indicated when patients with unstable angina cannot be stabilized with medical therapy. Intra-aortic balloon counterpulsation may be necessary for stabilization and is effective in relieving ischemic chest pain [67]. Revascularization with PTCA or CABG can be performed safely in these patients and is indicated, with the choice of procedure based on anatomical considerations and the experience and expertise of the institution.

Most patients who are stabilized with medical therapy will also require invasive testing with coronary angiography. Patients who have recurrence of symptoms or who are otherwise identified to be at high risk for future events should be revascularized during the same hospitalization if anatomy is suitable. The large randomized trials of unstable angina, however, suggest that patients can be continued on medical therapy and will be at no increased risk compared to a surgically treated group, except for those with depressed left ventricular function. This may be changing with widespread experience with PTCA and improved

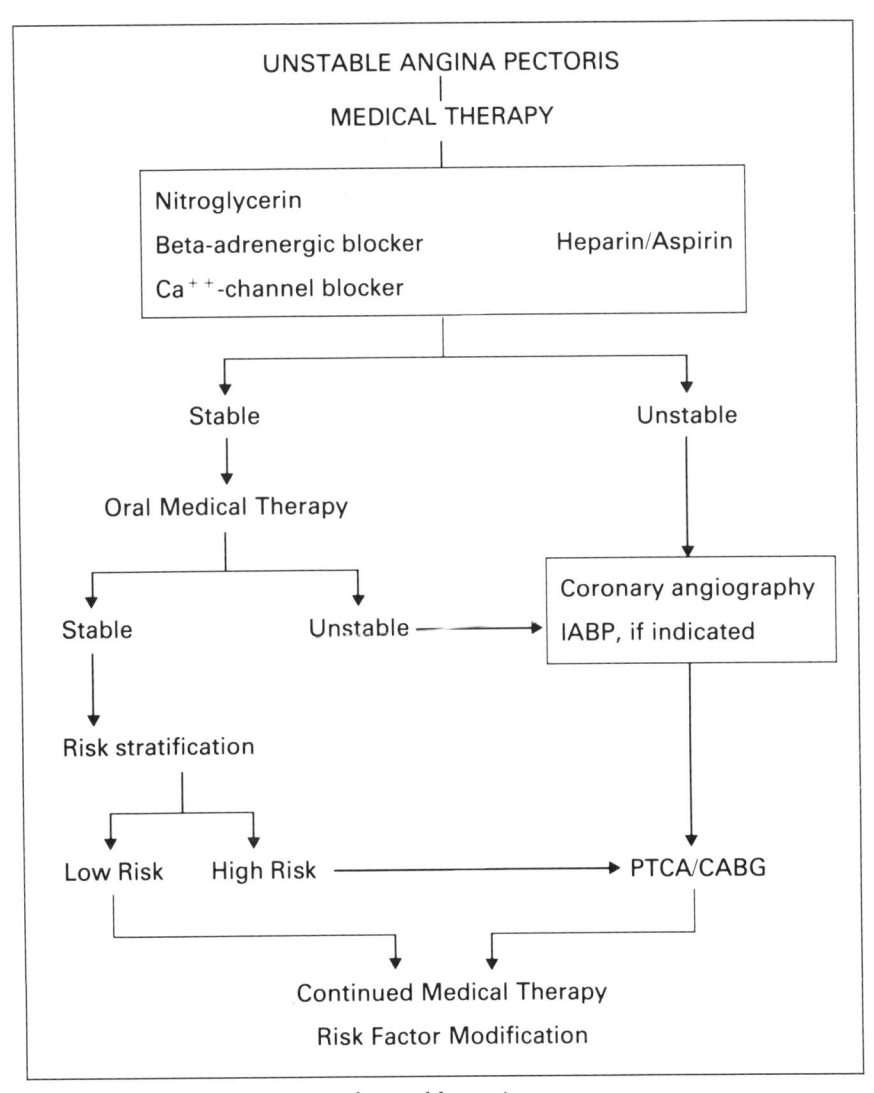

```
                    UNSTABLE ANGINA PECTORIS
                              |
                       MEDICAL THERAPY
                              |
        ┌─────────────────────────────────────────────┐
        │  Nitroglycerin                              │
        │  Beta-adrenergic blocker    Heparin/Aspirin │
        │  Ca⁺⁺-channel blocker                       │
        └─────────────────────────────────────────────┘
                    │                       │
                    ▼                       ▼
                 Stable                  Unstable
                    │                       │
                    ▼                       │
            Oral Medical Therapy            │
                    │                       │
            ┌───────┴───────┐               ▼
            ▼               ▼       ┌──────────────────────┐
          Stable         Unstable ──▶│ Coronary angiography │
            │                       │ IABP, if indicated   │
            ▼                       └──────────────────────┘
       Risk stratification                   │
            │                                │
        ┌───┴───┐                            │
        ▼       ▼                            │
     Low Risk  High Risk ──────────────▶ PTCA/CABG
        │       │                            │
        └───────┴────────────┬───────────────┘
                             ▼
                 Continued Medical Therapy
                  Risk Factor Modification
```

FIG. 2-2. Treatment strategy of unstable angina.

surgical techniques. Patients who have responded well to medical therapy and have no features identifying them as being at high risk can be followed and a decision regarding revascularization can be made based on their symptoms and anatomical findings, just as is done with patients who have chronic stable angina. As the pathophysiology of unstable angina and the contributions of endothelial disruption, thrombosis, platelet aggregation, and vasospasm become better understood, the approach to the patient with unstable angina will be further clarified.

MYOCARDIAL INFARCTION

Acute occlusion of an epicardial coronary artery is the usual cause of transmural myocardial infarction. Angiographic studies performed in the early stages of acute myocardial infarction have demonstrated thrombotic occlusion of 70 to 90 percent of the infarct-related coronary arteries and the remainder have severe stenoses [42, 113, 138]. The occluding thrombus usually develops at the site of a stenotic atherosclerotic plaque with disruption of the endothelium [24, 36]. When visualized angiographically after successful thrombolytic therapy, these ruptured plaques frequently appear as eccentric stenoses, with narrow necks or irregular borders; an appearance similar to that associated with unstable angina [4]. Coronary spasm has been suspected as a participating mechanism in the pathogenesis of acute myocardial infarction, although intracoronary administration of nitroglycerin or calcium channel antagonists only rarely opens an occluded infarct-related artery [139]. Platelet aggregation has also been implicated in the development of coronary thrombosis and acute myocardial infarction [176]. Although the presence or absence of Q waves on the electrocardiogram cannot reliably detect the presence or absence of transmural myocardial infarction, non-Q wave myocardial infarctions are not usually associated with total occlusion of an epicardial coronary artery [43].

Medical Therapy

In the past, the approach to therapy of acute myocardial infarction involved bed rest, electrocardiographic monitoring, oxygen, analgesia, and efforts to prevent and treat complications. The therapy of arrhythmias has produced a decrease in the mortality of acute myocardial infarction, but mortality from left ventricular dysfunction following infarction has been unaffected by this conventional approach.

In the 1960s it was recognized that the extent of left ventricular dysfunction is directly related to the amount of necrosis following acute myocardial infarction. It later became clear that survival was closely related to left ventricular function as measured by the ejection fraction [143]. As these concepts were established, a wide range of therapies were developed and evaluated in attempts to limit the size of myocardial infarcts, thereby hopefully improving the prognosis of survivors. Many of these early therapies were aimed at improving the balance between myocardial oxygen supply and demand. These therapies have included beta blockers, nitroglycerin, nitroprusside and other vasodilators, calcium channel antagonists, hyaluronidase, glucose-insulin-potassium infusion, corticosteroids, and intra-aortic balloon counterpulsation. Even though some benefit can be demonstrated with this approach, the amount of myocardium that can be salvaged is quite limited [143].

Reperfusion Strategies

As the pathophysiology of acute myocardial infarction became better understood and the role of coronary thrombosis in this disorder was again appreciated, strategies designed to reperfuse ischemic myocardium were developed and investigated. Use of reperfusion strategies has also been supported by experimental studies showing salvage of ischemic myocardium following reperfusion of an occluded coronary artery [62, 99, 137]. Thrombolytic therapy, percutaneous transluminal coronary angioplasty, and coronary artery bypass graft surgery are reperfusion therapies that address the underlying pathophysiology of acute myocardial infarction directly and have shown some promise in the treatment of this disorder. As these aggressive therapies have been evaluated, it has become apparent that reperfusion therapy must be instituted within a very limited time interval after the onset of coronary occlusion to be successful, usually within 6 hours [14].

Coronary Artery Bypass Graft Surgery (CABG)

No randomized trials comparing CABG to other forms of therapy for acute myocardial infarction have been performed. In retrospective studies, however, CABG has been performed safely and has been associated with improved survival in comparison to a nonrandomized control group [26, 41]. Other studies have shown no consistent benefit [37, 153]. Surgical revascularization has the potential advantage of restoring blood flow to normal in previously occluded coronary arteries, providing revascularization to other areas served by stenotic vessels, and providing successful revascularization to vessels where thrombolytic therapy or PTCA have failed or are not appropriate. CABG, however, is not applicable to most patients with acute myocardial infarction and has been used on a regular basis in only a few centers because of delays in initiating therapy, high costs, and lack of facilities. The widespread application of CABG for acute myocardial infarction, therefore, has been considered impractical.

Thrombolytic Therapy

Because the prevalence of thrombotic coronary artery occlusion in transmural myocardial infarction is high, thrombolytic therapy has been proposed and investigated as a means of achieving early reperfusion. Experimental studies of early reperfusion in the setting of coronary artery occlusion and the clinical reports of emergency surgical revascularization in acute myocardial infarction have given added support to the use of thrombolytic therapy.

Streptokinase

The first thrombolytic agent to be used in clinical trials was streptokinase. The early trials of intravenous streptokinase produced inconsistent results [1, 151], although some of these studies suggested improved survival [49].

The first report of the use of intracoronary streptokinase for acute myocardial infarction was by Chazov et al. in 1976 [25]. Intracoronary administration of thrombolytic therapy has the advantage of visualizing the thrombus and coronary artery stenosis and immediate assessment of the efficacy of therapy. Streptokinase by the intracoronary route has been proven to be successful in reperfusing occluded vessels in patients with acute myocardial infarction, achieving a reperfusion rate of 75 to 80 percent [33]. Despite the high reperfusion rate, the many randomized trials of intracoronary streptokinase have failed to show any clear improvement in survival [57]. The Western Washington trial of intracoronary streptokinase demonstrated a decreased 30-day and 6-month mortality, but at 1 year there was no longer a significant difference in mortality between treated and control groups. Some of these trials enrolled patients up to 12 hours after the onset of symptoms, when it may be too late to salvage myocardium by reperfusion. Very early administration of intracoronary streptokinase in the setting of ischemic chest pain and electrocardiographic findings of acute myocardial infarction can actually prevent the development of infarction, although even when administered within 1 to 2 hours it is not successful in reperfusing the vessel or preventing infarction in all cases [35]. In addition to showing no consistent beneficial effects in randomized trials, intracoronary streptokinase has the limitations of delay in instituting therapy, costs and risk of the invasive procedure, and lack of widespread applicability. The investigation of thrombolytic therapy, therefore, again focused on the use of intravenous agents.

Trials of intravenous streptokinase have utilized high doses (500,000–1,700,000 units) over a short period of 30 to 60 minutes in attempts to produce a high concentration of drug at the site of the thrombus but still limit the duration of a systemic fibrinolytic state. These studies have shown successful reperfusion in approximately 50 percent of patients when documented angiographically [148, 154]. Other studies investigating the very early use of intravenous streptokinase (within 3 hours) have suggested reperfusion in almost all patients if clinical and not angiographic criteria are used to assess reperfusion [59]. Assessing reperfusion with noninvasive clinical criteria would obviously include some patients with subtotal or incomplete occlusion of the infarct-related artery. In a comparison of intravenous streptokinase given less than 1½ hours and 1½ to 4 hours after the onset of symptoms of acute myocardial ischemia, Koren et al. demonstrated better ventricular function and less frequent progression to Q wave infarction in the patients treated within 1½ hours [100]. These studies have reconfirmed the concept that thrombolytic therapy is most effective in reperfusing the infarct vessel and in salvaging jeopardized myocardium when given very early in the course of acute myocardial infarction.

A number of trials have been designed to answer the question of whether thrombolytic therapy in acute myocardial infarction has a beneficial effect on survival. Pooled results from trials of intravenous streptokinase have suggested improved survival in patients treated up to 24 hours after onset of pain [155]. Two large trials of intravenous streptokinase have clearly shown improved survival in acute myocardial infarction when compared to conventional therapy. The GISSI study, performed by the Italian Group for the Study of Streptokinase in Myocardial Infarction, enrolled 11,606 patients equally divided between intravenous streptokinase and control groups and showed improvement in survival in patients treated up to 6 hours after the onset of symptoms of acute infarction [75]. The Second International Study of Infarct Survival, ISIS-2, enrolled 17,187 patients with suspected acute myocardial infarction and showed improved survival even in patients treated late after onset of symptoms (13–24 hours) [90]. This study revealed another important finding: aspirin alone improved survival when given to patients with suspected acute myocardial infarction and the combination of aspirin and streptokinase resulted in better survival than either therapy alone. Streptokinase also results in improved ventricular function compared to conventional therapy [155].

Despite these measurable beneficial effects on left ventricular function and survival, the use of streptokinase has some disadvantages. Streptokinase is antigenic and may cause allergic reactions. Hypotension may complicate acute administration. A significant incidence of reinfarction has been demonstrated. In addition, there is a small but important incidence of serious hemorrhagic complications. Intravenous administration of streptokinase has significant advantages over the intracoronary route, including its ease and rapidity of administration, low cost, relative safety, and lack of need for catheterization facilities. Intravenous use has a lower reperfusion success rate, however, and the inherent disadvantages of a lack of clot specificity, prolonged fibrinolysis, antigenicity, and possibility of hemorrhagic complications remain.

Tissue Plasminogen Activator

Tissue plasminogen activator is a relatively fibrin selective thrombolytic agent produced by recombinant DNA technology [127]. Randomized trials in acute myocardial infarction have shown tPA to be more successful than streptokinase when given intravenously, with recanalization rates of 60 to 79 percent [165, 168]. Even though a systemic fibrinolytic state can be avoided, hemorrhagic complications are frequent when combined with heparinization and invasive studies [177]. Most bleeding occurs at the catheterization site, although gastrointestinal bleeding, intracranial hemorrhage, and bleeding from other vascular puncture sites has also been observed. The incidence of intracranial hemorrhage is increased with a total dose of 150 mg (1.9 percent), but is similar to other agents with the now well-established standard dose of 100 mg (0.5 percent). Reocclusion of the reperfused infarct-related vessel is a significant problem with the use of tPA and is probably related to the short half-life of this agent [66]. Reocclusion rates can be reduced if the infusion of tPA is continued or combined with intravenous heparin therapy.

The effect of tPA on ventricular function has been assessed by a small number of clinical trials that show a modest but significant improvement in global ejection fraction when compared to conventional treatment [76, 121]. Survival is also improved with tPA therapy of acute myocardial infarction [175]. In nonconcordant studies that directly compare intravenous streptokinase with intravenous tPA, there is a trend toward better survival in the tPA-treated patients, although the largest trial comparing tPA and streptokinase done by the International Study Group in cooperation with the GISSI-2 trial showed no difference in survival between tPA- and streptokinase-treated patients [88].

Anisoylated Plasminogen Streptokinase Activator Complex (APSAC)

Anisoylated plasminogen streptokinase activator complex, or anistreplase, was developed to overcome some of the limitations of the streptokinase molecule as used for thrombolysis in acute myocardial infarction. The active enzymatic site of the plasminogen-streptokinase complex is temporarily protected by acylation, improving bioavailability at the site of clot, prolonging fibrinolytic action, and allowing for rapid intravenous injection. Similar to tPA and streptokinase, APSAC has been shown to improve both ventricular function and survival when given for acute myocardial infarction [3, 9]. Recanalization rates are intermediate between streptokinase and tPA, although patency rates are higher than for other agents and reocclusion rates are low.

Urokinase

Urokinase is a naturally occurring enzyme that is an effective thrombolytic agent when given for acute myocardial infarction, with recanalization and patency rates intermediate between streptokinase and tPA. It does not produce hypotension or allergic reactions, as streptokinase and APSAC can, but is relatively expensive; there is little information regarding ventricular function and survival.

Single Chain Urokinase-type Plasminogen Activator (Pro-urokinase)

Pro-urokinase is a naturally occurring plasminogen activator made by recombinant DNA technology. It is relatively fibrin specific and has recanalization and patency rates similar to tPA [45]. It is not currently available for widespread use.

Combination Strategies

Combinations of thrombolytic agents with possible synergism have been proposed because of the limitations of suboptimal efficacy, reocclusion, and hemorrhagic complications. Combined infusions of various doses of tPA and urokinase [163], tPA and pro-urokinase [32], and tPA and streptokinase [71] have been investigated. Even though reperfusion may not occur more frequently than with single agents, bleeding complications are not increased and reocclusion rates may be lower.

The use of antiplatelet antibodies in conjunction with tPA has provided encouraging results in an experimental model of acute myocardial infarction, with rapid and sustained recanalization of occluded coronary arteries [63].

Summary of Thrombolytic Therapy

Thrombolytic therapy is a safe and effective treatment in the setting of acute myocardial infarction. Successful reperfusion, when achieved early in the evolution of myocardial infarction, reduces myocardial damage and improves prognosis. The earlier that thrombolytic therapy is administered, the greater the likelihood of myocardial salvage. Intravenous administration is the most widely applicable method of administering thrombolytic therapy. Streptokinase, APSAC, and tPA have all been shown to improve ventricular function and survival when given for acute myocardial infarction. Many issues remain unresolved, however. Is there one thrombolytic agent or combination of agents that is best? What method of administration is best? Should all patients receive thrombolytic therapy the same way or should therapy be individualized? How can reocclusion after thrombolytic therapy be prevented? What is the role of PTCA and CABG, and when are these revascularization procedures optimally employed? Preliminary answers are available to some of these questions, but final solutions await further investigation.

Percutaneous Transluminal Coronary Angioplasty

Since the development of PTCA in 1977 by Grüntzig for the treatment of patients with stable angina, the indications for this form of therapy have been changing and broadening. Many centers experienced with

PTCA have expanded the role of PTCA to include therapy of acute myocardial infarction.

PTCA has a number of advantages over other forms of reperfusion therapy for acute myocardial infarction. These include visualization of the thrombus and stenosis with assessment of therapy, avoidance of systemic fibrinolysis, a high successful recanalization rate, and the potential for rapid restoration of blood flow to normal or near normal levels. Early studies also suggest that PTCA may result in a lower risk of reocclusion and reinfarction compared to thrombolytic therapy and a more significant beneficial effect on left ventricular function. The disadvantages of PTCA as a therapy for myocardial infarction are, for the most part, related to the need for cardiac catheterization. It is expensive, it is not applicable to many people because of lack of nearby facilities, there are potential delays in initiating therapy, and there are risks to the procedure, although these are small.

The early use of PTCA as primary therapy for acute myocardial infarction has been demonstrated to be safe in skilled hands and to result in successful recanalization of the infarct-related artery in a very high percentage of patients [81, 128]. These early observational studies reported improvement in left ventricular ejection fraction [81] and Killip classification [128] following successful reperfusion. Two randomized trials comparing PTCA to intracoronary streptokinase in acute myocardial infarction have been reported [48, 124]. These studies showed a high recanalization rate, which was similar with both reperfusion strategies. Ventricular function as assessed by global ejection fraction and regional wall motion, however, was significantly better after PTCA. The residual stenosis remaining after intervention was much less in the angioplasty groups, and it is thought that relief of the underlying stenosis results in better preservation of ventricular function. These studies were too small to make comparisons of survival.

Combination Therapy with Thrombolytic Agents and PTCA

Following successful thrombolytic therapy, residual severe stenosis often persists in the infarct-related artery. In addition, a minority of patients with evolving myocardial infarction have subtotal occlusions. In these instances there is a high likelihood of continued myocardial ischemia and reocclusion. PTCA is a logical therapy for these patients and in some centers is routinely performed after successful thrombolysis if a significant stenosis persists. PTCA has been performed in the setting of acute myocardial infarction following thrombolytic therapy with streptokinase [64, 81, 114] and tPA [76, 152, 164, 166]. Even though PTCA can be performed safely, with high recanalization rates both with successful and unsuccessful thrombolysis, immediate PTCA following thrombolytic therapy is associated with occasional transient or sustained reocclusion during the procedure, a significant incidence of recurrent ischemia following the procedure, and no improvement in ventricular function or survival when compared to thrombolytic therapy alone or delayed PTCA after thrombolytic therapy. A comparison of a conservative strategy and an invasive strategy including PTCA following treatment with tPA for acute myocardial infarction resulted in similar outcomes for these strategies, suggesting that routine PTCA after myocardial infarction is not necessary and that PTCA can be performed for those patients who have spontaneous or inducible ischemia [162].

Observational studies of PTCA in the subset of patients with cardiogenic shock suggest that survival is improved with PTCA [104].

Summary of PTCA in Acute Myocardial Infarction

PTCA is a technique that has proven benefit for selected patients with acute myocardial infarction. When performed early in the course of evolving myocardial infarction, 65 to 90 percent of occluded infarct-related arteries can be recanalized. Aggressive therapy that includes PTCA can improve myocardial function as compared to other reperfusion strategies involving only thrombolytic therapy. Although at least one study utilizing both thrombolytic therapy and PTCA in acute myocardial infarction has shown an improvement in survival over conventional therapy, more information is needed to assess the potential long-term benefit of PTCA. Patients with severe left ventricular dysfunction or cardiogenic shock during acute myocardial infarction may be benefited more with acute reperfusion with PTCA than those with more normal left ventricular function.

The major limitation of PTCA is the requirement of a skilled catheterization team and fully equipped cardiac catheterization laboratory available at all times. Availability of an experienced cardiothoracic surgical team is also important, although surgical standby during reperfusion of occluded vessels is not necessary.

As is the case with thrombolytic therapy, reperfusion with PTCA as primary therapy must be instituted within a very limited time interval after the onset of coronary occlusion to be successful. There is some suggestion, however, that this time interval may be longer with more complete reperfusion with PTCA as compared to thrombolytic therapy.

The role of PTCA as adjunctive therapy after thrombolysis has been clarified to a significant extent. Immediate PTCA following thrombolytic therapy for acute myocardial infarction has no advantage over delayed or deferred PTCA and may even lead to a poorer outcome. In addition, a strategy of routine PTCA at 18 to 48 hours following thrombolysis has no advantage over a more conservative strategy involving catheterization and PTCA done for spontaneous or inducible ischemia.

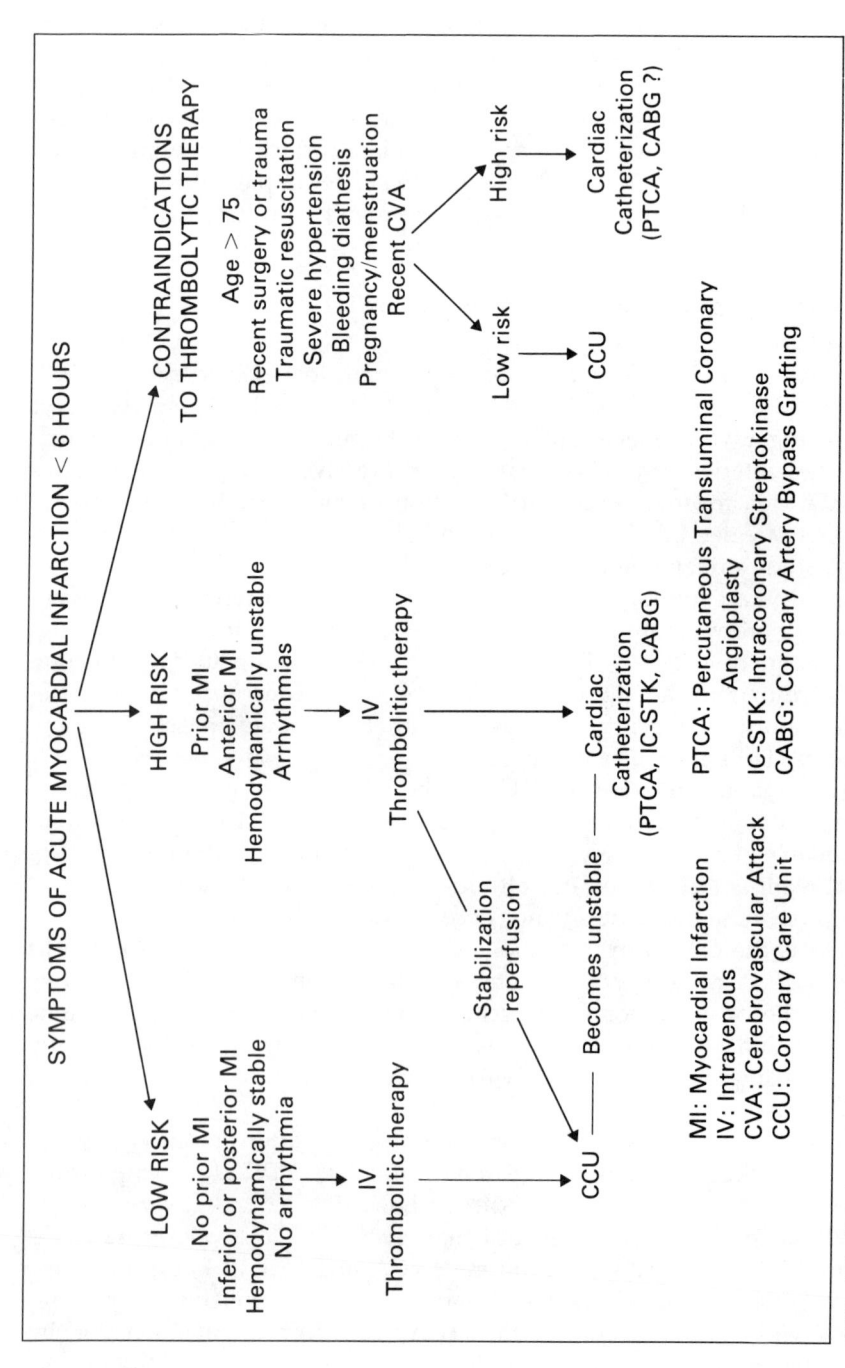

FIG. 2-3. Treatment strategy of acute myocardial infarction.

Treatment Strategy of Myocardial Infarction

The therapy of acute myocardial infarction has changed dramatically with the development of successful reperfusion therapies. Reperfusion therapy must be instituted within a very limited time interval after the onset of symptoms of acute myocardial infarction to have any significant beneficial effect on ventricular function and survival, usually within 6 hours, with salvage of threatened myocardium being inversely related to the time between onset of symptoms and institution of therapy.

The initial approach to the management of acute myocardial infarction is similar to the approach to unstable angina. Immediate attention by trained medical personnel, electrocardiographic monitoring, hospitalization in an intensive care setting, bed rest, oxygen, and analgesia are indicated. A trial of sublingual nitroglycerin should be given to patients with ongoing ischemic chest pain and no hypotension or signs of hypovolemia. Aspirin is of proven benefit and should be given if no contraindications exist. Efforts to decrease myocardial oxygen demand should be instituted if no contraindications exist. The complications of bradyarrhythmias, tachyarrhythmias, conduction abnormalities, right ventricular infarction, left ventricular dysfunction, and mechanical complications must be anticipated and aggressively treated.

Reperfusion therapy must be considered as early as possible in the course of myocardial infarction. It is helpful to stratify patients into low-risk and high-risk subsets (Fig. 2-3). Patients presenting within 6 hours after the onset of symptoms may benefit from intravenous thrombolytic therapy, especially if they present very early. Those patients who are high risk may also benefit from an aggressive approach including cardiac catheterization and other reperfusion strategies, although immediate PTCA following thrombolytic therapy does not have any advantage over delayed PTCA. Those patients who are low risk have a better prognosis and, in general, will not require emergent invasive procedures unless complications arise. If contraindication to thrombolytic therapy exists, consideration must be given to emergent cardiac catheterization and other reperfusion strategies if these therapies are available. With the development of newer and more effective thrombolytic agents and angioplasty technologies, the therapy of acute myocardial infarction will continue to change and improve.

REFERENCES

1. Aber, C. P., Bass, N. M., Berry, C. L., et al. Streptokinase in acute myocardial infarction; a controlled multicentre study in the United Kingdom. Br. Med. J. 2:1100–04, 1976.
2. Abrams, J. Nitroglycerin and long-acting nitrates. N. Engl. J. Med. 302:1234, 1980.
3. AIMS Trial Study Group. Long-term effects of intravenous anistreplase in

acute myocardial infarction: final report of the AIMS study. *Lancet* 335:427–31, 1990.
4. Ambrose, J. A., Winters, S. L., Arora, R. R., et al. Coronary angiographic morphology in myocardial infarction: a link between the pathogenesis of unstable angina and myocardial infarction. *J. Am. Coll. Cardiol.* 6:1233–38, 1985.
5. Ambrose, J. A., Winters, S. L., Stern, A., et al. Angiographic morphology and the pathogenesis of unstable angina pectoris. *J. Am. Coll. Cardiol.* 5:609–16, 1985.
6. Antman, E., Muller, J., Goldberg, S., et al. Nifedipine therapy for coronary-artery spasm. Experience in 127 patients. *N. Engl. J. Med.* 302:1269–73, 1980.
7. Armstrong, W. F. Echocardiography in coronary artery disease. *Prog. Cardiovasc. Dis.* 30:267–88, 1988.
8. Banks, D. C., Raftery, E. B., and Oram, S. Clinical significance of the coronary arteriogram. *Br. Heart J.* 33:863, 1971.
9. Bassand, J. P., Machecourt, J., Cassagues, J., et al., for the APSIM Study Investigators. Multicenter trial of intravenous anisoylated plasminogen streptokinase activator complex (APSAC) in acute myocardial infarction: effects on infarct size and left ventricular function. *J. Am. Coll. Cardiol.* 13:988–97, 1989.
10. Bates, E. R., Aueron, F. M., Legrand, V., et al. Comparative long-term effects of coronary artery bypass graft surgery and percutaneous transluminal coronary angioplasty on regional coronary flow reserve. *Circulation* 72:833–39, 1985.
11. Bertolasi, C. A., Tronge, J. E., Mon, G. A., et al. Clinical spectrums of unstable angina. *Clin. Cardiol.* 2:113, 1979.
12. Block, P. C. Percutaneous Transluminal Coronary Angioplasty. In W. E. Conner and J. D. Bristow (eds.), *Coronary Heart Disease: Prevention, Complications, and Treatment.* Philadelphia: Lippincott, 1985. Pp. 405–18.
13. Bourassa, M. G., Campeau, L., and Lesperance, J. Effects of bypass surgery on the coronary circulation: Incidence and effects of vein graft occlusion. In S. H. Rahimtoola (ed.), *Coronary Bypass Surgery.* Philadelphia: Davis, 1977. P. 107.
14. Braunwald, E. The aggressive treatment of acute myocardial infarction. *Circulation* 71(6):1087–92, 1985.
15. Bredlau, C. E., Roubin, G. S., Leimgraber, P. P., et al. In-hospital morbidity and mortality in patients undergoing elective coronary angioplasty. *Circulation* 72:1044–52, 1985.
16. Brown, K. A., Boucher, C. A., Okada, R. D., et al. Prognostic value of exercise thallium-201 imaging in patients presenting for evaluation of chest pain. *J. Am. Coll. Cardiol.* 1(4):994–1001, 1983.
17. Brunton, T. L. On the use of nitrate of amyl in angina pectoris. *Lancet* 2:97, 1867.
18. Bruschke, A. V., Proudfit, W. L., and Sones, F. M. Progress study of 490 consecutive nonsurgical cases of coronary diseases followed 5–9 years. I. Arteriographic correlations. *Circulation* 47:1147, 1973.
19. Cairns, J. A., Gent, M., Singer, J., et al. Aspirin, sulfinpyrazone or both in unstable angina. Results of a Canadian Multicenter Trial. *N. Engl. J. Med.* 313:1369–75, 1985.
20. Campeau, L., Enjalbert, M., Lesperance, J., et al. Comparison of late changes (closure and atherosclerosis at 10 years) in internal mammary artery and saphenous vein coronary artery grafts. (Abstract) *Circulation* 68 (Suppl III):114, 1983.

21. Campeau, L., Lesperance, J., Corbara, F., et al. Aortocoronary saphenous vein bypass graft changes 5–7 years after surgery. *Circulation* 59(Suppl I):1-117, 1978.
22. Campeau, L., Lesperance, J., Hermann, J., et al. Loss of the improvement of angina between 1 and 7 years after aortocoronary bypass surgery. *Circulation* 60(Suppl I):1, 1979.
23. CASS Principal Investigators and Their Associates. Coronary Artery Surgery Study (CASS): A randomized trial of coronary bypass surgery. Survival data. *Circulation* 68:939–50, 1983.
24. Chapman, I. Morphogenesis of occluding coronary artery thrombosis. *Arch. Pathol.* 80:256–61, 1965.
25. Chazov, E. I., Matava, L. S., Mazaw, A. V., et al. Intracoronary administration of fibrinolysin in acute myocardial infarction. *Ter. Arkh.* 48:8–19, 1976.
26. Cheanvechai, C., Effler, D. B., Loop, F. D., et al. Emergency myocardial revascularization. *Am. J. Cardiol.* 32:901, 1973.
27. Cheng, T. O. Physical diagnosis of coronary artery disease. *Am. Heart J.* 80:716, 1970.
28. Chierchia, S., Brinelli, C., Simonetta, I., et al. Sequence of events in angina at rest: Primary reduction in coronary flow. *Circulation* 61:759, 1980.
29. Chierchia, S., Lazzari, M., Freedman, B., et al. Impairment of myocardial perfusion and function during painless myocardial ischemia. *J. Am. Coll. Cardiol.* 1:924, 1983.
30. Christie, L. A., Jr., and Conti, C. R. Systematic approach to evaluation of angina-like chest pain: Pathophysiology and clinical testing with emphasis on objective documentation of myocardial ischemia. *Am. Heart J.* 102:897, 1981.
31. Cohen, L. S., Elliott, W. C., Klein, M. P., and Gorlin, R. Coronary heart disease: clinical, cine-arteriographic, and metabolic correlations. *Am. J. Cardiol.* 17:153, 1966.
32. Collen, D., Stump, D. C., and Van de Werf, F. Coronary thrombolysis in patients with acute myocardial infarction by intravenous infusion of synergic thrombolytic agents. *Am. Heart J.* 58:1083–84, 1986.
33. Cowley, M. J. Methodologic aspects of intracoronary thrombolysis: drugs, dosage, and duration. *Circulation* 68(Suppl I):I-90–95, 1983.
34. Curfman, G. D., Heinsimer, J. A., Lozner, E. C., and Fung, H. L. Intravenous nitroglycerin in the treatment of spontaneous angina pectoris. *Circulation* 67:276–82, 1983.
35. Davies, G. J., Chierchia, S., and Maseri, A. Prevention of myocardial infarction by very early treatment with intracoronary streptokinase: some clinical observations. *N. Engl. J. Med.* 311:1488–92, 1984.
36. Davies, M. J., and Thomas, A. Thrombosis and acute coronary artery lesions in sudden cardiac ischemic death. *N. Engl. J. Med.* 310:1137–40, 1984.
37. Dawson, J. T., Hall, R. J., Hallsman, G. L., and Cooley, D. A. Mortality in coronary artery bypass after previous myocardial infarction. *Am. J. Cardiol.* 31:128, 1973.
38. Deanfield, J. E., Shea, M. J., and Selwyn, A. P. Clinical evaluation of transient myocardial ischemia during daily life. *Am. J. Med.* 79(3A):18–24, 1985.
39. DeBakey, M., Garrett, H. E., and Dennis, E. W. Aorto-coronary bypass with saphenous vein graft. Seven-year follow-up. *J.A.M.A.* 233:792, 1973.
40. DeFeyter, P. J., Serrys, P. S., Vanden Brand, M., et al. Emergency coronary angioplasty in refractory unstable angina. *N. Engl. J. Med.* 313:342–46, 1985.

41. DeWood, M. A., Spore, J., Notske, R. N., et al. Medical and surgical management of myocardial infarction. *Am. J. Cardiol.* 44:1356–64, 1979.
42. DeWood, M. A., Spores, J., Notske, R., et al. Prevalence of total coronary occlusion during the early hours of transmural myocardial infarction. *N. Engl. J. Med.* 303:897–902, 1980.
43. DeWood, M. A., Stifter, W. F., Simpson, C. S., et al. Coronary arteriographic findings soon after non-Q-wave myocardial infarction. *N. Engl. J. Med.* 315:417–23, 1986.
44. Diamond, G.A., and Forrester, J. S. Analysis of probability as an aid in the clinical diagnosis of coronary artery disease. *N. Engl. J. Med.* 300:1350–58, 1979.
45. Diefenbach, C., Erbel, R., Pop, T., et al. Recombinant single-chain urokinase-type plasminogen activator during acute myocardial infarction. *Am. J. Cardiol.* 61:966–70, 1988.
46. Douglas, J. S., Jr., Grüntzig, A. R., King, S. B., III, et al. Percutaneous transluminal coronary angioplasty in patients with prior coronary bypass surgery. *J. Am. Coll. Cardiol.* 2:745, 1983.
47. Duncan, B., Fulton, M., Morrison, S. L., et al. Prognosis of new and worsening angina pectoris. *Br. Med. J.* 1:981, 1976.
48. Erbel, R., Pop, T., Henrichs, K., et al. Percutaneous transluminal coronary angioplasty after thrombolytic therapy: A prospective controlled randomized trial. *J. Am. Coll. Cardiol.* 8:485–95, 1986.
49. European Cooperative Study Group for Streptokinase Treatment in Acute Myocardial Infarction. Streptokinase in acute myocardial infarction. *N. Engl. J. Med.* 301:797–802, 1979.
50. European Coronary Surgery Study Group. Prospective randomized study of coronary artery bypass surgery in stable angina pectoris: A progress report on survival. *Circulation* 65(Part II):67, 1982.
51. European Coronary Surgery Study Group. Prospective randomized study of coronary artery bypass surgery in stable angina pectoris. Second Interim Report. *Lancet* 2:491, 1980.
52. Favaloro, R. G. Saphenous vein autograft replacement of severe segmental coronary occlusion. *Am. Thorac. Surg.* 5:334, 1968.
53. Faxon, D. P., Detre, K. M., McCabe, C. H., et al. Role of Percutaneous Transluminal Coronary Angioplasty in the Treatment of Unstable Angina. Report from the National Heart, Lung and Blood Institute Percutaneous Transluminal Coronary Angioplasty and Coronary Artery Surgery Study Registries. *Am. J. Cardiol.* 53:131C–135C, 1983.
54. Fielding, J. E. Smoking: Health effects and control. *N. Engl. J. Med.* 313(8):491, 1985.
55. Folts, J. D., Crowell, E. B., and Rowe, G. G. Platelet aggregation in partially obstructed vessels and its elimination with aspirin. *Circulation* 54:365–70, 1976.
56. Friesinger, G. C. The reasonable work-up before recommending medical or surgical therapy: An overall strategy. *Circulation* 65 (Suppl II):21, 1982.
57. Furberg, C. D. Clinical value of intracoronary streptokinase. *Am. J. Cardiol.* 53:626–27, 1984.
58. Fuster, V., Frye, R. L., Connolly, D. C., et al. Arteriographic patterns early in the onset of the coronary syndrome. *Br. Heart J.* 37:1250, 1975.
59. Ganz, W., Gelt, I., Shah, P. K., et al. Intravenous streptokinase in evolving acute myocardial infarction. *Am. J. Cardiol.* 53:1209–16, 1984.
60. Gazes, P. C., Mobley, E. M. Jr., Faris, H. M., et al. Preinfarction (unstable) angina—a prospective study. *Circulation* 48:331, 1973.
61. Gerstenblith, G., Ouyang, P., Achuff, S. C., et al. Nifedipine in unstable

angina. A double-blind, randomized trial. *N. Engl. J. Med.* 306:885–89, 1982.
62. Ginks, W. R., Sybers, P. R., Maroks, P. R., et al. Coronary artery reperfusion. II. Reduction of myocardial infarct size at 1 week after the coronary occlusion. *J. Clin. Invest.* 51:2717–23, 1972.
63. Gold, H. K., Coller, B. S., Yasuda, T., et al. Rapid and sustained coronary artery recanalization with combined bolus injection of recombinant tissue-type plasminogen activator and monoclonal antiplatelet GP IIb/IIIa antibody in a canine preparation. *Circulation* 77(3):670–77, 1988.
64. Gold, H. K., Cowley, M. J., Palaios, I., et al. Combined intracoronary streptokinase infusion and coronary angioplasty during acute myocardial infarction. *Am. J. Cardiol.* 53:122C–125C, 1984.
65. Gold, H. K., Johns, J. A., Leinbach, R. C., et al. A randomized, blinded, placebo-controlled trial of recombinant human tissue-type plasminogen activator in patients with unstable angina pectoris. *Circulation* 75(6):1192–99, 1987.
66. Gold, H. K., Leinbach, R. C., Garabedian, H. D., et al. Acute coronary reocclusion after thrombolysis with recombinant human tissue-type plasminogen activator: prevention by maintenance infusion. *Circulation* 73:347–52, 1986.
67. Gold, H. K., Leinbach, R. C., Sanders, C. A., et al. Intra-aortic balloon pumping for control of recurrent myocardial ischemia. *Circulation* 47:1197–1203, 1973.
68. Gottlieb, S. O., and Gerstenblith, G. Therapeutic choices in unstable angina. *Am. J. Med.* 80(4C):35–39, 1986.
69. Gottlieb, S. O., Weisfeldt, M. L., Ouyang, P., et al. Effect of the addition of propranolol to therapy with nifedipine for unstable angina: a randomized, double-blind, placebo-controlled trial. *Circulation* 73:331–37, 1986.
70. Gould, K. L. Assessing coronary stenosis severity—a recurrent clinical need. *J. Am. Coll. Cardiol.* 8:91–94, 1986.
71. Grimes, C. L., Nissen, S. E, Booth, D. C., et al., and the Kamit Study Group. A new thrombolytic regimen for acute myocardial infarction using combination half dose tissue-type plasminogen activtor with full dose streptokinase: a pilot study. *J. Am. Coll. Cardiol.* 14:573–80, 1989.
72. Grüntzig, A. R. Percutaneous Transluminal angioplasty: six years experience. *Am. Heart J.* 107:818, 1984.
73. Grüntzig, A. R. Transluminal dilatation of coronary artery stenosis. *Lancet* 1:263, 1978.
74. Grüntzig, A. R., and Meier, B. Percutaneous transluminal coronary angioplasty: The first five years and the future. *Int. J. Cardiol.* 2:319, 1983.
75. Gruppo Italiano Per Lo Studio Della Streptochinasi Nell' Infarcto Miocardio (GISSI). Effectiveness of intravenous thrombolytic treatment in acute myocardial infarction. *Lancet*, February 22, 1:397–401, 1986.
76. Guerci, A. D., Gerstenblith, G., Brinker, J. A., et al. A randomized trial of intravenous tissue plasminogen activator for acute myocardial infarction with subsequent randomization to elective coronary angioplasty. *N. Engl. J. Med.* 317:1613–18, 1987.
77. Guidelines for Exercise Testing. A report of the American College of Cardiology/American Heart Association Task Force on Assessment of Cardiovascular Procedures (Subcommittee on Exercise Testing.) *J. Am. Coll. Cardiol.* 8(3):725, 1986.
78. Hammermeister, K. E. The effect of coronary bypass surgery on survival. *Prog. Cardiovasc. Dis.* 25:297, 1983.
79. Harston, W. E., Tilley, S., Rodeheffer, R., et al. Safety and success of the

beginning percutaneous transluminal coronary angioplasty program using the steerable guidewire system. *Am. J. Cardiol.* 57:717–20, 1986.
80. Hartzler, G. O. Percutaneous Coronary Angioplasty in Patients with Multivessel Disease. In G. D. Jang (ed.), *Angioplasty.* New York: McGraw-Hill, 1986. P. 321.
81. Hartzler, G. O., Rutherford, B. D., and McConalray, D. R. Percutaneous transluminal coronary angioplasty: application for acute myocardial infarction. *Am. J. Cardiol.* 53:117C–121C, 1984.
82. Heberden, W. Some account of a disorder of the breast. *Med. Trans. Roy. Coll. Physicians* (London) 2:59, 1772.
83. Hjermann, I., Velve Byre, K., Holne, I. Effect of diet and smoking intervention on the incidence of coronary heart disease. *Lancet* 2:1303–10, 1981.
84. Holmes, D. R., and Vlietstra, R. E. Percutaneous transluminal coronary agioplasty: current status and future trends. *Mayo Clin. Proc.* 61:865–76, 1986.
85. Holmes, D. R., Von Raden, M. J., Reeder, G. S., et al. Return to work after coronary angioplasty. A report from the National Heart, Lung, and Blood Institute PTCA Registry. *Circulation* 53:48C, 1984.
86. Hultgren, H. N., Shettigar, U. R., and Miller, D. C. Medical versus surgical treatment of unstable angina. *Am. J. Cardiol.* 50:663–70, 1982.
87. Hypertension Detection and Follow-up Program Cooperative Group. Five-year findings of the hypertension detecting and follow-up program. *J.A.M.A.* 242:2562–77, 1977.
88. The International Study Group. In-hospital mortality and clinical course of 20,891 patients with suspected acute myocardial infarction randomized between alteplase and streptokinase with or without heparin. *Lancet,* 336:71–75, 1990.
89. The ISAM Study Group. A prospective trial of intravenous streptokinase in acute myocardial infarction (I.S.A.M.): Mortality, morbidity, and infarct size at 21 days. *N. Engl. J. Med.* 314:1465–71, 1986.
90. ISIS-2 (Second International Study of Infarct Survival) Collaborative Group. Randomized trial of intravenous streptokinase, oral aspirin, both, or neither among 17,187 cases of suspected acute myocardial infarction: ISIS-2. *Lancet,* August 13, 2:349–60, 1988.
91. Jang, G. C., Gruentzig, A. R., Block, P. C., et al. Work profile of patients following coronary angioplasty or coronary bypass surgery. *Circulation* 66(Suppl II):122, 1982.
92. Kannel, W. B. Update of cigarette smoking in coronary heart disease. *Am. Heart J.* 101:319–28, 1981.
93. Kaufmann, U.P., Garratt, K. N., Vlietstra, R. E., et al. Coronary atherectomy: first 50 patients at the Mayo Clinic. *Mayo Clinic Proc.* 64:747–52, 1989.
94. Kelly, M. E., Taylor, G. J., Moses, H. W., et al. Comparative cost of myocardial revascularization: percutaneous transluminal angioplasty and coronary artery bypass surgery. *J. Am. Coll. Cardiol.* 5:16–20, 1985.
95. Kennedy, J. W., Kaiser, G. C., Fisher, L. D., et al. Clinical and angiographic predictors of operative mortality from the collaborative study in coronary artery surgery (CASS). *Circulation* 63:793, 1981.
96. Kent, K. M., Bentivoglio, L., Block, P., et al. Percutaneous Transluminal Coronary Angioplasty: Report from the registry of the National Heart, Lung, and Blood Institute. *Am. J. Cardiol.* 49:2011–20, 1982.
97. Kent, K. M., Bonow, R. O., Rosing, D. R., et al. Improved myocardial function during exercise after successful percutaneous transluminal coronary angioplasty. *N. Engl. J. Med.* 306:441–46, 1982.
98. Kereiakes, D. H., Selmon, M. R., McAuley, B. H., et al. Angioplasty in

total coronary artery occlusion: experience in 76 consecutive patients. *J. Am. Coll. Cardiol.* 6:526–33, 1985.
99. Kloner, R. A., Ellis, S. G., Lange, R., and Braunwald, E. Studies of experimental coronary artery reperfusion: effects on infarct size, myocardial function, biochemistry, ultrastucture and microvascular damage. *Circulation* 68:(Suppl 1):I-8–15, 1983.
100. Koren, G., Weiss, A. T., Hasin, Y., et al. Prevention of myocardial damage in acute myocardial infarction by early treatment with intravenous streptokinase. *N. Engl. J. Med.* 313:1384–89, 1985.
101. Kouchoukas, N. T., Oherman, A., Kirklin, V. W., et al. Coronary bypass surgery: Analysis of factors affecting hospital mortality. *Circulation* 62(Suppl I):84, 1980.
102. Laffel, G. L., and Braunwald, E. Thrombolytic therapy: A new strategy for the treatment of acute myocardial infarction. *N. Engl. J. Med.* 311:710–17 and 311:770–76, 1984.
103. Lafin, E. S., Murray, J. A., Bruce, R. A., et al. Changes in maximal exercise performance in the evaluation of saphenous vein bypass surgery. *Circulation* 47:1164, 1973.
104. Lee, L., Bates, E. R., Pitt, B., et al. Percutaneous transluminal coronary angioplasty improves survival in acute myocardial infarction complicated by cardiogenic shock. *Circulation* 78:1345–51, 1988.
105. Lewis, H. D., Davis, J. W., Archibald, D. G., et al. Protective effects of aspirin against acute myocardial infarction and death in men with unstable angina. *N. Engl. J. Med.* 309:396–403, 1983.
106. Lindsey, H. E., and Cohn, P. E. "Silent" ischemia during and after exercise testing in patients with coronary artery disease. *Am. Heart J.* 95:441, 1978.
107. Lipid Research Clinics Program. The Lipid Research Clinics Coronary Primary Prevention Trial Results: I. Reduction in incidence of coronary heart disease. *J.A.M.A.* 251:121–29, 1984.
108. Luchi, R. J., Scott, S. M., Deupree, R. N., and the Principal Investigators and Their Associates of Veterans Administration Cooperative Study No. 28. Comparison of medical and surgical treatment for unstable angina pectoris: results of a Veterans Administration Cooperative Study. *N. Engl. J. Med.* 316:977–84, 1987.
109. Mandelkorn, J. B., Wolf, N. M., Singh, S., et al. Intracoronary thrombus in nontransmural myocardial infarction and in unstable angina pectoris. *Am. J. Cardiol.* 52:1–6, 1983.
110. Marder, V. J., Rothbard, R. L., Fitzpatrick, P. G., and Francis, C. W. Rapid lysis of coronary artery thrombi with anisoylated plasminogen: Streptokinase activator complex. *Ann. Intern. Med.* 104:304–10, 1986.
111. Maseri, A., L'Abbate, A., Baroldi, G., et al. Coronary vasospasm as a possible cause of myocardial infarction: A conclusion derived from the study of "preinfarction" angina. *N. Engl. J. Med.* 299:1271–77, 1978.
112. Mata, L. A., Bosch, X., David, P. R., et al. Clinical and angiographic assessment 6 months after double vessel percutaneous coronary angioplasty. *J. Am. Coll. Cardiol.* 6:1239–44, 1985.
113. Merx, W., Dorr, R., Rentrop, P., et al. Evaluation of the effectiveness of intracoronary streptokinase infusion in acute myocardial infarction: post procedure management and hospital course in 204 patients. *Am. Heart J.* 102:1181–87, 1981.
114. Meyer, J., Merx, W., Schmidtz, H., et al. Percutaneous transluminal coronary angioplasty immediately after intracoronary streptolysis of transmural myocardial infarction. *Circulation* 66:905–16, 1982.

115. Mock, M. B., Ringquist, I., Fisher, L. D., et al. Survival of medically treated patients in the Coronary Artery Surgery Study (CASS) registry. *Circulation* 66:562, 1982.
116. Moise, A., Theroux, P., Taeymans, Y., et al. Unstable angina and progression of atherosclerosis. *N. Engl. J. Med.* 309:685–89, 1983.
117. Murphy, M. L., Haltgren, H. N., Detre, K., et al. Treatment of chronic stable angina: A preliminary report of the randomized Veterans Administration Cooperative Study. *N. Engl. J. Med.* 297:621, 1977.
118. Myler, R. K., Grüntzig, A. R., Stertzer, S. H. Technique and Clinical Indications for Percutaneous Transluminal Coronary Angioplasty. In D. T. Mason, and J. J. Collins, Jr. (eds.), *Myocardial Revascularization*. New York: Yorke Medical Books, 1981. P. 431–44.
119. Namay, D. L., Hammermeister, K. E., Zia, M. S., et al. Effect of perioperative myocardial infarction on late survival in patients undergoing coronary artery bypass surgery. *Circulation* 65:1066, 1982.
120. National Cooperative Group to Compare Medical and Surgical Therapy. Unstable angina pectoris: 1. Report of protocol and patient population. *Am. J. Cardiol.* 37:896, 1976.
121. National Heart Foundation of Australia Coronary Thrombolysis Group. Coronary thrombolysis and myocardial salvage by tissue plasminogen activator given up to 4 hours after onset of myocardial infarction. *Lancet* 1:203–07, 1988.
122. 1990 Heart and Stroke Facts. American Heart Association, Dallas, 1989.
123. Okada, R. D., Boucher, C. A., Straus, H. W., and Pohost, G. M. Exercise radionuclide imaging approaches to coronary artery disease. *Am. J. Cardiol.* 46:1188, 1980.
124. O'Neill, W., Timmis, G. C., Bourdillon, P. D., et al. A prospective randomized clinical trial of intracoronary streptokinase versus coronary angioplasty for acute myocardial infarction. *N. Engl. J. Med.* 314:812–18, 1986.
125. Ouyang, P., Bulkley, B. H., Mellits, E. D., et al. A double-blind randomized trial of nifedipine in post infarction unstable angina. *Pract. Cardiol.* 3:30–38, 1983.
126. Peduzzi, P., and Hultgren, H. N. Effect of medical versus surgical treatment on symptoms in stable angina pectoris. The Veterans Administration Cooperative Study of Surgery for Coronary Artery Occlusive Disease. *Circulation* 60:888, 1979.
127. Pennica, D., Holmes, W. E., Kohr, W. J., et al. Cloning and expression of human tissue-type plasminogen activator cDNA in E. coli. *Nature* 301:214–20, 1983.
128. Pepine, C. V., Prida, X., Hill, J. A., et al. Percutaneous transluminal coronary angioplasty in acute myocardial infarction. *Am. Heart J.* 107:820–22, 1984.
129. Plotnick, G. D. Approach to the management of unstable angina. *Am. Heart J.* 98:243, 1979.
130. Proudfit, W. L., Bruschke, A. V. G., and Sones, F. M., Jr. Natural history of obstructive coronary artery disease: Ten year study of 601 non-surgical cases. *Prog. Cardiovasc. Dis.* 21:53, 1978.
131. Proudfit, W. L., Shirley, E. K., Sheldon, W. C., and Sones, F. M., Jr. Certain clinical characteristics correlated with the extent of obstructive lesions demonstrated by selective cine-coronary arteriography. *Circulation* 38:947, 1968.
132. Pugh, B., Platt, M. R., Mills, L. J., et al. Unstable angina pectoris. A randomized study of patients treated medically and surgically. *Am. J. Cardiol.* 41:1291, 1978.

133. Rahimtoola, S. H. Coronary bypass surgery for chronic angina—1981: A perspective. *Circulation* 65:225, 1982.
134. Reeder, G. S., Krishan, I., Nobrega, F. T., et al. Is percutaneous coronary angioplasty less expensive than bypass surgery? *N. Engl. J. Med.* 311:1157–62, 1984.
135. Reeves, T. J. Medical management of the patient with angina pectoris: An overview of the problem. *Circulation* 65 (Suppl II):3, 1982.
136. Reeves, T. J., Oberman, A., Jones, W. B., and Sheffield, L. T. Natural history of angina pectoris. *Am. J. Cardiol.* 33:423, 1974.
137. Reimer, K. A., Lower, J. E., Rasmussen, M. M., and Jennings, R. B. The wavefront phenomenon of ischemic cell death. I. Myocardial infarct size vs duration of coronary occlusion in dogs. *Circulation* 56:786–94, 1977.
138. Rentrop, P., Blanke, H., Karsch, K. R., et al. Selective intracoronary thrombolysis in acute myocardial infarction and unstable angina pectoris. *Circulation* 63:307–17, 1981.
139. Rentrop, K. P., Feit, F., Blanke, H., et al. Effects of intracoronary streptokinase and intracoronary nitroglycerin infusion on coronary angiographic patterns and mortality in patients with acute myocardial infarction. *N. Engl. J. Med.* 311:1457–63, 1984.
140. Report of the Inter-Society Commission for Heart Disease Resources. Optimal resources for coronary artery surgery. *Circulation* 46:325, 1972.
141. Robertson, R., Wood, A. J., Vaughn, W. K., and Robertson, D. Exacerbation of vasotonic angina pectoris by propranolol. *Circulation* 65:281–85, 1982.
142. Rozanski, A., Diamond, G. A., Berman, D., et al. The declining specificity of exercise radionuclide ventriculography. *N. Engl. J. Med.* 309:518–22, 1983.
143. Rude, R. E., Muller, J. E., and Braunwald, E. Efforts to limit the size of myocardial infarcts. *Ann. Intern. Med.* 95:736, 1981.
144. Russell, R. O., et al. Unstable angina pectoris: National Cooperative Study Group to Compare Surgical and Medical Therapy II. In-hospital experience and initial follow-up results in patients with one, two, and three vessel disease. *Am. J. Cardiol.* 42:839, 1978.
145. Russell, R. O., et al. Unstable angina pectoris: National Cooperative Study Group to Compare Surgical and Medical Therapy III. Results in patients with S-T segment elevation during pain. *Am. J. Cardiol.* 45:819, 1980.
146. Sanborn, T. A., Faxon, D. P., Kellett, M. A., and Ryan, T. J. Percutaneous coronary laser thermal angioplasty. *J. Am. Coll. Cardiol.* 8:1437–40, 1986.
147. Sanz, G., Castener, A., Betriu, A., et al. Determinants of prognosis in survivors of myocardial infarction. A prospective clinical angiographic study. *N. Engl. J. Med.* 306:1065–70, 1982.
148. Schroeder, R., Biamino, G., Enz-Rudiger, V. L., et al. Intravenous short-term infusion of streptokinase in acute myocardial infarction. *Circulation* 67:536–48, 1983.
149. Selden, R., Neill, W. A., Ritzmann, L. W., et al. Medical vs surgical therapy for acute coronary insufficiency. A randomized study. *N. Engl. J. Med.* 293:132, 1975.
150. Sherman, C. T., Litvack, F., Grundfest, W., et al. Coronary angioscopy in patients with unstable angina pectoris. *N. Engl. J. Med.* 315:913–19, 1986.
151. Simon, T. L., Ware, J. H., and Stengle, J. M. Clinical trials of thrombolytic agents in myocardial infarction. *Ann. Intern. Med.* 79:712–19, 1973.
152. Simoons, M. L., Arnold, A. E. R., Betriu, A., et al. Thrombolysis with tissue plasminogen activator in acute myocardial infarction: no additional

benefit from immediate percutaneous coronary angioplasty. *Lancet* 1:197–202, 1988.
153. Smullens, S. N., Weiner, L., Kasparian, H., et al. Evaluation and surgical management of acute evolving myocardial infarction. *J. Thorac. Cardiovasc. Surg.* 64:495, 1972.
154. Spann, J. F., Sherry, S., Carabello, B. A., et al. Coronary thrombolysis by intravenous streptokinase in acute myocardial infarction: acute and follow-up studies. *Am. J. Cardiol.* 53:655–61, 1984.
155. Stampfer, M. J., Goldhaber, S. Z., Yusuf, S., et al. Effect of intravenous streptokinase on acute myocardial infarction. Pooled results from randomized trials. *N. Engl. J. Med.* 307:1180–82, 1982.
156. Strauss, H. W., and Elmaleh, D. Musings on PET and SPECT. *Circulation* 73:611–14, 1986.
157. Takaro, T., Hultgren, H. N., Detre, K. M., et al. The Veterans Administration cooperative study of stable angina: Current status. *Circulation* 65(Suppl II):60, 1982.
158. Takaro, T., Hultgren, H. N., Lipton, M. J., et al. The Veterans Administration cooperative randomized study of surgery for coronary arterial occlusive disease. II. Subgroup with significant main left lesions. *Circulation* 54(Suppl III):107, 1976.
159. Tector, A. V., Schmahl, T. M., and Canino, V. R. The internal mammary artery graft: The best choice for bypass of the diseased left anterior descending coronary artery. *Circulation* 68 (Suppl II):214, 1983.
160. Telford, A. M., and Wilson, C. Trial of heparin vs. atenolol in prevention of myocardial infarction in intermediate coronary syndrome. *Lancet* 1:1225–28, 1981.
161. Theroux, P., Ouimet, H., McCans, J., et al. Aspirin, heparin or both to treat acute unstable angina. *N. Engl. J. Med.* 319:1105–11, 1988.
162. The TIMI Study Group. Comparison of invasive and conservative strategies after treatment with intravenous tissue plasminogen activator in acute myocardial infarction: Results of the Thrombolysis in Myocardial Infarction (TIMI) Phase II Trial. *N. Engl. J. Med.* 320:618–27, 1989.
163. Topol, E. J., Califf, R. M., George, B. S., et al., and the TAMI Study Group. Coronary arterial thrombolysis with combined infusion of recombinant tissue-type plasminogen activator and urokinase in patients with acute myocardial infarction. *Circulation* 77(5):1100–07, 1988.
164. Topol, E. J., Califf, R. M., George, B. S., et al., and the Thrombolysis and Angioplasty in Myocardial Infarcton Study Group. A randomized trial of immediate versus delayed elective angioplasty after intravenous tissue plasminogen activator in acute myocardial infarction. *N. Engl. J. Med.* 317:581–88, 1987.
165. Topol, E. J., Morris, D. C., Smalling, R. W., et al. A multicenter, randomized, placebo-controlled trial of a new form of intravenous recombinant tissue-type plasminogen activator (Activase) in acute myocardial infarction. *J. Am. Coll. Cardiol.* 9:1205–13, 1987.
166. Topol, E. J., Weiss, J. L., Brinker, J. A., et al. Regional wall motion. Improvement after coronary thrombolysis with recombinant tissue plasminogen activator: importance of coronary angioplasty. *J. Am. Coll. Cardiol.* 6:426–33, 1985.
167. Vandormael, M. G., Chaitman, B. R. Ischinger, T., et al. Immediate and short-term benefit of multilesion coronary angioplasty: influence of degree of revascularization. *J. Am. Coll. Cardiol.* 6:983–91, 1985.
168. Vestraete, M., Bernard, R., Borg, M., et al. Randomized trial of intravenous

recombinant tissue-type plasminogen activator versus intravenous streptokinase in acute myocardial infarction. *Lancet* 1:842, 1985.
169. Vetrovec, G. W., Leinbach, R. C., Gold, H. K., and Cowley, M. J. Intracoronary thrombolysis in syndromes of unstable ischemia; angiographic and clinical results. *Am. Heart J.* 104:946–52, 1982.
170. Walsh, W., Richards, A. F., and Balcon, R. Coronary arteriographic study of mild angina. *Br. Heart J.* 37:752, 1975.
171. Weber, K. T., and Janicki, J. S. The metabolic demand and oxygen supply of the heart: physiologic and clinical considerations. *Am. J. Cardiol.* 44:722, 1979.
172. Weiner, D. A., Ryan, T. J., McCabe, C. H., et al. Exercise stress testing; correlations among history, ST-segment response and prevalence of coronary-artery disease in the Coronary Artery Surgery Study (CASS). *N. Engl. J. Med.* 301:230–35, 1979.
173. Welch, C. C., Proudfit, W. L., and Sheldon, W. C. Coronary arteriographic findings in 1000 women under age 50. *Am. J. Cardiol.* 35:211, 1975.
174. White, C. W., Wright, C. B., Doty, D. B., et al. Does visual interpretation of the coronary arteriogram predict the physiologic importance of a coronary stenosis? *N. Engl. J. Med.* 310:819, 1984.
175. Wilcox, R. G., Von der Lippe, G., Olsson, C. G., et al., for the ASSET Study Group. Trial of tissue plasminogen activator for mortality reduction in acute myocardial infarction. Anglo-Scandinavian Study of Early Thrombolysis (ASSET). *Lancet*, September 3, 2:525–30, 1988.
176. Willerson, J. T., and Buja, L. M., Cause and course of acute myocardial infarction. *Am. J. Med.* 69:903–04, 1980.
177. Williams, D. O., Borer, J., Braunwald, E., et al. Intravenous recombinant tissue-type plasminogen activator in patients with acute myocardial infarction: a report from the NHLBI thrombolysis in myocardial infarction trial. *Circulation* 73:338–46, 1986.
178. Williams, D. O., Riley, R. S., Singh, A. K., and Mort, A. S. Coronary circulatory dynamics before and after coronary angioplasty. *J. Am. Coll. Cardiol.* 1:1268, 1983.
179. Williams, D. O., Riley, R. S., Singh, A. K., et al. Evaluation of the role of coronary angioplasty in patients with unstable angina pectoris. *Am. Heart J.* 102:1, 1981.
180. Williams, D. O., Topol, E. J., Califf, R. M., et al. Intravenous recombinant tissue-type plasminogen activator in patients with unstable angina pectoris. *Circulation* 72:376–83, 1990.
181. Wilson, R. F., Laughlin, D. E., Ackell, P. H., et al. Transluminal subselective measurement of coronary artery blood flow velocity and vasodilator reserve in man. *Circulation* 72:82–92, 1985.
182. Yasuno, M., Saito, Y., Ishida, M., et al. Effects of percutaneous transluminal coronary angioplasty: intracoronary thrombolysis with urokinase in acute myocardial infarction. *Am. J. Cardiol.* 53:1217–20, 1984.

CHAPTER 3

MECHANISM OF ACTIONS OF NITRATES

JONATHAN ABRAMS

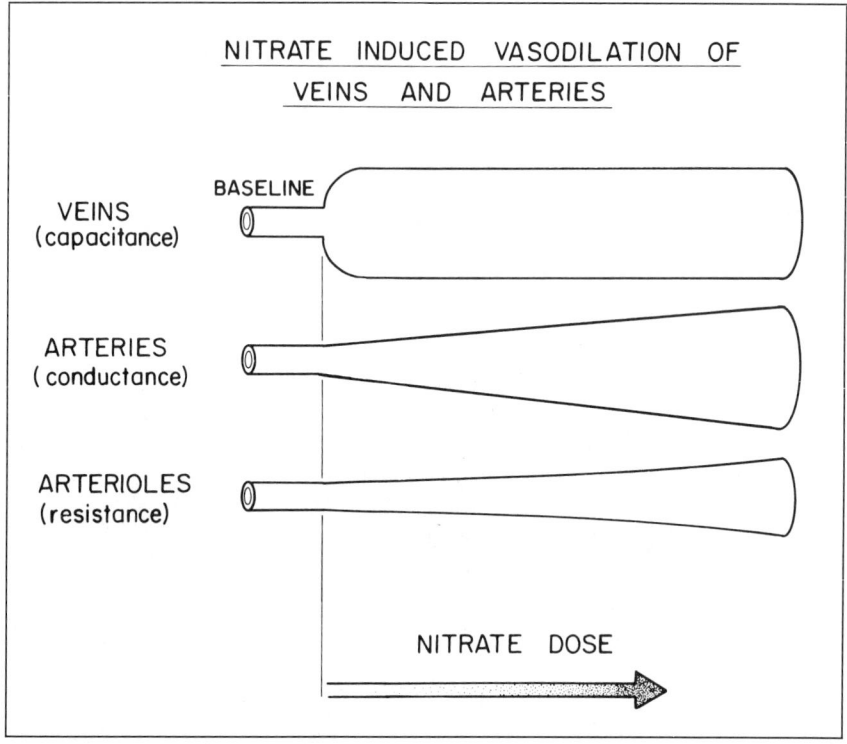

NITRATE INDUCED VASODILATION OF VEINS AND ARTERIES

FIG. 3-1. This schematic indicates the dose-response actions of nitrates on the various components of the peripheral circulation. Note that venodilation occurs with small amounts of nitrate and there is relatively little additional increase in venous capacity with larger doses. The arteries begin to develop conductance and compliance alterations with low nitrate concentrations, which increase in a dose-dependent fashion. The muscular resistance vessels or arterioles significantly vasodilate only in the presence of high nitrate concentrations. (From Ref. 2, with permission.)

Nitroglycerin (NTG) and all organic nitrate esters are dilators of vascular smooth muscle and exert their beneficial clinical effects through this basic action. There remains considerable uncertainty as to which vascular beds are most important with respect to nitrate vasodilation. Veins, arteries, and arterioles all undergo dilation after acute nitrate administration in a dose-dependent fashion [2, 5] (Fig. 3-1). Venodilation is a unique feature of nitrates; the other antianginal agents available in the United States, the beta blockers and calcium channel antagonists, do not produce any increase in venous capacitance. The predictable decrease in right and left heart filling pressures and intracardiac volumes after NTG, associated with a redistribution of the circulating blood volume within the venous circulation (Fig. 3-2), has been an important

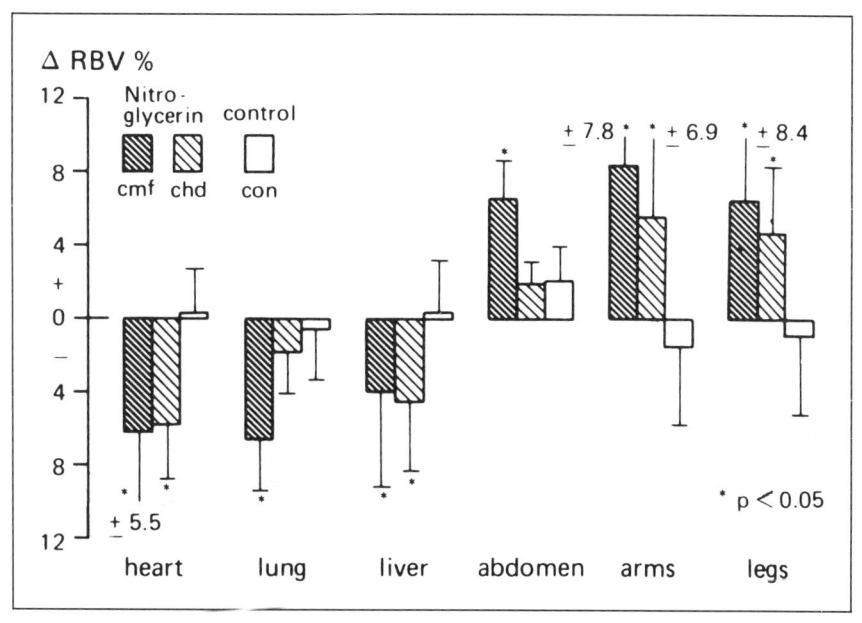

FIG. 3-2. Effects of sublingual nitroglycerin on regional circulations. These data are derived from a radionuclear blood pool study in patients with normal ventricular function and coronary artery disease (CAD) and another group of subjects with congestive heart failure (CHF). All subjects were given 1.6 mg of sublingual nitroglycerin and underwent serial radionuclear scanning with a gamma camera to detect changes in regional blood volume (RBV). Control indicates repeat radionuclear studies without the administration of nitroglycerin. Percent changes ±1 SD in regional redistribution are indicated. Note that there is a significant redistribution of circulating blood volume away from the heart, lungs, and liver toward the splanchnic and abdominal circulations and extremities. The redistribution of blood volume appears to be quantitatively greater in patients with heart failure than those with intact ventricular function (CHD). (From Ref. 18, with permission.)

and consistent hemodynamic observation that has convinced most investigators that the peripheral vasodilatory properties of nitrates (e.g., systemic veins and arteries) are the primary determinants of nitrate action in the relief of angina. The decrease in arterial pressure and systemic resistance enhances the beneficial response to nitrates and contributes to an additional reduction in cardiac work and myocardial oxygen consumption in patients with angina pectoris. The classic hypothesis has been that nitrates exert their beneficial actions in ischemic heart disease by reducing myocardial energy requirements through simultaneous venous and arterial vasodilation [18, 31].

In addition to the traditional view of nitrate action, a substantial body of work suggests that NTG effects on the central circulation or coronary bed itself may be of significance in the alleviation of myocardial ischemia, at least in some subjects [7]. Evidence for nitrate-induced vasodilation of large epicardial coronary arteries, smaller coronary resistance arteries, and coronary collaterals has been documented in numerous studies [7, 11, 13, 39]. In addition, it is now known that many coronary atherosclerotic stenoses can dilate, resulting in the hypothesis that stenosis dilation may play a major role in relief of ischemia [7, 9]. Animal work has confirmed that during conditions of ischemia, nitrates improve abnormal subendocardial oxygenation in zones of impaired perfusion. The mechanism for this improvement is not clear; both the peripheral and central actions of nitrates could play a role in alleviating regional ischemia.

Reversal and prevention of coronary vasoconstriction or overt coronary vasospasm is another important mechanism of ischemia relief with nitrates in those individuals who have a primary or secondary component of enhanced coronary arterial tone as an exacerbating factor in the ischemic syndrome. A recent report suggests that exercise can induce additional stenosis constriction at the site of significant coronary lesions and that this can be reversed or prevented by NTG [16] (Fig. 3-3). Other work indicates that abnormal vasomotion in coronary arteries may be common in atherosclerotic arteries [28]. Nitrates augment coronary flow by vasodilating vessels that are both normal as well as abnormally constricted, even in the absence of endothelial relaxing factor (ERDF) [45].

Other work suggests that nitrates may exert their actions by altering the pressure-volume relationship of the heart, decreasing myocardial compressive forces, and improving diastolic coronary blood flow [44].

It is thus apparent that a variety of mechanisms can be invoked to explain the consistent improvement in ischemia after NTG administration. It is likely that there is no one single pathway but that different actions are important in different patients, in part related to the underlying pathogenesis of the angina syndrome itself. Table 3-1 lists most of the potential actions of nitrates in alleviating myocardial ischemia.

CELLULAR MECHANISMS OF NITRATE ACTION

Nitroglycerin and the organic nitrates are direct acting vasodilators of vascular tissue. The smooth muscle in the media of veins and arteries relaxes on exposure to organic nitrate in vivo and in vitro. It had been postulated in the early 1970s that NTG induces vasodilation by reacting with a nitrate receptor on the surface of smooth muscle cells [36]. It is now recognized that nitrates are actively taken up by vascular tissue and undergo a sequence of intracellular alterations [21] (Fig. 6-2). The final mediator of nitrate vasodilation is an increase in intracellular cyclic

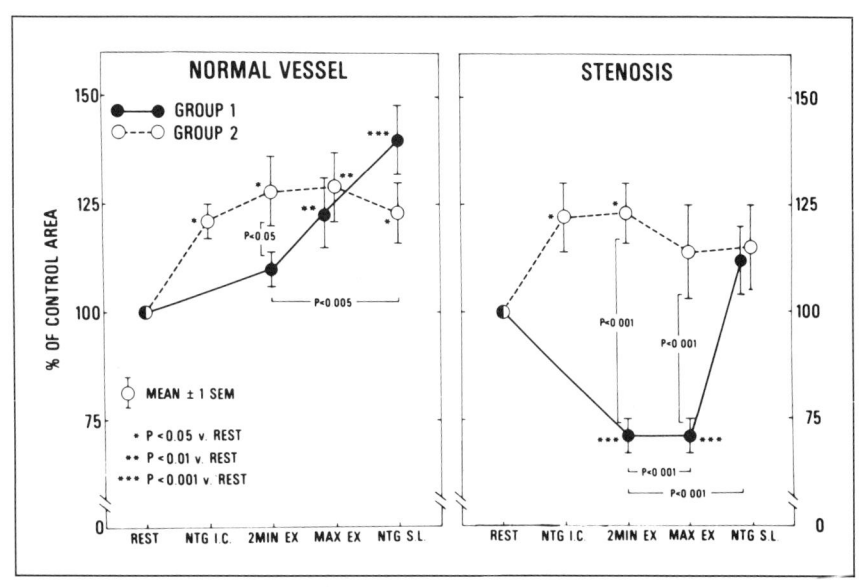

FIG. 3-3. Coronary artery and atherosclerotic stenosis caliber changes with exercise in patients with angina. In this study, patients with severe angina pectoris were exercised on a bicycle in the catheterization laboratory to the onset of chest pain. Coronary arteriography was carried out using careful methodology to isolate a normal coronary vessel as well as the maximal atherosclerotic narrowing in a diseased artery. Group 1 patients were exercised to the point of angina pectoris and were then given sublingual nitroglycerin. Repeat arteriograms were obtained at peak exercise and after NTG. Group 2 individuals were pretreated with intracoronary NTG immediately prior to exercise. Note that in group 1 subjects there was a modest but definite enlargement of the normal coronary artery caliber during exercise, which was further increased with the administration of sublingual NTG. On the contrary, there was a significant reduction in the coronary stenosis diameter area during exercise as well as at peak exercise. This was reversed with the administration of sublingual NTG. In the NTG pretreated patients (Group 2), intracoronary NTG produced coronary vasodilation that increased slightly during exercise. Pretreatment with intracoronary NTG completely prevented the decrease in atherosclerotic stenosis diameter; the stenosis area increased prior to exercise. This study is consistent with exercise-induced stenosis constriction in angina pectoris, which is preventable or reversed by nitroglycerin. (From Ref. 16, with permission.)

TABLE 3-1. *Potential Mechanisms for Relief of Myocardial Ischemia with Nitrates*

Systemic or peripheral effects
Venodilation
  Decreased left and right ventricular volumes and filling pressures (preload)
  Decreased left ventricular diastolic compressive forces
Arterial and arteriolar dilation
  Decreased systemic arterial pressure
  Decreased systemic vascular resistance, high doses
  Decreased left ventricular afterload and impedance
*Coronary or central effects**
  Brief increase in global coronary blood flow followed by late reduction as myocardial oxygen requirements decrease
  Dilation of epicardial (conduit) coronary arteries
  Dilation of coronary collateral arteries and enhanced collateral blood flow
  Dilation of atherosclerotic coronary artery stenoses (eccentric lesions)
  Reversal and prevention of coronary spasm and vasoconstriction
  Redistribution of myocardial blood flow to zones of ischemia

*Most studies documenting beneficial coronary actions of nitrates have been performed with sublingual or intravenous nitroglycerin.
Source: From Ref. 25, with permission.

GMP levels that triggers vascular relaxation [21, 23, 35]. Sulfhydryl (SH) groups are necessary for NTG to exert its effects. Ignarro et al. have demonstrated that NTG and the organic nitrates, as well as sodium nitroprusside, are converted to S-nitrosothiols, short-lived compounds that appear to be activators of guanylate cyclase, the enzyme responsible for cGMP formation [21] (Fig. 6-2). It is uncertain if formation of nitrosothiols is obligatory for guanylate cyclase activation; nitric oxide (NO) derived from organic nitrate (RONO$_2$) may directly stimulate the enzyme (see discussion in Chapter 6).

The sequence of events appears to be as follows (see Fig. 6-2): organic nitrates are converted to NO$_2-$, which is subsequently transformed to nitrous acid, and in turn is reduced to nitric oxide (NO) (also a direct end product of sodium nitroprusside metabolism) [21]. NO reacts with thiol or SH moieties to form S-nitrosothiols, which activate guanylate cyclase, or NO may directly activate the enzyme. Thiol groups are also involved in the initial rate-limiting reaction of the organic nitrate with the oxidation of cysteine, the SH-component of gluthathione (R'SH conversion to R'SSR', Fig. 6-2). Nitrate tolerance is currently thought to be related in part to a depletion of available intracellular SH groups responsible for the initial denitration of the organic nitrate and subsequent formation of NO, possibly due to a decreased availability of cysteine and gluthathione molecules. Administration of exogenous thiol donors, such as N-acetylcysteine or methionine, has been shown to enhance NTG action as well as reverse nitrate tolerance, consistent with the current hypothesis of nitrate intracellular transformation [19, 26,

32]. (See Chapters 6 and 16 for a more detailed discussion of nitrate intracellular metabolism and nitrate tolerance.)

Nitrates and Prostaglandins

Several years ago a number of studies suggested that the actions of NTG might be modulated through the prostaglandin system. It was demonstrated that NTG can induce the release of prostacycline from vascular endothelium, possibly inhibiting thromboxane A_2 generation and platelet aggregation as well [25, 42]. More recent studies have convincingly demonstrated that nitrate vasodilation does not appear to occur through the stimulation of prostacycline formation [41, 37, 43] (see also Chapter 6).

Changes in Intracellular Ionized Calcium

There is some evidence that NTG-induced vascular smooth muscle relaxation may result in efflux of intracellular free-Ca^{++} from smooth muscle cells. This may be related to the increase of cGMP previously described [38].

SPECIFIC MECHANISMS OF NITRATE ACTION IN ISCHEMIC HEART DISEASE

As stressed in the introductory section, a number of potential effects of NTG and long acting nitrates contribute to relief of myocardial ischemia in patients with angina pectoris (Table 3-1) [1]. Some of these actions are also important when nitrates are used for the treatment of other cardiovascular conditions, such as in vasodilator therapy of congestive heart failure, the lowering of systolic blood pressure during surgical procedures, and the treatment of pulmonary hypertension of diverse etiology. McGregor has reviewed this subject and has emphasized the diversity of mechanisms of nitrate action, including relief of coronary vasospasm, decreased coronary tone, and systemic vasodilatory actions on veins, arteries, and arterioles [33]. Others have subsequently stressed the role of coronary stenosis dilation, a fascinating hypothesis that is not yet fully understood [7, 16, 39]. Finally, Smith and coworkers have stressed the action of nitrates in decreasing left ventricular size as well as diminishing pericardial pressure due to a downward shift of the left ventricular pressure-volume relationship [44].

This discussion will emphasize the commonly accepted mechanisms of action of NTG.

Peripheral Effects of NTG

VENODILATION

Nitrates are potent venodilators. Changes in venous compliance are seen at low doses; this results in venous pooling, a decrease in systemic venous pressure, and redistribution of the circulating blood volume providing a decrease in venous return to the heart and a fall in cardiac output. Right and left heart pressures and intracardiac volumes decrease. If reflex tachycardia is not excessive, myocardial energy costs are considerably lowered by the smaller heart [10, 18, 31, 40].

Nitrates act as venodilators at very low plasma concentrations [2, 5] (Fig. 3-1). Increasing the amount of administered nitrate does not usually result in substantial additional venodilation; near maximal changes in venous vasodilation occur with relatively small amounts of NTG or other organic nitrates. Patients in whom the venodilating effect is particularly important in alleviating ischemia may be very sensitive to nitrate action; this may in part explain the mechanism of angina relief with low doses of transdermal NTG or oral nitrates. It has been suggested that such individuals would have typical exertional angina with a nonvariable angina threshold.

CHANGES IN REGIONAL CIRCULATIONS

Nitrates cause a redistribution of the total circulating blood volume from intrathoracic sites into extrathoracic regions as a result of systemic venodilation (Fig. 3-2). Recent radionuclide measurements of regional blood volume have demonstrated indirect evidence for venodilation of the splanchnic bed as well as the veins of the arms and legs [27, 29]. Another study using abdominal ultrasound demonstrates direct NTG-induced dilation of the portal, mesenteric, and splenic veins [46]. Interestingly, the inferior vena cava may decrease in caliber after NTG administration, probably due to the substantial decrease in systemic venous pressure and venous return.

In contrast to venous pooling in the splanchnic circulation and limbs, the heart, lungs, and liver demonstrate a reduction of blood volume after NTG. Such changes in regional blood volume after NTG may be more pronounced in congestive heart failure, emphasizing the important role of organic nitrates in this syndrome (Fig. 3-2). The decrease in intracardiac dimensions, contributing to a fall in myocardial energy costs, is of major benefit in the relief of myocardial ischemia (Fig. 3-4).

ARTERIAL VASODILATION

Conventional doses of nitrates induce systemic and regional vasodilation of muscular arteries. Even small doses will increase the compliance of large arteries. McGregor has emphasized the potential benefits of this little-recognized component of NTG action [33]. Arterial conductance, compliance, and the Windkessel capacity are all increased by NTG without an accompanying fall in systemic vascular resistance [41]. Forearm arteries have been shown to dilate after NTG [30].

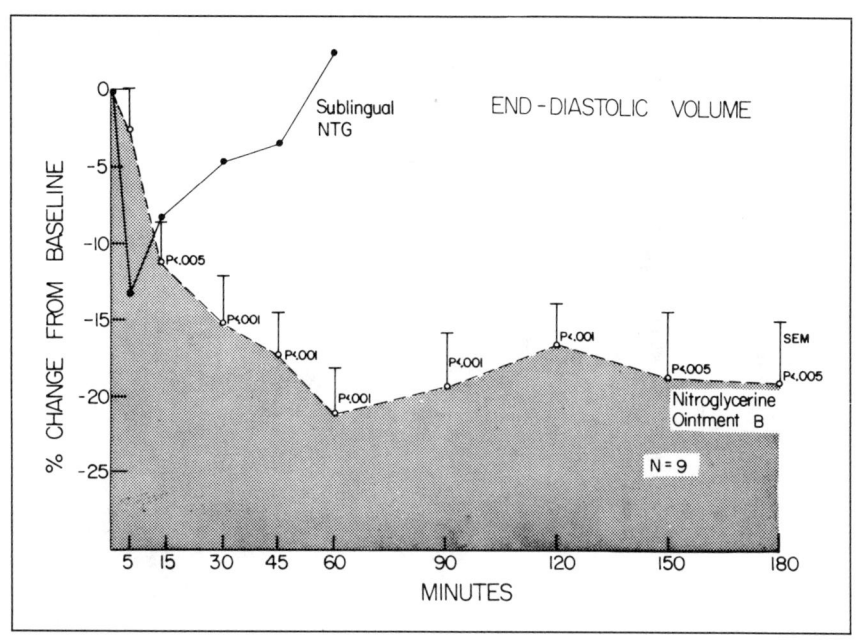

FIG. 3-4. Reduction of left ventricular cavity size with nitroglycerin. This study represents data obtained in normal volunteers using serial M-mode echocardiography following administration of sublingual NTG as well as NTG ointment in a placebo-controlled trial. The calculated end-diastolic volume reductions derive from the decrease in left ventricular end-diastolic diameter following NTG administration. Note the marked diminution in left ventricular cavity size, which is sustained at least after three hours following NTG ointment application. (From Ref. 3, with permission.)

ARTERIOLAR VASODILATION

At high nitrate concentrations arteriolar vasodilation may occur, resulting in a decrease in systemic vascular resistance. This may be of particular importance for afterload reduction therapy in congestive heart failure, where a decrease in systemic vascular resistance is desirable and results in an augmentation of stroke volume in the failing heart [3, 9].

REDUCTION IN MYOCARDIAL OXYGEN DEMANDS

The combination of venous and arterial vasodilation after nitrate administration results in a cardiovascular system that functions with lower pressures and diminished cardiac chamber size [10, 27, 40] (see Fig. 3-4). Left ventricular wall tension is reduced and myocardial oxygen consumption decreases. Total coronary blood flow actually decreases after an initial rise following sublingual NTG administration, as there

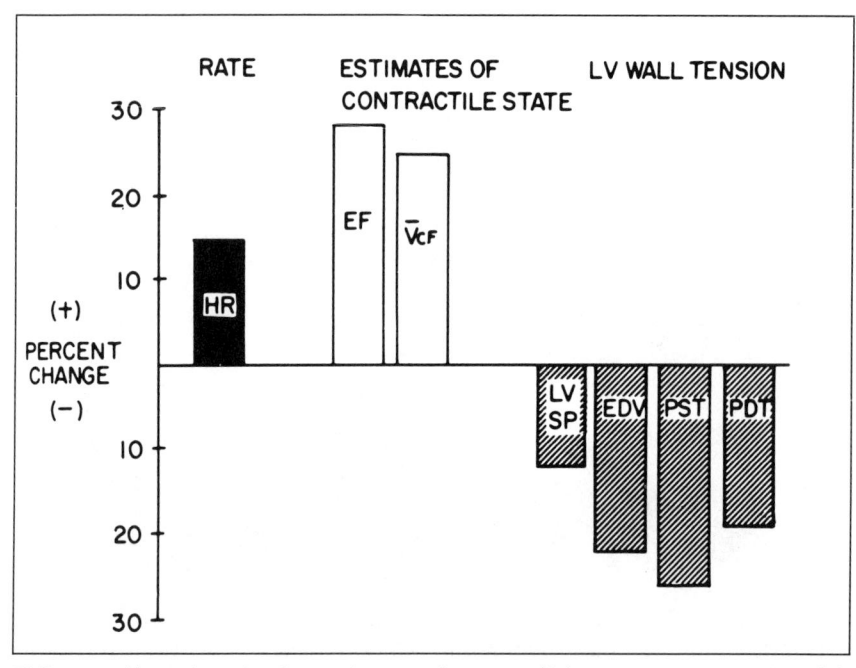

FIG. 3-5. Alterations in determinants of myocardial oxygen consumption following nitroglycerin. Left ventricular angiography was performed before and 3 to 6 minutes after 0.6 mg of sublingual NTG. Note the substantial decreases in those parameters contributing to left ventricular wall tension, including reductions in ventricular size and pressure. There was a decrease in PDT and a fall of 57 percent in calculated end-diastolic wall tension. Heart rate, ejection fraction, and VCF are augmented because of reflex sympathetic discharge following the fall in systolic blood pressure. LVSP = left ventricular systolic pressure; EDV = end diastolic volume; PST = peak systolic tension; PDT = peak developed tension. (From Ref. 18, with permission.)

is less need for energy substrates. In a classic study, Greenberg and colleagues directly measured the determinants of oxygen consumption after sublingual nitroglycerin (see Fig. 3-5) [18]. They observed an 18 percent decrease in peak developed left ventricular wall tension that correlated with reductions in left ventricular end-diastolic volumes and systolic pressure. These authors also noted a 57 percent decline in end-diastolic wall tension and postulated that in some patients NTG may enhance diastolic coronary blood flow by reducing diastolic compressive forces that could limit coronary flow during ischemia. Contractility and heart rate often increase after nitroglycerin is given, due to reflex sympathetic discharge resulting from a decrease in systemic arterial pressure.

Most experts agree that the dominant role of nitrates in relieving myocardial ischemia is a result of a major decrease in myocardial oxygen requirements. This fundamental nitrate action operates to some degree in all patients with cardiovascular disease.

Central or Coronary Arterial Effects of Nitroglycerin

Nitroglycerin and the organic nitrate esters exert effects in the normal and abnormal coronary circulation that are likely to be important in the treatment of myocardial ischemia. In recent years, a number of experts have speculated that some of these actions may play a major role in the relief of anginal pain or improvement of the hemodynamics in acute myocardial infarction.

NORMAL CORONARY CIRCULATION

NTG is a potent vasodilator of the large epicardial conductance vessels, resulting in increased vessel diameter and a transient increase in coronary blood flow (Fig. 3-6). These changes can be documented with small doses of NTG that do not induce systemic hemodynamic changes. Studies by Brown et al. and Conti et al. indicate that smaller coronary arteries dilate relatively more than larger vessels [7, 11]. As myocardial oxygen consumption (M$\dot{V}$O$_2$) decreases following the reduction of left ventricular size and pressure, coronary blood flow falls, paralleling the diminished myocardial energy needs. Thus, there is a biphasic coronary blood flow response, with an initial increase and then a decline in flow in concert with the NTG-induced decrease in M$\dot{V}$O$_2$. Reflex coronary vasoconstriction resulting from sympathetic activation due to a fall in systemic arterial pressure may further reduce coronary blood flow following NTG administration.

At high nitrate concentrations NTG induces coronary arteriolar relaxation, and at least in an animal model, an increase in coronary sinus venous oxygen saturation [5, 6]. This phenomenon represents a relaxation of the coronary resistance vessels; whether such effect is achieved in humans following conventional nitrate doses is unknown, but coronary arteriolar vasodilation would represent an additional role for nitrates in the relief of myocardial ischemia.

ABNORMAL CORONARY CIRCULATION

Nitrates dilate abnormal epicardial arteries in patients with coronary atherosclerosis [7, 11]. In addition, coronary collateral vessels dilate following NTG administration [13]. It has been recently demonstrated that the coronary artery stenosis itself may dilate after NTG or isosorbide dinitrate (ISDN) administration [7, 8, 11, 16, 39] (Fig. 3-6). The degree of stenosis enlargement is unpredictable; not all lesions respond. For such an effect to occur, there must be sufficient intact smooth muscle

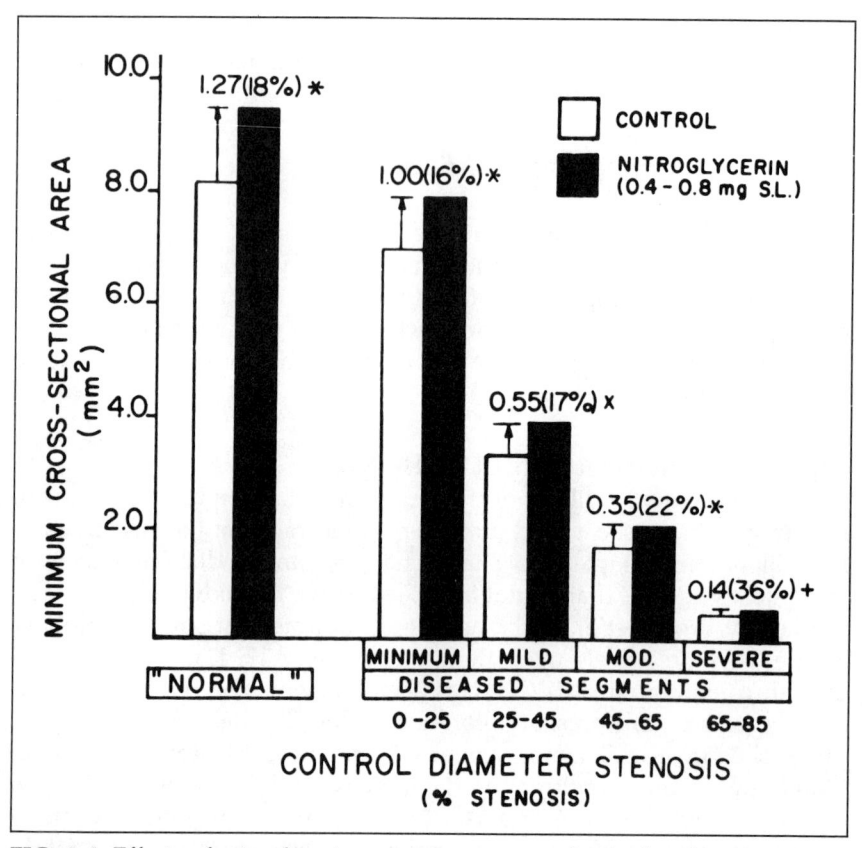

FIG. 3-6. Effects of nitroglycerin on coronary artery luminal and stenosis area. Quantitative computer-assisted coronary angiography was carried out before and after 0.4 to 0.8 mg of sublingual NTG. Coronary arterial stenoses were carefully isolated and were visualized in multiple projections. The actual diameter and calculated area of the normal appearing artery and the maximal stenosis were calculated. Nitroglycerin increased the area of the epicardial coronary arteries in the normal arteries by 18 percent over control. Stenosis enlargement occurred in most lesions, with increases in stenosis area proportional to stenosis severity. Thus, minimally diseased segments dilated by 1.0 mm^2, or 16 percent of the initial area; severely diseased segments dilated by only 0.4 mm^2, although this calculated to a 36 percent increase in stenosis area. The reduction in coronary stenosis resistance was 38 percent in the most severe lesions. (From Ref. 7, with permission.)

in the diseased vessel wall to be able to respond with vasodilation. Some have suggested that eccentrically shaped lesions identified on coronary arteriography are most likely to vasodilate [7, 8, 11, 16, 39]. Conti's work suggests that very "tight" lesions are less likely to respond to NTG [11]. Brown et al., however, have demonstrated that the magnitude of stenosis dilation and decrease in calculated stenosis resistance is greater in more severely narrowed lesions [7]. Feldman and Conti have discussed the issue of stenosis vasodilation and its putative role in ischemic heart disease in an elegant editorial [14]. A recent study has suggested that NTG may prevent exertion-related constriction of coronary atherosclerotic lesions in patients with stable exertional angina (Fig. 3-3) [16]. The relatively new concept of stenosis dilation occurring at rest or during exercise provides a fresh insight into the relief or prevention of myocardial ischemia with nitrates.

NITRATE EFFECTS DURING ISCHEMIA

A variety of studies in animals and humans suggest that nitrates can improve myocardial ischemia by increasing flow and subendocardial oxygenation in regional zones of ischemia, augmenting coronary collateral flow, and decreasing myocardial compressive forces restricting coronary blood flow during diastole [13, 17, 20, 33, 34, 44]. Whether or not stenosis dilation or an increase in coronary resistance vessel diameter also plays a role during ischemia remains unclear, but Brown et al. present a convincing argument that these mechanisms are important, at least in some patients [7, 8].

CORONARY VASOCONSTRICTION AND SPASM

Nitroglycerin and ISDN are effective in reversing or preventing coronary vasospasm, whether provoked in the laboratory or during spontaneous attacks (Prinzmetal's angina). Whether or not coronary vasoconstriction is a common element in stable or unstable angina syndromes is unknown. On the other hand, exercise-induced coronary vasoconstriction has been demonstrated in patients with chest pain with normal and abnormal arteries [47]. Thus, nitrates are useful in preventing or reversing increases in coronary vasomotor tone. In patients with normal coronary arteries (e.g., Prinzmetal's or variant angina) or those with underlying coronary atherosclerosis and a propensity to undergo coronary vasoconstriction (mixed angina), administration of nitrates should be extremely beneficial. It now seems likely that disordered vasomotion is common in vessels with impaired endothelial function, contributing to increased coronary vasomotor tone. Nitroglycerin is effective in the presence of endothelial dysfunction and impaired EDRF release [45].

In summary, the diverse effects of nitrates on normal and abnormal coronary arteries, dilating both the large conductive vessels and perhaps the small resistance vessels, offer a number of additional modes of action for prevention or relief of myocardial ischemia in anginal syndromes or acute myocardial infarction. Table 3-1 lists these mechanisms in addition to the traditional actions of decreased preload and afterload. It is not known how important any particular coronary action might be; it is likely that the mode of anginal relief after nitrate administration varies from patient to patient [1].

The interested reader is referred to several excellent discussions dealing with this complex but still unresolved subject [7, 14, 33].

ANTIPLATELET ACTIVITY OF NITRATES

It has been long recognized that the organic nitrates exert an in vitro antiaggregatory effect on platelets, usually with pharmacologic doses. The clinical implications of this phenomenon have remained uncertain. Recent data suggest that NTG may have an important antiplatelet action in humans [12, 15, 22, 24] and that such effects may contribute to nitrate-induced arterial vasodilation in the presence of arterial injury [24]. It is unlikely that these actions are mediated through the prostaglandin system [4, 37, 43], as has been previously suggested [25, 42]. The putative role of nitrates in preventing or reversing platelet aggregation and thrombosis is controversial and remains to be elucidated further. However, these new findings are quite promising, particularly with respect to NTG's ability to exert such actions in the absence of functional endothelium [45]. Some recent work suggests that thiol groups may enhance the antithrombotic actions of nitroglycerin [15].

REFERENCES

1. Abrams, J. A reappraisal of nitrate therapy. *J.A.M.A.* 259:396, 1988.
2. Abrams, J. Hemodynamic effects of nitroglycerin and long acting nitrates. *Am. Heart J.* 110:216, 1985.
3. Abrams, J. Pharmacology of nitroglycerin and long-acting nitrates and their usefulness in the treatment of chronic congestive heart failure. In L. Gould and C. V. R. Reddy (eds.), *Vasodilator Therapy for Cardiac Disorders.* Mount Kisco, NY: Futura Publishing Co., 1979, P. 129.
4. Abrams, J., Raizada, V. R., Schroeder, K., et al. Prostaglandins do not modulate the actions of nitroglycerin. *J. Clin. Pharmacol.* 24:414, 1984 (abstr).
5. Bassenge, E., Holtz, J., Kindater, H., and Kolin, A. Threshold dosages of nitroglycerin for coronary artery dilatation, afterload reduction, and venous pooling in conscious dogs. In P. R. Lichtlen, H. J. Engle, A. Schrey, and J. H. C. Swan (eds.), *Nitrates III. Cardiovascular Effects.* Berlin, Springer-Verlag: 1981. P. 238.
6. Bassenge, E., and Strein, K. Dose-dependent effects of isosorbide-5-mononitrate on the venous, arterial and coronary arterial system of conscious dogs. *Naumyn-Schmiedeberg's Arch. Pharmaco.* 334:100, 1986.
7. Brown, B. G., Bolson, E., Petersen, R. B., et al. The mechanisms of nitroglycerin action. Stenosis vasodilatation as a major component of drug response. *Circulation* 65:1089, 1981.

8. Brown, B. G., Lee, A. B., Bolson, E. L., and Dodge, H. T. Reflex constriction of significant coronary stenosis as a mechanism contributing to ischemic left ventricular dysfunction during isometric exercise. *Circulation* 70:18–25, 1984.
9. Chatterjee, K., and Parmley, W. W. Vasodilator therapy for acute myocardial infarction and chronic congestive heart failure. *J.A.C.C.* 1:133, 1983.
10. Choong, C. Y. P., Roubin, G. S., Bautovich, G. J., et al. Antianginal effects of nitroglycerin during exercise-induced angina: hemodynamic and left ventricular function changes related to indexes of myocardial consumption. *Am. J. Cardiol.* 60:10H, 1987.
11. Conti, C. R., Feldman, R. L., Pepine, C. J., et al. Effect of glyceryl trinitrate on coronary and systemic hemodynamics in man. *Am. J. Med.* 74(6R):28, 1983.
12. Diodati, J., Theroux, P., Latour, J.-G., et al. Nitroglycerin at therapeutic doses inhibits platelet aggregation in man. *J.A.C.C.* 11:54A, 1988 (abstr).
13. Fam, W. M., and McGregor, M. Effect of coronary vasodilator drugs on retrograde flow in areas of chronic myocardial ischemia. *Circ. Res.* 15:355, 1964.
14. Feldman, R. L., and Conti, C. R. Relief of myocardial ischemia with nitroglycerin: what is the mechanism? *Circulation* 64:1098, 1981.
15. Folts, J. D., Stamler, J., and Loscalzo, J. N-acetylcysteine potentiates IV nitroglycerin in inhibiting periodic platelet thrombus formation in stenosed dog coronary arteries. *J.A.C.C.* 1989; 13:145A.
16. Gage, J. E., Hess, O. M., Murakami, T., et al. Vasoconstriction of stenotic coronary arteries during dynamic exercise in patients with classic angina pectoris: reversibility by nitroglycerin. *Circulation* 73:865, 1986.
17. Gorman, M. W., and Sparks, H. V. Nitroglycerin causes vasodilatation within ischemic myocardium. *Cardiovasc. Res.* 14:515, 1980.
18. Greenberg, H., Dwyer, E. M., Jameson, A. G., and Pinkernell, B. M. Effects of nitroglycerin on the major determinants of myocardial oxygen consumption. An angiographic and hemodynamic assessment. *Am. J. Cardiol.* 36:426, 1975.
19. Horowitz, L. D., Antman, E. M., Lorell, B. H., et al. Potentiation of the cardiovascular effects of nitroglycerin by N-acetylcysteine. *Circulation* 687:1247, 1983.
20. Horwitz, L. D., Gorlin, R., Taylor, W. J., and Kemp, H. Effects of nitroglycerin on regional myocardial blood flow in coronary artery disease. *J. Clin. Invest.* 50:1578, 1971.
21. Ignarro, L. J., Lippton, H., Edwards, J. C., et al. Mechanism of vascular smooth muscle relaxation by organic nitrates, nitrites, nitroprusside and nitric oxide: evidence for the involvement of s-nitrosothiols as active intermediates. *J. Pharmacol. Exp. Ther.* 218:739, 1981.
22. Johnstone, M., Lam, J. Y. T., and Waters, D. The antithrombotic action of nitroglycerine: cyclic GMP as a potential mediator. *J.A.C.C.* 13:231A, 1989.
23. Kukovetz, W. R., and Holzmann, S. Mechanism of nitrate-induced vasodilatation and tolerance. *Z. Kardiol.* 73(Suppl 3):14, 1983.
24. Lam, J. Y. T., Chesebro, J. H., and Fuster, V. Platelets, vasoconstriction and nitroglycerin during arterial wall injury. *Circulation* 78:712–16, 1988.
25. Levin, R. I., Jaffe, E. A., Weksler, B. B., and Tack-Goldman, K. Nitroglycerin stimulates synthesis of prostaglandin by cultured human endothelial cells. *J. Clin. Invest.* 67:762, 1981.
26. Levy, W. S., Katz, R. J., and Wasserman, A. G. Methionine reverses tolerance to transdermal nitroglycerin. *J.A.C.C.* 13:230A, 1989.
27. Loos, D., Schneider, R., and Schorner, W. Changes in regional body blood volume caused by nitroglycerin. *Z. Kardiol.* 72(Suppl 3):29, 1983.

28. Ludmer, P. L., Selwyn, A. P., Shook, T. L., et al. Paradoxical vasoconstriction induced by acetylcholine atherosclerotic arteries. *N. Engl. J. Med.* 315:1046–51, 1986.
29. Manyari, D. E., Smith, E. R., and Spragg, J. Isosorbide dinitrate and glyceryl trinitrate: Demonstration of cross tolerance in the capacitance vessels. *Am. J. Card.* 55:927, 1985.
30. Mason, D. T., and Braunwald, E. The effects of nitroglycerin and amyl nitrite on arteriolar and venous tone in the human forearm. *Circulation* 32:755, 1965.
31. Mason, D.T., Zelis, R., and Amsterdam, E. A. Actions of the nitrates on the peripheral circulation and myocardial oxygen consumption: Significance in the relief of angina pectoris. *Chest* 59:296, 1971.
32. May, D. C., Popma, J. J., Black, W. H., et al. In vivo induction and reversal of nitroglycerin tolerance in human coronary arteries. *N. Engl. J. Med.* 317:805, 1987.
33. McGregor, M. Pathogenesis of angina pectoris and role of nitrates in relief of myocardial ischemia. *Am. J. Med.* 74(6B):21, 1983.
34. Moir, T. W. Subendocardial distribution of coronary blood flow and the effects of antianginal drugs. *Circulation Res.* 30:621, 1972.
35. Murad, F. Cyclic guanosine monophosphase as a mediator of vasodilation. *J. Clin. Invest.* 78:1, 1987.
36. Needleman, P., and Johnson, E. M. The pharmacological and biochemical interaction of organic nitrates with sulfhydryls: possible correlations with the mechanism for tolerance development, vasodilation and mitochondrial and enzyme reactions. In P. Needleman (ed), *Organic Nitrates. Handbook Exp. Pharmacol.*, Vol 40, New York: Springer-Verlag, 1975. Pp. 97–114.
37. Panzenbeck, M. J., Baez, A., and Kaley, G. Nitroglycerin and nitroprusside increase coronary blood flow in dogs by a mechanism independent of prostaglandin release. *Am. J. Cardiol.* 53:936, 1984.
38. Popescu, L. M., Foril, C. P., Minescu, M., et al. Nitroglycerin stimulates the sarcolemmal Ca^{2+} extrusion of coronary smooth muscle cells. *Biochem. Pharmacol.* 34:1857, 1985.
39. Rafflenbeul, W., and Lichtlen, P. R. Quantitative coronary angiography: evidence of a sustained increase in vascular smooth muscle tone in coronary artery stenoses. *Z. Kardiol.* 72(Suppl 3):87, 1983.
40. Ritchie, J. L., Sorenson, S. G., Kennedy, J. W., and Hamilton, G. W. Radionuclide angiography: noninvasive assessment of hemodynamic changes after administration of nitroglycerin. *Am. J. Card.* 43:278, 1979.
41. Sauer, G., Willia, H. H., Tebbe, V., et al. Influence of nitroglycerin on aortic compliance, capacity of the Windkessel, and peripheral resistance. In P. R. Lichtlen, H. J. Engel, A. Schrey, and J. H. C. Swan, (eds.), *Nitrates III. Cardiovascular Effects.* Berlin: Springer-Verlag, 1981. P. 251.
42. Schafer, A. I., Alexander, R. W., and Handlin, R. I. Inhibition of platelet function by organic nitrate vasodilators. *Blood* 55:649, 1980.
43. Simonetti, I., DeCaterina, R., Marzilli, M., et al. Coronary vasodilation by nitrates is not mediated by the prostaglandin system: an angiographic and hemodynamic study. *Z. Kardiol.* 72 (Suppl 3):40–45, 1983.
44. Smith, E. R., Smiseth, O. A., Kingma, I., et al. Mechanisms of action of nitrates. Role of changes in venous capacitance and in the left ventricular diastolic pressure–volume relation. *Am. J. Med.* 76(6A):14, 1984.
45. Stewart, D. J., Holtz, J., and Bassenge, E. Long-term nitroglycerin treatment and effect on direct and endothelium-mediated large coronary artery dilation in conscious dogs. *Circulation* 75:847–56, 1987.

46. Strohm, W. D., Rahn, R., Cordes, H. J., et al. Diameters of abdominal veins and arteries during nitrate therapy. *Z. Kardiol.* 72 (Suppl 3):56–61, 1983.
47. Yasue, H., Omote, S., Takizawa, A., et al. Exertional angina pectoris caused by coronary arterial spasm. Effects of various drugs. *Am. J. Cardiol.* 43:647–52, 1979.

CHAPTER 4

MECHANISM OF ACTIONS OF BETA BLOCKERS

EDWIN G. OLSON
STEPHEN F. HAMILTON
UDHO THADANI

The beta-adrenergic blocking agents are one of the most versatile groups of drugs available today. These agents are useful for angina pectoris, hypertension, and arrhythmias. They have been shown to improve survival following myocardial infarction, and they have the potential to limit the size of myocardial infarction. In addition, these agents are useful for hyperthyroidism, migraine prophylaxis, tremor, stage fright, and alcohol withdrawal.

The primary mechanism of action of all these agents is a competitive inhibition of the beta-adrenergic receptor. In the cardiovascular system, inhibition of the beta receptor produces decreases in heart rate, contractility, and blood pressure, which are the major determinants of myocardial oxygen consumption. However, the beta blockers also have individual properties. These properties include relative selectivity for the beta-1 or beta-2 receptor, alpha-adrenergic blockade, intrinsic sympathomimetic activity, lipid solubility, and nonspecific membrane effects.

To understand the actions of beta blocking drugs it is important to understand both the common properties of beta blockade and the individual properties of each drug. This chapter will begin with a brief review of the adrenergic nervous system and the physiology of the beta-adrenergic receptor. Regulation of the beta receptor will be outlined, with special emphasis on the effects of ischemia, congestive heart failure, and chronic beta blockade. The relationship between the structure and activity of the beta blockers will be discussed. Finally, the effects of beta blockade on hemodynamics, myocardial oxygen demands, coronary blood flow, platelet function, arrhythmias, and metabolism will be reviewed.

ADRENERGIC NERVOUS SYSTEM

The adrenergic nervous system has widespread effects, with adrenergic receptors found in almost every tissue. The naturally occurring mediators of the adrenergic system are the catecholamines, epinephrine and norepinephrine. Epinephrine is released systemically by the adrenal medulla and functions primarily as a hormone. Norepinephrine is released locally by the sympathetic nerve endings and functions primarily as a neurotransmitter. The magnitude of response depends on the concentration of the catecholamine, the affinity of the receptor for the catecholamine, and the number of active receptors. The magnitude of response is further determined by the coupling of the receptor to the intracellular mediator adenylate cyclase.

The present concept of alpha- and beta-adrenergic receptors was presented by Ahlquist in 1948 [2]. He evaluated the effects of a series of catecholamines on the responses of various tissues. He found two orders of potency. For alpha receptor functions such as constriction of vascular smooth muscle, the potency order was epinephrine greater than norepinephrine greater than isoproterenol. For beta receptor functions such as excitation of the heart and relaxation of vascular smooth muscle, the potency order was isoproterenol greater than epinephrine greater than norepinephrine.

The adrenergic receptors have been further subdivided into alpha-1 and alpha-2 and beta-1 and beta-2. The two types of beta receptors were first described by Lands in 1967 [45]. He also examined the order of potency of various catecholamines on various tissue responses and found two different patterns for beta receptors. In tissues with predominantly beta-1 receptors such as cardiac tissue, epinephrine and norepinephrine were about equal in potency. In tissues with predominantly beta-2 receptors, epinephrine was more potent than norepinephrine.

The distribution of beta receptors is outlined in Table 4-1, adapted from Lefkowitz et al. [47]. In general, beta-1 receptors predominate on cardiac tissue and stimulate heart rate and contractility. Beta-1 receptors are also present on fat cells and stimulate lipolysis. Beta-2 receptors predominate on bronchial and vascular smooth muscle and inhibit contraction. Beta-2 receptors are also present in the liver and promote glycogenolysis.

Although it is convenient to associate one type of beta receptor with each tissue, it is important to realize that combinations of $beta_1$ and $beta_2$ receptors are present in many tissues. Recent studies have verified the presence of $beta_2$ receptors in cardiac tissue, although some of these $beta_2$ receptors may be located on vascular smooth muscle cells of arterioles within the myocardium.

THE RECEPTOR ADENYLATE CYCLASE SYSTEM

Most of the effects of beta-adrenergic stimulation are mediated by cyclic AMP. Activation of the beta receptor results in activation of adenylate cyclase and production of cyclic AMP. Cyclic AMP activates a group of protein kinases. The protein kinases phosphorylate a diverse group of substrates that mediate the final responses attributed to beta-adrenergic stimulation. Thus, cyclic AMP is the second messenger, which links activation of the beta receptor to its physiologic effects.

The receptor adenylate cyclase system consists of three separate components: the receptor (R), the guanine regulatory protein (N or G), and the catalyst (C) adenylate cyclase (Fig. 4-1). The regulatory protein associated with the beta receptor is stimulatory (Ns), but regulatory proteins associated with other receptors may also be inhibitory (Ni). Activation of the system occurs in a stepwise fashion. Hormone is bound by a specific receptor; in this case, the beta-adrenergic receptor. The hormone-receptor complex (H-R) interacts with the regulatory pro-

TABLE 4-1. Distribution of Alpha Receptors and Beta Receptors

	Alpha Receptors		Beta Receptors	
	Alpha-1	Alpha-2	Beta-1	Beta-2
Agonist potency series	E > NE >> PE > I	E > NE >> PE >> I	I > E ≥ NE > PE	I > E >> NE > PE
Specific antagonists	Prazosin	Yohimbine Rauwolseine	Propranolol Nadolol Pindolol Metoprolol Atenolol Esmolol Acebutolol	Propranolol Nadolol Pindolol ICI 118.551
Physiologic responses	Smooth-muscle contraction in blood vessels and genitourinary tract Activation of glycogenolysis (rat liver)	Smooth-muscle relaxation in gastrointestinal tract Smooth-muscle contraction in selected vascular beds Inhibition of norepinephrine release from sympathetic-nerve terminals	Stimulation of rate and force of cardiac contraction Stimulation of lipolysis	Smooth-muscle relaxation in bronchi, blood vessels, and genitourinary and gastrointestinal tracts Facilitation of norepinephrine release Increased glycogenolysis and gluconeogenesis in liver

4. MECHANISM OF ACTIONS OF BETA BLOCKERS

	Inhibition of lipolysis in adipose cells (human, hamster)	Stimulation of amylase secretion by salivary glands	Increased glycogenolysis in muscle
	Platelet aggregation (human, rabbit)		Increased insulin and glucagon secretion by pancreatic cells
	Inhibition of renin release from juxtaglomerular cells of the kidney		Stimulation of renin release by juxtaglomerular cells
	Stimulation of potassium and water secretion by salivary glands		
	Inhibition of insulin release by pancreatic islet cells		
Location	Presynaptic, postsynaptic, and nonsynaptic (e.g., platelets)	Postsynaptic	Presynaptic and postsynaptic; also present on lymphocytes, and polymorphonuclear leukocytes
Mechanism	Inhibition of adenylate cyclase	Alterations of cellular calcium-ion fluxes	Stimulation of adenylate cyclase

Adapted from Lefkowitz et al., *N. Engl. J. Med.* 310:1571, 1984.

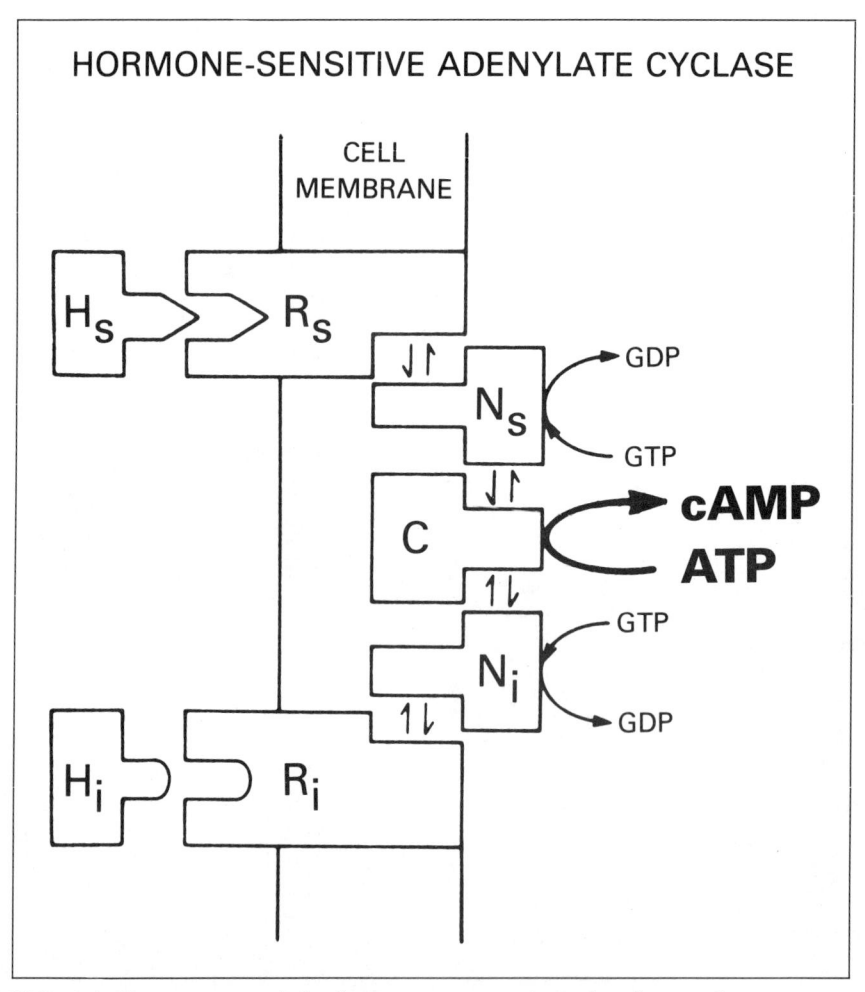

FIG. 4-1. Components of the hormone responsive adenylate cyclase system. (Adapted from Ref. 47.)

tein to form a complex (H-R-Ns). This complex promotes the binding of the guanine nucleotide (GTP) to the guanine regulatory protein (Ns). The activated regulatory protein (Ns-GTP) is able to activate adenylate cyclase. Activated adenylate cyclase catalyzes the production of cyclic AMP. Activation of adenylate cyclase proceeds until GTP is hydrolyzed to GDP, inactivating the guanine regulatory protein (Ns-GTP → Ns-GDP).

Beta Receptor

Initially, beta receptors were evaluated by analyzing the physiologic responses of various tissues to adrenergic agonists and antagonists. An important advance in the evaluation of beta receptors was the development of radiolabeled ligand binding studies [56, 79]. These studies allow quantification of both receptor number and receptor affinity for hormone in various tissues. Binding studies are performed with an agonist or antagonist that is highly specific for the receptor and is radiolabeled. Most studies have been performed with [^{3}H] dihydroalprenolol, [^{125}I] hydroxybenzylpindolol, or [^{125}I] cyanopindolol. Various concentrations of hormone are incubated with either whole cells or membrane preparations. The incubations are performed in the presence or absence of an unlabeled hormone, such as propranolol. Binding of the labeled ligand in the absence of propranolol is called total binding. Binding in the presence of excess propranolol is called nonspecific binding. Specific binding to the beta receptor is determined as the difference between total and nonspecific binding. Figure 4-2 displays the amount of specifically bound hormone plotted against the concentration of hormone. The specific binding reaches a plateau, which approximates the total number of receptors (B_{max}). The calculated dissociation constant (K_D) represents the affinity of the receptor for the hormone.

The binding characteristics of beta receptors have also been analyzed using competitive binding techniques [56]. These techniques determine the ability of various compounds to compete with a radiolabeled ligand for binding to the beta receptor. Membrane preparations are incubated with a fixed concentration of the radiolabeled ligand and various concentrations of the competing compounds. The percent displacement of the radiolabeled ligand from maximum is plotted against the concentration of the other compound (Fig. 4-3). These competitive binding studies are extremely useful for studying relative affinities of different hormones for the receptor. Computer analysis of these studies has also been used to determine the relative proportions of beta$_1$ and beta$_2$ receptors and the presence of high-affinity and low-affinity receptor binding states.

Competitive binding studies have revealed important differences in the binding characteristics among agonists, partial agonists, and antagonists [42]. When competitive binding studies are performed in the absence of a guanine nucleotide, analysis of the binding curve for an antagonist, such as alprenolol, reveals a single population of receptors with a single binding state (Fig. 4-4). Analysis of the binding curve for an agonist, such as isoproterenol, reveals two populations of receptors, one with high-affinity binding for the agonist and one with low-affinity binding for the agonist (Fig. 4-5). The binding curve for the partial agonist soterenol reveals an intermediate-affinity binding state (Fig. 4-6). Thus, only agonists and partial agonists are able to form high-affinity binding complexes with receptors. Further, only agonists and partial agonists are capable of activating the receptor. The high-affinity binding state is necessary for receptor activation.

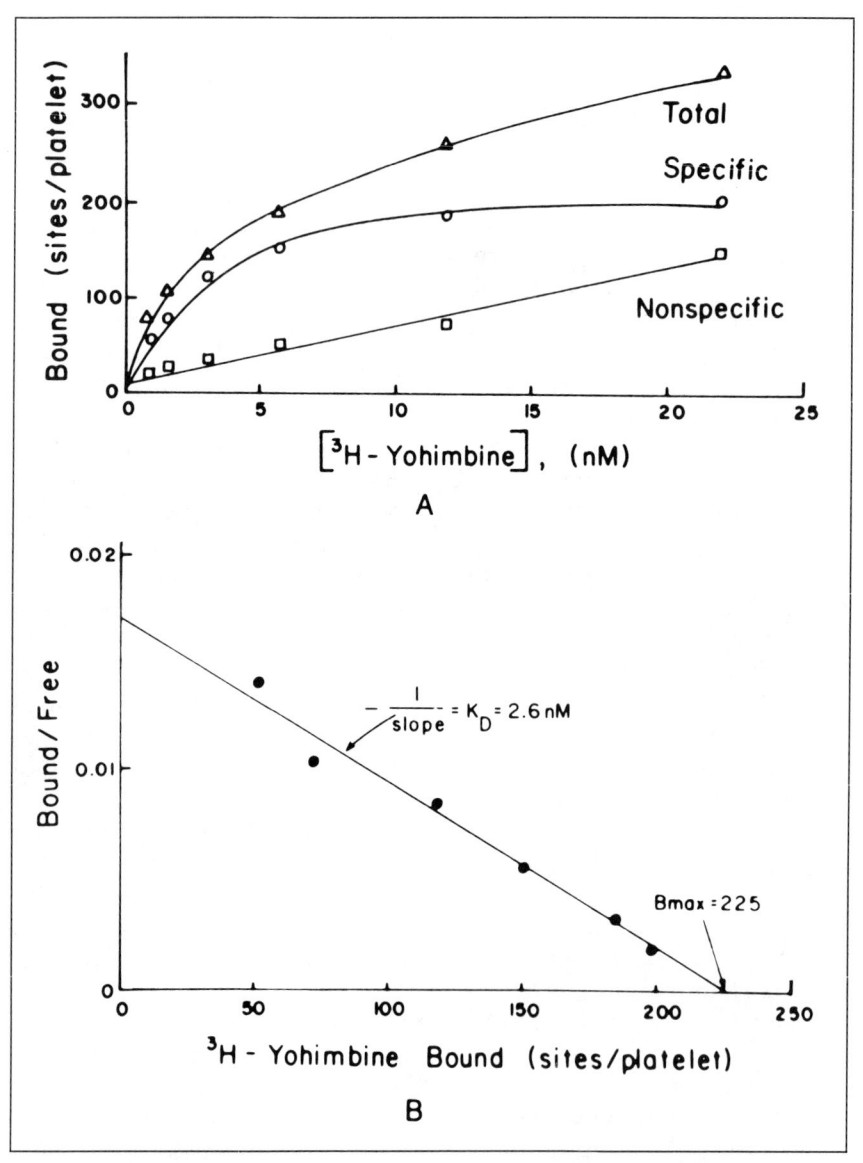

FIG. 4-2. Radiolabeled ligand binding study. *A* displays the amount of ligand binding (total, nonspecific, and specific) as a function of the total concentration of ligand. *B* shows the data rearranged into a Scatchard plot. The ratio of bound ligand to free ligand is plotted as a function of bound ligand. This format yields a straight line. The *x*-intercept (B_{max}) represents the maximum number of binding sites. The negative reciprocal of the slope (K_D) represents the dissociation constant. (From Ref. 56, with permission.)

4. MECHANISM OF ACTIONS OF BETA BLOCKERS

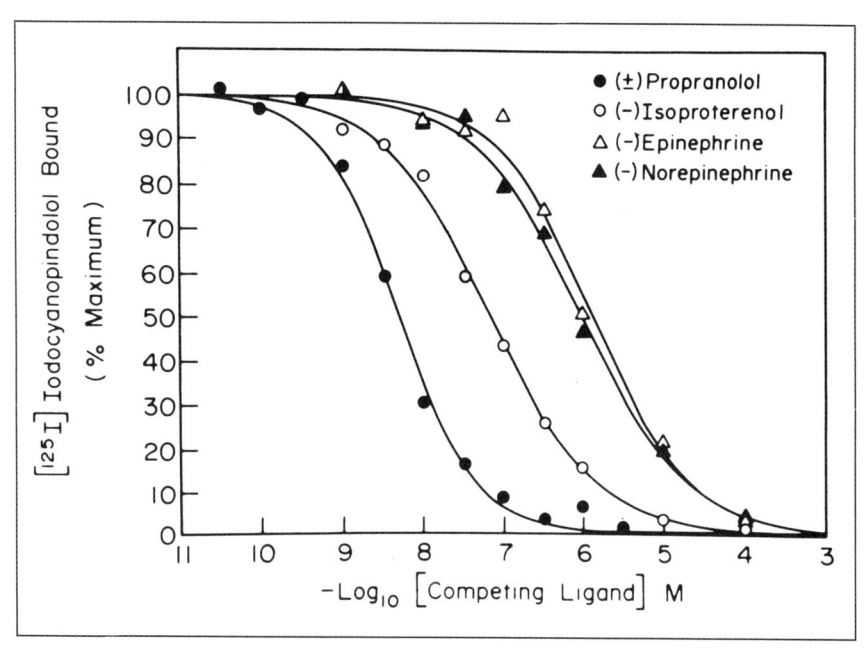

FIG. 4-3. Competitive binding curves between a fixed concentration of [^{125}I] idocyanopindolol and various concentrations of propranolol, isoproterenol, epinephrine, and norepinephrine. The membranes were derived from human left ventricles and consist of predominantly beta-1 receptors. The order of potency was propranolol > isoproterenol > epinephrine = norepinephrine, which is consistent with the beta-1 receptor classification. (From Stiles et al., *Life Sciences* 33:469, 1983, with permission.)

The high-affinity binding state between hormone and receptor is maintained until the regulatory protein binds GTP. Once GTP is bound to the regulatory protein, the receptor is dissociated from the regulatory protein and reverts to the low-affinity binding state. Hormone is released from the receptor. The receptor and the regulatory protein can only form another high-affinity binding complex after the bound GTP is hydrolyzed to GDP.

New techniques have allowed the isolation and purification of the beta$_2$-adrenergic receptor [47]. The mammalian beta$_2$-receptor appears to be a single glycoprotein with a molecular weight of about 60,000 to 65,000 Daltons [69]. Recently the DNA strand that encodes the human beta$_2$ receptor has been isolated and sequenced [44]. The amino acid sequence of the beta receptor has been deduced, and it appears to contain seven clusters of hydrophobic amino acids. These clusters are believed to form helices that span the plasma membrane.

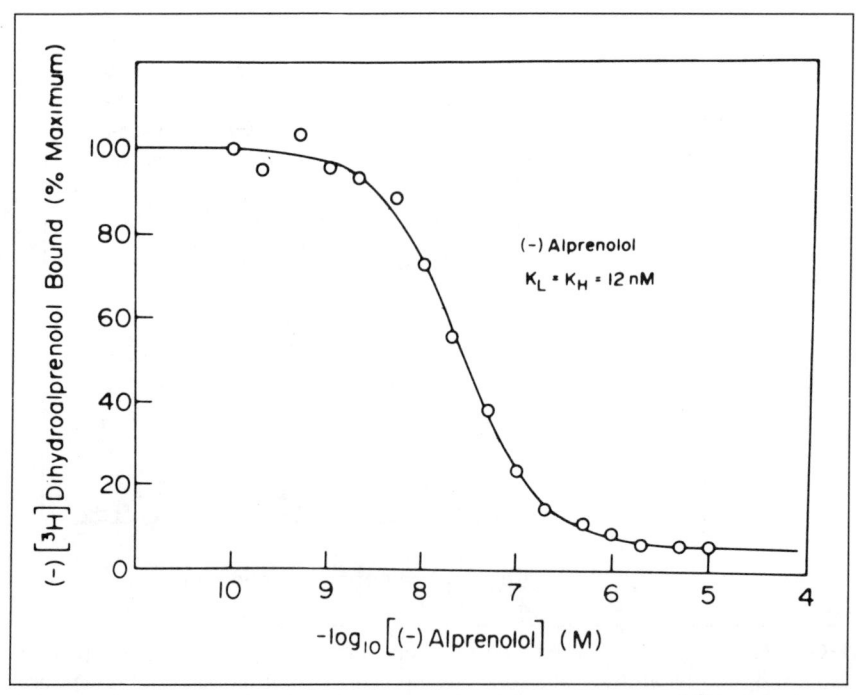

FIG. 4-4. Competitive binding between a fixed concentration of [^{3}H] dihydroalprenolol and various concentrations of unlabeled alprenolol, an antagonist. The displacement of [^{3}H] DHA from maximum binding is plotted against the concentration of alprenolol. The curve is the same both in the presence and absence of guanine nucleotides (not shown). Computer analysis of the curve reveals a homogeneous population of receptors with one binding affinity ($K_L = K_H$ = dissociation constant). (From Ref. 42, with permission.)

Regulatory Protein

The guanine nucleotide regulatory protein (N) is a large protein located on the inner surface of the cell membrane [30]. It has been isolated and found to consist of three subunits: alpha, beta, and gamma. The alpha subunit has a molecular weight of 41,000 to 42,000; the beta subunit 35,000; and the gamma subunit 5,000 [70]. The regulatory protein is activated by binding GTP to the alpha subunit. During activation, the alpha subunit is cleaved from the complex. The alpha subunit is the active component capable of stimulating adenylate cyclase. The alpha subunit is also capable of hydrolyzing GTP to GDP, which results in its own inactivation.

Adenylate Cyclase

The catalyst adenylate cyclase has been partially purified. It appears to be a glycoprotein with a molecular weight of approximately 150,000. It

4. MECHANISM OF ACTIONS OF BETA BLOCKERS

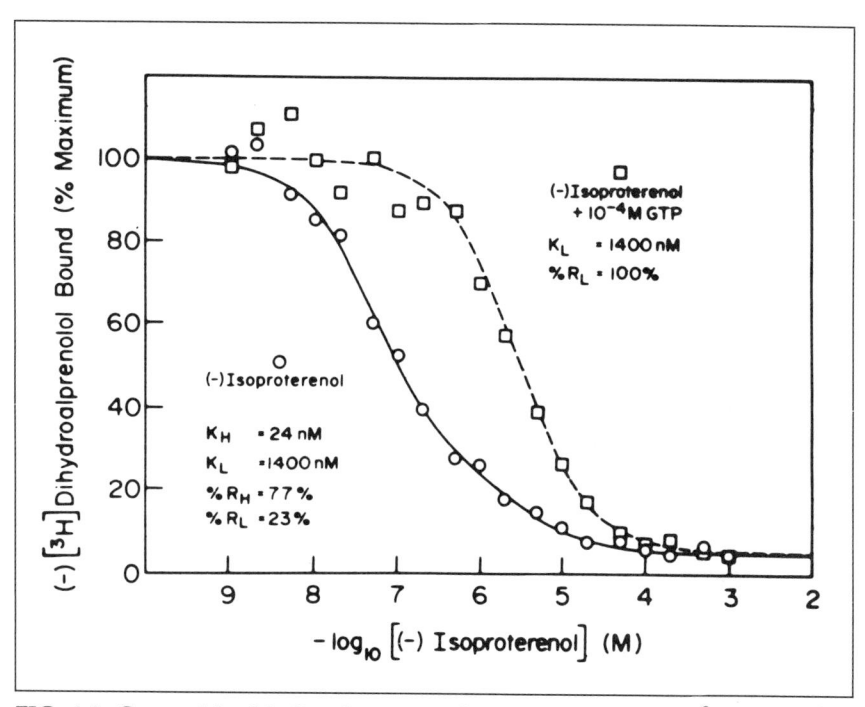

FIG. 4-5. Competitive binding between a fixed concentration of [^{3}H] dihydroalprenolol and various concentrations of unlabeled isoproterenol, a strong agonist. The displacement of [^{3}H] DHA is plotted against the concentration of isoproterenol. In the presence of a guanine nucleotide (GTP), computer analysis reveals a single population of receptors with a low-affinity binding state (R_L = 100%). In the absence of GTP, computer analysis reveals two populations of receptors, with 77% in the high-affinity state and 23% in the low-affinity state. The dissociation constants of the high-affinity state (K_H) and low-affinity state (K_L) are markedly different. (From Ref. 42, with permission.)

resides on the inside surface of the cell membrane. Purified adenylate cyclase has little enzymatic activity, but it can be stimulated directly by forskolin.

The ability to purify the beta receptor (R), the regulatory protein (N_s), and adenylate cyclase (C) has allowed in-depth study of the entire system. Recently developed techniques have allowed the insertion of each component into phospholipid vesicles. Further, the vesicles can be reconstituted with any combination of components or fully reconstituted with all the components. These studies have verified the functional integrity of the purified components, have clarified the interactions between the components, and have shed light on the regulation of the system [48].

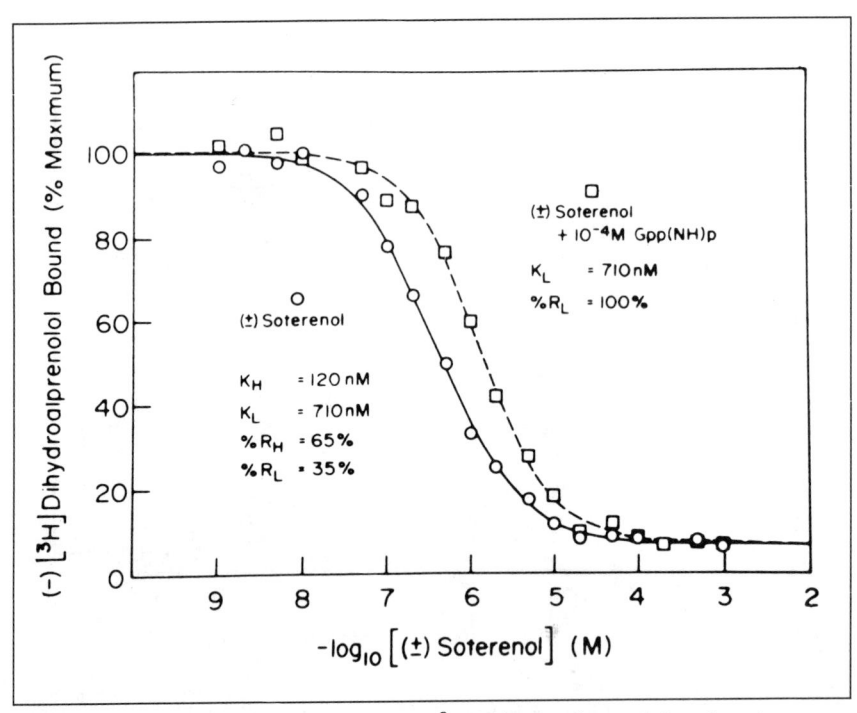

FIG. 4-6. Competitive binding between [^{3}H] dihydroalprenolol and various concentrations of soterenol, a partial agonist. In the absence of guanine nucleotide, computer analysis reveals two populations of receptors (R_H = 65% and R_L = 35%). Compared to a strong agonist like isoproterenol (Figure 4-5), there are fewer receptors in the high-affinity state (65% versus 77%). The dissociation constants of the high- and low-affinity states are closer together than with isoproterenol. (From Ref. 42, with permission.)

REGULATION OF RECEPTORS

Sensitivity to beta-adrenergic stimulation may be regulated upward or downward [70]. Desensitization is seen after chronic treatment with beta agonists, such as isoproterenol, and is manifested by resistance to increasing doses of the drug (tachyphylaxis). Hypersensitization is seen after chronic beta blockade and is manifested by an increased sensitivity to catecholamines after withdrawal of beta blockade.

Desensitization of the beta receptor has been extensively studied in animal models. The two basic mechanisms proposed for desensitization include uncoupling of the receptor from the adenylate cyclase system and decreasing the density of receptors on the cell surface (Fig. 4-7).

The initial step in desensitization is the uncoupling of the beta receptor from the guanine nucleotide regulatory protein. Uncoupling is manifested as a decreased responsiveness to hormone stimulation, without

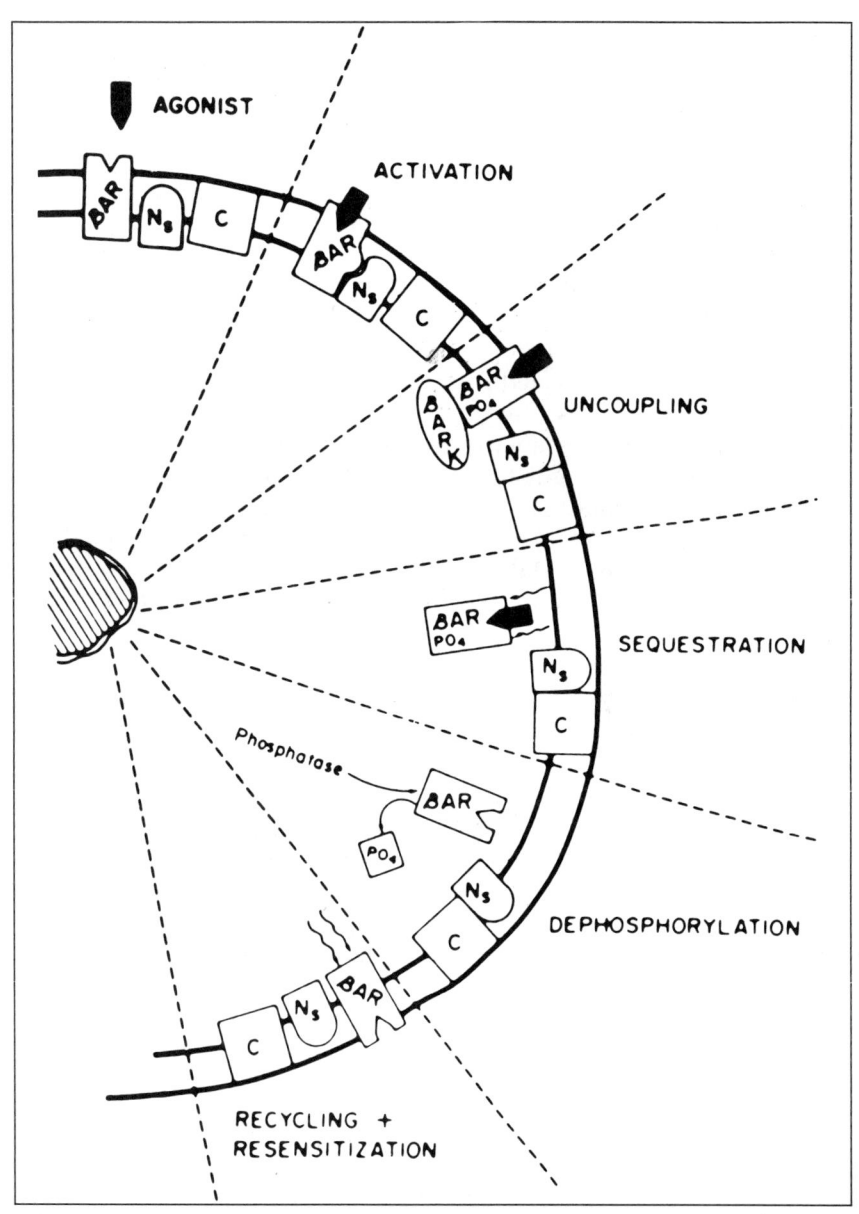

FIG. 4-7. Mechanisms of desensitization of the beta-adrenergic receptor. BAR denotes beta-adrenergic receptor, BARK denotes beta-adrenergic receptor kinase, N_s denotes the regulatory protein, and C denotes the catalytic unit, adenylate cyclase. (From Ref. 71, with permission.)

a change in receptor number on the plasma membrane. Uncoupling can be documented as a decrease in the number of receptors capable of the high-affinity binding state. Uncoupling generally requires hormone stimulation. It can occur rapidly and reversibly. Two mechanisms of uncoupling have been proposed: (1) sequestration of the receptor and (2) chemical alteration of the receptor. Sequestration involves movement of the receptor within the cell membrane so that it is chemically hidden from the rest of the adenylate cyclase system. Chemical alteration involves a small change in the receptor that may not prevent recognition of the receptor by hormones but prevents the receptor from activating the adenylate cyclase system.

Sibley et al. have suggested that phosphorylation of the beta receptor is the primary mechanism for uncoupling [71]. Phosphorylation does not affect the receptor's ability to bind hormones but does limit its ability to activate the regulatory protein. Phosphorylation can be produced by protein kinase A, which is activated by cyclic AMP, and by protein kinase C, which is independent of cyclic AMP [7]. Benovic et al. have described an additional kinase, the beta-adrenergic receptor (BAR) kinase [4]. Phosphorylation by protein kinase A and BAR kinase has been shown to be facilitated by agonist occupancy of the receptor. Thus, they are likely mediators of homologous desensitization. Lefkowitz's group has suggested that phosphorylation of the beta receptor is likely to be the first step common to all types of desensitization and down-regulation [71].

The next major step in the desensitization process is down-regulation, decreasing the density of receptors on the plasma membrane. This process is less rapid and generally requires chronic beta-adrenergic stimulation. The most likely mechanism is the internalization of receptors from the plasma membrane to an intracellular compartment. Several experimental techniques support the concept of internalization. Receptor numbers have been determined for various membrane fractions of broken cells [11]. During desensitization, the decrease in receptors on the plasma membrane is paralleled by an increase in receptors on light membrane fractions believed to represent intracellular vesicles. In another technique using intact cells, receptor numbers have been determined both within the cell and on the cell surface using radiolabeled ligands that are either permeable or impermeable to the plasma membrane. However, recent studies on whole cells have suggested that some of the supposedly internalized receptors are actually redistributed within the cell membrane and are just chemically hidden from impermeable hormones [50].

The final step in down-regulation is the permanent chemical degradation of old receptors. Degradation probably occurs after receptors have been internalized and sequestered in intracellular vesicles. Similarly, receptor number can be increased by the synthesis of new recep-

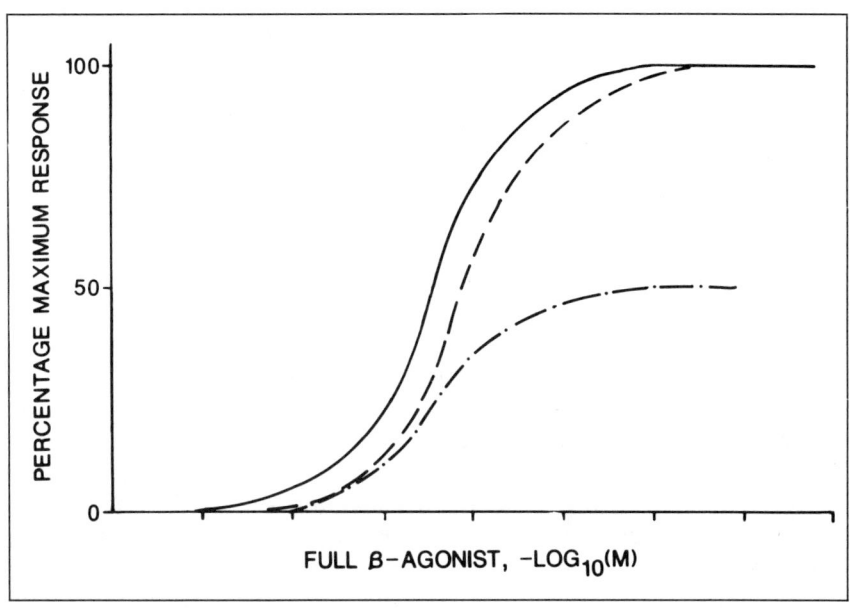

FIG. 4-8. Hypothetical dose response curves for a receptor-mediated activity. The percentage of the maximum response is plotted as a function of the concentration of agonist. For the first curve (–) the receptors are present in full complement. For the second curve (– –), the receptors are decreased but spare receptors are still present. The curve is shifted to the right, but a maximum response is still achievable with a higher concentration of agonist. For the third curve (– · –), the receptors are decreased and there are no spare receptors. The curve is shifted to the right, and a maximum response is no longer achievable. (From Bristow et al., *J. Mol. Cell Cardiol.* 17 (Suppl 2):45, 1985, with permission.)

tors. New receptors are synthesized within the cell and are probably stored within intracellular vesicles. They can be externalized to the plasma membrane as needed.

Spare Receptors

Crucial to understanding the relationship between receptor number and responsiveness of the beta-adrenergic system is the concept of spare receptors. Spare receptors are the additional or extra receptors that are not necessary for maximal physiologic response. However, spare receptors have an important effect on the dose-response curve of any hormone-receptor system. As the number of spare receptors is decreased, the dose-response curve is shifted downward and to the right (Fig. 4-8). Thus, any given response will require a higher dose of hormone. However, the maximal response can still be achieved by giving higher doses of hormone.

If there are no spare receptors, then decreasing the number of receptors has two effects on the dose-response curve (Fig. 4-8). The curve will be shifted downward and to the right, as in the case with spare receptors. In addition, the maximal response will be limited, even when extremely high doses of hormone are given.

Congestive Heart Failure

Patients with chronic congestive heart failure have a decreased responsiveness to beta-adrenergic stimulation. This decreased responsiveness is in part due to down-regulation of beta-adrenergic receptors [25]. The density of beta receptors is decreased in both circulating lymphocytes and the myocardium. This desensitization is probably the result of chronic beta-adrenergic stimulation. Serum levels of catecholamines are mildly increased in patients with congestive heart failure. Local release of catecholamines by the myocardium is also increased, as evidenced by the depletion of myocardial catecholamine stores. Treatment with beta-adrenergic agonists produces even greater down-regulation of the beta receptor and greater tolerance [13].

The combination of down-regulation of beta receptors and depletion of catecholamine stores further limits the ability of the failing myocardium to respond to stress. Bristow and colleagues have concluded that the down-regulation of receptors in the failing myocardium is severe enough to eliminate "spare receptors" [8]. The elimination of spare receptors means that the maximal inotropic response to beta-adrenergic stimulation is decreased even at very high levels of catecholamines.

Down-regulation of beta receptors in the failing myocardium appears to be selective for the beta-1 receptor [8]. Bristow et al. demonstrated a 61 percent decrease in beta-1 receptors and only a 21 percent decrease in beta-2 receptors in failing left ventricular myocardium. The selective down-regulation produces a shift in the ratio of beta-1 to beta-2 receptors from 77:23 in nonfailing myocardium to 60:39 in failing myocardium. The remaining beta-2 receptors appear to assume greater importance in mediating the inotropic response to beta-adrenergic stimulation. Bristow et al. have demonstrated an inotropic response to stimulation of these beta-2 receptors with a relatively selective beta-2 agonist, zinterol.

Up-regulation of beta receptors should help restore the inotropic response of the failing myocardium to beta-adrenergic stimulation. Theoretically, low dose beta blockade could prevent the down-regulation of beta receptors produced by constant low levels of catecholamines without preventing the stimulation produced by transient high levels of catecholamines. Low dose beta blockade could also limit myocardial damage produced by chronic adrenergic stimulation. Although still controversial, several studies have demonstrated improvement in patients with congestive cardiomyopathy following long-term treatment with metoprolol [19, 74]. The use of a beta-1 selective beta blocker such as metoprolol has a theoretical advantage. Beta-1 selective blockade could allow up-regulation of the beta-1 receptors. Stimulation of the beta-2 receptors could produce some inotropic response and also some peripheral vasodilation.

Chronic Beta Blockade and Withdrawal

Beta blockers can prevent the desensitization of beta receptors produced by beta agonists. In addition, beta blockers can produce hypersensitization of beta receptors. Aarons et al. documented a 43 percent increase in beta receptor density in lymphocytes of humans treated with propranolol for 1 week [1]. They also documented hypersensitivity of the cardiac beta receptors by demonstrating an augmentation of the orthostatic change in heart rate during the first 48 hours of propranolol withdrawal.

The chronic effects of treatment with cardioselective and nonselective beta blockers have been compared. Both agents appear to have similar effects on myocardial beta receptor density. Golf and Hansson showed that the degree of up-regulation and the ratio of beta-1 to beta-2 receptors were not different in atrial specimens from patients taking atenolol, metoprolol, timolol, or propranolol [32].

The chronic effects of beta blockers with ISA are poorly understood. Pindolol appears to have complex effects on beta receptor density. Hedberg et al. found that rats treated with pindolol for 7 days actually had a decreased density of beta-2 receptors in lymphocytes, lung tissue, and ventricular myocardium [34]. The density of beta-1 receptors in the ventricular myocardium was unchanged. On the other hand, Golf and Hansson showed an increased density of beta-1 receptors in atrial myocardium of patients treated with pindolol [32]. Confirmatory studies are needed, but it appears that pindolol causes down-regulation of beta-2 receptors and either up-regulation or no change in beta-1 receptors.

The up-regulation of beta receptors caused by chronic beta blockade is probably responsible for the adrenergic hypersensitivity seen after sudden withdrawal. Beta receptor density is probably increased for 2 to 4 days following withdrawal of beta blockade, while serum concentrations of most beta blockers are negligible 24 hours after withdrawal [6, 62].

Several studies have indicated an increased frequency of ischemic events following abrupt withdrawal of large doses of propranolol [3, 55]. The ischemic events have included increased angina, unstable angina, myocardial infarction, and sudden death. The risk of developing withdrawal phenomena is greatly reduced by gradually tapering the dose of beta blocker. The risk of serious withdrawal phenomena is also very low in hospitalized patients with restricted activity and other antianginal therapy [15, 55].

Hormonal Regulation

Abnormalities in thyroid function have been closely linked to abnormalities in adrenergic responsiveness. Hyperthyroid patients have increased cardiac sensitivity to catecholamines and have improvement in symptoms with beta blockade. Several investigators have documented an increased beta receptor density in animals made hyperthyroid. Hammond et al. have recently shown an 83 percent increase in beta receptor density in atrial myocardium from hyperthyroid pigs [33]. The increased density of beta receptors was directly related to an increased sensitivity of heart rate to isoproterenol infusion.

Numerous studies have documented a decreased density of beta receptors in hypothyroid animals. The decreased density of beta receptors has been shown to correlate with decreased adenylate cyclase activity and decreased levels of intracellular cyclic AMP.

Corticosteroids have also been shown to affect beta-adrenergic receptor regulation. Davies and Lefkowitz demonstrated that humans treated with cortisone acetate for 4 hours had an increase in granulocyte beta receptors and a decrease in lymphocyte beta receptors [16]. After 24 hours, both the granulocyte and lymphocyte beta receptors were increased.

Corticosteroids also limit the down-regulation of beta receptors produced by agonists. Asthmatics treated with beta-adrenergic agonists, such as terbutaline, have been shown to have down-regulation of beta receptors on peripheral leukocytes. This down-regulation probably explains the resistance that develops to beta-adrenergic stimulation. Corticosteroids have been shown to limit down-regulation and to accelerate up-regulation following withdrawal of the agonist [9].

ADRENERGIC SYSTEM IN MYOCARDIAL ISCHEMIA

During myocardial infarction, changes in the adrenergic nervous system occur both systemically and locally within the myocardium. Systemically, epinephrine and norepinephrine are released into the circulation. Locally, norepinephrine stores are released into the myocardium and myocardial beta-adrenergic receptors are altered.

Bertel et al. compared catecholamine levels in patients admitted to the cardiac care unit for possible myocardial infarction with those in a normal control group [5]. In 11 patients, myocardial infarction was excluded. These 11 patients had significantly higher serum levels of epinephrine and norepinephrine than the control group. The 30 patients with documented infarctions had higher catecholamine levels than either the controls or the 11 patients in whom infarction was excluded. Of the 30 patients with infarction, 9 had an episode of ventricular fibrillation. The 9 patients with ventricular fibrillation had higher serum levels of epinephrine and norepinephrine than the 21 patients without ventricular fibrillation.

Concomitant with the elevation of serum catecholamines, there is a local release of catecholamines within the ischemic zone of the myocardium. Norepinephrine, the major catecholamine of the heart, is stored in sympathetic nerve terminals. During severe ischemia, norepinephrine is released from the sympathetic nerve terminals. In dog hearts, Muntz et al. have demonstrated the diffusion of catecholamines from nerve endings and have documented a decrease in the catecholamine content of the nerve endings within 1 hour of coronary occlusion [59]. They concluded that catecholamines are shifted from the nerve endings to the tissue compartments. Thus, local tissue levels are transiently increased. However, the tissue eventually becomes depleted as the catecholamines are washed out. Muntz found that total tissue catecholamines in the ischemic zone were decreased by 76 to 83 percent 3 hours after coronary occlusion.

Changes in beta receptors have also been documented in the ischemic dog heart. Mukherjee et al. have demonstrated that beta receptors are increased in the ischemic zone as early as 1 hour and as late as 8 hours following coronary occlusion [58]. The increase in beta receptors with ischemia is probably not a generalized nonspecific response since muscarinic cholinergic receptors are not changed. In a follow-up study, the same group showed that the increased number of beta receptors are still responsive to stimulation with a beta agonist at 1 hour after coronary occlusion [57].

If confirmed in patients with myocardial infarctions, the combination of increased beta receptors and increased levels of serum and tissue catecholamines could have several deleterious effects. The increased sympathetic activity could increase myocardial oxygen demands, increase ischemia, and increase infarct size. The increased sympathetic activity and increased ischemia could also facilitate ventricular arrhythmias.

If sympathetic hypersensitivity occurs in the ischemic myocardium, it is a transient phenomenon. Tissue catecholamines are quickly depleted by over 75 percent within 8 hours of infarction in the dog. Further, recent studies indicate that the beta receptors are uncoupled from the adenylate cyclase complex within a short period [17].

Finally, beta receptors are probably not increased chronically after myocardial infarction. Karliner et al. found no change in the number of beta receptors in the ischemic zone of dogs 3 weeks following coronary occlusion [40].

BETA-ADRENERGIC ANTAGONISTS
Structure Activity Relationships
The interaction between hormone and receptor is highly specific. Both the binding to the receptor and the activation of the receptor are dependent on the specific structure of the hormone [31]. Beta agonists and antagonists have a very similar structure. The basic structure consists of a benzene ring and an ethylamine side chain (Fig. 4-9). The activity is determined by substitutions on the aromatic ring, the alpha and beta carbon atoms, and the terminal amino group. Compounds have been developed that are: (1) pure agonists that bind to the receptor and fully activate the receptor, (2) partial agonists (antagonists with intrinsic sympathomimetic activity) that bind to the receptor but only partially activate the receptor, and (3) pure antagonists that bind to the receptor and prevent its activation.

The ability to bind to the beta-adrenergic receptor is largely determined by substitutions on the amino group. Generally speaking, increasing the size of the alkyl group on the amino terminal will increase the affinity for beta receptors and decrease the affinity for alpha receptors. Isoproterenol has a large isopropyl group on the amino terminal and has maximal affinity for both beta-1 and beta-2 receptors.

The ability to activate the beta receptor is largely determined by substitutions on the benzene ring. Maximal activation of both alpha and beta receptors generally requires hydroxyl groups at the 3 and 4 positions of the benzene ring. Blockade of beta receptors requires substitutions for the hydroxyl groups. Propranolol has an aromatic ring substitution and is a potent beta blocker. Of interest, substitutions on the benzene ring also determine the relative affinity for beta-1 and beta-2 receptors.

The hydroxyl group at the beta carbon atom is necessary for binding to both alpha and beta receptors. The hydroxyl group at the beta carbon gives the molecule optical activity. For both beta agonists and antagonists, the levo stereoisomer has much greater affinity for the receptor and is considered the active form. The dextro isomer binds weakly to the beta receptor but possesses all the other chemical properties. Thus, the presence of two stereoisomers of drugs such as propranolol has allowed investigators to distinguish between the beta blocking effects and the nonspecific effects. Beta blockers used clinically are generally supplied as racemic mixtures; however, the stereoisomers can be purified for research applications. The dextro isomer is especially useful for studying local anesthetic activity, nonspecific effects on arrhythmias, and effects on platelet function.

To summarize, beta antagonists are very similar in structure to beta agonists such as isoproterenol. The affinity for the beta receptor is determined by the large alkyl group on the amino terminal. The ability

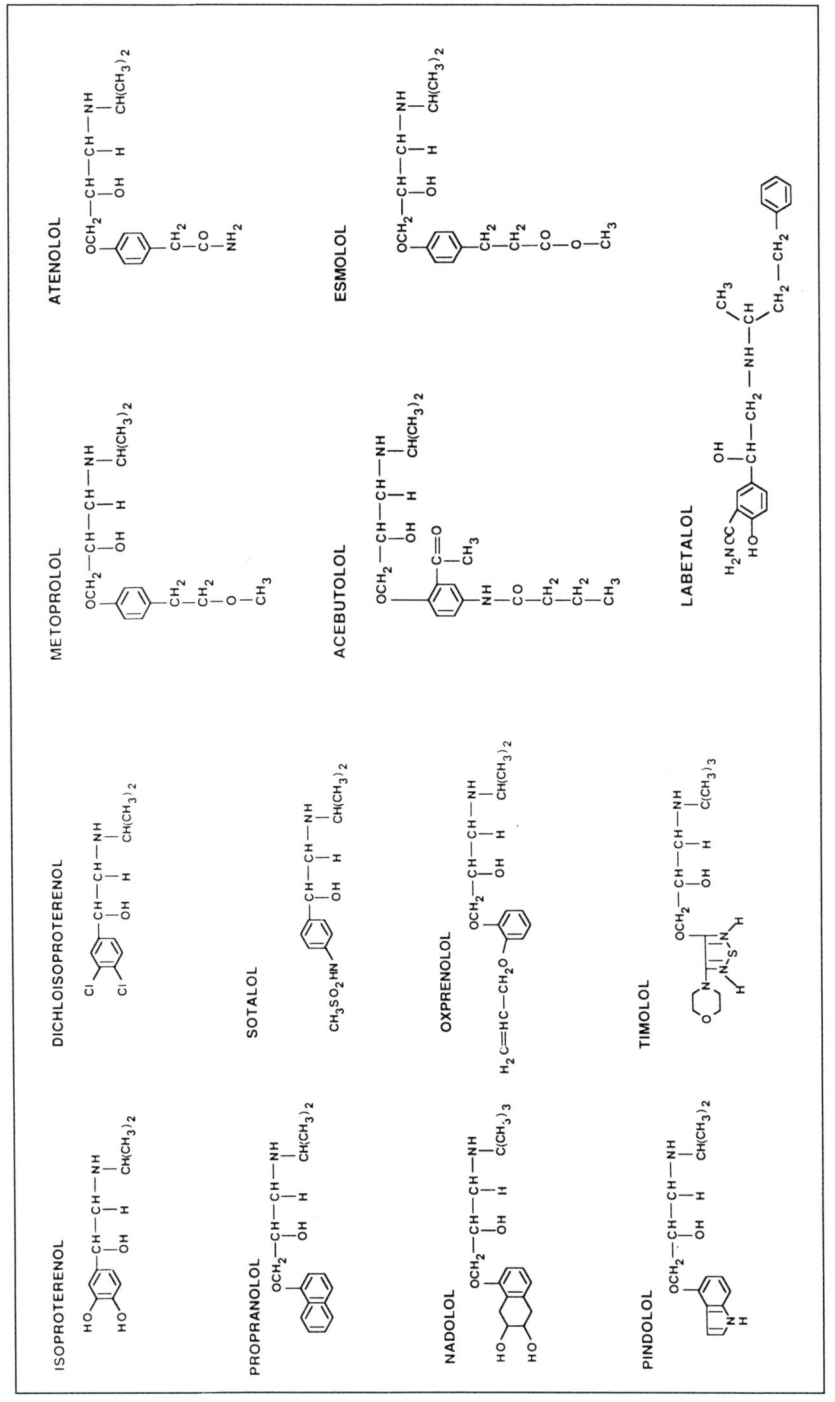

FIG. 4-9. Molecular structures of isoproterenol and some beta blockers.

to block the receptor is determined by substitutions on the benzene ring. Substitutions on the benzene ring also affect the relative affinity for beta-1 and beta-2 receptors. The hydroxyl group on the beta carbon gives the molecule optical activity. The levo isomer is much more potent as a beta blocker than the dextro isomer.

Intrinsic Sympathomimetic Activity (ISA)

Drugs with intrinsic sympathomimetic activity (ISA), such as pindolol, are really partial agonists of the beta receptor. These drugs bind to the beta receptor, but they are less able to form the high-affinity binding state produced by full agonists. Thus, these drugs elicit a partial response even at very high concentrations. Further, at high concentrations these drugs occupy the receptors and inhibit further stimulation by full agonists. When adrenergic activity is low and the beta receptor is unoccupied, the partial agonists will stimulate beta receptors. However, when adrenergic activity is high, the partial agonists will compete with the full agonists and will prevent full stimulation of the beta receptors. When sympathetic tone is increased by exercise, stress, or disease, partial agonists produce beta blockade that is almost indistinguishable from full antagonists.

Beta blockers with ISA have theoretical advantages in patients dependent on small amounts of adrenergic tone. These agents limit the resting bradycardia, the decrease in resting cardiac output, and the increase in filling pressure produced by full antagonists [51, 63, 75]. They may be advantageous in patients with congestive heart failure. However, Man In't Veld et al. found that pindolol and propranolol had identical effects on left ventricular ejection fraction at rest and exercise in patients with angina and normal ventricular function [51].

Beta blockers with ISA such as pindolol are relatively strong beta-2 agonists. Pindolol decreases systemic vascular resistance, whereas beta blockers without ISA increase vascular resistance [51]. The decrease in vascular resistance, a vasodilator effect, may be a theoretical advantage in patients with hypertension. In addition, these agents may be better tolerated in patients with peripheral vascular disease and Raynaud's phenomenon.

Although there are possible advantages to ISA, there are also possible disadvantages. The increase in resting sympathetic tone can potentially increase myocardial oxygen consumption. Thus, these agents may increase ischemia in patients with unstable angina or myocardial infarction. The increase in sympathetic tone and the resulting increase in resting heart rate may also limit their effectiveness as antiarrhythmic agents.

Thus, the beta blockers with intrinsic sympathomimetic activity have theoretical advantages and disadvantages. For most patients with hypertension or exertional angina, their effectiveness is equivalent to full antagonists. For certain select patients, they may have a slight advantage. It is probably prudent to limit their use to patients with specific indications for intrinsic sympathomimetic activity.

Beta Receptor Selectivity

Several beta blockers are now available with a higher affinity for the beta-1 than the beta-2 receptor. These agents include metoprolol, atenolol, and acebutolol. Cardioselective agents have possible advantages in patients with reactive airway disease, diabetes mellitus, peripheral vascular disease, and congestive heart failure.

Patients with reversible obstructive lung disease may require beta-adrenergic stimulation to maintain adequate air flow. Most of the beta receptors in the bronchi are the beta-2 type. Therefore, cardioselective agents are less likely to aggravate bronchospasm [41].

In patients with diabetes mellitus, catecholamines are released in response to insulin-induced hypoglycemia. Beta-2 receptors in the liver mediate glycogenolysis and gluconeogenesis. Cardioselective agents are less likely to inhibit rapid recovery from insulin-induced hypoglycemia [41].

Cardioselective agents may have an advantage in patients with hypertension and peripheral vascular disease. Nonselective blockade of the beta-2 receptors in vascular smooth muscle may permit unopposed alpha-mediated vasoconstriction. During adrenergic stimulation, nonselective agents may permit greater increases in blood pressure. Floras et al. demonstrated that the increase in blood pressure during bicycling was less with the selective agents atenolol and metoprolol than with the nonselective agents pindolol and propranolol [23]. However, the difference was small and may not be important clinically.

There are theoretical disadvantages to cardioselective agents. One disadvantage is the failure to block catecholamine-induced hypokalemia. Hypokalemia appears to be mediated by beta-2 receptors on skeletal muscle [66]. Patients on diuretics may develop prominent hypokalemia during an acute myocardial infarction [38]. In this setting, hypokalemia may aggravate ventricular arrhythmias precipitated by ischemia and stress [38].

Another possible disadvantage of cardioselective agents is the failure to block fully the chronotropic response to catecholamine stimulation [10, 53]. Recent studies have demonstrated a small population of beta-2 receptors in both the atria and ventricles. The atrial beta-2 receptors may mediate part of the chronotropic response to adrenergic stimulation. Cardioselective agents are not as effective in reducing heart rate during infusions of isoproterenol or epinephrine.

Most of the advantages and disadvantages of cardioselectivity are probably lost at the doses commonly used to treat angina and hypertension. However, the cardioselective agents are preferred in patients with reversible obstructive lung disease, diabetes mellitus, and peripheral vascular disease.

Alpha-Adrenergic Blockade

Labetalol is a nonselective beta blocker with the additional properties of alpha blockage and direct vasodilation. The beta blocking potency of labetalol is 4 to 16 times the alpha blocking potency [27].

Labetalol produces a reduction in heart rate both during rest and exercise [27]. The reduction is less than that produced by pure beta blockers. Both systolic and diastolic blood pressure are reduced. Systemic vascular resistance is significantly reduced and cardiac output is maintained at control levels [54]. The vasodilatory properties are prominent, despite the relatively weak potency as an alpha blocker.

The addition of alpha blockade to beta blockade may offer several advantages. Labetalol is effective in both the acute and chronic treatment of hypertension. Because vascular resistance is decreased and cardiac output is maintained, labetalol may be better tolerated in patients with mild congestive heart failure. Studies have documented less deterioration in left ventricular function with labetalol than with pure beta blockers [27]. Because labetalol has alpha blockade and direct vasodilatory activity, it may also be better tolerated in patients with peripheral vascular disease or Raynaud's phenomenon. Unlike pure beta blockers, labetalol does not increase coronary vascular resistance [54]. Whether labetalol will have an advantage in patients with coronary spasm is unknown. Finally, labetalol does not appear to have any deleterious effects on serum lipids [46].

HEMODYNAMIC EFFECTS OF BETA BLOCKERS

The hemodynamic effects of beta blockers are directly related to the competitive inhibition of beta-adrenergic receptors [22]. Therefore, the magnitude of effect is directly related to the underlying level of adrenergic tone. The only exceptions are drugs that have intrinsic sympathomimetic activity and are capable of stimulating beta receptors under conditions of low adrenergic tone. Beta blockers without ISA have minimal effects when adrenergic tone is low. In the normal patient resting in the supine position, beta blockade produces minimal hemodynamic effects. When the adrenergic tone is increased by assuming the upright posture, stress, or exercise, then the effects of beta blockade are magnified [36].

Heart Rate

Beta blockers produce a significant decrease in heart rate by competitive inhibition of beta receptors [82]. In the resting supine state, adrenergic

HEMODYNAMIC EFFECTS OF BETA ADRENERGIC BLOCKERS BY SELECTIVITY, ISA, AND ALPHA BLOCKADE

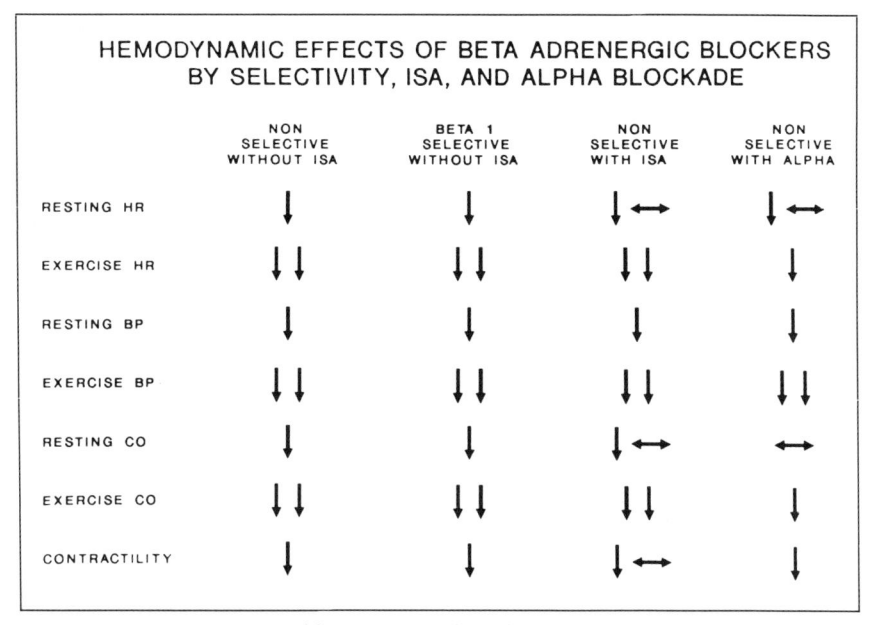

	NON SELECTIVE WITHOUT ISA	BETA 1 SELECTIVE WITHOUT ISA	NON SELECTIVE WITH ISA	NON SELECTIVE WITH ALPHA
RESTING HR	↓	↓	↓↔	↓↔
EXERCISE HR	↓↓	↓↓	↓↓	↓
RESTING BP	↓	↓	↓	↓
EXERCISE BP	↓↓	↓↓	↓↓	↓↓
RESTING CO	↓	↓	↓↔	↔
EXERCISE CO	↓↓	↓↓	↓↓	↓
CONTRACTILITY	↓	↓	↓↔	↓

FIG. 4-10. The response of heart rate to beta blockade as influenced by cardioselectivity and intrinsic sympathomimetic activity (ISA).

tone is minimal and the reduction in heart rate with beta blockade is minimal. Beta blockade produces a marked decrease in heart rate at any given level of exercise and also in the maximal attainable heart rate at peak exercise [12, 20].

The response of heart rate to beta blockade is partially influenced by the ancillary properties of the specific agent—namely, beta receptor selectivity and intrinsic sympathomimetic activity (Fig. 4-10). Drugs with and without beta-1 specificity appear to reduce heart rate equally during rest and exercise states [76]. However, during isoproterenol infusions, nonselective beta blockers such as propranolol produce a greater reduction in heart rate than cardioselective agents such as atenolol [10, 53]. The mechanism for this disparity probably involves the recent discovery that both beta-1 and beta-2 receptors can mediate chronotropic responses.

Beta blockers with ISA have different effects depending on the underlying adrenergic tone. During periods of low tone such as sleep they can stimulate beta receptors; during periods of high tone they inhibit receptors [73]. Beta blockers with ISA have been shown to block the normal diurnal variations of heart rate [21]. Rather than the normal decrease at night and increase during the day, heart rate tends to remain steady during therapy with beta blockers with ISA. Drugs without ISA tend to produce a more consistent decrease in heart rate throughout the day. During exercise, beta blockers with and without ISA reduce heart rate equally [21, 76].

Cardiac Output

At rest, when adrenergic tone is very low, beta blockade produces a small decrease in cardiac output. During exercise, when adrenergic tone is increased, beta blockade produces a large decrease in cardiac output. The change in cardiac output produced by beta blockade seems to parallel the change in heart rate. The reason for the close correlation between cardiac output and heart rate is the relatively small change in stroke volume with beta blockade. Stroke volume tends to remain unchanged or decrease with beta blockade at rest and to increase slightly with beta blockade during exercise. The small increase in stroke volume with beta blockade is not sufficient to compensate for the decrease in heart rate [12].

Beta blockers without ISA produce the greatest reduction in cardiac output. At rest, beta blockers with potent ISA may produce little or no reduction in resting cardiac output. However, during exercise, all beta blockers appear to reduce cardiac output similarly. This includes drugs with and without ISA and with and without beta-1 selectivity [64, 73].

At any fixed level of exercise, beta blockers produce a reduction in both heart rate and cardiac output. Despite the reduction of cardiac output, the systemic oxygen consumption is unchanged [20, 28]. Systemic oxygen consumption is the product of cardiac output and arteriovenous oxygen content (AVO_2) difference. Systemic oxygen consumption is maintained by increasing the arteriovenous oxygen content difference [28]. More oxygen is extracted from the blood, and the mixed venous oxygen content is reduced. This compensatory mechanism is operative at all levels of submaximal exercise.

In normal subjects, the level of maximal exercise is reduced by beta blockade [20]. The level of maximal exercise is dependent on the maximal systemic oxygen consumption. The AVO_2 difference has already been increased to compensate for the decreased cardiac output at submaximal levels of exercise. The AVO_2 difference cannot increase enough to compensate fully the reduced cardiac output at maximal exercise.

In patients with ischemic heart disease, the level of maximal exercise may be limited either by maximal systemic oxygen consumption or by the onset of cardiac ischemia. If exercise is limited by maximal oxygen consumption, then beta blockade will probably reduce the level of maximal exercise. If exercise is limited by cardiac ischemia, then beta blockade will probably increase the level of maximal exercise.

Blood Pressure

In the resting state, the acute oral administration of a beta blocker has little effect on systemic blood pressure [36]. During exercise, all the beta blockers produce a moderate decrease in systolic and mean blood pressure [76]. The decrease in blood pressure is probably related to the decrease in cardiac output. Systemic vascular resistance is unchanged or slightly increased with acute beta blockade during exercise.

Effects of chronic beta blockade on systemic blood pressure are less well understood. Beta blockers without ISA appear to lower pressure through several mechanisms. Cardiac output may be modestly reduced. Renin release from the kidney is inhibited. Systemic vascular resistance does not appear to be decreased.

Beta blockers with ISA appear to reduce resting blood pressure through additional mechanisms. Resting systemic vascular resistance is significantly reduced, and cardiac output is usually maintained. The reduction in resistance is secondary to stimulation of peripheral beta-2 receptors and subsequent arterial vasodilation.

Ventricular Diastolic Function

Beta blockers have some deleterious effects on ventricular diastolic function. Beta blockers decrease the rate of relaxation of the ventricle [35]. The decreased rate of ventricular relaxation can prolong the isovolumic phase of relaxation and decrease the rate of filling in early diastole. Beta blockers also decrease ventricular contractility and heart rate, which tend to cause increases in ventricular diastolic filling pressures. However, beta blockers do not appear to have any direct effects on ventricular compliance during acute administration [35].

Beta blockers may improve diastolic filling in patients with certain conditions such as mitral stenosis and hypertrophic cardiomyopathy. Beta blockers prolong the diastolic filling period by decreasing heart rate. Thus, diastolic filling may occur at lower flow rates and lower atrial pressures. In patients with mitral stenosis, the pressure gradient across the mitral valve is directly proportional to the flow rate across the valve. These patients benefit from decreased heart rate and often improve significantly following beta blockade. Similarly, patients with hypertrophic cardiomyopathy may benefit from longer diastolic filling periods.

Chronic beta blockade may improve diastolic function in hypertensive patients with left ventricular hypertrophy. Fouad et al. have documented improvement in diastolic filling after control of blood pressure [24]. Apparently, the improvement in diastolic function is not a direct effect but is related to regression of left ventricular hypertrophy. Patients without regression of hypertrophy may have no improvement in diastolic function [72].

Myocardial Oxygen Demand

Myocardial oxygen demand is determined by heart rate, blood pressure, and to a lesser extent contractility. The major determinants of myocardial oxygen consumption are reduced by beta blockade [39, 76]. At rest, when adrenergic tone is low, myocardial oxygen consumption is only reduced slightly. At any given level of exercise, myocardial oxygen consumption is reduced significantly. This reduction occurs despite the maintenance of systemic oxygen consumption. As previously stated, systemic oxygen consumption is maintained despite the decreased cardiac output by increasing the systemic arteriovenous oxygen content (AVO_2) difference. Thus, systemic oxygen consumption is maintained while myocardial oxygen consumption is decreased. In patients with coronary blood flow limited by atherosclerosis and maximal exertion limited by myocardial ischemia, beta blockers may improve the level of maximal exertion. In patients without myocardial ischemia, beta blockers may limit the level of maximal exertion by limiting maximal cardiac output and maximal systemic oxygen consumption [12, 20].

Myocardial Oxygen Supply

Myocardial oxygen supply is determined by the product of myocardial blood flow and the myocardial oxygen extraction (AVO_2 difference). Since myocardial oxygen extraction is near maximal levels at rest, myocardial blood flow is the most important determinant of myocardial oxygen supply. Myocardial blood flow is determined by coronary vascular resistance, the pressure gradient across the coronary bed, and the length of diastole. Coronary vascular resistance is affected by hormones, neurotransmitters, and local metabolic products, as well as intraventricular pressure.

Beta receptors are present in high concentrations on the smooth muscle cells of coronary resistance arterioles. The receptors on arterioles are predominantly of the beta-2 subtype [60]. Blockade of these beta receptors would be expected to block catecholamine-induced vasodilation and promote unopposed alpha vasoconstriction. In fact, most studies have documented a decrease in coronary blood flow with beta blockade, both at rest and during stress [39, 64, 82].

However, there are several lines of evidence that indicate that the decrease in coronary blood flow is not detrimental: (1) myocardial oxygen extraction is not increased with beta blockade; (2) myocardial lactate production is decreased; and (3) clinical signs of ischemia, such as chest pain and ST changes, are decreased with beta blockade. Thus, beta blockade appears to improve the balance between myocardial oxygen supply and demand. Myocardial oxygen demand is decreased more than supply.

How is the decrease in coronary blood flow tolerated by the myocardium? In the nonischemic myocardium, the flow may be appropriate for the decreased demands produced by beta blockade. In the ischemic myocardium, the flow is probably preserved by local metabolic control.

These hypotheses have been investigated by studying regional myocardial blood flow using radiolabeled microspheres.

Studies have shown that coronary blood flow to the subepicardial region of both the ischemic and nonischemic zones is decreased by beta blockade. However, blood flow to the subendocardial regions has a more varied response to beta blockade. Flow to the nonischemic subendocardial regions is decreased. Flow to the border zone is decreased slightly. However, flow to the ischemic subendocardium is unchanged. These alterations produce an apparent redistribution of coronary flow to the ischemic zone. This redistribution is produced by appropriate reductions in flow to nonischemic areas and maintenance of flow to ischemic areas by local metabolic control. Although the overall balance of supply and demand is improved, the decrease of blood flow to the border zones may still be detrimental. It is unknown whether further benefit could be derived from preventing the coronary vasoconstriction of beta blockade. The effects of beta blockade on collateral flow are also unknown.

The distribution of beta receptors on large coronary arteries is still controversial. As previously stated, small coronary arterioles have a high density of beta receptors, which are predominantly of the beta-2 subtype. Large coronary arteries have a lower density of beta receptors, which are predominantly of the beta-1 subtype. Purdy and Stupecky examined the ratio of beta-1 and beta-2 receptors in the left anterior descending artery of the cow [65]. They prepared isolated vessel rings and tested the response to various concentrations of beta agonists and antagonists. They concluded that bovine large coronary arteries contain a homogeneous population of beta-1 receptors. Vatner et al. used both physiologic studies of vasodilation and competitive membrane binding studies to analyze the ratio of beta receptors in bovine circumflex coronary arteries [77]. They concluded that bovine large coronary arteries contain both beta-1 and beta-2 receptors with a ratio of 1.5–2.0:1.0.

The response of large coronary arteries to beta blockade is also controversial. Most authorities believe that beta blockade can aggravate coronary spasm by producing unopposed alpha vasoconstriction. There are numerous reports of Prinzmetal's angina being exacerbated by beta blockade. Kern et al. demonstrated that propranolol could potentiate the coronary vasoconstriction produced by cold pressor testing in patients with coronary artery disease [43]. Although beta blockers may be detrimental in patients with Prinzmetal's angina, they are often beneficial in patients with rest pain and unstable angina. Perhaps the simultaneous administration of nitrates and calcium antagonists prevents an increase in coronary vasomotor tone.

Gaglione et al. have demonstrated that intracoronary propranolol does not decrease coronary artery size in patients with coronary artery disease and exercise-induced angina [29]. They analyzed the change in coronary artery lumen area both at rest and exercise after the administration of 1 mg of intracoronary propranolol. At rest, intracoronary propranolol did not decrease coronary lumen area of either the normal segments or the stenotic segments. At exercise, intracoronary propranolol prevented the exercise-induced decrease in coronary lumen area of the stenotic segment. The mechanism of the prevention of exercise-induced coronary vasoconstriction is unknown. The role of the prevention of exercise-induced vasoconstriction in alleviating angina is also not known.

Effects on Platelets

Since platelet aggregation is important in the pathogenesis of both unstable angina and myocardial infarction, the effects of beta blockers on platelet function have been investigated. Most evidence indicates that beta blockade per se has minimal effects but that individual agents may have significant effects on platelet function.

Several investigators have characterized beta receptors on human platelets. Cook et al. determined both the density of binding sites (B_{max} = 5.54 ± 0.7 fmol/mg protein) and the equilibrium dissociation constant (KD = 24.27 ± 1.36 pM) using Scatchard analysis of levo [^{125}I] pindolol binding to human platelet membranes [14]. Competitive binding curves performed with highly selective beta antagonists practolol (beta-1 selective) and ICI[118,551] (beta-2 selective), indicated the receptors were all of the beta-2 type.

In support of these findings, Winther et al. found that isoproterenol stimulated platelets to form cyclic AMP [80]. Further, cyclic AMP formation was blocked by nonselective beta blockers such as propranolol and timolol but not by beta-1 selective blockers such as atenolol and metoprolol. Since cyclic AMP is known to inhibit platelet aggregation, nonselective beta blockers might act to potentiate platelet aggregation. However, beta blockers have not been shown to increase platelet aggregation significantly.

Individual agents such as propranolol have actually been shown to reduce platelet aggregation [26]. Propranolol inhibits aggregation induced by adenosine diphosphate (ADP), epinephrine, collagen, and thrombin. Propranolol mainly affects the secondary phase of aggregation and may function by interfering with calcium mobilization.

The effects of propranolol on platelet aggregation are nonspecific and not the result of beta blockade [26]. The stereoisomers of propranolol appear to inhibit platelet function equally, despite the relative lack of beta blockade by the dextro isomer of propranolol. Further, certain beta blockers without membrane stabilizing effects do not inhibit platelet aggregation. Since many of these agents are also useful for angina, arrhythmias, and prevention of sudden death following myocardial infarction, the importance of propranolol's inhibition of platelet aggregation is unclear.

Metabolic Effects

Beta blockers can have important effects on lipid metabolism, carbohydrate metabolism, and potassium homeostasis. Metabolic changes may occur after acute or chronic administration of beta blockers.

Acute metabolic changes produced by beta blockers may be beneficial during myocardial ischemia. Beta blockers inhibit the rise in serum free fatty acids produced by adrenergic stimulation. They subsequently decrease the myocardial uptake of free fatty acids [67]. Free fatty acids are the predominant fuel source for the myocardium under normal conditions. However, glucose becomes the preferred fuel source during ischemia. By reducing the utilization of free fatty acids, beta blockers may further reduce myocardial oxygen demands and ischemia.

Chronic treatment with beta blockers may produce deleterious effects on serum lipids [46, 61]. Nonselective beta blockers produce a significant elevation of serum triglycerides and a reduction of high density lipoprotein (HDL) cholesterol. Total cholesterol is not significantly changed. Selective beta blockers such as metoprolol and atenolol produce similar changes in lipids but of less magnitude than nonselective agents. Pindolol, a beta blocker with ISA, does not produce a significant elevation of serum triglycerides during chronic treatment [46]. Further, pindolol appears to produce an elevation of HDL cholesterol. Labetalol, an agent with combined alpha and beta blockade, does not appear to produce significant changes in serum lipids [46].

Beta blockers have important consequences on carbohydrate metabolism [31]. Nonselective blockers inhibit the release of insulin by catecholamines. However, serum levels of glucose and insulin are not significantly affected in normals. More importantly, nonselective blockers inhibit the rebound of serum glucose following insulin-induced hypoglycemia. These effects are due to blockade of beta-2 receptors, which stimulate glycogenolysis and gluconeogenesis. Beta blockers should be used cautiously in patients treated with insulin, especially those prone to hypoglycemia.

ELECTROPHYSIOLOGIC EFFECTS OF BETA BLOCKERS

The electrophysiologic effects of beta blockers are due both to the specific inhibition of the beta receptor, a property shared by all drugs of this class, and to the nonspecific effects produced by individual drugs [78, 81]. The nonspecific effects include the quinidinelike or local anesthetic effects of drugs such as propranolol and the class III effects of sotalol.

In the following sections, the electrophysiologic effects of beta-adrenergic stimulation and blockade will be outlined for pacemaker tissue, atrioventricular nodal tissue, and working myocardium. The nonspecific effects of individual drugs will be discussed briefly.

Pacemaker Tissue

The sinus node, the atrioventricular node, and the His-Purkinje system are capable of spontaneous depolarization. This pacemaker activity is the result of a slow, steady rise in the resting potential during phase 4. When the resting potential achieves threshold, then spontaneous depolarization occurs. Beta-adrenergic stimulation increases the rate of phase 4 depolarization and thus increases the spontaneous rate of pacemaker tissue [81]. Beta-adrenergic stimulation of the sinus node produces sinus tachycardia. Beta-adrenergic stimulation of the atrium, AV junction, and ventricle can produce ectopic arrhythmias due to increased automaticity.

Beta-adrenergic blockade prevents the increase in automaticity produced by beta-adrenergic stimulation [81]. The magnitude of effect is directly related to the underlying adrenergic tone. Thus, beta blockers produce a marked decrease in heart rate during exercise and stress but little change during recumbent rest.

Atrioventricular Node

The atrioventricular node delays conduction between the atrium and the His-Purkinje system. The relatively slow rate of rise of phase 0 of the cardiac action potential is a major factor in delaying conduction. Beta-adrenergic stimulation of the AV node increases the rate of rise of the action potential and increases the conduction velocity through the node [81]. Beta-adrenergic stimulation also decreases the relative and absolute refractory periods of the AV node.

Beta blockade of the AV node slows the velocity of conduction and increases the refractory period [81]. During atrial tachycardia, atrial fibrillation, and atrial flutter, beta blockers may slow the rate of ventricular response. Beta blockers may also be useful for treatment and prophylaxis of paroxysmal supraventricular tachycardia (PSVT). PSVT is usually the result of either atrioventricular nodal reentry utilizing dual pathways for the reentry circuit or atrioventricular reentry utilizing an accessory pathway. Both forms of reentry utilize the AV node in the antegrade limb of the circuit. Beta blockade may terminate reentry by increasing the AV node refractory period and thus producing block in the antegrade limb. Unfortunately, beta blockers also have the potential to aggravate these reentry supraventricular tachycardias by slowing antegrade conduction in the AV node and allowing a longer recovery time for the retrograde pathway.

His-Purkinje System

In the His-Purkinje system, beta-adrenergic stimulation has little effect on cellular electrophysiology [78, 81]. The action potential duration and the refractory period are both shortened. Most significantly, beta-adrenergic stimulation increases the rate of phase 4 depolarization and thus enhances automaticity of the Purkinje fibers.

Beta blockers have little direct effect on the His-Purkinje system [81]. They prevent the slight shortening of the refractory period produced by adrenergic stimulation. They also inhibit the increase in automaticity of the Purkinje system produced by adrenergic stimulation.

Working Myocardium

In normal myocardial tissue, beta-adrenergic stimulation has little direct effect on cellular electrophysiology [78, 81]. Resting membrane potential, upstroke velocity and amplitude, and conduction velocity are all unchanged. Phase 4 diastolic depolarization is not induced. However, adrenergic stimulation may shorten the monophasic action potential duration and the ventricular effective refractory period.

Sympathetic stimulation may produce marked electrocardiographic changes in the T wave, U wave, and QTU interval. The changes are especially prominent in patients with the congenital long Q–T syndrome. In these patients, stress can amplify the T wave and U wave abnormalities, even producing alternation of the T wave. In animal models, the syndrome can be reproduced by stimulating the left stellate ganglion or suppressing the right stellate ganglion. Two theories have been proposed to explain the ventricular arrhythmias seen in the long Q–T syndrome: (1) uneven sympathetic stimulation may result in dispersion of ventricular refractoriness and subsequent reentry arrhythmias or (2) sympathetic stimulation may enhance delayed after-depolarizations and produce triggered arrhythmias [37]. The arrhythmias have been successfully treated with beta blockers and left sympathectomy.

Ventricular Arrhythmias

Beta-adrenergic stimulation may initiate ventricular arrhythmias through several other mechanisms: (1) the ventricular fibrillatory threshold is decreased by adrenergic stimulation, (2) automaticity is enhanced in Purkinje fibers, (3) the ventricular refractory period is decreased and may help propagate reentry tachycardias, and (4) inhomogeneous adrenergic stimulation, such as seen in the congenital long Q–T syndrome, may produce ventricular arrhythmias through dispersion of refractoriness or possibly delayed after-depolarizations. Finally and most importantly, beta-adrenergic stimulation may aggravate ventricular arrhythmias by metabolic changes such as increased ischemia and hypokalemia.

Beta blockers are not generally considered potent agents against ventricular arrhythmias, but they have proven effective in several specific syndromes. Beta blockers are the agents of choice in patients with exercise-induced ventricular tachycardia and with the congenital long Q–T syndrome. They may be effective in patients with mitral valve prolapse, hypertrophic cardiomyopathy, hyperthyroidism, and digitalis toxicity. In patients with a previous myocardial infarction, several beta blockers have been shown to prolong survival and reduce the incidence of sudden death, presumably by reducing lethal ventricular arrhythmias [49, 68].

The mechanisms of action of beta blockers in ventricular arrhythmias are poorly understood. Beta blockers probably act both directly on cellular electrophysiology and indirectly on metabolic parameters such as ischemia and hypokalemia. The direct effects of beta blockers include the following: (1) Beta blockers increase the ventricular fibrillatory threshold [78]. (2) Beta blockers suppress automatic arrhythmias by decreasing phase 4 spontaneous depolarization in Purkinje fibers. (3) Beta blockers suppress certain triggered arrhythmias by reducing heart rate and decreasing delayed after-depolarizations. (4) Beta blockers may prevent dispersion of refractoriness caused by uneven adrenergic stimulation of the ventricular myocardium. (5) Beta blockers may prevent reentry by prolonging refractoriness in Purkinje fibers and working myocardium. (6) In the ischemic zone, beta blockers appear to prolong ventricular conduction and may prevent reentry [78].

Ancillary Properties of Beta Blockers

Many of the beta blockers have ancillary properties that are unrelated to adrenergic blockade but may be related to their antiarrhythmic effects. Propranolol has membrane stabilizing activity, which has been referred to as a quinidinelike effect and a local anesthetic effect. This activity resides equally in both stereoisomers of propranolol, despite the relative lack of beta blocking activity in the dextro isomer. At high doses, dextropropranolol reduces both the rate of rise and the overshoot of the cardiac action potential. These class I effects result from suppression of the inward fast sodium channels. In experimental preparations, dextropropranolol has been effective in the suppression of ventricular arrhythmias produced by digitalis intoxication and ischemia. Membrane stabilizing activity has also been demonstrated in acebutolol, oxprenolol, and pindolol.

Membrane stabilizing activity is felt to have limited clinical significance. The activity is only demonstrated at drug levels significantly higher than those routinely obtained in clinical practice. In addition, beta blockers without membrane stabilizing activity appear to be equally effective against most clinical arrhythmias. However, some patients with ventricular arrhythmias have responded to very high doses of propranolol [18]. Presumably, the response was due to a nonspecific effect of propranolol and was not seen at lower doses.

Sotalol is a beta blocker with unique class III electrophysiologic activity [52]. Sotalol has been shown to prolong the duration of the cardiac action potential without affecting the rate of rise or overshoot. This prolongation of the cardiac action potential results in lengthening of the refractory periods of both atrial and ventricular myocardium. The prolongation of the cardiac action potential also results in lengthening of the Q–T and QTc intervals on the surface electrocardiogram. Sotalol has proven effective against both atrial and ventricular arrhythmias. Sotalol has been shown to suppress complex ventricular ectopy, sustained ventricular tachycardia, and ventricular fibrillation.

REFERENCES

1. Aarons, R. D., Nies, A. S., Gal, J., et al. Elevation of beta-adrenergic receptor density in human lymphocytes after propranolol administration. *J. Clin. Invest.* 65:949, 1980.
2. Ahlquist, R. P. A study of the adrenotropic receptors. *Am. J. Physiol.* 163:586, 1948.
3. Alderman, E. L., Coltart, D. J., Wettach, G. E., and Harrison, D. C. Coronary artery syndromes after sudden propranolol withdrawal. *Ann. Intern Med.* 81:625, 1974.
4. Benovic, J. L., Strasser, R. H., Caron, M. G., and Lefkowitz, R. J. Beta-adrenergic receptor kinase: Identification of a novel protein kinase that phosphorylates the agonist-occupied form of the receptor. *Proc. Natl. Acad. Sci. USA* 83:2797, 1986.
5. Bertel, O., Buhler, F. R., Baitsch, G., et al. Plasma adrenaline and noradrenaline in patients with acute myocardial infarction: Relationship to ventricular arrhythmias of varying severity. *Chest* 82:64, 1982.
6. Boudoulas, H., Lewis, R. P., Kates, R. E., and Dalamagas, G. Hypersensitivity to adrenergic stimulation after propranolol withdrawal in normal subjects. *Ann. Intern. Med.* 87:433, 1977.
7. Bouvier, M., Leeb-Lundberg, L. M. F., Benovic, J. L., et al. Regulation of adrenergic receptor function by phosphorylation. II. Effects of agonist occupancy on phosphorylation of alpha$_1$ and beta$_2$-adrenergic receptors by protein kinase C and the cyclic AMP-dependent protein kinase. *J. Biol. Chem.* 262:3106, 1987.
8. Bristow, M. R., Ginsburg, R., Umans, V., et al. Beta-1 and beta-2-adrenergic-receptor subpopulations in nonfailing and failing human ventricular myocardium: Coupling of both receptor subtypes to muscle contraction and selective beta-1-receptor down-regulation in heart failure. *Circ. Res.* 59:297, 1986.
9. Brodde, O. E., Brinkmann, M., Schemuth, R., et al. Terbutaline-induced desensitization of human lymphocyte beta-2-adrenoceptors: Accelerated restoration of beta-adrenoceptor responsiveness by prednisone and ketotifen. *J. Clin. Invest.* 76:1096, 1985.
10. Brown, J. E., McLeod, A. A., and Shand, D. G. In support of cardiac chronotropic beta$_2$ adrenoceptors. *Am. J. Cardiol.* 57:11F, 1986.
11. Chuang, D., and Costa, E. Evidence for internalization of the recognition

site of beta-adrenergic receptors during receptor subsensitivity induced by (-)-isoproterenol. *Proc. Natl. Acad. Sci. USA* 76:3024, 1979.
12. Bruce, R. A., Hossack, K. F., Kusumi, F., and Clarke, L. J. Acute effects of oral propranolol on hemodynamic responses to upright exercise. *Am. J. Cardiol.* 44:132, 1979.
13. Colucci, W. S., Alexander, R. W., Williams, G. H., et al. Decreased lymphocyte beta-adrenergic-receptor density in patients with heart failure and tolerance to the beta-adrenergic agonist pirbuterol. *N. Engl. J. Med.* 305:185, 1981.
14. Cook, N., Nahorski, S. R., and Barnett, D. B. $(-)[^{125}I]$ Pindolol binding to the human platelet beta-adrenoceptor: Characterisation and agonist interactions. *Eur. J. Pharmacol.* 113:247, 1985.
15. Croft, C. H., Rude, R. E., Gustafson, N., et al. Abrupt withdrawal of beta-blockade therapy in patients with myocardial infarction: Effects on infarct size, left ventricular function, and hospital course. *Circulation* 73:1281, 1986.
16. Davies, A. O., and Lefkowitz, R. J. Corticosteroid-induced differential regulation of beta-adrenergic receptors in circulating human polymorphonuclear leukocytes and mononuclear leukocytes. *J. Clin. Endocrinol. Metab.* 51:599, 1980.
17. Devos, C., Robberecht, P., Nokin, P., et al. Uncoupling between beta-adrenoceptors and adenylate cyclase in dog ischemic myocardium. *Naunyn-Schmiedeberg's Arch. Pharmacol.* 331:71, 1985.
18. Duff, H. J., Mitchell, L. B., and Wyse, D. G. Antiarrhythmic efficacy or propranolol: Comparison of low and high serum concentrations. *J. Am. Coll. Cardiol.* 8:959, 1986.
19. Engelmeier, R. S., O'Connell, J. B., Walsh, R., et al. Improvement in symptoms and exercise tolerance by metroprolol in patients with dilated cardiomyopathy: A double-blind, randomized, placebo-controlled trial. *Circulation* 72:536, 1985.
20. Epstein, S. E., Robinson, B. F., Kahler, R. L., and Braunwald, E. Effects of beta-adrenergic blockade on the cardiac response to maximal and submaximal exercise in man. *J. Clin. Invest.* 44:1745, 1965.
21. Fitscha, P., Tiso, B., Meisner, W., and Spitzer, D. The effect of intrinsic sympathomimetic activity of beta-adrenoceptor blockers in circadian heart rate. *Br. J. Clin. Pharmacol.* 13:211S, 1982.
22. Fitzgerald, J. D., Wale, J. L., and Austin, M. The haemodynamic effects of ($\pm$)-propranolol, dextropropranolol, oxprenolol, practolol, and sotalol in anaesthetised dogs. *Eur. J. Pharmacol.* 17:123, 1972.
23. Floras, J. S., Hassan, M. O., Jones, J. V., and Sleight, P. Cardioselective and nonselective beta-adrenoceptor blocking drugs in hypertension: A comparison of their effect on blood pressure during mental and physical activity. *J. Am. Coll. Cardiol.* 6:186, 1985.
24. Fouad, F. M., Slominski, M. J., Tarazi, R. C., and Gallagher, J. H. Alterations in left ventricular filling with beta-adrenergic blockade. *Am. J. Cardiol.* 51:161, 1983.
25. Fowler, M. B., Laser, J. A., Hopkins, G. L., et al. Assessment of the beta-adrenergic receptor pathway in the intact failing human heart: Progressive receptor down-regulation and subsensitivity to agonist response. *Circulation* 74:1290, 1986.
26. Frishman, W. H. Beta-adrenergic blockade for the treatment of angina pectoris. In D. A. Weiner and W. H. Frishman (eds.), *Therapy of Angina Pectoris: A Comprehensive Guide for the Clinician.* New York: Marcel Dekker, 1986. P. 83.
27. Frishman, W. H., Strom, J. A., Kirschner, M., et al. Labetalol therapy in

patients with systemic hypertension and angina pectoris: Effects of combined alpha and beta adrenoceptor blockade. *Am. J. Cardiol.* 48:917, 1981.
28. Furberg, C., and Schmalensee, G. V. Beta-adrenergic blockade and central circulation during exercise in sitting position in healthy subjects. *Acta Physiol. Scand.* 73:435, 1968.
29. Gaglione, A., Hess, O. M., Corin, W. J., et al. Is there coronary vasoconstriction after intracoronary beta-adrenergic blockade in patients with coronary artery disease? *J. Am. Coll. Cardiol.* 10:299, 1987.
30. Gilman, A. G. Guanine nucleotide-binding regulatory proteins and dual control of adenylate cyclase. *J. Clin. Invest.* 73:1, 1984.
31. Gilman, A. G., Goodman, L. S., and Gilman, A. *The Pharmacological Basis of Therapeutics.* New York: Macmillan, 1980.
32. Golf, S., and Hansson, V. Effects of beta blocking agents on the density of beta adrenoceptors and adenylate cyclase response in human myocardium: Intrinsic sympathomimetic activity favors receptor upregulation. *Cardiovasc. Res.* 20:637, 1986.
33. Hammond, H. K., White, F. C., Buxton, I. L. O., et al. Increased myocardial beta-receptors and adrenergic responses in hyperthyroid pigs. *Am. J. Physiol.* 252:H283, 1987.
34. Hedberg, A., Gerber, J. G., Nies, A. S., et al. Effects of pindolol and propranolol on beta adrenergic receptors on human lymphocytes. *J. Pharmacol. Exp. Ther.* 239:117, 1986.
35. Hess, O. M., Grimm, J., and Krayenbuehl, H. P. Diastolic function in hypertrophic cardiomyopathy: Effects of propranolol and verapamil on diastolic stiffness. *Eur. Heart J.* 4(Suppl F):F-47, 1983.
36. Iskandrian, A. S., Nestico, P. F., Hakki, A. H., et al. Effects of beta blockade on systolic and diastolic left ventricular function at rest and during exercise in patients with chronic stable angina pectoris. *Am. Heart J.* 113:791, 1987.
37. Jackman, W. M., Friday, K. J., Anderson, J. L., et al. The long QT syndrome: A critical review. New clinical observations and a unifying hypothesis. *Progr. Cardiovasc. Dis.* 31(2):115, 1988.
38. Johansson, B. W. Effect of beta blockade on ventricular fibrillation- and ventricular tachycardia-induced circulatory arrest in acute myocardial infarction. *Am. J. Cardiol.* 57:34F, 1986.
39. Jorgensen, C. R., Wang, K., Wang, Y., et al. Effect of propranolol on myocardial oxygen consumption and its hemodynamic correlates during upright exercise. *Circulation* 48:1173, 1973.
40. Karliner, J. S., Stevens, M., Grattan, M., et al. Beta-adrenergic receptor properties of canine myocardium: Effects of chronic myocardial infarction. *J. Am. Coll. Cardiol.* 8:349, 1986.
41. Kendall, M. J. Impact of beta$_1$ selectivity and intrinsic sympathomimetic activity on potential unwanted noncardiovascular effects of beta blockers. *Am. J. Cardiol.* 59:44F, 1987.
42. Kent, R. S., DeLean, A., and Lefkowitz, R. J. A quantitative analysis of beta-adrenergic receptor interactions: Resolution of high and low affinity states of the receptor by computer modeling of ligand binding data. *Mol. Pharmacol.* 17:14, 1980.
43. Kern, M. J., Ganz, P., Horowitz, J. D., et al. Potentiation of coronary vasoconstriction by beta-adrenergic blockade in patients with coronary artery disease. *Circulation* 67:1178, 1983.
44. Kobilka, B. K., Dixon, R. A. F., Frielle, T., et al. cDNA for the human beta$_2$-adrenergic receptor: A protein with multiple membrane-spanning domains and encoded by a gene whose chromosomal location is shared with that of

the receptor for platelet-derived growth factor. *Proc. Natl. Acad. Sci. USA* 84:46, 1987.
45. Lands, A. M., Arnold, A., McAuliff, J. P., et al. Differentiation of receptor systems activated by sympathomimetic amines. *Nature* 214:597, 1967.
46. Lardinois, C. K., and Newman, S. L. The effects of antihypertensive agents on serum lipids and lipoproteins. *Arch. Intern. Med.* 148:1280, 1988.
47. Lefkowitz, R. J., Caron, M. G., and Stiles, G. L. Mechanisms of membrane-receptor regulation: Biochemical, physiological, and clinical insights derived from studies of the adrenergic receptors. *N. Engl. J. Med.* 310:1570, 1984.
48. Lefkowitz, R. J., Cerione, R. A., Codina, J., Birnbaumer, L., and Caron, M. G. Reconstitution of the beta-adrenergic receptor. *J. Membr. Biol.* 87:1, 1985.
49. Lichstein, E., Morganroth, J., Harrist, R., and Hubble, E. Effects of propranolol on ventricular arrhythmias: The beta-blocker heart attack trial experience. *Circulation* 67(Suppl I):I-5, 1983.
50. Mahan, L. C., Motulsky, H. J., and Insel, P. A. Do agonists promote rapid internalization of beta-adrenergic receptors? *Proc. Natl. Acad. Sci. USA* 82:65–66, 1985.
51. Man In't Veld, A. J. Effect of beta blockers on vascular resistance in systemic hypertension. *Am. J. Cardiol.* 59:21F, 1987.
52. McComb, J. M., McGovern, B., McGowan, J. B., Ruskin, J. N., and Garan, H. Electrophysiologic effects of d-sotalol in humans. *J. Am. Coll. Cardiol.* 10:211, 1987.
53. McDevitt, D. G. Pharmacologic aspects of cardioselectivity in a beta-blocking drug. *Am. J. Cardiol.* 59:10F, 1987.
54. Mehta, J., Feldman, R. L., Marx, J. D., and Kelly, G. A. Systemic, pulmonary, and coronary hemodynamic effects of labetalol in hypertensive subjects. *Am. J. Med.* 75:32, 1983.
55. Miller, R. R., Olson, H. G., Amsterdam, E. A., and Mason, D. T. Propranolol-withdrawal rebound phenomenon: Exacerbation of coronary events after abrupt cessation of antianginal therapy. *N. Engl. J. Med.* 293:416, 1975.
56. Motulsky, H. J., and Insel, P. A. Adrenergic receptors in man: Direct identification, physiologic regulation, and clinical alternations. *N. Engl. J. Med.* 307:18, 1982.
57. Mukherjee, A., Bush, L. R., McCoy, K. E., et al. Relationship between beta-adrenergic receptor numbers and physiological responses during experimental canine myocardial ischemia. *Circ. Res.* 50:735, 1982.
58. Mukherjee, A., Wong, T. M., Buja, L. M., et al. Beta adrenergic and muscarinic cholinergic receptors in canine myocardium: Effects of ischemia. *J. Clin. Invest.* 64:1423, 1979.
59. Muntz, K. H., Hagler, H. K., Boulas, H. J., Willerson, J. T., and Buja, L. M. Redistribution of catecholamines in the ischemic zone of the dog heart. *Am. J. Pathol.* 114:64, 1984.
60. Muntz, K. H., Olson, E. G., Lariviere, G. R., et al. Autoradiographic characterization of beta adrenergic receptors in coronary blood vessels and myocytes in normal and ischemic myocardium of the canine heart. *J. Clin. Invest.* 73:349, 1984.
61. Murphy, M. B., Sugrue, D., Trayner, I., et al. Effects of short term beta adrenoreceptor blockade on serum lipids and lipoproteins in patients with hypertension or coronary artery disease. *Br. Heart J.* 51:589, 1984.
62. Nattel, S., Rangno, R. E., and Van Loon, G. Mechanism of propranolol withdrawal phenomena. *Circulation* 59:1158, 1979.

63. Prichard, B. N. C. Pharmacologic aspects of intrinsic sympathomimetic activity in beta-blocking drugs. *Am. J. Cardiol.* 59:13F, 1987.
64. Prida, X. E., Feldman, R. L., Hill, J. A., and Pepine, C. J. Comparison of selective (beta₁) and nonselective (beta₁ and beta₂) beta-adrenergic blockade on systemic and coronary hemodynamic findings in angina pectoris. *Am. J. Cardiol.* 60:244, 1987.
65. Purdy, R. E., and Stupecky, G. L. Bovine anterior desending coronary artery possesses a homogeneous population of beta-1 adrenergic receptors. *J. Pharmacol. Exp. Ther.* 239:634, 1986.
66. Reid, J. L., Whyte, K. F., and Struthers, A. D. Epinephrine-induced hypokalemia: The role of beta adrenoceptors. *Am. J. Cardiol.* 57:23F, 1986.
67. Rousseau, M. F., Hanet, C., Pardonge-Lavenne, E., et al. Changes in myocardial metabolism during therapy in patients with chronic stable angina: A comparison of long-term dosing with propranolol and nicardipine. *Circulation* 73:1270, 1986.
68. Ryden, L., Ariniego, R., Arnman, K., et al. A double-blind trial of metoprolol in acute myocardial infarction: Effects on ventricular tachyarrhythmias. *N. Engl. J. Med.* 308:64, 1983.
69. Shorr, R. G. L., McCaslin, D. R., Strohsacker, M. W., et al. Molecular structure of the beta-adrenergic receptor. *Biochemistry* 24:68–69, 1985.
70. Sibley, D. R., and Lefkowitz, R. J. Molecular mechanisms of receptor desensitization using the beta-adrenergic receptor-coupled adenylate cyclase system as a model. *Nature* 317:124, 1985.
71. Sibley, D. R., Strasser, R. H., Benovic, J. L., et al. Phosphorylation/dephosphorylation of the beta-adrenergic receptor regulates its functional coupling to adenylate cyclase and subcellular distribution. *Proc. Natl. Acad. Sci. USA* 83:9408, 1986.
72. Smith, V. E., White, W. B., Merran, M. K., and Karimeddini, M. K. Improved left ventricular filling accompanies reduced left ventricular mass during therapy of essential hypertension. *J. Am. Coll. Cardiol.* 8:1449, 1986.
73. Svendsen, T. L., Trap-Jensen, J., Carlsen, J. E., and McNair, A. Immediate central hemodynamic effects of five different beta-adrenoceptor-blocking agents, acebutolol, atenolol, pindolol, practolol, and propranolol, in patients with ischemic heart disease. *Am. Heart J.* 109:1145, 1985.
74. Swedberg, K., Hjalmarson, A., Waagstein, F., and Wallentin, I. Beneficial effects of long-term beta-blockade in congestive cardiomyopathy. *Br. Heart J.* 44:117, 1980.
75. Taylor, S. H. Role of cardioselectivity and intrinsic sympathomimetic activity in beta-blocking drugs in cardiovascular disease. *Am. J. Cardiol.* 59:18F, 1987.
76. Thadani, U., Davidson, C., Singleton, W., and Taylor, S. H. Comparison of the immediate effects of five beta-adrenoreceptor-blocking drugs with different ancillary properties in angina pectoris. *N. Engl. J. Med.* 300:750, 1979.
77. Vatner, D. E., Knight, D. R., Homcy, C. J., et al. Subtypes of beta-adrenergic receptors in bovine coronary arteries. *Circ. Res.* 59:463, 1986.
78. Venditti, F. J., Jr., Garan, H., and Ruskin, J. N. Electrophysiologic effects of beta blockers in ventricular arrhythmias. *Am. J. Cardiol.* 60:3D, 1987.
79. Williams, L. T., and Lefkowitz, R. J. *Receptor Binding Studies in Adrenergic Pharmacology.* New York: Raven Press, 1978.
80. Winther, K., Klysner, R., Geisler, A., and Anderson, P. H. Characterization of human platelet beta-adrenoceptors. *Thromb. Res.* 757, 1985.

81. Wit, A. L., Hoffman, B. F., and Rosen, M. R. Electrophysiology and pharmacology of cardiac arrhythmias, IX. Cardiac electrophysiologic effects of beta adrenergic receptor stimulation and blockade. Part A, B, and C. *Am. Heart J.* 90:521, 665, 795, 1975.
82. Wolfson, S., Heinle, R. A., Herman, M. V., et al. Propranolol and angina pectoris. *Am. J. Cardiol.* 18:345, 1966.

CHAPTER 5

MECHANISM OF ACTIONS OF CALCIUM ANTAGONISTS

CHARLES R. LAMBERT
CARL J. PEPINE

Calcium channel antagonists comprise a heterogeneous class of compounds that modulate physiological processes primarily by altering calcium flux through interactions with membrane elements. These compounds can be divided into five classes based on chemical derivation; however, a precise structure-activity relationship cannot be defined. Verapamil and tiapamil are papaverine derivatives, while nifedipine, nicardipine, and nimodipine are examples of dihydropyridine derivatives. Diltiazem is a benzothiazepine derivative and piperazine derivatives include lidoflazine and flunarizine. A miscellaneous category includes such compounds as bepredil and prenylamine. As one might expect, based on the chemical heterogeneity of these compounds and the lack of a definite structure-activity relationship, there is evidence that the different classes of calcium channel antagonists may act to modulate calcium flux by different mechanisms at the molecular and cellular levels. In this chapter we will consider the mechanism of actions of the various calcium channel antagonists at the receptor, organ, and system levels with particular regard to cardiovascular effects. Emphasis will be placed on consideration of these mechanisms as they apply to treatment of the patient with ischemic heart disease.

CALCIUM CHANNELS

A *calcium channel* is generally held to be a glycoprotein macromolecular structure residing in the cell membrane that is approximately cylindrical in shape with a central aqueous pore [13]. The permeation of calcium through such a channel is accomplished by several discrete steps that begin with reversible interaction at a coordination site. The basic functional characteristics of the calcium channel in this regard can be described using classical stochastic principles and kinetic theory. Within the aqueous pore of the calcium channel, there appears to be a molecular selectivity filter that confers the relative calcium specificity of the pore. This filter also sets the limit in terms of absolute ionic current flow that can be achieved by regulating the speed of passage for a given ionic species through the channel. Calcium channels seem to exist in one of three possible states: the open or activated state, the deactivated state, and the inactivated state. Calcium channels may be further subdivided by the type of stimulus that causes conversion to the activated state. In this light there are voltage-sensitive channels that activate in response to a change in transmembrane potential and receptor-sensitive channels that are activated by hormones, neurotransmitters, or drugs. Most excitable tissues in the cardiovascular system possess both types of calcium channels.

Bean and coworkers have recently utilized patch clamping techniques to describe the characteristics of calcium channels in myocardial and vascular smooth muscle cells [2, 3]. These investigations have shown that atrial myocardium contains channels for calcium current of two types. The first component of calcium current is only present if cells are held at negative potentials, is most prominent for small depolarizations, and is inactivated quickly. The second, slower component is present even at positive holding potentials, requires greater depolarizations for maximal current, and is inactivated more slowly. The latter component is sensitive to calcium blocking drugs. Findings in mesenteric vascular smooth muscle cells were similar to those in myocardium with respect to calcium channel activation.

Possible primary sites of action for calcium channel antagonists include the exterior, interior, and inner surface of the cell membrane. Numerous radioligand binding studies have been performed in order to characterize the membrane subunit with which the calcium channel antagonists interact. In general, such studies have identified two groups of membrane sites; a low-affinity high-capacity group and a high-affinity low-capacity group. Quantitation of calcium blocking drug binding to these sites and functional calcium channel blockade may or may not yield a good correlation depending on the particular study and tissue used. On the basis of binding studies, Glossmann [10] suggested that calcium antagonists could be divided into three groups based on site of action. Dihydropyridines, such as nifedipine, as well as the papaverine derivatives tiapamil and fendiline appeared to interact with the outer mouth of the membrane-bound calcium channels. Verapamil and D600 appeared to interact with the inner mouth of the calcium channels and compounds such as diltiazem appeared to have some other site of interaction. This schema is supported by the experiments of Payet and coworkers [36], who demonstrated that a hydrophilic highly polar form of D600 (D890) did not exhibit calcium blocking effects unless applied intracellularly. This was not the case for the lipophilic parent compound D600, which was able to cross the cell membrane and had effects when applied either intra- or extracellularly. These observations are consistent with the requirement for transmembrane diffusion or transport of this class of compounds to an active site on the interior of the cell membrane in order to produce calcium channel antagonism.

As noted earlier, high-affinity binding sites for dihydropyridine compounds have been described in membrane fragments by multiple investigators. Verapamil, D600, and diltiazem are several hundred times weaker than nifedipine for binding to such sites, and the binding of verapamil is not of a simple competitive type [9, 28]. In other studies, diltiazem was found to stimulate dihydropyridine binding to cardiac microsomes [7]. Such interactions between the various classes of calcium channel antagonists have led to the concept of allosterically linked receptor sites for the dihydropyridines and other agents allowing interaction and cross-modulation of calcium flux between groups of compounds with dissimilar chemical derivation [29]. This theory is especially attractive since it allows for the existence of dihydropyridine compounds that have dose-dependent calcium channel agonistic-antagonistic activity as well as compounds such as Bay 8644, which is a dihydropyridine calcium agonist. Electrophysiologic studies also suggest differences in the manner in which various calcium antagonists interact with calcium channels. The effects of nifedipine in such studies appear to be consistent with a reduction in the number of functioning calcium channels while verapamil seems to alter the kinetics of the channels [25, 32]. It has also been suggested that calcium blocking agents may simply exert their effects through a nonspecific membrane action on calcium channels similar to that of local anesthetics on sodium channels in nerve tissue [1].

Thus, calcium channel antagonists appear to have several dissimilar modes of interaction with membrane elements governing transmembrane calcium flux. As summarized by Andersson [1], these differences may be due to heterogeneity in chemical structure and physiochemical properties of the drugs, differences in structure between or distribution of calcium channels or binding sites, or differences in modes of calcium-dependent activation between tissues. This latter observation may be especially germane to consideration of calcium blockade in vascular smooth muscle where multiple calcium-dependent activational mechanisms are known to be functional. In this instance both tonic and phasic activational systems are found, the latter being highly sensitive to calcium channel antagonists and possibly important in generation of arterial spasm in vivo through generation of complex propagated constrictor activity [19].

In addition to the sites of action outlined earlier, the possibility that calcium channel antagonists may interact with intracellular calcium-dependent processes is suggested by work using sarcoplasmic reticulum and calmodulin preparations [5, 14]. Evidence also exists suggesting that calcium channel antagonists may interact with adrenergic receptors. The precise role of such interactions in the overall pharmacology of the calcium channel antagonists remains to be defined by further study.

USE-DEPENDENT CALCIUM BLOCKADE

Use dependence is a prominent feature in the action of many calcium blocking compounds on excitable cells. This phenomenon is manifested by an increasing degree of inhibition with each successive depolarization until a steady-state is reached. Use-dependent blockade occurs if an inhibitor has little or no affinity for a given ion channel in the deactivated state but will interact with the channel in the activated and/or inactivated state [12]. Use dependency may be visualized by considering that a membrane depolarization, if long enough, will allow interaction between the ion channel complex and the inhibitor that will lead to blockade for a finite period of time. With return of the membrane potential to resting conditions, dissociation of inhibitor begins. However, if a second depolarization occurs rapidly enough, some inhibitor will be retained and more will be bound during the second cycle. This process can repeat itself, leading to increasing inhibition to a point where frequency of stimulation, as well as association and dissociation of inhibitor, yield a steady-state level of inhibition. From these basic considerations, it is obvious that demonstration of use-dependent blockade is highly frequency-dependent and must also be influenced by the resting membrane potential since the state of calcium channels is dependent on the latter. With these constraints, use dependency of inhibition has been demonstrated for a number of calcium channel antagonists, most notably verapamil and diltiazem [8, 15].

UNIQUE PROPERTIES OF DIHYDROPYRIDINES

As noted earlier, the dihydropyridine calcium channel antagonists have many different pharmacologic properties when compared to the other calcium antagonists. Indeed, certain dihydropyridines have markedly different effects on calcium-dependent phenomena when compared to other agents in the same class. In contrast to verapamil and diltiazem, the dihydropyridines nifedipine, nitrendipine, and nisoldipine, among others, do not exhibit more than minimal use dependency as defined earlier [11, 16, 21]. This may be due to rapid dissociation of these compounds from their binding sites, which suggests that use-dependent inhibition might become apparent at higher frequencies. Whether this is true and, further, whether the presence or absence of use-dependent inhibition has direct clinical relevancy remains to be determined.

The unique dihydropyridine Bay 8644 enhances calcium channel current and thus behaves as a calcium agonist [45]. This effect appears to be due to prolongation of the mean open time for the calcium channel, thus increasing the percentage of the calcium channel population in the open or activated state at any given time [41]. The agonistic activity of this compound has been shown to become antagonistic at high concentrations and with high stimulation rates [40]. On the basis of these observations, it has been termed a partial agonist. Interestingly, nifedipine and nicardipine have been shown to exhibit similar, although less potent, calcium channel agonistic activity to that occurring at low doses only [45]. This may be due to a possible multiple molecule receptor complex, which, when occupied by one inhibitor molecule, promotes calcium flux, and when fully occupied by multiple molecules, inhibits it. The importance of partial or complete calcium channel agonistic activity of the various dihydropyridine compounds at the level of the intact animal or human remains to be determined.

NEUROHORMONAL INFLUENCES

As noted earlier, calcium channel activation can also be accomplished or modified by receptor-based neurohormonal influences. These effects are generally felt to be due to modulation of voltage-dependent calcium channel operation. Examples of such activity include increase of membrane depolarization-induced calcium current by excitation of beta-adrenergic receptors [17]. In contrast, activation of muscarinic cholinergic receptors decreases the magnitude of membrane depolarization-dependent calcium current [44]. The interaction of drugs or humoral agents, adrenergic receptors, and calcium channel activation is mediated via the adenylate cyclase system. Activation of this system is felt to culminate in calcium channel activation through phosphorylation of membrane proteins, which are a part of the calcium channel receptor complex [34]. Similarly, the reduction of calcium current induced by cholinergic agonists mentioned above may be related to the cyclic GMP system.

GENERAL CARDIOVASCULAR EFFECTS

Having outlined the functional characteristics of calcium channels and related activational mechanisms, we will now consider the effects calcium channel antagonists have on the cardiovascular system at the tissue and organ system level. It is generally held that all calcium channel antagonists have a negative inotropic effect on myocardial tissue. Although at most doses this is true, recent studies have demonstrated a small but definite calcium channel agonistic effect of certain dihydropyridines in vitro [45]. This agonistic effect can be manifested as a small increase in left ventricular contractility seen at low doses of drug. Possible mechanisms for such an effect have been mentioned in the preceding section. It is not known whether such an effect can be demonstrated in humans or whether it has any clinical importance. Studies in which calcium channel antagonists are given by the intravenous, buccal, or oral routes may be difficult to interpret with regard to effects on myocardial function due to reflex sympathetic mechanisms and alterations in loading. This is especially true with dihydropyridines, which are potent peripheral vasodilators. In terms of in vitro studies on currently available calcium channel antagonists, the most potent negative inotropic influence is exerted by nifedipine, which is followed by verapamil and diltiazem. Studies using unsedated, instrumented animals and intracoronary infusion of calcium channel antagonists offer the best data for comparison of in vivo myocardial depression. Walsh and coworkers found dose-related myocardial depression with intracoronary administration of calcium channel antagonists that was greatest with nifedipine and least with diltiazem [47]. Nakaya and coworkers similarly found diltiazem least and verapamil most depressant. However, they noted a small positive inotropic response to nifedipine [30]. Whether this was due to differences in measurement times and relative sympathetic reflexes or possibly to the calcium channel agonism that has been shown in vitro for low-dose nifedipine [45] is not clear.

In general, myocardial depression is not a problem with clinical use of calcium channel antagonists since ventricular afterload reduction and/or reflex sympathetic tone serve to offset this effect in the absence of overt heart failure. However, great interpatient variability in this regard can be anticipated and myocardial depression can be abrupt and profound with administration of calcium channel antagonists. This subject will be discussed in more detail elsewhere in this volume.

The effects of calcium channel antagonists on systemic and coronary blood flow as well as blood pressure are all a manifestation of vascular smooth muscle contractile inhibition. Just as for depression of myocardial contraction, nifedipine is the most potent of the available agents in this regard, followed by diltiazem and verapamil. Animal studies suggest that nifedipine dilates all vascular beds to a similar degree while diltiazem may have some coronary specificity in this regard [31]. In humans, an effective increase in coronary blood flow out of proportion to peripheral vasodilator action is difficult to demonstrate with direct measurement techniques for any of the clinically available agents. Relative coronary selectivity with regard to vasodilation has, however, been demonstrated with newer calcium channel antagonists such as nicardipine in humans [20]. The vasodilator potency of the various calcium channel antagonists in humans appears to parallel results of studies in animals as noted earlier.

The mechanisms by which calcium channel antagonists influence exercise-related hemodynamic changes appear, in general, to be similar in both human and animal models. These alterations have been described in a study by Cleary and coworkers in instrumented dogs [4]. Intravenous administration of equihypotensive doses of verapamil, nifedipine, and diltiazem was carried out before and after beta blockade with propranolol. None of the agents altered the heart rate response to exercise before beta blockade. Verapamil administration was associated with a slight increase in preload and decrease in contractile state while nifedipine and diltiazem had no net effect with regard to these variables. After beta blockade, both diltiazem and verapamil attenuated the heart rate response to exercise and all agents decreased the contractile response to exercise. Although most human studies offer similar findings with regard to exercise hemodynamics, a radionuclide angiocardiographic study of left ventricular function in normal men showed no depression of left ventricular function at rest or with exercise during administration of intravenous verapamil [6]. Further discussion of calcium channel antagonists and exercise hemodynamics in patients with myocardial ischemia is included later in this volume.

EFFECTS ON DIASTOLIC VENTRICULAR FUNCTION

Since the kinetics of activator calcium sequestration and myofilament interaction dictates the physiology of ventricular relaxation, it would be expected that calcium channel antagonists might influence diastolic ventricular function. Just as for ventricular systolic function, it is often difficult to sort out direct versus afterload or reflex-mediated changes in diastolic function in studies where calcium channel antagonists are administered by other than the intracoronary route. In order to circumvent these problems, Walsh and O'Rourke studied awake, instrumented dogs during administration of equihypotensive doses of calcium channel antagonists [46]. Diastolic function was monitored by calculating the time constant for isovolumic relaxation during the various infusions. When studied in this manner, equidepressant doses of nifedipine, verapamil, and diltiazem impaired relaxation to a similar degree when given by the intracoronary route. In contrast, when administered intravenously in equihypotensive doses, nifedipine improved relaxation while verapamil and diltiazem exerted no effect. After beta blockade, intravenous infusion of nifedipine produced no augmentation of relaxation, suggesting that the previously noted improvement was reflexly mediated. The combination of intravenous verapamil and beta-adrenergic blockade impaired relaxation. Thus the direct effects of calcium channel antagonists on diastolic function appear to parallel their negative inotropic effect (i.e., to impair relaxation). This effect may be altered, however, by reflex sympathetic responses as well as by altered loading produced by peripheral vasodilation.

It should be noted that these experiments reflect the direct and indirect effects of calcium channel antagonists on diastolic processes in normal hearts. In pathological conditions where relaxation is impaired or altered in some way, these agents may exert different effects. Ventricular diastolic pathophysiology is especially complex in patients with coronary artery disease where regional contraction and relaxation abnormalities occur [37]. Although diastolic function may be improved in patients with coronary artery disease after sublingual administration of nifedipine [23], intracoronary administration impairs relaxation and produces a negative inotropic effect [38]. These observations again emphasize the importance of taking load-dependent and reflexly mediated phenomena into account when considering studies of systolic or diastolic contractile function during calcium channel antagonist administration.

The influences of different calcium channel antagonists on diastolic function in other cardiovascular disorders also appear to be variable. Sublingual nifedipine has been shown to affect diastolic function favorably in patients with hypertrophic cardiomyopathy without evidence of any depression of systolic function [22]. In contrast, acute administration of verapamil in patients with hypertrophic cardiomyopathy did not improve left ventricular relaxation, as evidenced by prolongation of the time constant for isovolumetric relaxation [43].

ELECTROPHYSIOLOGIC EFFECTS

Although all calcium channel antagonists have electrophysiologic effects mediated by mechanisms described earlier in this chapter, the net effects seen in vivo reflect a composite of direct drug action and reflex- or load-dependent phenomena as outlined earlier. The primary mechanism by which calcium channel antagonists exert their electrophysiologic effects is by altering the kinetics of the slow calcium current in excitable tissues. Since the tissues most dependent on the slow calcium current for normal activity are the sinoatrial and atrioventricular nodes, these regions are most affected by calcium channel blockade. Effects of calcium channel antagonists on these tissues are manifested by a decrease in the rate of sinoatrial discharge and an increase in the conduction time through the atrioventricular (AV) node. The effects are readily demonstrated by intracoronary injection of the various calcium channel antagonists in vivo or in situ [18] and can also be assessed using a variety of in vitro preparations [33]. When studied in such preparations, the available compounds appear to be of similar potency in suppressing calcium-dependent action potential activity.

As noted earlier, in vivo electrophysiologic effects of the various agents are greatly modified by reflex influences just as are the hemodynamic and mechanical effects discussed earlier. Administration of either verapamil, nifedipine, or diltiazem to animals with intact autonomic reflexes produces a relative tachycardia [27, 30, 47]. In contrast, acute administration of verapamil to humans produces a variable change, diltiazem produces a slight decrease, and nifedipine an increase in heart rate [27]. Calcium channel antagonists have little effect on sinus node recovery time or sinoatrial conduction time in humans unless there is preexisting sinus node disease. In this latter circumstance, verapamil and diltiazem prolong these parameters while nifedipine has little net effect [24].

Studies of atrioventricular nodal function in humans reveal that verapamil and diltiazem both prolong the A-H interval modestly in clinical doses while nifedipine shortens it secondary to reflex sympathetic influences [39, 42, 48]. Both verapamil and diltiazem prolong the effective and functional refractory periods of the AV node in humans, the former to a greater degree [39, 42, 48]. As might be expected, nifedipine has opposite effects on AV nodal refractoriness [35]. In general, calcium channel antagonists do not cause significant effects on fast channel-dependent electrophysiologic processes in vivo. Thus, changes in H-V conduction or in the surface electrocardiographic QRS complex are not seen in humans. Clinical implications with regard to the electrophys-

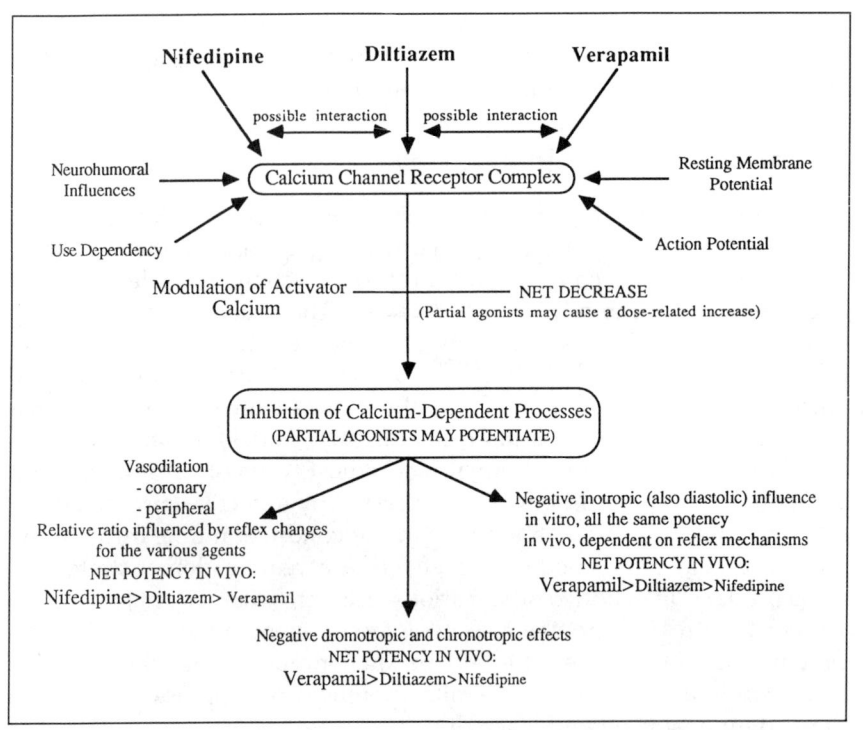

FIG. 5-1. A schematic representation of mechanisms and interactions operant in cardiovascular actions of calcium antagonists. Net potencies in vivo are estimated from data in humans with intact sympathetic reflexes.

iologic properties of calcium channel antagonists will be covered elsewhere in this volume.

CONCLUSIONS

Calcium channel antagonists are a heterogeneous class of compounds from both the chemical and pharmacologic standpoint. Although a final common pathway for drug action is modulation of cellular activator calcium, this may occur by a variety of mechanisms. These mechanisms may involve different types of calcium-receptor complexes, intracellular processes, and a variety of other activational systems that function in striated and smooth muscle as well as specialized conduction tissues. In addition, the net effects of calcium channel antagonists in vivo may be dramatically altered by reflex and possibly direct interactions with the sympathetic nervous system. Manifestations of calcium channel blockade on cardiovascular function with regard to the three of the agents available currently in the United States are illustrated in Figure 5-1.

The goals of treatment with the various calcium channel antagonists in the patient with cardiovascular disease must be considered in light of their complex pharmacology and diverse mechanisms of action in order to derive maximum therapeutic benefit.

REFERENCES

1. Andersson, K. E. Calcium entry blockers. A heterogeneous family of compounds. *Acta Med. Scand.* 694:142, 1984.
2. Bean, B. P. Two kinds of calcium channels in canine atrial cells. *J. Gen. Physiol.* 86:1, 1985.
3. Bean, B. P., et al. Calcium channels in muscle cells isolated from rat mesenteric arteries: Modulation by dihydropyridine drugs. *Circ. Res.* 59:229, 1986.
4. Cleary, F., Walsh, R. A., and O'Rourke, R. A. Relative effects of calcium antagonists on exercise hemodynamics in dogs. *Circulation* 107-II:235, 1984.
5. Colvin, R. A., Pearson, N., and Messineo, F. C. Effects of calcium channel blockers on calcium transport and Ca-ATPase in skeletal and cardiac sarcoplasmic reticulum vesicles. *J. Cardiovasc. Pharmacol.* 4:935, 1982.
6. D'Agostino, H. J., et al. Effect of verapamil on left ventricular function at rest and during exercise in normal men. *J. Cardiovasc. Pharmacol.* 5:812, 1983.
7. Depover, A., Matlib, M. A., and Lee, S. W. Specific binding of ^{3}H nitrendipine to membranes from coronary arteries and heart in relation to pharmacological effects. Paradoxical stimulation by diltiazem. *Biochem. Biophys. Res. Commun.* 108:110, 1982.
8. Ehara, T., and Kaufmann, R. The voltage and time dependent effects of (−I)-verapamil on the slow inward current in isolated cat ventricular myocardium. *J. Pharmacol. Exp. Therap.* 207:49, 1978.
9. Ehlert, F. J., et al. The interaction of ^{3}H nitrendipine with receptors for calcium antagonists in the cerebral cortex and heart of rats. *Biochem. Biophys. Res. Commun.* 104:937, 1982.
10. Glossmann, H., et al. Identification of voltage operated calcium channels by binding studies: Differentiation of subclasses of calcium antagonist drugs with ^{3}H-nimodipine radioligand binding. *J. Recep. Res.* 3:177, 1983.
11. Hachisu, M., and Pappano, A. J. A comparative study of the blockade of calcium dependent action potentials by verapamil, nifedipine, and nimodipine in ventricular muscle. *J. Pharmacol. Exp. Ther.* 225:112, 1983.
12. Hondeghem, L. M., and Katzung, B. G. Antiarrhythmic agents: The modulated receptor mechanism of action of sodium and calcium channel-blocking drugs. *Ann. Rev. Pharmacol.* 24:387, 1984.
13. Hurwitz, L. Pharmacology of calcium channels and smooth muscle. *Ann. Rev. Pharmacol.* 26:225, 1986.
14. Johnson, J. D., Vaghy, P. L., and Crouch, T. An hypothesis for the mechanism of action of some of the calcium antagonist drugs: Calcodulin as a receptor. *Adv. Pharmacol. Chemother.* 3:121, 1982.
15. Kanaya, S., et al. Diltiazem and verapamil preferentially block inactivated calcium channels. *J. Mol. Cell Cardiol.* 15:145, 1983.
16. Kass, R. S. Nisoldipine: A new, more selective, calcium current blocker in cardiac Purkinje fibers. *J. Pharmacol. Exp. Ther.* 223:446, 1982.
17. Kass, R. S., and Wiegers, S. E. Ionic basis of concentration related effects of neoadrenalin on the action potential of cardiac Purkinje fibers. *J. Physiol.* 322:541, 1982.

18. Kawai, C., Konishi, T., and Matsuyama, E. Comparative effects of three calcium antagonists, diltiazem, verapamil, and nifedipine, on the sinoatrial and atrioventricular nodes: Experimental and clinical studies. *Circulation* 63:1035, 1981.
19. Lambert, C. R., and Pepine, C. J. Tetraethylammonium-induced phasic arterial constriction: Temporal and spatial characteristics. *Am. J. Physiol.* 251:H436, 1986.
20. Lambert, C. R., et al. Effects of nicardipine on left ventricular function and energetics in man. *Int. J. Cardiol.* 10:237, 1986.
21. Lee, K. S., and Tsien, R. W. Mechanism of channel blockade by verapamil, D600, diltiazem and nitrendipine in single dialysed heart cells. *Nature* 302:790, 1983.
22. Lorell, B. H., et al. Modification of abnormal left ventricular diastolic properties by nifedipine in patients with hypertrophic cardiomyopathy. *Circulation* 65:499, 1982.
23. Ludbrook, P. A., et al. Acute hemodynamic responses to sublingual nifedipine: Dependence on left ventricular function. *Circulation* 65:489, 1982.
24. McCall, D., et al. Calcium entry blocking drugs: Mechanisms of action, experimental studies and clinical uses. *Curr. Prob. Cardiol.* 10:1, 1985.
25. McDonald, T. F., Pelzer, D., and Trautwein, W. On the mechanisms of slow calcium channel block in heart. *Pfluegers Arch.* 385:175, 1980.
26. Millard, R. W., Lathrop, D. A., and Grupp, G. Differential cardiovascular effects of calcium channel blocking agents: Potential mechanisms. *Am. J. Cardiol.* 49:499, 1982.
27. Mitchell, B. L., Schroeder, J. S., and Mason, J. W. Comparative clinical electrophysiologic effects of diltiazem, verapamil and nifedipine: A review. *Am. J. Cardiol.* 49:629, 1982.
28. Murphy, K. M. M., and Snyder, S. H. Calcium antagonist receptor binding sites labelled with ^{3}H nitrendipine. *Eur. J. Pharmacol.* 77:201, 1982.
29. Murphy, K. M. M., et al. A unitary mechanism of calcium antagonist drug action. *Proc. Nat. Acad. Sci.* 80:860, 1983.
30. Nakaya, H., Schwartz, A., and Millard, R. W. Reflex chronotropic and inotropic effects of calcium channel blocking agents in conscious dogs: diltiazem, verapamil, and nifedipine compared. *Circ. Res.* 52:302, 1983.
31. Nago, T., Sato, M., and Nakajina, H. Studies on a new 1,5-benzothiazepine derivative (CRD-401): II Vasodilator actions. *Jap. J. Pharmacol.* 22:1, 1972.
32. Nawrath, H., et al. On the mechanisms underlying the action of D600 on slow inward current and tension in mammalian myocardium. *Circ. Res.* 40:408, 1977.
33. Okada, T., and Konishi, T. Effects of verapamil and SA and AV nodal action potentials in the isolated rabbit heart. *Jap. Circ. J.* 39:913, 1975.
34. Osterrieder, W., et al. Injection of subunits of cyclic AMP-dependent protein kinase into cardiac myocytes modulates Ca current. *Nature* 298:576, 1982.
35. Padeletti, L., Franchi, F., and Brat, A. The cardiac electrophysiological effects of nifedipine. *Int. J. Clin. Pharmacol. Ther. Toxicol.* 17:290, 1979.
36. Payet, M. D., et al. Inhibitory activity of blockers of the slow inward current in rat myocardium, a study in steady state and rate of action. *J. Mol. Cell. Cardiol.* 12:187, 1980.
37. Pouleur, H., et al. Assessment of regional left ventricular relaxation in patients with coronary artery disease: Importance of geometric factors and changes in wall thickness. *Circulation* 69:696, 1984.
38. Rousseau, M. F., et al. Impaired early left ventricular relaxation in coronary artery disease: Effects of intracoronary nifedipine. *Circulation* 62:764, 1980.

39. Rowland, E., Evans, T., and Krikler, D. Effect of nifedipine on atrioventricular conduction as compared with verapamil: Intracardiac electrophysiologic study. *Br. Heart J.* 42:124, 1979.
40. Sanguinetti, M. C., and Kass, R. S. Voltage selects activity of the calcium channel modulator Bay K8644. *Biophys. J.* 47:513a, 1985.
41. Schramm, M., et al. Novel dihydropyridines with positive inotropic action through activation of calcium channels. *Nature* 303:535, 1983.
42. Sugimoto, T., Ishikawa, T., and Kaseno, K. Electrophysiologic effects of diltiazem, a calcium antagonist, in patients with impaired sinus or atrioventricular node function. *Angiology* 31:700, 1980.
43. TenCate, F., et al. Effects of short term administration of verapamil on left ventricular relaxation and filling dynamics measured by a combined hemodynamic ultrasonic technique in patients with hypertrophic cardiomyopathy. *Circulation* 68:1274, 1983.
44. TenEick, R., et al. On the mechanism of the negative inotropic effect of acetylcholine. *J. Physiol.* 361:207, 1976.
45. Thomas, G., Grob, R., and Schramm, M. Calcium channel modulation: Ability to inhibit or promote calcium influx resides in the same dihydropyridine molecules. *J. Cardiovasc. Pharmacol.* 6:1170, 1984.
46. Walsh, R. A., and O'Rourke, R. A. Direct and indirect effects of calcium entry blocking agents on isovolumic relaxation in conscious dogs. *J. Clin. Invest.* 75:1426, 1985.
47. Walsh, R. A., Badke, F. R., and O'Rourke, R. A. Differential effects of systemic and intracoronary calcium channel blocking agents on global and regional left ventricular function in conscious dogs. *Am. Heart J.* 102:341, 1981.
48. Wellens, H. J. J., Tan, S. L., and Bar, F. W. H. Effect of verapamil studied by programmed electrical stimulation of the heart in patients with paroxysmal re-entrant supraventricular tachycardia. *Br. Heart J.* 39:1058, 1977.

CHAPTER 6

PHARMACOLOGY AND PHARMACOKINETICS OF NITRATES

ELIZABETH KOWALUK
HO-LEUNG FUNG

The nitrates are a group of powerful vasodilators that have been found useful in treating ischemic heart disease. The most well-known member of this group of compounds is nitroglycerin, which was first introduced into clinical use by Murrell in 1879 [82]. Now, more than one hundred years later, the popularity of this drug (and its chemical family) has increased considerably. Yet, the mechanisms of action and the problems associated with the therapeutic use of these drugs still remain largely unresolved. Important questions about the optimal mode and rate of administration are still unanswered. The eventual solution of these uncertainties requires a comprehensive and integrated understanding of the physiologic, biochemical, pharmacokinetic, and pharmacodynamic aspects of these compounds. It is the purpose of this chapter to examine the biochemical pharmacology and pharmacokinetics of these drugs and to determine how these phenomena might relate to nitrate therapy now and possibly in the future. The physiological components of nitrate action are discussed in Chapter 3.

There are three major nitrates in clinical use today: nitroglycerin, isosorbide dinitrate (ISDN), and isosorbide-5-mononitrate (5-ISMN). The last compound has not yet been approved for use in the United States but it has been widely used in Europe. Two other compounds, molsidomine and nicorandil, exert a spectrum of pharmacologic activity similar to that of nitrates. However, neither of these compounds has been approved in this country. The structures of these vasodilators are shown in Figure 6-1.

BIOCHEMICAL MECHANISM OF NITRATE ACTION

Metabolic Activation to Nitric Oxide

The nitrate esters have been termed direct-acting vasodilators, in that they are thought to elicit their effects by a direct action on the vasculature, not through neuroendocrine interactions. The mechanism of nitrate-induced vasodilation is not clearly understood. However, current hypotheses of nitrate action require vascular metabolism of nitrate either prior to or as a result of vasodilation. These views are consistent with the known nitrate metabolizing activity of the vasculature [41] and the recent finding that nitroglycerin biotransformation to the dinitrometabolites occurs concurrently with relaxation of rabbit aortic strips [18].

Needleman and Johnson [84] first suggested that denitration of the nitrate might accompany vascular relaxation and proposed a critical role for intracellular sulfhydryl groups in this process. They had found that

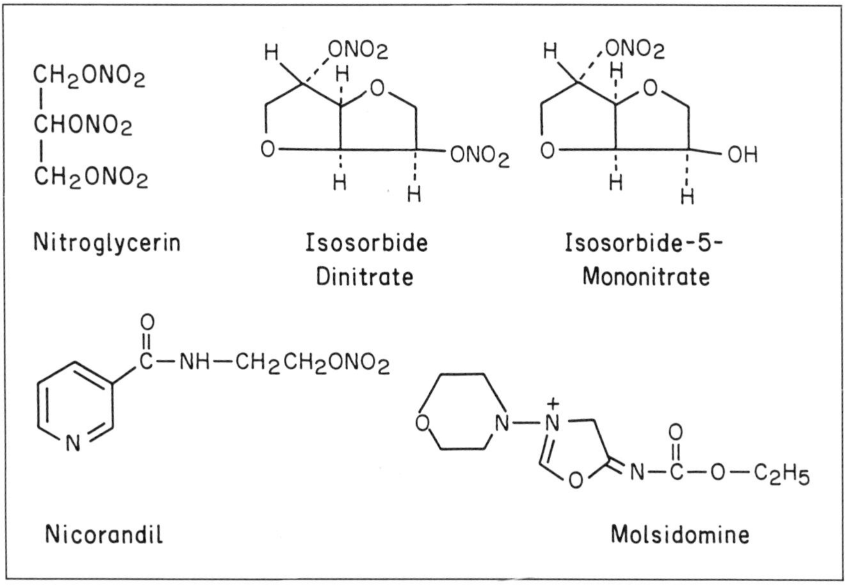

FIG. 6-1. Chemical structures of selected nitrovasodilators.

tissue sulfhydryl groups decreased upon induction of vascular tolerance to the effects of nitroglycerin and that tolerance was reversed by treating the tissue with dithiothreitol, a sulfhydryl reducing agent. Needleman and coworkers also reported that the sulfhydryl alkylating agent ethacrynic acid reduced nitroglycerin-induced relaxation in vascular smooth muscle [83]. Such findings were consistent with their proposed hypothesis that the nitrate reacted with a critical sulfhydryl group associated with a nitrate receptor in the vascular smooth muscle cell. Relaxation ensued as a consequence of this reaction, accompanied by denitration of the nitrate and oxidation of the receptor to the disulfide form.

More recent investigations suggest that nitrates are first converted intracellularly to nitric oxide and/or a chemically related intermediate, which activates the enzyme guanylate cyclase, catalyzing cyclic GMP formation and causing vascular relaxation. The evidence for the involvement of cyclic GMP in nitrate-induced vascular relaxation is strong: elevated cyclic GMP levels in vascular smooth muscle are seen after nitrate exposure [9, 27, 44, 48, 60, 67] and the extent and time-course of cyclic GMP formation correlate closely with relaxation [7]. In addition, both relaxation and cyclic GMP formation are inhibited by the oxidant methylene blue, an antagonist of guanylate cyclase activation [44, 48, 60].

Experiments with cell-free preparations of guanylate cyclase from various tissues revealed that nitrate activation of the enzyme is tissue-specific and occurs only poorly, if at all, without the presence of thiols [53, 55, 59]. These findings suggest that nitrates may require conversion to a more active species in order to activate guanylate cyclase and stimulate cyclic GMP formation [53]. That nitric oxide may be the reactive intermediate was originally proposed by Murad and coworkers [59, 81]. In early studies of the role of cyclic GMP in smooth muscle function, these authors and others [6, 26, 102] found that, in addition to nitroglycerin, several other agents capable of forming or releasing nitric oxide under appropriate conditions also activated guanylate cyclase and elevated cyclic GMP levels in tissue incubations. These included sodium nitroprusside, sodium nitrite, azide, hydroxylamine, certain nitrosamines, tobacco smoke, and nitric oxide gas itself. Subsequent studies showed that, like nitrates, several of these agents cause vascular relaxation due to accumulation of tissue cyclic GMP [47, 48]. As a consequence of the postulated common role of nitric oxide in the action of these agents, this class of compounds has been termed *nitrogen oxide-containing vasodilators* [54] or *nitrovasodilators* [80].

The common intermediary role of nitric oxide in nitrovasodilator-induced relaxation is further supported by data showing that certain hemoproteins and the oxidants methylene blue and ferricyanide inhibit activation of cell-free guanylate cyclase by these agents [47, 48]. Interestingly, these antagonists were found to have varying inhibitory effects in intact arterial strips [47, 48]: thus, the relaxant effects of all nitrovasodilators were blocked by methylene blue, which readily permeates the vascular smooth muscle cell, but not by ferricyanide, which remains in the extracellular space. In addition, methemoglobin, which binds nitric oxide avidly but cannot penetrate into the intracellular space, abolished the relaxation elicited by exogenously applied nitric oxide but not by the other nitrovasodilators. These observations suggest that the nitrovasodilators examined release or form nitric oxide intracellularly [47, 54].

That organic nitrates enter the vascular smooth muscle cell to liberate nitric oxide intracellularly seems reasonable in view of their relative lipophilic nature. Indeed, the hemodynamic potency of a series of nitrates, determined using an isolated heart preparation, has been shown to correlate well with the degree of lipophilicity of the compounds [85]. In contrast, nitroprusside seems less likely to permeate readily into the cell since it is a large divalent anion. However, the nitric oxide (NO) group may confer sufficient lipophilicity upon the molecule to permit passive diffusion into the cell. Alternatively, nitroprusside may spontaneously release nitric oxide near the cell membrane, enabling rapid movement of nitric oxide into the cell [55].

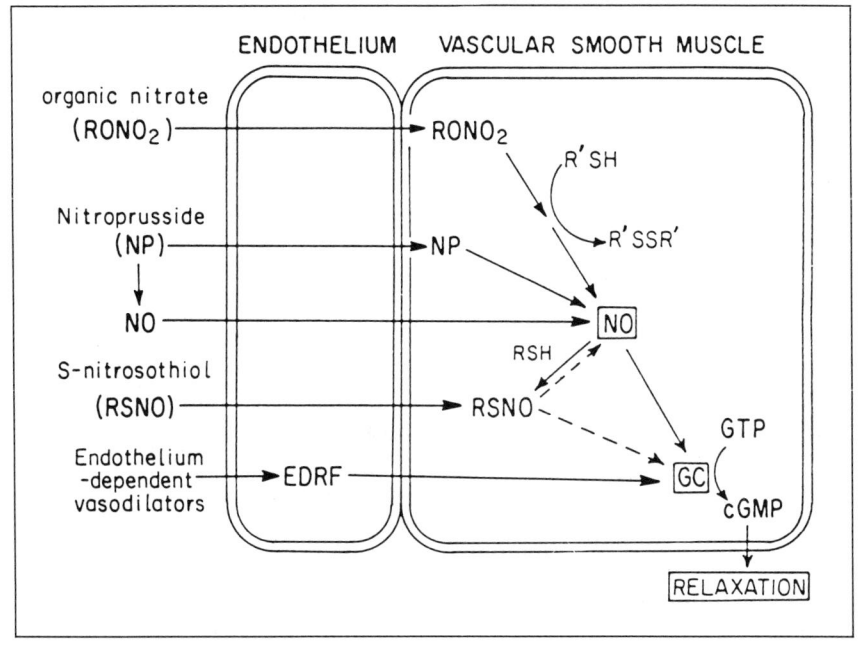

FIG. 6-2. Proposed mechanisms by which nitrovasodilators and endothelium-dependent vasodilators relax vascular smooth muscle. Abbreviations: NO, nitric oxide; EDRF, endothelium-derived relaxing factor; R'SH and RSH, two distinct pools of intracellular sulfhydrl groups; R'SSR', disulfide groups; GC, guanylate cyclase. (Adapted from Refs. 52 and 73.)

Role of S-Nitrosothiols as Obligatory Intermediates

The precise nature of the intermediary role of nitric oxide and the mechanisms by which nitrates and other nitrovasodilators generate nitric oxide are not clearly understood. Studies to evaluate the activation of unpurified soluble guanylate cyclase from coronary artery by nitrovasodilators revealed that enzyme activation either requires or is enhanced by the addition of certain exogenous thiols [53]. On the basis of these observations and reports that thiols react with nitric oxide to form S-nitrosothiols [101], Ignarro and coworkers [53, 55] suggested that S-nitrosothiols may be active intermediates for nitrovasodilator-induced relaxation. They proposed that nitric oxide was formed within the vascular smooth muscle cell by a sulfhydryl-dependent process (from nitrates) or spontaneously (from sodium nitroprusside). The nitric oxide then reacts with intracellular sulfhydryl groups to form the S-nitrosothiol, which, in turn, activates guanylate cyclase, catalyzing cyclic GMP formation (Fig. 6-2). In support of the S-nitrosothiol hypothesis, Ignarro and coworkers [53, 55] showed that: (1) the nitrovasodilators react with cysteine to form S-nitrosocysteine; (2) S-nitrosothiols are potent activators of guanylate cyclase (without further thiol additions); (3) S-nitrosothiols mimic the hemodynamic, vasodilator, and cyclic GMP-elevating effects of nitroglycerin and nitroprusside; and (4) these effects of S-nitrosothiols are blocked by methylene blue. Further, the unstable nature of S-nitrosothiols is consistent with the short duration of action of nitrates. The role for sulfhydryl groups embodied in the S-nitrosothiol hypothesis of nitrate action is consistent with the critical role of sulfhydryl groups in nitroglycerin-induced relaxation originally proposed by Needleman and coworkers [83, 84].

While the S-nitrosothiol hypothesis is an attractive one and has provided a useful framework for the further understanding of the mechanism of nitrate action, the role of S-nitrosothiols as obligatory intermediates is uncertain. S-nitrosothiols are unstable in solution and degrade to form nitric oxide [101, 112]. Recently, Craven and DeRubertis [23] showed that solutions containing completely degraded S-nitrosocysteine could stimulate guanylate cyclase, raising the possibility that S-nitrosothiols are not the proximate species responsible for enzyme activation. They and others [52] have found that guanylate cyclase activation by nitroso compounds is mediated by the formation of a nitrosyl-heme complex with enzyme-bound heme, suggesting that nitric oxide is the proximate species. Thus, in common with other nitrovasodilators, S-nitrosothiols may exert their activity via the generation of nitric oxide.

In addition to sulfhydryl compounds, intracellular heme and perhaps other cellular constituents (which remain to be identified) may be involved in interactions with nitrates to form nitric oxide. Bennett and coworkers [11] showed that nitroglycerin can be converted to its dinitrometabolites through an interaction with reduced hemoglobin and postulated that a direct interaction of nitroglycerin with guanylate cyclase–bound heme may lead to the formation of nitric oxide or a nitrosyl intermediate [18]. More recently, Chung and Fung [21] have investigated the generation of nitric oxide by various subcellular fractions of the bovine cardiac circumflex artery incubated with nitroglycerin. Nitric oxide–generating activity appeared to be well correlated with the activities of marker enzymes of the plasma membrane but not with those of the endoplasmic reticulum, mitochondria, and cytosol. Thus, the metabolic activation of nitrates may be catalyzed by an enzyme(s) located in the plasma membrane of the vascular smooth muscle cell.

Nitrates and the Endothelium-derived Relaxing Factor

Recent evidence suggests that the nitrovasodilators may represent prodrugs of an endogenous endothelium-dependent relaxing factor

(EDRF), which is released from the vascular endothelium in response to acetylcholine, the calcium ionophore A23187, and various other chemical and physical stimuli [42, 72, 110] (Fig. 6-2). Like nitrovasodilators, EDRF-mediated relaxation responses are associated with accumulation of cyclic GMP in vascular smooth muscle [97]. The effects of both nitrovasodilators and endothelium-dependent vasodilators are inhibited by similar agents, such as hemoglobin and methylene blue [66]. In addition, the cascade of events distal to cyclic GMP synthesis appears to be identical for both classes of vasodilators [80]. The many observations of close similarities in chemical and pharmacologic properties between nitrovasodilators, nitric oxide, and endothelium-dependent vasodilators have culminated in the recent identification of at least one of the endothelium-derived relaxing factors as nitric oxide [51, 91].

Nitrates and Prostaglandins

Although much attention has been focused on cyclic GMP as the mediator of nitrate-induced vascular relaxation, several reports have also suggested that the release of vasoactive prostaglandins may, in part, be responsible for the pharmacologic actions of nitrovasodilators. Nitroglycerin, at therapeutically relevant concentrations, was shown to cause release of prostacyclins from cultured human endothelial cells [65] and isolated bovine coronary arteries [100]. During intravenous infusion of nitroglycerin to anesthetized open-chest dogs, the expected fall in systemic blood pressure and coronary vascular resistance was found to be accompanied by increased myocardial prostaglandin production [73]. These effects were attenuated by indomethacin, an inhibitor of prostaglandin synthesis. On the other hand, several studies have demonstrated that local prostaglandin release is not important in mediating the effects of nitrates in specific vascular beds. Thus, indomethacin and other inhibitors of prostaglandin synthesis do not alter responses to nitrovasodilators in the coronary circulation of open-chest dogs [92], in certain feline and canine peripheral vascular beds [29, 57], in isolated rabbit mesenteric and celiac rings [12], or in the human coronary circulation [105]. Thus, at present, the prostaglandin system does not appear to be responsible for the vascular actions of nitrates, although this remains controversial.

PHARMACOKINETICS OF NITRATES

Pharmacokinetics has been described as "the study of the time course of drug absorption, distribution, metabolism and excretion" and, further, as concerning "the relationship of these processes to the intensity and time course of pharmacologic (therapeutic and toxicologic) effects

TABLE 6-1. *Summary of Pharmacokinetic Parameters of Nitroglycerin, Isosorbide Dinitrate, Isosorbide-5-Mononitrate in Humans After Intravenous Dosing*

	Nitroglycerin	ISDN	5-ISMN
Intravenous Administration			
$t_{1/2}$(min) α	3	10	276
β		65	
Venous clearance (ℓ/min)	50	4	0.1
Apparent V_d (ℓ/kg)	3	4	0.6
Arteriovenous extraction	60%	Small	Not known
Estimated Bioavailability (%)			
Sublingual	2–100	31–59	Low
Oral	0	20–25	100%
Transdermal	75	10–30	Low

of drugs" [46]. In this context, it should be stated at the outset that the relationships between plasma concentrations of nitrates and their therapeutic action are extremely complex and that no clear-cut therapeutic concentration ranges have been established for these compounds. However, it is clear that plasma nitrate concentration reflects the rates and extents of drug absorption, distribution, and elimination in the body. These pharmacokinetic processes undoubtedly play a role (although not exclusively so) in governing the pharmacologic activities of nitrates. A thorough understanding of the pharmacokinetic properties of the nitrates appears to be essential if optimization of nitrate therapy can eventually be successfully implemented. It is not our intent here to provide a comprehensive review of all the pharmacokinetic data that have been published for nitrates. Several recent publications might have already answered this need [2, 15, 16, 24, 30, 31].

Although nitroglycerin, ISDN, and 5-ISMN are similar in terms of their mode and scope of cardiovascular action, their pharmacokinetic properties are different from one another. A summary of their basic characteristics is presented in Table 6-1. As was pointed out elsewhere [33], the observed plasma concentrations of nitrates in patients are dependent not only on the intrinsic pharmacokinetic properties of the parent drug but also on a number of coexisting factors. These include, for example, the route of drug administration and the pharmaceutical dosage form used, the presence of different disease states, food ingestion, and possible pharmacokinetic interaction with other drugs. These interactive factors must be taken into consideration when interpreting pharmacokinetic data for nitrates.

Pharmacokinetics of Nitroglycerin

INTRAVENOUS ADMINISTRATION

The most outstanding pharmacokinetic feature of nitroglycerin is its very large systemic clearance, which is contributed by rapid elimination and extensive tissue distribution (Table 6-1). Upon intravenous infusion of therapeutic doses, nitroglycerin rapidly reaches steady-state in the plasma, but the observed concentrations normally only reach the nanogram/ml range. This low concentration level makes quantitative analysis extremely difficult; it is only in the last decade that plasma nitroglycerin concentrations in humans could be reliably determined. Several methodological problems arising from the physicochemical and biochemical properties of nitroglycerin further complicate the estimation and interpretation of its plasma concentrations. Nitroglycerin is rapidly degraded by red blood cells (half-life of several minutes, depending on the concentration), thus immediate separation of nitroglycerin from the erythrocytes is essential if in vivo plasma concentrations are to be obtained. Nitroglycerin is highly adsorptive to plastics, and drug loss to infusion bags and delivery sets can reduce the dose administered significantly [69]. The high volatility of nitroglycerin often leads to substantial lowering of drug content in sublingual tablets, causing uncertainties in the dose administered.

A direct consequence of the rapid clearance of nitroglycerin is the high intra- and intersubject variability in the plasma concentrations observed for this drug. It is not unusual to observe a change of severalfold in magnitude in the (presumed) venous steady-state concentrations of nitroglycerin after intravenous and transdermal administration in humans [70, 93]. Part of the reason for this variability derives from the low fractional presence of nitroglycerin in the plasma compartment: it has been estimated that only 1 percent of the total body load of nitroglycerin exists in plasma [70]. Thus, if tissue binding decreases from 99 to 98 percent of total body load (a small change), the corresponding change in the systemic circulation would be from 1 to 2 percent of total body load (a twofold increase). It is, therefore, not surprising to see that plasma nitroglycerin concentrations are highly variable and that they might even increase paradoxically after termination of intravenous infusion [70].

The venous plasma clearance of nitroglycerin in humans has been variably reported to be between 10 to 50 liters/min [16], which far exceeds the normal liver blood flow and even cardiac output. This result is difficult to reconcile with an earlier belief that intravenously introduced nitroglycerin is predominantly metabolized by the liver [64]. In this regard, a recent study showed that rats with portal-systemic shunts exhibited essentially the same systemic clearance as sham-operated controls [14], indicating that intravenously administered nitroglycerin is primarily cleared by extrahepatic tissues. As was pointed out earlier, recent data have appeared documenting the presence of vascular metabolism of nitrates [18, 41]. This vascular metabolism appears not only important for the initiation of the vasodilator action of nitroglycerin but also in explaining its vast systemic clearance.

The large venous systemic clearance of nitroglycerin is contributed by two other pharmacokinetic phenomena unusual among drugs: that there is a substantial arterial-venous gradient in the plasma concentration and that the plasma clearance (on both the arterial and venous sides) is dependent on the cardiac output. Armstrong et al. [5] showed that arterial plasma concentrations of nitroglycerin in patients with chronic heart failure are three to four times higher than the corresponding venous concentrations, suggesting an arterial-venous extraction of about 60 percent. In the presence of this extraction, it is pharmacokinetically inappropriate to compare the values of the venous clearance directly with those of blood flow. Fung et al. [35] recently examined the relationship between cardiac output and the pharmacokinetics of nitroglycerin in rats and showed that arterial nitroglycerin clearance is approximately 75 percent of cardiac output. Thus, 75 percent of the drug in the arterial blood is cleared with each passage through the circulation. These data suggest that the pharmacokinetics of nitroglycerin are intimately related to systemic hemodynamics and that proper control of these physiological parameters is essential if the pharmacokinetic parameters of nitroglycerin are to be reproducibly determined.

A recent report [88] suggested that the pharmacokinetics of intravenous nitroglycerin in normal volunteers might be both dose- and time-dependent. These workers infused nitroglycerin at 10, 20, 40, and 10 µg/min over successive periods of 40 minutes each and showed nitroglycerin clearance to decrease with respect to both increasing dose and time of infusion. Armstrong et al. [4] showed earlier that patients with congestive heart failure who did not respond to intravenous nitroglycerin therapy (and therefore who were receiving higher doses) also exhibited slower venous plasma nitroglycerin clearance than responders. This dose dependency, however, was not seen by Imhof et al. [56], who infused nitroglycerin at 4.8 and 10.6 µg/min over 75 minutes. Zimrin et al. [113] recently infused nitroglycerin for 24 hours in ten patients with stable angina pectoris (at a constant rate for each patient) but did not observe any time-dependency in nitroglycerin kinetics. Given the high variability in plasma nitroglycerin concentrations, it is possible that in some instances the manifestation of either dose- or time-dependency might have been masked. However, the existence of these pharmacokinetic phenomena is still uncertain.

OTHER ROUTES OF ADMINISTRATION
Transdermal delivery of nitroglycerin has become a major dosing mode for nitrate therapy in recent years. The rationale for this route of ad-

ministration is that it can provide constant plasma concentrations over much of the dosing period (e.g., from 2 to 24 hours after application). It was therefore reasoned that sustained action against angina pectoris or congestive heart failure can also be maintained for this duration. There are now considerable data [1] showing that the latter conclusion is incorrect, although there is no dispute regarding the ability of all transdermal patches to deliver a constant plasma concentration of nitroglycerin. At a 10 cm^2 surface area of application, the plasma concentration of nitroglycerin usually reaches a steady-state of about 0.2 ng/ml. Increasing the surface area of application (and thereby the dose) usually brings about some increase in the plasma concentration, although such an increase is not always proportional to the dose [3, 78, 93]. About 75 percent of the quantity of nitroglycerin released by the transdermal system passes into the systemic circulation [56]. The skin is the rate-limiting barrier for the absorption of transdermal nitroglycerin; thus, there is little difference in the bioavailability of the different transdermal preparations. Interindividual absorption of transdermal nitroglycerin can vary greatly [45, 58], although the application site (chest, upper arm, and pelvic regions) appears not to be critical in determining absorption [45]. Increased physical exercise and high ambient temperatures have been shown to produce higher nitroglycerin plasma concentrations than controls [10].

Nitroglycerin ointment can be used as an alternate dosage form for transdermal application. Moe and Armstrong [71] showed recently that there was no apparent difference in drug absorption from three application sites—arm, chest and thigh. Arterial plasma concentrations were still in the range of 3 to 4 ng/ml at 6 hours after application. Curry et al. [25] compared the absorption of nitroglycerin from an ointment (applied every 8 hours) to that of a 20 cm^2 patch designed to release 10 mg of nitroglycerin per day. Their data can be analyzed to suggest that 1 inch of 2 percent ointment over an application area of 50 cm^2 every 8 hours would be roughly equivalent in nitroglycerin delivery to a transdermal patch releasing 20 mg/day [32].

Both sublingual and buccal nitroglycerin have been shown to give prompt absorption, although the plasma concentrations obtained can still be highly variable [20, 86] and can be indicative of incomplete absorption [86]. A lingual spray has recently become available; this preparation is essentially identical to the sublingual tablet but without the latter's problem of chemical instability. The advantage of nitroglycerin absorption through the buccal/mucosal membrane is that the absorbed drug is not significantly subjected to hepatic first-pass metabolism. Sublingual nitroglycerin usually induces a rapid rise in nitroglycerin plasma concentration concomitant with the appearance of beneficial therapeutic effects, sometimes even in the presence of nitrate tolerance [95]. It is not known whether the burst absorption of nitroglycerin from this mode of administration causes this phenomenon.

Because of extensive presystemic metabolism, oral nitroglycerin dosing in humans leads to low plasma concentrations of the intact drug. Much of the nitrates present in plasma are the denitrated metabolites of nitroglycerin, namely, the 1,2- and 1,3-glyceryl dinitrates, and the 1- and 2-mononitrates [87]. These lower nitrates might have contributed to the observed antianginal activities seen after high-dose oral nitroglycerin therapy.

Pharmacokinetics of Isosorbide Dinitrate

INTRAVENOUS ADMINISTRATION

The systemic plasma clearance of ISDN is about 3 to 4 liters/min [2]. Morrison and Fung [74] determined the in vitro erythrocyte to plasma partitioning ratio of ISDN to be 0.13 at 37°. When corrected for this distribution, the systemic (blood) clearance of ISDN can be calculated to be between 5 to 6 liters/min, approaching normal cardiac output. Interestingly however, the plasma concentrations of ISDN are considerably less fluctuating than those of nitroglycerin, and arterial-venous extraction only occurs to a small extent [77].

Like nitroglycerin, in vivo elimination of ISDN occurs exclusively through metabolism to its denitrated metabolites. The apparent elimination half-life of ISDN has been variably reported to be between 18 to 79 minutes [2] after intravenous administration. It is likely that this variability reflects the ability of the various studies to detect a short elimination phase ($t_{1/2}$ of about 10 minutes) prior to a terminal decay with a half-life of about 1 hour. There is no evidence to suggest that the pharmacokinetics of ISDN are either dose- or time-dependent after short-term intravenous infusion.

OTHER ROUTES OF ADMINISTRATION

Transdermal delivery of ISDN also produces significant ISDN plasma concentrations and therapeutic effects. Morrison et al. [76] showed that after percutaneous application of a topical formulation of ISDN (at a dose of 100 mg over an area of 400 cm^2), steady-state plasma concentrations of about 7 ng/ml were maintained from 6 to 24 hours. These workers estimated the bioavailability of the topical application to be about 30 percent. Parker et al. [95] showed that significant improvement in exercise tolerance occurs after the first dose of a transdermal ISDN cream, but the short-term beneficial effects (up to 8 hours) were not seen at 24 hours, even though similar plasma ISDN concentrations were maintained over the entire period. After sustained therapy with the same preparation for 7 to 10 days, plasma concentrations of both ISDN and 5-ISMN were elevated, but the antianginal effects were totally abolished (Fig. 6-3). This seemingly paradoxical relationship between

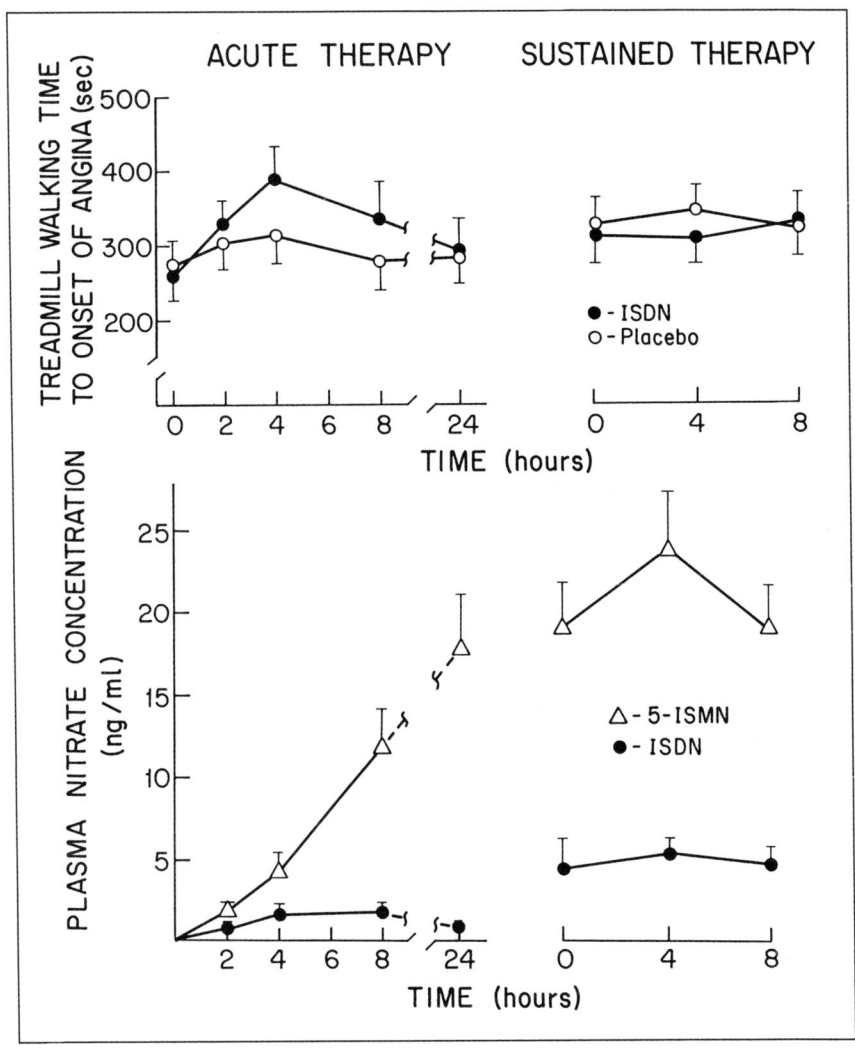

FIG. 6-3. Lack of correlation between plasma nitrate concentration and antianginal effects after transdermal ISDN application (Adapted from Ref. 95).

nitrate concentration and antianginal effects will be addressed in a later discussion of nitrate tolerance.

Sublingual ISDN is variably and incompletely absorbed; a 5 mg dose has a mean bioavailability of about 60 percent but the range of absorption relative to an intravenous dose is wide (19–93 percent).

Oral ISDN is the preferred route of administration for this nitrate. Absorption is normally rapid and results in a bioavailability of about 20 to 25 percent. Fung et al. [37] showed that the area under the plasma

ISDN concentration versus time curve is proportional to the oral dose between 15 to 120 mg. Thus, within this dose range, ISDN absorption appears independent of the dose.

The apparent half-life of elimination after oral ISDN normally is shown to be about 1 hour if plasma samples were monitored up to 4 hours after dosing. Fung and Parker [38] showed, however, that a terminal disappearance half-life (of about 8 hours) was observed if plasma concentrations were determined for 24 hours after dosing. The physiological reason for this prolonged disappearance phase is not known but the following speculation has been put forward: the in vitro degradation half-life of ISDN in human blood at 37° is about 1.5 hours, some five times faster than this in vivo half-life. This would suggest that the terminal decline phase of ISDN is not rate-limited by metabolism or elimination but by an input process, namely, redistribution of ISDN from the peripheral tissues back to the systemic circulation or an extremely prolonged absorption process of the oral dose [38].

Chronic oral ISDN administration, at four times daily, leads to extensive accumulation of plasma ISDN and loss of therapeutic effect [37, 108], a situation similar to that previously discussed for transdermal ISDN. The accumulation of plasma ISDN concentration cannot be totally explained by the elimination half-life of the compound. In animal studies, Fung and associates [75, 107] showed that the mononitrate metabolites of ISDN inhibited the clearance of the parent drug, thus suggesting that product inhibition might have been the cause for the observed accumulation of ISDN after chronic dosing.

Pharmacokinetics of Isosorbide-5-Mononitrate

INTRAVENOUS ADMINISTRATION
The pharmacokinetics of 5-ISMN is the least complex of the three nitrates discussed [2]; this property forms the basis on which therapeutic use of this compound has been argued, even though the pharmacologic potency of 5-ISMN is considerably less than those of nitroglycerin and ISDN. 5-ISMN has an elimination half-life of about 4.6 hours, and because of its polar nature, it is primarily distributed in plasma water. This compound is almost completely eliminated via metabolism, either through denitration to isosorbide or through glucuronidation to form the 2-glucuronide conjugate.

OTHER ROUTES OF ADMINISTRATION
In contrast to nitroglycerin and ISDN, 5-ISMN is not subjected to presystemic metabolism. Thus, an oral dose of this nitrate is totally bioavailable. This property is shared by its positional isomer, isosorbide-2-

mononitrate. Oral absorption of 5-ISMN is neither dose- nor time-dependent. Because of its chemical polarity, absorption through the sublingual or transdermal routes is anticipated to be poor. However, there is no good reason to employ these routes of administration for this nitrate since oral doses are rapidly and completely absorbed.

Effects of Disease States on the Pharmacokinetics of Nitrates

The pharmacokinetics of nitroglycerin are not substantially different in various patient groups [15]. This is understandable since this drug is eliminated by the entire body and the involvement of disease in a particular organ is unlikely to produce a significant alteration in the overall kinetics. A notable exception to this general conclusion is the finding of Armstrong et al. [4], who showed that patients with a greater venous congestion in congestive heart failure exhibited a reduced nitroglycerin plasma clearance compared to the less congested group. These investigators attributed this difference to the presence of impaired hepatic metabolism secondary to increasing venous congestion. However, the more congested patient group also received a much larger intravenous nitroglycerin dose. Thus, the observed alteration in pharmacokinetics could have been influenced by the dose rather than the disease.

Fung et al. [40] have compared the pharmacokinetics and hemodynamics of sublingual and oral ISDN in patients with advanced congestive heart failure versus those with angina pectoris. They showed that the relative bioavailability of oral ISDN, when compared to the sublingual route, is not changed in heart failure, but the circulatory effects are less marked in this patient group. It is therefore possible that this difference is derived from a decreased hemodynamic responsiveness to ISDN in heart failure.

Liver disease has a major impact on the bioavailability of oral nitroglycerin and ISDN (but not 5-ISMN) since the first two compounds are subjected to extensive presystemic hepatic metabolism. Bogaert [15] has shown that plasma concentrations of ISDN are higher in cirrhotic patients. In a more detailed study, Blei et al. [13] examined ISDN pharmacokinetics and its effect on portal hypertension in patients with stable alcoholic cirrhosis. These workers showed that a 20 mg dose of oral ISDN produced a peak reduction of the hepatic venous gradient of about 25 percent, and significant reductions in this parameter were seen over 4 hours after dosing. There was no correlation between the hepatic extraction of ISDN and the portal hypotensive effect seen. The effect of liver disease on the pharmacokinetics of nitroglycerin is not as well characterized. Porchet and Bircher [96], however, proposed to exploit the complete presystemic hepatic metabolism of nitroglycerin through a healthy liver to devise a noninvasive method for the measurement of portal-systemic shunting in a cirrhotic liver. In this procedure, cirrhotic patients are given both oral and intravenous solutions of nitroglycerin, and the pharmacologic bioavailability (as assessed by computer-assisted digital plethysmography) is equated to the fraction of portal-systemic shunting in these patients.

Since only a small fraction of nitrates is excreted unchanged through the kidney, the effect of renal disease on their pharmacokinetics is expected to be minimal. This has been confirmed for both ISDN and 5-ISMN [15, 98].

Pharmacokinetic Interaction with Other Drugs

Ochs et al. [89] have shown that therapeutic doses of beta blockers did not influence the pharmacokinetics of oral ISDN or 5-ISMN or those of the dinitrates after oral nitroglycerin administration. This finding was expected since the metabolic pathways of nitrates (principally denitration via glutathione S-transferases) do not overlap with those of beta blockers (principally hydroxylation and glucuronidation). For a similar reason, Boje et al. [17] found little pharmacokinetic interaction between oral nifedipine and sublingual nitroglycerin. Nitrates are not extensively bound to plasma proteins [35, 37]. Thus, pharmacokinetic interaction arising from protein-binding displacement has not been seen with nitrates. Nitrates, however, can cause moderate changes in liver blood flow. For example, Feely [28] has reported that sublingual nitroglycerin reduced hepatic blood flow by 18 percent at 5 minutes after drug administration. Thus, the pharmacokinetics of drugs with high intrinsic hepatic clearance could be affected by concomitant nitrate administration.

NITRATE TOLERANCE

Biochemical Mechanism

The clinical controversy regarding nitrate tolerance will be discussed in detail in Chapter 15. Our focus here is to examine the biochemical sequence of events that occur during pharmacologic tolerance. As reported earlier, tolerance to the antianginal effects of nitrates occurs after chronic therapy when plasma nitrate concentrations are either similar to or even more elevated than those seen after acute dosing. Thus, it is clear that nitrate tolerance is not due to a systemic dispositional change that reduces the total amount of drug exposed to the systemic circulation.

The most extensively investigated mechanisms of nitrate tolerance assume that the locus of tolerance resides within the vascular smooth muscle cell. There is considerable supportive evidence for this deduction. Blood vessels obtained from animals made tolerant to the in vivo hypotensive effects of nitroglycerin also exhibit decreased in vitro vascular nitrate sensitivity [60, 84, 106]. This suggests that nitrate tolerance cannot be mediated entirely through a systemic mechanism, at least at the experimental doses used. In addition, tolerance can be successfully induced in vitro by incubating vascular segments with high concentrations of nitrate at either alkaline [8, 84] or physiologic pH [49, 60, 109].

Vascular tolerance to nitrates may arise from decreased metabolic activation of the nitrate to nitric oxide in vascular tissues (Fig. 6-2). Fung and Poliszczuk [39] have shown that in nitrate-tolerant rats, total metabolite production from nitroglycerin in aortic tissues is reduced. This reduction is primarily due to a decrease in the production of 1,2-glyceryl dinitrate, suggesting that the denitration step to this particular metabolite might be the pharmacologically productive pathway.

Reduced metabolic activation within the smooth muscle cell during nitrate tolerance could be brought about by depletion of critical cofactor(s) necessary for this conversion. Needleman and Johnson [84] postulated that, during prolonged nitrate exposure, sulfhydryl groups in the nitrate receptor are oxidized to the disulfide form, which has a lesser affinity for the drug. More recently, Ignarro and coworkers [55] modified this hypothesis by suggesting that sulfhydryl depletion diminishes the formation of the requisite intermediates—the S-nitrosothiols.

Evidence in support of the sulfhydryl depletion hypothesis is mixed. In support of this mechanism, it has been shown that the induction of nitrate tolerance was associated with a decrease in tissue sulfhydryl groups [84] and that tolerance could be partially reversed with the potent sulfhydryl reducing agent dithiothreitol [8, 84] and the sulfhydryl donor N-acetylcysteine [109]. N-acetylcysteine was also reported to reverse tolerance to the in vivo effects of intravenous nitroglycerin [68, 90]. However, Greutter and Lemke [49, 50] found that nitrate tolerance can be slightly reversed by mercaptoethanol but not by dithiothreitol, N-acetylcysteine, or cysteine. Other workers have also been unable to reverse in vitro nitrate tolerance with cysteine and glutathione [8, 84]. Fung et al. [36] showed recently that reversal of nitrate tolerance by sulfhydryl donors may be mediated by formation of active S-nitrosothiols in plasma. This finding suggests that the ability of sulfhydryl donors to reverse nitrate tolerance is not, by itself, sufficient evidence to implicate intracellular sulfhydryl depletion during nitrate tolerance.

An alternate hypothesis of vascular tolerance toward nitrates has emerged in recent years, namely, that tolerance may be due to conformational changes in the enzyme guanylate cyclase, rendering it less responsive to activation by nitrovasodilators [8, 111]. In support of this mechanism, it has been shown that guanylate cyclase prepared from nitroglycerin-tolerant vessels is less responsive to activation by nitroglycerin/cysteine, nitroprusside, and nitric oxide than enzyme prepared from control vessels [8, 111]. However, this hypothesis appears at present to be inconsistent with the reported lack of cross-tolerance between nitroglycerin-tolerant vessels and S-nitroso-N-acetylpenicillamine [62], SIN-1 [63], and nitric oxide itself [61]. Recently, Mulsch and coworkers [79] found that soluble guanylate cyclase, prepared from nitroglycerin-tolerant rabbit aorta, was desensitized to stimulation by nitroglycerin and sodium nitroprusside, while only the relaxation responses to nitroglycerin were attenuated in intact aorta. These data suggest that although alterations in guanylate cyclase activity can be demonstrated in nitrate-tolerant vessels, these mechanisms may not contribute substantially to nitroglycerin relaxation tolerance.

In addition to a vascular mechanism, neurohormonal compensation may contribute to the phenomenon of in vivo nitrate tolerance. Thus, Packer and coworkers [90] have shown that tolerance to intravenous nitroglycerin in a group of heart failure patients was accompanied by increased plasma renin activity and body weight. It has also been found that chronic transdermal therapy resulted in decreased hematocrit and blood viscosity [19]. The delineation of the contributions of diminished vascular metabolic activation of nitrate and neurohormonal changes to in vivo nitrate tolerance awaits further investigation.

Avoidance of Nitrate Tolerance Through Dosage Regimen Manipulation

Whatever the mechanism of nitrate tolerance, avoidance of it through manipulation of dosing regimen would have a chance of success only if the refractory period of reduced nitrate sensitivity is relatively short. Recent data suggest that omission of the evening dose of nitrate may be sufficient to restore reactivity to a new dose given the next morning. This approach has seen success in early trials with oral ISDN [99, 104], buccal nitroglycerin [95], and transdermal nitroglycerin in stable angina [22] and chronic congestive heart failure [103]. A detailed review of the current status of this interval therapy has appeared. At present, there does not appear to be any relationship between the time needed for regeneration of pharmacologic reactivity by a particular nitrate and any of its pharmacokinetic parameters, nor can a critical nitrate plasma concentration be defined that would reflect the presence or absence of nitrate tolerance [34].

CONCLUSIONS

Both the pharmacologic and pharmacokinetic aspects of nitrates are extremely complex, particularly in relation to nitrate tolerance. Although significant strides have been made in the understanding of the mechanisms of nitrate action in the last few years, much remains to be done.

REFERENCES

1. Abrams, J. Interval therapy to avoid nitrate tolerance: Paradise regained? *Am. J. Cardiol.* 64:931, 1989.
2. Abshagen, U. Pharmacokinetics of ISDN, sustained-release ISDN, and IS-5-MN. In J. N. Cohn and R. Rittinghausen (eds.), *Mononitrates*. Berlin: Springer-Verlag, 1985. P. 53.
3. Armstrong, P. W. Pharmacokinetic-hemodynamic studies of transdermal nitroglycerin in congestive heart failure. *J. Amer. Coll. Cardiol.* 9:420, 1987.
4. Armstrong, P. W., Armstrong, J. A., and Marks, G. S. Pharmacokinetic hemodynamic studies of intravenous nitroglycerin in congestive cardiac failure. *Circulation* 62:160, 1980.
5. Armstrong, P. W., Moffat, J. A., and Marks, G. S. Arterial-venous nitroglycerin gradient during intravenous infusion in man. *Circulation* 66:1273, 1982.
6. Arnold, W. P., Aldred, R., and Murad, F. Cigarette smoke activates guanylate cyclase and increases guanosine 3', 5'-monophosphate in tissues. *Science* 198:934, 1977.
7. Axelsson, K. L., Andersson, R. G. G., and Wikberg, J. E. S. Correlation between vascular smooth muscle relaxation and increase in cyclic GMP induced by some organic nitro esters. *Acta pharmacol. et toxicol.* 49:270, 1981.
8. Axelsson, K. L., Andersson, R. G. G., and Wikberg, J. E. S. Vascular smooth muscle relaxation by nitro compounds: Reduced relaxation and cGMP elevation in tolerant vessels and reversal of tolerance by dithiothreitol. *Acta pharmacol. et toxicol.* 50:350, 1982.
9. Axelsson, K. L., Wilkberg, J. E. S., and Andersson, R. G. G. Relationship between nitroglycerin, cyclic GMP and relaxation of vascular smooth muscle. *Life Sci.* 24:1779, 1979.
10. Barkve, T. F., Langseth-Manrique, K., Bredesen, J. E., and Gjesdal, K. Increased uptake of transdermal glyceryl trinitrate during physical exercise and during high ambient temperature. *Amer. Heart J.* 112:537, 1986.
11. Bennett, B. M., Kobus, S. M., Brien, J. F., et al. Requirement for reduced, unliganded hemoprotein for the hemoglobin and myoglobin-mediated biotransformation of glyceryl trinitrate. *J. Pharmacol. Exp. Ther.* 237:629, 1986.
12. Bennett, B. M., Moffat, J. A., Armstrong, P. W., and Marks, G. S. Investigation of the role of prostaglandins in nitroglycerin-induced relaxation of isolated rabbit blood vessels. *Can. J. Physiol. Pharmacol.* 61:554, 1983.
13. Blei, A. T., Garcia-Tsao, G., Groszmann, R. J., et al. A hemodynamic evaluation of isosorbide dinitrate in alcoholic cirrhosis: Pharmacokinetic-hemodynamic interactions. *Gastroenterology* 93:576, 1987.
14. Blei, A. T., Gottstein, J., and Fung, H.-L. The role of the liver in the disposition of intravenous nitroglycerin in the rat. *Biochem. Pharmacol.* 33:2681, 1984.
15. Bogaert, M. G. Clinical pharmacokinetics of organic nitrates. *Clin. Pharmacokin.* 8:410, 1983.
16. Bogaert, M. G. Clinical pharmacokinetics of glyceryl trinitrate following the use of systemic and topical preparations. *Clin. Pharmacokin.* 12:1, 1987.
17. Boje, K. M., Fung, H.-L., Yoshitomi, K., and Parker, J. O. Hemodynamic

effects of combined oral nifedipine and sublingual nitroglycerin in patients with chronic stable angina. *Eur. J. Clin. Pharmacol.* 349, 1987.
18. Brien, J. F., McLaughlin, B. E., Breedon, T. H., et al. Biotransformation of glyceryl trinitrate occurs concurrently with relaxation of rabbit aorta. *J. Pharmacol. Exp. Ther.* 237:608, 1986.
19. Brugger, W., Imhof, P., Muller, P., et al. Effect of nitroglycerin on blood rheology in healthy subjects. *Eur. J. Clin. Pharmacol.* 29:331, 1985.
20. Bussmann, W.-D., Kromm, W., Reifart, N., and Fung, H.-L. Acute hemodynamic and pharmacokinetic effects of buccal nitroglycerin. In W.-D. Bussmann, R.-R. Dries, and W. Wagner (eds.), *Advances in Pharmacotherapy.* Basel: Karger, 1982. Pp. 64–72.
21. Chung, S. J., and Fung, H.-L. Identification of the subcellular site for nitroglycerin metabolism to nitric oxide in bovine coronary smooth muscle cells. *J. Pharmacol. Exp. Ther.* 253:614, 1990.
22. Cowan, C., Bourke, J., Reid, D., and Julian, D. G. Tolerance to glyceryl trinitrate patches: Prevention by intermittent dosing. *Brit. Med. J.* 294:544, 1987.
23. Craven, P. A., and DeRubertis, F. R. Requirement for heme in the activation of purified guanylate cyclase by nitric oxide. *Biochim. Biophys. Acta* 745:310, 1983.
24. Curry, S. H., and Aburawi, S. M. Analysis, disposition and pharmacokinetics of nitroglycerin. *Biopharm. Drug Disp.* 6:235, 1985.
25. Curry, S. H., Kwon, H.-R., Perrin, J. H., et al. Plasma nitroglycerin concentrations and hemodynamic effects of sublingual, ointment, and controlled-release forms of nitroglycerin. *Clin. Pharmacol. Ther.* 36:765, 1984.
26. DeRubertis, F. R., and Craven, P. A. Calcium-independent modulation of cyclic GMP and activation of guanylate cyclase by nitrosamines. *Science* 193:897, 1976.
27. Diamond, J., and Blisard, K. S. Effects of stimulant and relaxant drugs on tension and cyclic nucleotide levels in canine femoral artery. *Mol. Pharmacol.* 12:688, 1976.
28. Feely, J. Nifedipine increases and glyceryl trinitrate decreases apparent liver blood flow in normal subjects. *Br. J. Clin. Pharmacol.* 17:83, 1984.
29. Feigen, L. P., Chapnick, B. M., Flemming, J. E., and Kadowitz, P. J. Prostaglandins: Renal vascular responses to bradykinin, histamine, and nitroglycerin. *Am. J. Physiol.* 234:H496, 1978.
30. Fung, H.-L. Pharmacokinetics of nitroglycerin and long acting nitrate esters. *Am. J. Med.* 74(Suppl 6B):13, 1983.
31. Fung, H.-L. Pharmacokinetic determinants of nitrate action. *Am. J. Med.* 76(Suppl 6A):22, 1984.
32. Fung, H.-L. Nitrate formulations and drug delivery systems—An overview. *Z. Kardiol.* 74(Suppl 4):4, 1985.
33. Fung, H.-L. Pharmacokinetics and pharmacodynamics of organic nitrates. *Am. J. Cardiol.* 60:4H, 1987.
34. Fung, H.-L. Pharmacokinetics of organic nitrates and their metabolites: Are they relevant in therapy? In D. G. Julian, R. Rittinghausen, and H. J. Uberbacher (eds.), *Mononitrates II.* Berlin: Springer-Verlag, 1987. Pp. 47–52.
35. Fung, H.-L., Blei, A., and Chong, S. Cardiac output is an apparent determinant of nitroglycerin pharmacokinetics in rats. *J. Pharmacol. Exp. Ther.* 239:701, 1986.
36. Fung, H.-L., Chong, S., Kowaluk, E., et al. Mechanisms for the pharmacologic interaction of organic nitrates with thiols. Existence of an extracel-

lular pathway for the reversal of nitrate vascular tolerance by N-acetylcysteine. *J. Pharmacol. Exp. Ther.* 245:524, 1988.
37. Fung, H.-L., McNiff, E. F., Ruggirello, D., et al. Kinetics of isosorbide dinitrate and relationships to pharmacological effects. *Brit. J. Clin. Pharmacol.* 11:579, 1981.
38. Fung, H.-L., and Parker, J. O. Prolonged plasma half-life after oral isosorbide dinitrate in patients with angina pectoris. *Brit. J. Clin. Pharmacol.* 15:746, 1983.
39. Fung, H.-L., and Poliszczuk, R. Nitrosothiol and nitrate tolerance. *Z. Kardiol.* 75(Suppl 3):25, 1986.
40. Fung, H.-L., Ruggirello, D., Stone, J. A., and Parker, J. O. Effects of cardiovascular disease, smoking and food on the pharmacokinetics and circulatory effects of sublingual and oral isosorbide dinitrate. *Z. Kardiol.* 72(Suppl 3):5, 1983.
41. Fung, H.-L., Sutton, S. C., and Kamiya, A. Blood vessel uptake and metabolism of organic nitrates in the rat. *J. Pharmacol. Exp. Ther.* 228:334, 1984.
42. Furchgott, R. F. Role of endothelium in responses of vascular smooth muscle. *Circ. Res.* 53:557, 1983.
43. Furchgott, R. F., and Zawadzki, J. V. The obligatory role of endothelial cells in the relaxation of arterial smooth muscle by acetylcholine. *Nature* 288:373, 1980.
44. Galvas, P. E., and DiSalvo, J. Concentration and time-dependent relationships between isosorbide dinitrate-induced relaxation and formation of cyclic GMP in coronary arterial smooth muscle. *J. Pharmacol. Exp. Ther.* 224:373, 1983.
45. Gerardin, A., Gaudry, D., Moppert, J., et al. Glycerol trinitrate (nitroglycerin) plasma concentrations achieved after application of transdermal therapeutic systems to healthy volunteers. *Arzneim. Forsch./Drug Res.* 35:530, 1985.
46. Gibaldi, M., and Perrier, D. *Pharmacokinetics.* New York: Marcel Dekker, Inc., 1975.
47. Gruetter, C. A., Barry, B. K., McNamara, D. B., et al. Relaxation of bovine coronary artery and activation of coronary arterial guanylate cyclase by nitric oxide, nitroprusside and a carcinogenic nitrosamine. *J. Cycl. Nucl. Res.* 5:211, 1979.
48. Gruetter, C. A., Gruetter, D. Y., Lyon, J. E., et al. Relationship between cyclic guanosine 3', 5' monophosphate formation and relaxation of coronary arterial smooth muscle by glyceryl trinitrate, nitroprusside, nitrite and nitric oxide: Effects of methylene blue and methemoglobin. *J. Pharmacol. Exp. Ther.* 219:181, 1981.
49. Gruetter, C. A., and Lemke, S. M. Dissociation of cysteine and glutathione levels from nitroglycerin-induced relaxation. *Eur. J. Pharmacol.* 111:85, 1985.
50. Gruetter, C. A., and Lemke, S. M. Effects of sulfhydryl reagents on nitroglycerin-induced relaxation of bovine coronary artery. *Can. J. Physiol. Pharmacol.* 64:1395, 1986.
51. Ignarro, L. J., Byrns, R. E., Buga, G. M., and Wood, K. S. Endothelium-dependent relaxing factor from pulmonary artery and vein possesses pharmacologic and chemical properties identical to those of nitric oxide radical. *Circ. Res.* 61:866, 1987.
52. Ignarro, L. J., Degnan, J. N., Baricos, W. H., et al. Activation of purified guanylate cyclase by nitric oxide requires heme: Comparison of heme-deficient, heme-reconstituted and heme-containing forms of soluble enzyme from bovine lung. *Biochim. Biophys. Acta* 718:45, 1982.

53. Ignarro, L. J., and Gruetter, C. A. Requirement of thiols for activation of coronary arterial guanylate cyclase by glyceryl trinitrate and sodium nitrite. Possible involvement of S-nitrosothiols. *Biochim. Biophys. Acta* 631:221, 1980.
54. Ignarro, L. J., and Kadowitz, P. J. The pharmacological and physiological role of cyclic GMP in vascular smooth muscle relaxation. *Ann. Rev. Pharmacol. Toxicol.* 25:171, 1985.
55. Ignarro, L. J., Lippton, H., Edwards, J. C., et al. Mechanism of vascular smooth muscle relaxation by organic nitrates, nitrites, nitroprusside and nitric oxide: Evidence for the involvement of S-nitrosothiols as active intermediates. *J. Pharmacol. Exp. Ther.* 218:739, 1981.
56. Imhof, P. R., Vuillemin, T., Gerardin, A., et al. Studies of the bioavailability of nitroglycerin from a transdermal therapeutic system (Nitroderm TTS). *Eur. J. Clin. Pharmacol.* 27:7, 1984.
57. Kadowitz, P. J., Armstead, W. M., Hyman, A. L., et al. Cyclooxygenase-independent vascular responses to nitroglycerin, nitroprusside and nicorandil. *Fed. Proc.* 42:500, 1983.
58. Karim, A. Transdermal absorption of nitroglycerin from microseal drug delivery (MDD) system. *Angiology* 34:11, 1983.
59. Katsuki, S., Arnold, W., Mittal, C., and Murad, F. Stimulation of guanylate cyclase by sodium nitroprusside, nitroglycerin and nitric oxide in various tissue preparations and comparison to the effects of sodium azide and hydroxylamine. *J. Cycl. Nucl. Res.* 3:23, 1977.
60. Keith, R. A., Burkman, A. M., Sokoloski, T. D., and Fertel, R. H. Vascular tolerance to nitroglycerin and cyclic GMP generation in rat aortic smooth muscle. *J. Pharmacol. Exp. Ther.* 221:525, 1982.
61. Kowaluk, E. A., and Fung, H.-L. Effect of nitroglycerin tolerance on nitrovasodilator-induced and endothelium-dependent relaxation of isolated rat aorta. *FASEB J.* 2:A381, 1988.
62. Kowaluk, E. A., Poliszczuk, R., and Fung, H.-L. Tolerance to relaxation in rat aorta: Comparison of an S-nitrosothiol with nitroglycerin. *Eur. J. Pharmacol.* 144:379, 1987.
63. Kukovetz, W. R., and Holzmann, S. Cyclic GMP as the mediator of molsidomine-induced vasodilatation. *Eur. J. Pharmacol.* 122:103, 1986.
64. Lang, S., Johnson, E. M., Jr., and Needleman, P. Metabolism and vascular response of glyceryl trinitrate in the eviscerated rat. *Biochem. Pharmacol.* 21:422, 1972.
65. Levin, R. I., Jaffe, E. A., Weksler, B. B., and Tack-Goldman, K. Nitroglycerin stimulates synthesis of prostacyclin by cultured human endothelial cells. *J. Clin. Invest.* 67:762, 1981.
66. Martin, W., Villani, G. M., Jothianandan, D., and Furchgott, R. F. Selective blockade of endothelium-dependent and glyceryl trinitrate induced relaxation by hemoglobin and by methylene blue in the rabbit aorta. *J. Pharmacol. Exp. Ther.* 233:708, 1985.
67. Matsuoka, I., Sakurai, K., and Nakanishi, H. Isosorbide-5-mononitrate effects on isolated rabbit aorta and vena cava: Relationship between cyclic GMP and relaxation of vascular smooth muscle. *Eur. J. Pharmacol.* 118:155, 1985.
68. May, D. C., Popma, J. J., Black, W. H., et al. In vivo induction and reversal of nitroglycerin tolerance in human coronary arteries. *N. Engl. J. Med.* 317:805, 1987.
69. McNiff, E. F., Lai, C. M., Iook, Z. M., et al. Effect of infusion administration set on the delivery rate and plasma concentration of nitroglycerin in dogs. *J. Pharm. Sci.* 74:774, 1985.

70. McNiff, E. F., Yacobi, A., Young-Chang, F. M., et al. Pharmacokinetics of nitroglycerin after intravenous infusion in normal subjects. *J. Pharm. Sci.* 70:1054, 1981.
71. Moe, G., and Armstrong, P. W. Influence of skin site on bioavailability of nitroglycerin ointment in congestive heart failure. *Amer. J. Med.* 81:765, 1986.
72. Moncada, S., Radomski, M. W., and Palmer, R. M. J. Endothelium-derived relaxing factor. Identification as nitric oxide and role in the control of vascular tone and platelet function. *Biochem. Pharmacol.* 37:2495, 1988.
73. Morcillio, E., Reid, P. R., Dubin, N., et al. Myocardial prostaglandin E release by nitroglycerin and modification by indomethacin. *Am. J. Cardiol.* 45:53, 1980.
74. Morrison, R. A., and Fung, H.-L. Determination of the partitioning, stability and metabolite formation of isosorbide dinitrate in human and rat blood using an improved gas chromatographic assay. *J. Chromat.* (Biomed. Applic.), 308:153, 1984.
75. Morrison, R. A., and Fung, H.-L. Isosorbide dinitrate disposition in the rat. Metabolite pharmacokinetics and interactions. *J. Pharmacol. Exp. Ther.* 231:124, 1984.
76. Morrison, R. A., Wiegand, U.-W., Jahnchen, E., et al. Isosorbide dinitrate kinetics and dynamics after intravenous, sublingual, and percutaneous dosing in angina. *Clin. Pharmacol. Ther.* 33:747, 1983.
77. Morrison, R. A., Wiegand, U.-W., Jahnchen, E., et al. Determination of hepatic extraction of isosorbide dinitrate in cardiac patients. *Clin. Pharmacol. Ther.* 34:724, 1983.
78. Muller, P., Imhof, P. R., Burkart, F., et al. Human pharmacologic studies of a new transdermal system containing nitroglycerin. *Eur. J. Clin. Pharmacol.* 22:473, 1982.
79. Mulsch, A., Busse, R., and Bassenge, E. Desensitization of guanylate cyclase in nitrate tolerance does not impair endothelium-dependent responses. *Eur. J. Pharmacol.* 158:191, 1988.
80. Murad, F. Cyclic guanosine monophosphate as a mediator of vasodilation. *J. Clin. Invest.* 78:1, 1986.
81. Murad, F., Mittal, C. K., Arnold, W. P., et al. Guanylate cyclase: Activation by azide, nitro compounds, nitric oxide, and hydroxyl radical and inhibition by hemoglobin and myoglobin. *Adv. Cycl. Nucl. Res.* 9:145, 1978.
82. Murrell, W. Nitroglycerine as a remedy for angina pectoris. *Lancet* 80, 1879.
83. Needleman, P., Jakschik, B., and Johnson, E. M. Sulfhydryl requirement for relaxation of vascular smooth muscle. *J. Pharmacol. Exp. Ther.* 187:324, 1973.
84. Needleman, P., and Johnson, E. M. Mechanism of tolerance development to organic nitrates. *J. Pharmacol. Exp. Ther.* 184:709, 1973.
85. Noack, E. Investigation on structure-activity relationship in organic nitrates. *Meth. and Find. Exptl. Clin. Pharmacol.* 6:583, 1984.
86. Noonan, P. K., and Benet, L. Z. Incomplete and delayed bioavailability of sublingual nitroglycerin. *Am. J. Cardiol.* 55:184, 1985.
87. Noonan, P. K., and Benet, L. Z. The bioavailability of oral nitroglycerin. *J. Pharm. Sci.* 75:241, 1986.
88. Noonan, P. K., Williams, R. L., and Benet, L. Z. Dose dependent pharmacokinetics of nitroglycerin after multiple intravenous infusions in healthy volunteers. *J. Pharmacok. Biopharm.* 13:143, 1985.
89. Ochs, H. R., Neugetauer, G., Greenblatt, D. J., and Labedzki, L. Influence of beta-blocker coadministration on the kinetics of isosorbide mononitrate and dinitrate. *Klin. Wochenschr.* 64:1213, 1986.

90. Packer, M., Lee, W. H., Kessler, P. D., et al. Prevention and reversal of nitrate tolerance in patients with congestive heart failure. *N. Engl. J. Med.* 317:799, 1987.
91. Palmer, R. M. J., Ferrige, A. G., and Moncada, S. Nitric oxide release accounts for the biological activity of endothelium-derived relaxing factor. *Nature* 327:524, 1987.
92. Panzenbeck, M. J., Baez, A., and Kaley, G. Nitroglycerin and nitroprusside increase coronary blood flow in dogs by a mechanism independent of prostaglandin release. *Am. J. Cardiol.* 53:936, 1984.
93. Parker, J. O., and Fung, H.-L. Transdermal nitroglycerin in angina pectoris. *Am. J. Cardiol.* 54:471, 1984.
94. Parker, J. O., Vankoughnett, K. A., and Farrell, B. Comparison of buccal nitroglycerin and oral isosorbide dinitrate for nitrate tolerance in stable angina pectoris. *Am. J. Cardiol.* 56:724, 1985.
95. Parker, J. O., Vankoughnett, K. A., and Fung, H.-L. Transdermal isosorbide dinitrate in angina pectoris. Effect of acute and sustained therapy. *Am. J. Cardiol.* 54:8, 1984.
96. Porchet, H., and Bircher, J. Non-invasive assessment of portal systemic shunting: Evaluation of a method to investigate systemic availability of oral nitroglycerin by digital plethysmography. *Gastroenterology* 82:629, 1982.
97. Rapoport, R. M., and Murad, F. Agonist-induced endothelium-dependent relaxation in rat thoracic aorta may be mediated through cGMP. *Circ. Res.* 53:557, 1983.
98. Raue, F., Ritz, E., Akpan, W., et al. Kinetics of IS-5-MN and its glucuronide in patients with renal failure. In J. N. Cohn and R. Rittinghausen (eds.), *Mononitrates.* Berlin: Springer-Verlag, 1985.
99. Rudolph, W., Blasini, R., Reiniger, G., and Brugmann, U. Tolerance development during isosorbide dinitrate treatment: Can it be circumvented? *Z. Kardiol.* 73:195, 1983.
100. Schror, K., Grodzinska, L., and Darius, H. Stimulation of coronary vascular prostacyclin and inhibition on human platelet thromboxane A2 after low-dose nitroglycerin. *Thromb. Res.* 23:59, 1981.
101. Schulz, U., and McCalla, D. R. Reactions of cysteine with N-methyl-N-nitroso-p-toluene sulfonamide and N-methyl-N'-nitro-N-nitrosoguanidine. *Can. J. Chem.* 47:2021, 1969.
102. Schultz, K.-D., Schultz, K., and Schultz, G. Sodium nitroprusside and other smooth muscle relaxants increase cyclic GMP levels in rat ductus deferens. *Nature* 265:750, 1977.
103. Sharpe, N., Coxon, R., Webster, M., and Luke, R. Hemodynamic effects of intermittent transdermal nitroglycerin in chronic congestive heart failure. *Am. J. Cardiol.* 59:895, 1987.
104. Silber, S. Clinical relevance of nitrate tolerance. In J. N. Cohn and R. Rittinghausen (eds.), *Mononitrates.* Berlin: Springer-Verlag, 1985.
105. Simonetti, I., DeCaterina, R., Michelassi, C., et al. Coronary vasodilation is not mediated by the prostaglandin system: A quantitative cineangiographic study. *J. Am. Coll. Cardiol.* 8:1263, 1986.
106. Sutton, S. C., and Fung, H.-L. Effect of dosage regimen on the development of tolerance to nitroglycerin in rats. *J. Cardiovasc. Pharmacol.* 5:1086, 1983.
107. Sutton, S. C., and Fung, H.-L. Metabolites decrease the plasma clearance of isosorbide dinitrate in rats. *Biopharm. Drug Disp.* 5:85, 1984.
108. Thadani, U., Fung, H.-L., Darke, A. C., and Parker, J. O. Oral isosorbide dinitrate in angina pectoris. Comparison of duration of action and dose

response relationship during acute and sustained therapy. *Am. J. Cardiol.* 49:411, 1982.
109. Torresi, J., Horowitz, J. D., and Dusting, G. J. Prevention and reversal of tolerance to nitroglycerin with N-acetylcysteine. *J. Cardiovasc. Pharmacol.* 7:777, 1985.
110. Vanhoutte, P. M., Rubanyi, G. M., Miller, V. M., and Houston, D. S. Modulation of vascular smooth muscle contraction by the endothelium. *Ann. Rev. Physiol.* 48:307, 1986.
111. Waldman, S. A., Rapoport, R. M., Ginsburg, R., and Murad, F. Desensitization to nitroglycerin in vascular smooth muscle from rat and human. *Biochem. Pharmacol.* 35:3525, 1986.
112. Williams, D. L. H. S-Nitrosation and the reactions of S-nitroso compounds. *Chem. Soc. Reviews* 14:171, 1985.
113. Zimrin, D., Reichek, N., Bogin, K. T., et al. Antianginal effects of intravenous nitroglycerin over 24 hours. *Circulation* 77:1376, 1988.

CHAPTER 7

PHARMACOLOGY AND PHARMACOKINETICS OF BETA BLOCKERS

STEPHEN F. HAMILTON
BETH H. RESMAN-TARGOFF
EDWIN G. OLSON
UDHO THADANI

The beta blockers exert their action by competitive inhibition of the beta-adrenergic receptor. This effect is discussed in detail in Chapter 4. Primary emphasis will be given here to the beta blocking agents used in ischemic heart disease. The official Food and Drug Administration (FDA) indications for the beta blockers are listed in Table 7-1. The pharmacokinetic and pharmacodynamic properties of these agents will be discussed and an attempt will be made to relate these properties to clinically relevant issues. A discussion of practical dosing considerations will conclude the chapter. The beta blockers are listed along with their ancillary properties in Table 7-2 on pages 180–181 and on text pages 187–191. There are numerous investigational drugs with various combinations of beta blockade and ancillary properties. Available data on these agents are also presented in Table 7-2.

PHARMACOKINETIC PARAMETERS

Absorption

A distinction must be made between the extent of absorption and bioavailability. All beta blockers except the least lipid soluble agents, nadolol and atenolol, are rapidly (within 1 hour) and almost completely (90 percent or greater) absorbed. Bioavailability, however, is the percent of the dose reaching the systemic circulation. It may be low and highly variable with up to a fourfold difference in bioavailability between individuals for most of these drugs. This is due to extensive first-pass hepatic extraction. However, most of these agents achieve peak serum concentrations within 1 to 3 hours, except for formulations designed for slow release. Since the duration of action of beta blockers is longer than would be predicted on the basis of serum half-life (Table 7-2), the use of the extended release products seems to offer little advantage for their increased expense.

For the beta blockers with high intrinsic hepatic clearance, as much as 50 to 70 percent of the dose is inactivated during the first pass through the liver before reaching the systemic circulation. Therefore, bioavailability for the lipophilic beta blockers is inversely proportional to the hepatic clearance, which is a product of the hepatic extraction ratio and hepatic blood flow. The beta blockers with the highest hepatic clearance can show dose-dependent bioavailability. Therefore, the serum concentrations and the pharmacologic effects may increase disproportionately to the increase in dose. This has been shown for propranolol and to a lesser extent for metoprolol [44, 61, 75, 115], but could be possible for other lipophilic beta blockers. Many factors, such as food and inter- and intrapatient variability may be important to this observation.

The bioavailability of propranolol and metoprolol has been shown to be increased by up to 20 to 50 percent by high protein meals [94, 98, 137, 156]. This may be partly a result of a transient increase in post-

TABLE 7-1. *United States Food and Drug Administration Approved Indications for Beta Blockers*

Drug	Indications
Propranolol	Hypertension
	Angina pectoris
	Cardiac arrhythmias
	Paroxysmal atrial tachycardia
	Persistent sinus tachycardia
	Tachycardia and arrhythmias of thyrotoxicosis
	Persistent atrial extrasystoles
	Atrial flutter and fibrillation
	Ventricular tachycardia
	Premature ventricular extrasystoles
	Tachyarrhythmias of digitalis intoxication
	Resistant tachyarrhythmias of excess catecholamine action during anesthesia
	Reduction of mortality after myocardial infarction
	Migraine headache prophylaxis
	Hypertrophic subaortic stenosis
	Pheochromocytoma
Metoprolol	Hypertension
	Angina pectoris
	Reduction of mortality after myocardial infarction
Nadolol	Angina pectoris
	Hypertension
Acebutolol	Hypertension
	Ventricular premature beats
Atenolol	Hypertension
	Angina pectoris
	Reduction of mortality after myocardial infarction
Timolol	Hypertension
	Reduction of mortality after myocardial infarction
	Topically to reduce intraocular pressure
Pindolol	Hypertension
Labetalol	Hypertension
Esmolol	Supraventricular tachycardia
	Sinus tachycardia (noncompensatory)
Betaxolol	Hypertension
	Topically to reduce intraocular pressure
Levobunolol	Topically to reduce intraocular pressure
Oxprenolol	Hypertension (not marketed)
Carteolol	Hypertension
Penbutolol	Hypertension

TABLE 7-2. Properties of Beta Blockers

Drug	Beta Receptor Blocked (Cardiac Selectivity)	Membrane Stabilizing Activity	Intrinsic Sympathomimetic Activity	Lipid Solubility	Serum Half-Life (HR)	Duration of Action (HR)	Protein Binding (%)	Usual Oral Dosage Range (Mg/Day)
Acebutolol	1[e,f]	+	+	Low	7–10	24	26	400–1800
Alprenolol[a]	1 & 2	+	+	High	2–3	NA	85	200–800
Atenolol	1[e]	—	—	Low	5–9	24	6–16	100–200
Betaxolol[c]	1[e]	—	—	Mod	12–22	23–25	50–60	10–40
Bevantolol[a,b]	1[e]	±	—	Mod	2	>24	NA	150–400
Bisoprolol[a]	1[e]	—	—	NA	10–12	24	NA	2.5–40
Bopindolol[a]	1 & 2	±	+	Mod	4–5	72–96	NA	4[g]
Bufentolol[a]	1 & 2	+	—	Low	NA	NA	NA	30
Bupranolol[a]	1 & 2	+	—	Mod	2	NA	80–90	60
Carteolol	1 & 2	—	+	Low	5–7	72	NA	15–30
Celiprolol[a,b]	1[e]	NA	+	Mod	4–6	24	NA	200–600
Esmolol	1[e]	—	—	Low	9(min)	10–20(min)	55	None
Labetalol[b]	1 & 2	+	—	Mod	3–4	8–12	50	150–1200
Levobunolol[c]	1 & 2	—	—	High	6.1	>24	NA	2–4
Mepindolol[a]	1 & 2	+	+	Mod	4	>24	50–60	10

7. PHARMACOLOGY AND PHARMACOKINETICS OF BETA BLOCKERS

Drug	Beta Receptor Blocked (Cardiac Selectivity)	Membrane Stabilizing Activity	Intrinsic Sympathomimetic Activity	Lipid Solubility	Serum Half-Life (HR)	Duration of Action (HR)	Protein Binding (%)	Usual Oral Dosage Range (Mg/Day)
Metoprolol	1[e]	±	—	Mod	2–6	10–12	13	150–400
Nadolol	1 & 2	—	—	Low	14–24	39	20	80–240
Oxprenolol[a]	1 & 2	+	++	Mod	2–5	13	80	160–320
Penbutolol	1 & 2	+	+	High	12–20	>24	99	40–60
Pindolol	1 & 2	±	+++	Low	3–4	8	57	10–20
Practolol[a,d]	1[e]	—	++	Low	6–8	12–24	NA	400–800
Propranolol	1 & 2	++	—	High	3.5–6	11	90	160–320
Sotalol[a]	1 & 2	—	—	Low	5–13	24	5	240–480
Timolol[c]	1 & 2	—	—	Mod	3–4	15	10	15–45
Tolamolol[a,b]	1[e]	—	+	High	2–3	10–12	NA	200–400

+ Present
— Absent
± Weak to variable response
Mod Moderate
NA Data not available
[a] Not currently marketed in the United States
[b] Has postsynaptic alpha-1-adrenergic blocking ability
[c] Available in the United States as ophthalmic dosage form
[d] Withdrawn from European market because of toxicity
[e] Blocks beta-2 receptors at higher doses of therapeutic range
[f] The major metabolite diacetolol may not be cardioselective (see text)
[g] Has been dosed effectively as one 12 mg oral dose per week for hypertension

TABLE 7-3. *Absorption Characteristics of Beta Blockers*

Drug	Absorption (% of Dose)	Bioavailability (% of Dose)	Time to Peak Concentration (HR)
Acebutolol	90	40	3–4
Atenolol	50	40	2–4
Metoprolol	95	50	0.5–1.5
Nadolol	30	30	1–4
Pindolol	>90	>90	1.5–2
Propranolol	90	30	1–3
Timolol	90	50	1–3
Oxprenolol	90	30	0.5–1
Labetalol	>90	25	1–2

prandial hepatic blood flow resulting in saturation of the first-pass metabolism [137]. However, the magnitude of these effects was insufficient to explain fully the increase in bioavailability. The oral absorption characteristics of the beta blockers are given in Table 7-3.

Timolol is administered topically to the eye for the treatment of chronic open angle glaucoma (Timoptic, MSD). After instillation into the conjunctival sac, timolol is absorbed through the conjunctival capillaries and mucous membranes of the nasal and gastrointestinal tract [2]. Serum concentrations of timolol ranging from 3 to 10 ng/ml were found with prolonged ophthalmic use every 12 hours for 5 days in a minority of the subjects [3]. These concentrations are approximately equal to the values obtained at 6 to 8 hours after an oral dose of 10 mg of timolol [144, 159].

Distribution

All of the beta blockers are rapidly and widely distributed, as evidenced by apparent volumes of distribution in excess of physiologic volumes. The volume of distribution is a proportionality constant relating the amount of drug in the body to the serum concentration. The smaller the serum concentration for a given dose, the larger the volume of distribution, suggesting accumulation in peripheral tissues. The more lipid soluble the beta blocker, the larger the volume of distribution. The volume of distribution for propranolol and metoprolol, for example, is approximately 5.6 l/kg [59, 115], while less lipid soluble beta blockers such as atenolol and nadolol have apparent volumes of distribution of 0.17 and 0.31 l/kg, respectively [88, 126].

Distribution of beta blockers to the central nervous system deserves special consideration. Lipid solubility, as defined by drug partitioning into octanol:water (pH 7), is well correlated with spinal fluid:serum concentration ratios. This indicates that lipid solubility is a major determinant of, at least, initial central nervous system penetration. Studies of propranolol in animal models show that concentrations in the serum and central nervous system follow a similar time sequence, indicating that lipid solubility may also be a major determinant of removal of beta blockers from the central nervous system [79]. Less lipid soluble agents, such as atenolol and nadolol, may penetrate the central nervous system more slowly but show more accumulation. Atenolol continues to accumulate in the cerebrospinal fluid for 4 days after initiating therapy [138]. When taken on a chronic basis, all beta blockers can be expected to accumulate in the central nervous system. Clinical and animal studies suggest that the concentrations of the least lipid soluble agents are adequate to produce near maximal central nervous system pharmacologic responses [57, 120]. Whether the less lipid soluble beta blockers offer a significant advantage by decreasing central nervous system side effects in clinical practice remains to be proven.

Metabolism (Biotransformation) and Elimination

The metabolism of the beta blockers is relevant to dosing considerations, and the agents will be discussed individually. The more lipophilic agents undergo extensive hepatic metabolism and show low bioavailability despite almost complete absorption. Agents with low lipid solubility are much less dependent on hepatic biotransformation, while pindolol is eliminated relatively equally by hepatic and renal mechanisms. The hepatic metabolism of the beta blockers is a result of biotransformation by the cytochrome P-450 mixed oxidase function enzymes, which accounts for the large first-pass metabolism of the lipophilic beta blockers. Some patients can be identified as rapid or slow metabolizers of the lipid soluble beta blockers based on their ability to metabolize debrisoquine. The ability to hydroxylate debrisoquine is polymorphically distributed and inherited as an autosomal recessive trait [42, 112]. The percentage of poor debrisoquine metabolizers is 1 percent in Arabs, 9 percent in the caucasian population of Britain, and may be up to 30 percent of Hong Kong Chinese [42, 83]. Poor hydroxylators of debrisoquine are poor metabolizers of many of the lipophilic beta blockers. Therefore, these agents will show greater bioavailability and reduced clearance, which could result in excessive pharmacologic action with usual dosage regimens (Fig. 7-1).

Acebutolol is metabolized to diacetolol. Both of these are present as enantiomers but neither appears to undergo stereoselective metabolism [121]. Diacetolol is pharmacologically active and of equal potency to acebutolol in some animal models [11] and accumulates to levels two to three times that of the parent compound during chronic oral dosing [158, 160]. Both acebutolol and diacetolol are eliminated in the bile and

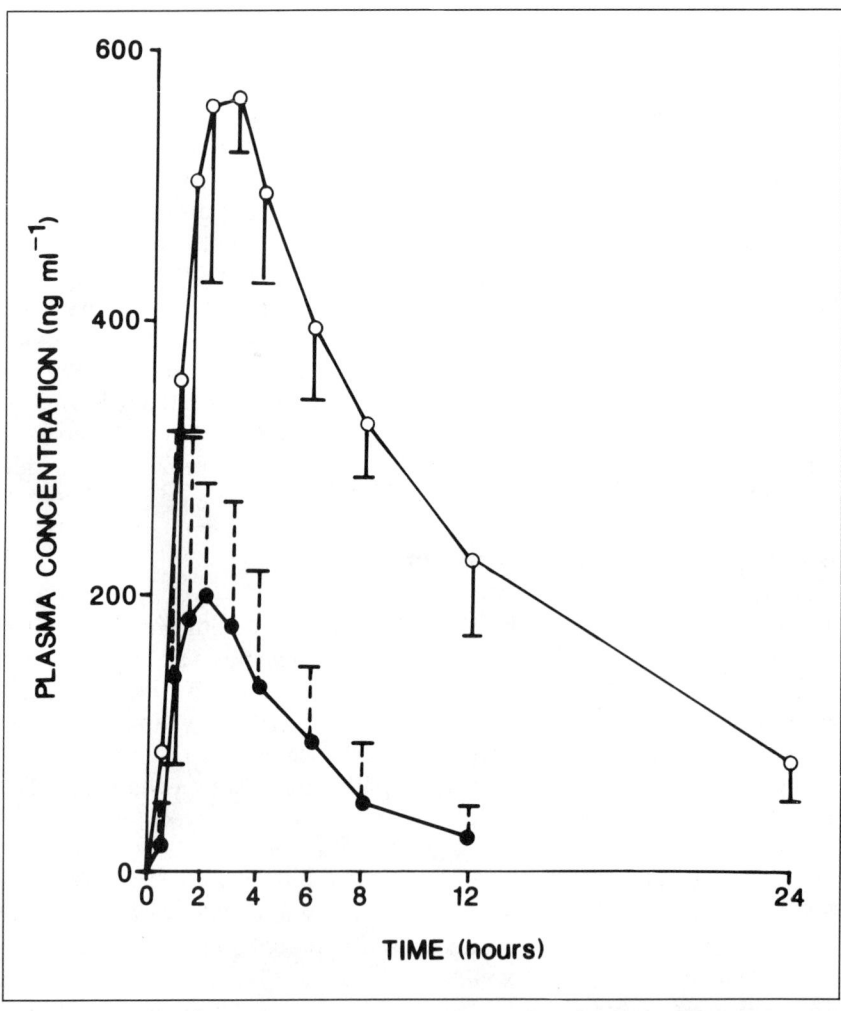

FIG. 7-1. Plasma metoprolol concentrations as a function of time in extensive (○) and poor (●) hydroxylators of debrisoquine. Data represented are mean with vertical bars for standard deviation. (From Ref. 83, with permission.)

perhaps actively transported across the intestinal wall [6, 54, 58, 72, 97]. These multiple routes of elimination may explain why there is no accumulation of these substances in renal failure [118].

Atenolol is metabolized to only a small extent by hydroxylation and subsequent conjugation with glucuronic acid [114]. The interindividual variation in the relationship between the serum concentration and the dose is four- to sixfold, which is much less than with many other beta blockers. Atenolol can accumulate in renal failure since its renal clearance correlates well with creatinine clearance [90]. The half-life of atenolol in renal failure is 70 to 100 hours, but it declines to 7.5 hours during hemodialysis [46, 90].

Nadolol metabolism is negligible [34, 150]. Up to 60 to 80 percent of nadolol appears in the urine and feces as unchanged drug after oral dosing. Excretion of nadolol in the bile may account for elimination of as much 40 percent of the dose [38]. The half-life of elimination for nadolol in functionally anephric patients was found to have a mean of 44.7 hours with a range of 32.2 to 68.6 hours and was probably dependent largely on biliary excretion [62]. The renal clearance of nadolol correlates with creatinine clearance for patients with varying degrees of renal dysfunction [62].

Timolol is metabolized by the cytochrome P-450 system, which accounts for up to 80 percent of the elimination of an oral dose [7, 65, 143]. The clearance of timolol is reduced in slow metabolizers of debrisoquine [7]. Since only 20 percent of the parent compound is excreted by nonhepatic pathways, the renal elimination of timolol has not been extensively studied. No dosage changes are required in renal failure [85].

Esmolol is unique in that the ester linkage is hydrolyzed by blood esterases, resulting in an elimination half-life of 9 minutes. The acid metabolite has 1/1500 the activity of the parent compound and an elimination half-life of 3.7 hours. The esterases responsible for the metabolism of esmolol are found in the cytosol of the red blood cells; however, plasma components are needed for full expression of metabolic efficiency. Within 24 hours of termination of an intravenous infusion, 73 to 88 percent of the dosage was excreted in the urine. Less than 2 percent of the unchanged parent compound was recovered from the urine [133].

Propranolol is eliminated almost exclusively by hepatic biotransformation, with the total body clearance being directly related to hepatic blood flow and intrinsic clearance or activity of the cytochrome P-450 system [75, 131]. The high-affinity low-capacity cytochrome P-450 enzyme system can become saturated during oral absorption resulting in nonlinear kinetic profiles [43, 89, 127, 153]. Another factor that could contribute to the dose-dependent nonlinear absorption kinetics of propranolol is propranolol's ability to inhibit its own metabolism through a decreased cardiac output and reduced hepatic blood flow [103]. A reduction in the activity of hepatic enzymes by propranolol or one of the many metabolites could be another explanation [122]. Some debate surrounds these models since other investigators have failed to reproduce the results [19, 25, 155]. This confusion may result from the dose-dependent kinetics described as linear kinetics for propranolol doses of 160 to 960 mg/day and nonlinear for doses between 40 and 160 mg/day

[147, 153]. The possibility of real nonlinear kinetics is supported by the accumulation of propranolol in clinical studies [43]. The interpatient variability of the dose to serum concentration relationship of propranolol may be as high as twentyfold following oral administration [26, 141, 145]. Patients greater than 65 years of age have diminished clearance of propranolol compared to younger patients [22, 24, 147]. Both decreased hepatic blood flow and intrinsic clearance may be responsible [22, 147]. Smoking is a known inducer of the cytochrome P-450 system and increases the intrinsic clearance of propranolol [146, 147]. Oxidation by the cytochrome P-450 system produces 4-hydroxypropranolol [151]. However, accumulation of metabolites does not occur [105, 153] except, perhaps, in renal disease [142, 154]. The ability to metabolize propranolol to 4-hydroxypropranolol is directly related to ability to hydroxylate debrisoquine [112]. As much as 20 percent of a dose of propranolol may be eliminated via nonrenal routes. Total urinary recovery of unchanged propranolol is less than 1 percent of the dose [67] and is decreased further by increasing the urine pH from 5 to 8 [73]. Elimination of propranolol is decreased in renal insufficiency [123, 146]. There may be as much as a tenfold increase in the glucuronide form of the metabolites with decreased renal function [15, 123]. The half-life of propranolol does not change in renal impairment [142], but the bioavailability appears to increase [15, 84]. This is seen in patients with renal failure who have a two- to threefold increase in serum concentration and a longer time to peak concentrations when compared to dialysis patients [15]. However, there appears to be little increase in effect from the parent drug or metabolites in renal failure, and dosage adjustments are not required. This may be because 4-hydroxypropranolol does not show altered kinetics in renal failure [142].

Metoprolol metabolism is similar to that of propranolol; however, it is not as extensively metabolized hepatically. Also, like propranolol, metoprolol has very large intrapatient variations in the relation between dose and serum concentration [47, 74, 125, 149]. The evidence for nonlinearity of metoprolol kinetics is less well documented than with propranolol [70, 149]. The effects of age and smoking on metoprolol metabolism are not well established. Slow debrisoquine metabolism predicts slow metoprolol metabolism [82, 83]. The alpha hydroxy metabolite appears as the major metabolite of metoprolol and is the only one of the eight metabolites to have been extensively studied [18]. The elimination of this metabolite appears to be correlated with creatinine clearance [64]. Only 3 to 5 percent of the oral dose is eliminated as unchanged metoprolol [116]. The bioavailability of metoprolol does not appear to be increased in renal failure, as is seen with propranolol [70]. However, the half-life of each of the metabolites of metoprolol is prolonged when the creatinine clearance falls below 5 ml/min. The metabolites of metoprolol are cleared by dialysis [64]. As with propranolol, there appears to be little need to adjust dosage regimens for renal failure [70].

ANCILLARY PROPERTIES

The following sections discuss the ancillary properties of beta blockers (see Table 7-2).

Cardiac Selectivity
Some of the marketed beta blockers, acebutolol, atenolol, betaxolol, esmolol, and metoprolol, show relative cardioselectivity. There is, however, controversy concerning the cardioselectivity of diacetolol, the major metabolite of acebutolol. In a double-blind crossover study, two doses of both propranolol and acebutolol were evaluated in ten men with reversible airway disease and hypertension. After 5 days of continuous treatment, no difference was found in the beta-1 or beta-2 blocking properties of the two drugs. This absence of cardioselectivity could possibly have been due to lack of beta-1 selectivity of diacetolol, which accumulated to two to three times the concentration of acebutolol [158].

Patients with any component of reactive airway disease are at risk for severe bronchospasm, and any beta blocker is at least relatively contraindicated [55, 69, 113, 128, 129, 130]. Bronchospasm has occurred in asthmatics [95] and some normal subjects [77, 96]. Patients with chronic obstructive lung disease are also at risk. It can be shown that cardioselective agents reduce forced expiratory volumes less than the nonselective agents in asthmatic patients [69]. However, there have been reports of bronchospasm with even low doses of selective agents, perhaps because of blockade of beta-1 receptors in the lung. The pulmonary effects of beta-adrenergic stimulants are blocked less with selective agents [31, 39, 69], and it may be beneficial to treat patients with a combination of a cardioselective beta blocker and a beta-2 selective agonist such as albuterol.

Membrane Stabilizing Activity
Membrane stabilizing activity is also referred to as local anesthetic or quinidine-like activity, and the effects on the action potential of the myocardial cell are shared by the type I antiarrhythmic agents. Propranolol is the beta blocker with the most membrane stabilizing activity; however, acebutolol, metoprolol, pindolol, oxprenolol, and labetalol all have some degree of membrane stabilizing activity. Unlike the beta blocker activity, the membrane stabilizing activity does not show stereoselectivity.

It has been found that high plasma concentrations of beta blockers show electrophysiological effects in humans that are unrelated to their beta blocker properties. The effects observed were shortening of both the ventricular refractory period and the nonphasic action potential. The overall effect was to increase the ratio of the ventricular effective refractory period to the monophasic action potential duration [36]. Total (free + plasma protein bound) propranolol concentrations of 200 to 1000 ng/ml have antiarrhythmic effects that are not seen with the usual doses. In a study by Woosley et al. [163], 40 percent of the patients who had ventricular tachyarrhythmias responsive to propranolol had serum concentrations of at least 150 ng/ml. It is conceivable that these concentrations may be achievable in clinical practice. The electrophysiologic effects of high concentrations of d-propranolol have been compared to lower concentrations of the racemic mixture (d,l-propranolol). Concentrations of approximately 980 ng/ml of d-propranolol possessed greater electrophysiological effects than d,l-propranolol at concentrations of 34 ng/ml, while the degree of beta blockade was similar [37]. These studies are of great interest and suggest that the membrane stabilizing activity of beta blockers may be exploitable in the treatment of ventricular tachyarrhythmias.

The ocular effects of membrane stabilizing activity of beta blockers chronically applied to the eye may have clinical relevance. The three beta blockers marketed for the reduction of intraocular pressure (timolol, levobunolol, and betaxolol) lack significant membrane stabilizing activity when compared to propranolol. However, timolol may have more membrane stabilizing or local anesthetic activity than levobunolol or betaxolol, and this could be important with chronic daily use for glaucoma. The local anesthetic action of timolol has been implicated in cases of reduced corneal sensitivity after continuous long-term use. More extensive use of levobunolol or betaxolol will be required to demonstrate a significantly lower incidence of this topical reaction.

Intrinsic Sympathomimetic Activity

Intrinsic sympathomimetic activity is an ancillary property of the beta blockers that has recently been evaluated. There are three beta blockers with intrinsic sympathomimetic activity. In decreasing order of potency, they are pindolol, oxprenolol, and acebutolol [28, 91].

In norepinephrine-depleted animals at rest and supine, some beta blockers have partial beta-adrenergic agonist activity [91]. This seemingly paradoxical property can be explained on the basis of current understanding of the beta receptor model (Chapter 4).

The value of beta blockers with intrinsic sympathomimetic activity in patients prone to congestive heart failure has been discussed. Subjects at rest and in the supine position showed less decrease in cardiac output when given beta blockers with intrinsic sympathomimetic activity [110, 136]. However, the degree to which cardiac output is dependent on increased sympathetic tone is higher in patients with congestive heart failure and any beta blocker would act more as an antagonist than as a partial agonist under these conditions. The increase in sympathetic tone is a compensatory condition in congestive heart failure; whether interruption of this mechanism is beneficial remains controversial.

Beta blockers without intrinsic sympathomimetic activity have been shown to produce a decrease in ejection fraction in patients with normal cardiac function at rest while pindolol did not cause such a decrease [76]. Whether this is a result of decreased total peripheral resistance or beta-1 intrinsic sympathomimetic activity is not clear. Further, the implication that pindolol is advantageous in patients with congestive heart failure is an extrapolation beyond these data generated in normal subjects.

Propranolol, a beta blocker without intrinsic sympathomimetic activity, causes an increase in pulmonary capillary wedge pressure and cardiopulmonary blood volume, whereas oxprenolol and pindolol caused only slight or no increases in these parameters when hypertensive patients were studied [86].

The hemodynamic effects of intravenous acebutolol were studied in seven patients with normal cardiac innervation who had undergone coronary artery bypass surgery and four who had received cardiac transplants and had denervated hearts. Similar mean responses were observed in all parameters measured except cardiac output, which decreased only in the bypass group [87]. The magnitude of the decrease in cardiac output seen with acebutolol is between that seen with propranolol and pindolol [135].

The intrinsic sympathomimetic activity of some of the beta blockers may be an advantage in some subjects who require a beta blocker but have some component of reactive airway disease. A multicenter trial showed that the reported incidence of dyspnea for pindolol [117] was less than has been reported for atenolol [125]. However, the comparison of reported incidences of side effects in different trials should be interpreted with caution. While some authors report benefits of intrinsic sympathomimetic activity in patients with reactive airway disease [14, 23], others disagree [1]. There has been a report of the successful use of pindolol for treatment of supraventricular tachycardia in patients who experienced bronchospasm while taking propranolol [52]. However, since the beta-2 intrinsic sympathomimetic activity affinity for pindolol is higher than the beta-1 affinity, it could require higher doses of a beta agonist to reverse bronchospasm if it should occur.

The use of beta blockers with intrinsic sympathomimetic activity for secondary intervention of myocardial infarction has raised concern. Recent trials of beta blockers with intrinsic sympathomimetic activity have shown little effect on the reduction of morbidity or mortality [10, 41, 139]. Further, a recent retrospective review that pooled all the data from trials of beta blockers after myocardial infarction suggests that, overall, there is a 30 percent reduction in the incidence of death after a myocardial infarction when using a beta blocker without intrinsic sympathomimetic activity and only a 10 percent reduction with drugs possessing intrinsic sympathomimetic activity [164]. These studies have been small; however, it seems prudent to choose agents with proven benefit for use in postmyocardial infarction. There are theoretical advantages to selecting beta blockers with intrinsic sympathomimetic activity rather than those lacking it for other indications. Blood flow in extremities may be decreased less when beta blockers with intrinsic sympathomimetic activity are used [104]. Acebutolol decreases total peripheral resistance more than propranolol whether given orally or intravenously [71, 161]. Pindolol is well known to decrease blood pressure by decreasing total peripheral resistance without changing cardiac output, while other beta blockers, such as metoprolol, decrease blood pressure by lowering cardiac output and may even increase total peripheral resistance in hypertensive patients [136]. This reduction in total peripheral resistance appears to be a significant advantage in the treatment of hypertension in subjects who cannot tolerate a decrease in cardiac output. Also, the decrease in birth weight of neonates born to mothers treated with beta blockers may result from a decrease in placental blood flow [78]. Further, neonatal bradycardia may be less of a problem when the mother is treated with beta blockers with intrinsic sympathomimetic activity [35, 119]. Whether intrinsic sympathomimetic activity is also of significant benefit in patients with Raynaud's phenomenon also remains to be proven. Lastly, some beta blockers are known to increase serum lipoproteins [30]. This does not appear to be the case with acebutolol in hypertensive patients treated for 6 months [80].

Protein Binding and Lipophilicity

Together, the properties of plasma protein binding and lipophilicity determine the volume of distribution of the beta blocker drugs. Protein binding and lipophilicity do not depend on each other, however. For example, metoprolol and propranolol are both lipophilic drugs but are about 10 and 90 percent protein bound, respectively [29].

The plasma protein binding of these drugs cannot be attributed solely to serum albumin binding [44]. Beta blockers are weak bases that bind to acute phase reactants such as alpha-1-acid glycoprotein (AAG). This is being recognized as an important characteristic of the beta blockers [13, 107]. While serum albumin concentrations can be altered, the change takes a relatively long period compared to the change of AAG. A change of AAG can acutely change the free fraction of the beta blockers and alter their pharmacologic action [108]. The plasma protein binding of propranolol and oxprenolol is greater than 90 percent for both drugs. When each is incubated with AAG alone, they are approximately 70 percent bound, but with albumin alone, propranolol is 55 percent bound and oxprenolol is 23 percent bound [13]. The extent of binding of metoprolol and atenolol is not greatly affected by AAG since they bind only slightly to either serum albumin or AAG [13].

Since propranolol is widely used, highly protein bound in plasma, and has its pharmacologic response determined by its free fraction, changes in protein binding may be significant, especially with intravenous use where plasma concentrations may be high. It has been reported that the free fraction of propranolol, which is difficult to determine, is inversely proportional to AAG concentrations [108]. Increases in AAG have been determined to decrease the free fraction of propranolol in acute trauma, inflammatory diseases such as rheumatoid arthritis, and during surgery [48, 106]. Further, the active l-isomer of propranolol appears to bind to a greater extent than the d-isomer to AAG [4, 157]. Both these effects could decrease the action of propranolol. Renal failure and liver dysfunction both increase the free fraction of propranolol and could lead to an exaggerated response. Although these changes will be difficult to measure, they can be managed by the judicious monitoring of heart rate and blood pressure.

Alpha Blockade

Labetalol has been reviewed in depth elsewhere [50]. It is unique among the available beta blockers in that it also possesses the ability to block alpha-adrenergic receptors. It has been suggested that the increase in total peripheral resistance seen with administration of beta blockers is a result of unopposed alpha activity. With its additional property, labetalol has the ability to act as a vasodilator and does not decrease cardiac output. Labetalol has about one-tenth the activity of phentolamine as an alpha blocker and one-fourth the activity of propranolol as a beta blocker [50]. Labetalol is, therefore, a more potent beta blocker than alpha blocker.

The addition of alpha blockade to beta blockers has been described as a potential benefit in the treatment of angina [63, 101]. The intravenous administration of labetalol has increased the treadmill walking time of patients [16]. Further, administration of 300 to 1200 mg daily of labetalol to hypertensive patients with angina has been shown to produce a significant reduction in blood pressure and heart rate. A significant reduction in angina frequency and a significant increase in treadmill walking time were apparent at a mean dose of 1050 mg per day compared to placebo [53].

PHARMACODYNAMICS

Dose- or Plasma-Concentration Relationships

The study of pharmacokinetics attempts to relate the action (efficacy or adverse effects) of drugs to measurable pharmacokinetic parameters.

The closer the relationship between the drug action and the parameters, the more useful the therapeutic drug monitoring is in predicting therapeutic success or failure. Therapeutic drug monitoring is critical for drugs with a narrow therapeutic index and without easy clinical parameters to monitor. For the beta blockers, the relationship between the response and the serum concentration is far from optimal, but there are readily available clinical monitoring parameters (i.e., heart rate and blood pressure). These monitoring parameters, however, have no relationship to other actions of the beta blockers, such as membrane stabilizing ability. The study of pharmacokinetics has revealed information relevant to the understanding of these drugs and the processes involved in disease.

A clear result of pharmacokinetic studies is that the duration of action for the beta blockers far exceeds that which would be predicted on the basis of the serum half-life [8, 9, 21, 27, 45, 68]. There is also a large variation in the plasma concentration needed to produce most effects of the beta blockers [49, 149]. The explanation for these observations relates to several factors. First, individual patients have different levels of sympathetic tone [51]. In fact, the level of sympathetic tone is dynamic and is expected to vary. Second, the dose-response curve for many beta blockers is flat for many effects [67]. An explanation that may relate to the flat dose-response curves is that some beta blockers produce active metabolites that may accumulate [67, 126]. Quantification of metabolites is not always done and the ratio of active to inactive isomers is rarely measured. The 4-hydroxy metabolite of propranolol is active but it does not accumulate [123, 152, 153]. On the other hand, the active metabolite of acebutolol (diacetolol) has a half-life two to four times longer than the parent drug, accumulates to two to three times the parent's concentration, and is more active [6, 160, 166]. Another possible explanation for the flat dose-response curves that have been investigated for propranolol is differences in free and bound drug [132]. Since drug effects are determined by free drug concentrations, if the free concentrations do not increase in proportion to increases in total dose, the response curve could flatten.

Beta Blockade

A relationship has been described for serum concentration and negative chronotropic effects during conditions of increased sympathetic tone for several beta blockers. These studies show a relationship between the serum concentration of the beta blockers and suppression of the increase in heart rate during exercise or after administration of isoproterenol [8, 27, 60, 66, 165]. The results of these studies are not identical since the increase in sympathetic tone is not equivalent following these different methods. Further, a lower dose of isoproterenol is required to increase heart rate after selective beta blockers since the nonselective agents block isoproterenol-induced vasodilation. This correlation is in contrast to the lack of such a relationship at rest [109, 145], probably because of variable resting sympathetic tone. The correlation between free drug concentration and beta blockade response is superior to that with total drug concentration for propranolol [92]. While most studies show a far longer duration of action than would be predicted by serum half-life, some investigators have found a relationship between duration of effect and serum concentration during chronic dosing [148]. This is especially true for beta blockers that show accumulation such as propranolol and metoprolol as opposed to atenolol, timolol, and pindolol, which do not accumulate. The result of increasing serum concentrations beyond that required for maximal beta blockade would be to increase the duration of action. For metoprolol, the duration of effect was found to be 13.2 hours and 19.2 hours for 50 mg and 200 mg doses, respectively. Similar effects have been described for timolol [17], propranolol [93], and pindolol [56]. However, there is a linear relationship between the serum concentration and beta blockade for pindolol under the condition of increased sympathetic tone after isoproterenol administration [56].

Antianginal Effects

The mechanism of action for the beta blockers in angina is to decrease heart rate and contractility, thereby decreasing myocardial oxygen demand. Therefore, one would expect a similar relationship between serum concentration and antianginal effect as is seen with beta blockade. This appears to be the case. There is a linear relationship between the serum concentration and the increase in treadmill walking time or frequency of angina [5, 66, 140]. For propranolol, the antianginal effects are apparent at 30 ng/ml [5, 109]. Others have found that the maximal antianginal effects are seen at 14 to 90 ng/ml [109], while a flat dose-response relationship was found for doses of propranolol of 160 versus 80 ng [141]. A sustained duration of action beyond what would be predicted on the basis of serum half-life has been shown for propranolol [140, 141]. This effect has been of value clinically since propranolol can be dosed twice daily for angina [140, 141]. However, once daily dosing may be less effective [12].

The dose-effect relationship for beta blockers and myocardial contractility has received little attention because of the difficulty of assessment and the contraindication of beta blockers in patients with poor systolic function. No correlation of ejection fraction or regional wall motion was found for doses of 160 or 480 ng/day of propranolol [100]. However, velocity of circumferential fiber shortening, assessed by echocardiography, was related to the serum concentration of propranolol and indicates that both the inotropic and chronotropic blockade were important in increasing exercise duration in angina patients [20].

Hypertension

The duration of antihypertensive effect for beta blockers is longer than would be expected on the basis of serum half-life [27, 32] and often lasts as long as 24 hours. There generally is a poor concentration-response relationship for the beta blockers in hypertension [81, 82, 102, 149], although some investigators show a good correlation [40]. Whether a beta blocker drug has a flat or steep dose-response curve for hypertension is a function of the drug. The dose-response relationship for atenolol in hypertension is flat [33, 102] between doses of 75 and 600 mg [102]. The dose-response relationship for propranolol is steeper [81]. Labetalol was studied between doses of 300 and 1200 mg; it was found that maximal reduction in blood pressure was at 900 mg/day, while maximal negative chronotropic effect was at 600 mg/day [53].

Antiarrhythmic Effects

The use of beta blockers as antiarrhythmic agents is covered earlier in this chapter. Serum concentration- or dose-response relationships for complex ventricular tachyarrhythmias will be discussed here. Blockade of catecholamines, which are arrhythmogenic, occurs at low doses while the membrane stabilizing activity occurs at high plasma concentrations. A complete suppression of ventricular arrhythmias in 10 of 15 patients revealed that 4 of 15 responded below 100 ng/ml of propranolol while 6 of 15 required concentrations greater than 300 ng/ml [163]. Further studies comparing propranolol to placebo showed that 24 of 32 patients had a 70 to 100 percent suppression of ventricular arrhythmias between 12 and 100 ng/ml [162]. For metoprolol, suppression of complex ectopy was seen at 72 ng/ml [111]. No serum concentration-response relationship could be shown for atenolol in a mixed group of patients with simple or complex ventricular ectopy [99].

Adverse Effects

No relationship for dose or serum concentration has been established for adverse effects of the beta blockers. Few prospective studies are done with pharmacokinetics of adverse effects. The occurrence of adverse effects with beta blockers seems to be highly patient-specific.

Dosing Guidelines

This section will cover practical dosing guidelines for beta blockers with primary emphasis on ischemic heart disease. The beginning dosage regimen will be followed by the titration schedule and recommendations will be given for usually accepted maximal dosages. Not all beta blockers have identical indications. Therefore, when in question, agents with well-documented evidence in the literature of efficacy should be chosen for any given indication. It is important to remember that maximal and optimal dosages are not necessarily the same. When patients are already taking medication with similar actions or if the patient is intolerant, lower drug dosages will be required. Where appropriate, guidelines will be discussed for alteration of dosage regimens in special physiologic conditions such as renal failure. When beta blockers are to be discontinued, the dose should be tapered over 1 to 2 weeks with close supervision.

The most often used parameter to monitor the beta blockers is the heart rate. However, the effect of beta blockade on the heart rate will not necessarily reflect antihypertensive effects or antiarrhythmic effects. When decreased heart rate is used to optimize dosage regimens for antianginal effects, differing effects on resting and exercise heart rate should be considered. Generally, the goal in angina is to decrease the resting heart rate to 60 beats per minute or lower while maintaining an adequate cardiac output. When this is done, the increase in heart rate with modest exercise will be 20 percent or less. When a patient's heart rate increases to 80 beats per minute or greater with modest exercise, such as walking the halls, the dosage is not optimized. It is usually possible to increase the dosage and see a greater decrease in the exercise heart rate than in the resting heart rate. The heart rate during sleep is under vagal control and is not relevant to optimization of the beta blocker dosage.

Beta blockers are used in combination and as monotherapy for appropriate patients with hypertension. The maximal doses of beta blockers are usually not required to optimize combination antihypertensive regimens. The blood pressure should be taken at the end of a dosing interval to assure optimal control is maintained.

The use of beta blockers in prevention of secondary complications of myocardial infarction deserves special note. The studies of the empirical use of beta blockers as secondary intervention of myocardial infarction have shown a significant reduction in morbidity and mortality. However, it is important to realize that the mechanism of action is yet to be elucidated and there are no reliable parameters to monitor to ensure beneficial outcomes. Therefore, it is prudent to use only those agents approved for use after myocardial infarction, employing the recommended dosage.

Dosing Schedule

PROPRANOLOL (INDERAL)
The initial dosage regimen for propranolol for angina is 10 to 20 mg three to four times daily; for hypertension, 40 mg twice daily; for secondary intervention in myocardial infarction, 40 to 80 mg three to four times daily; and for IHSS, 20 to 40 mg three to four times daily is used. The titration schedules used for dosage adjustments are: for angina,

increases of 10 to 40 mg per day every 3 to 7 days; for hypertension, increases of 10 to 40 mg per day every 1 to 4 weeks; and for arrhythmias and IHSS, the adjustment schedule used for angina is appropriate. The maximal recommended dosage per day of propranolol is: for angina, 320 mg; for hypertension, 640 mg; and for myocardial infarction intervention, 240 mg. There is no established maximum for propranolol in the treatment of arrhythmias or IHSS.

Intravenous propranolol is used in the treatment of life-threatening arrhythmias. Doses of 1 to 3 mg may be given intravenously at a rate not to exceed 1 mg/min, while monitoring blood pressure and electrocardiogram. More specifically, a test dose of 0.1 to 0.15 mg may be given intravenously followed by doses of 0.5 to 0.75 mg every 1 to 2 minutes. The maximum intravenous dose recommended is 5 mg in anesthetized patients and 10 mg in conscious patients.

METOPROLOL (LOPRESSOR)

For angina, 50 to 100 mg two to three times daily is a reasonable initial dosage regimen for angina. The dosage adjustments are 50 mg to 100 mg per day every 3 to 7 days.

For hypertension, 100 mg per day is given, but may be divided into 50 mg twice daily. Dosage adjustments are made by increasing the dose by 50 to 100 mg daily every 1 to 4 weeks, up to a maximum of 450 mg per day.

For early intervention in myocardial infarction, three intravenous bolus injections of 5 mg each are given at 2-minute intervals, while heart rate, blood pressure, and ECG are monitored. If the patient tolerates the full 15 mg dose, the maintenance dose is begun 15 minutes after the last intravenous dose. For the first 48 hours, 50 mg orally every 6 hours is given, followed by 100 mg twice daily. If the patient is unable to tolerate the full 15 mg dose (i.e., develops bradycardia or hypotension), the maintenance dose is begun 15 minutes after last intravenous dose with 25 to 50 mg orally every 6 hours for 48 hours. If the patient reaches the end points of bradycardia or hypotension with the first intravenous dose, 25 mg orally every 6 hours should be used. There are no guidelines for patients who reach these end points with the second dose; however, the authors have seen central nervous system toxicity with the larger maintenance dose and tend to use the lower dosage, depending on the degree of intolerance. If a patient becomes severely intolerant (symptomatic), treatment is discontinued.

For late intervention in myocardial infarction, 100 mg is given orally twice daily.

ATENOLOL (TENORMIN)

Atenolol is useful for angina, at doses of 50 or 100 mg given once daily by the oral route. This is similar to use in hypertension where 50 mg orally is given daily. If the response is not adequate after 14 days, the dose is doubled. The dose-response schedule is flat, and there is rarely a need for doses greater than 100 mg per day. Dosage adjustments are recommended for patients with renal dysfunction. For a creatinine clearance of 15 to 35 ml/min/1.73m^2, 50 mg per day is recommended. For a creatinine clearance of less than 15 ml/min/1.73m^2, 50 mg every other day is recommended. For patients undergoing hemodialysis, 50 mg after each dialysis session is given under hospital supervision.

The intravenous form of atenolol (5mg/ml) may be used for treatment of an acute myocardial infarction. Treatment is begun by giving 5 mg intravenously over 5 minutes followed by a second 5 mg dose in 10 minutes with continuous monitoring of heart rate and blood pressure. If the patient tolerates the full 10 mg intravenous dose, 50 mg should be given orally 10 minutes after the second intravenous dose. Another 50 mg oral dose should be given in 12 hours. Thereafter 100 mg daily or 50 mg twice daily should be given for 6 to 9 days or until time of hospital discharge. An alternative to use of the intravenous product is to give oral doses of 100 mg daily or 50 mg twice daily.

NADOLOL (CORGARD)
Nadolol is indicated for both angina and hypertension. The initial dosage regimen for both conditions is 40 mg orally daily and may be increased by 40 to 80 mg per day every 3 to 7 days. The maximum dosage recommended for angina is 240 mg per day and for hypertension is 320 mg per day. The dosage should be altered in renal failure by increasing the dosing interval. For a creatinine clearance of 50 ml/min/1.73m^2 or greater, the dosage interval is 24 hours. For creatinine clearances between 50 and 31 ml/min/1.73m^2, 24 to 36 hours is recommended for a dosage interval. For a creatinine clearance between 30 and 10 ml/min/1.73m^2, 24 to 48 hours is recommended. For a creatinine clearance less than 10 ml/min/1.73m^2, a dosage interval of 40 to 60 hours is recommended.

TIMOLOL (BLOCADREN)
The initial dosage for angina, hypertension, and myocardial infarction intervention is 10 mg orally twice daily. Dosages are adjusted by 10 to 20 mg per day every 7 days for angina and hypertension. The maximum dosage recommended for hypertension is 30 mg twice daily. The only dose studied in intervention of myocardial infarction is 10 mg orally twice daily.

ESMOLOL (BREVIBLOC)
Esmolol is given by intravenous infusion, with continuous monitoring of blood pressure and electrocardiogram, for the treatment of supraventricular tachycardia. The end point of a heart rate less than 100 beats/minute or normal sinus rhythm is used for efficacy and hypotension for toxicity.

Usually 5 g of esmolol is diluted in 500 ml of 5% dextrose or normal saline, yielding a final concentration of 10 mg/ml. The initial infusion rate is 500 mcg/kg/min for 1 minute followed by 50 mcg/kg/min for 4 minutes. If there is not an adequate response, the initial loading infusion rate of 500 mcg/kg/min is repeated for an additional minute and the maintenance infusion is increased by 50 mcg/kg/min. This procedure is repeated every 5 minutes until the desired response is achieved or a maintenance infusion of 200 mcg/kg/min is reached. If the heart rate slows dramatically or approaches the desired rate or if the patient becomes hypotensive, the loading dose may be omitted and/or the maintenance dose may be increased by 25 mcg/kg/min or less or the titration interval may be increased to 10 minutes.

The majority of patients respond at 200 mcg/kg/min or less and tolerate a 24-hour infusion well [134].

OXPRENOLOL

Doses of 160 mg twice daily have been shown to be effective in chronic stable angina. Daily doses of 160 to 300 mg per day are used for hypertension. Patients without adequate response to 200 mg per day are unlikely to respond to higher doses. However, doses up to 1260 mg per day have been used.

BETAXOLOL (KERLONE)

Betaxolol is another beta blocker used for systemic treatment of ischemic heart disease. Single doses of 5, 10, and 20 mg have been shown to be effective in increasing treadmill walking time and decreasing anginal pain.

REFERENCES

1. Addis, G. J., and Thorp, J. M. Effects of oxprenolol on the airways of normal and bronchitic subjects. *Eur. J. Clin. Pharmacol.* 9:259, 1976.
2. Adler, A. G., McElwain, G. E., Merli, G. J., and Martin, J. H. Systemic effects of eye drops. *Arch. Intern. Med.* 142:2293, 1982.
3. Affrime, M. B., Lowenthal, D. T., Tolbert, J. A., et al. Dynamics and kinetics of ophthalmic timolol. *Clin. Pharmacol. Ther.* 27:471, 1980.
4. Albani, F., Riva, R., Contin, M., and Baruzzi, A. Stereoselective binding of propranolol enantiomers to human alpha-1-acid glycoprotein and human plasma. *Br. J. Clin. Pharmacol.* 18:244, 1984.
5. Alderman, E. L., Davies, R. O., Crowley, J. J., et al. Dose response effectiveness of propranolol for the treatment of angina pectoris. *Circulation* 51:964, 1975.
6. Alexander, M. S., and Bianchine, J. R. Acebutolol kinetics following oral and intravenous administration in man. *Clin. Pharmacol. Ther.* 35:225, 1984.
7. Alvan, G., von Bahr, C., Seideman, P., and Sjoqvist, F. High plasma concentrations of beta-receptor blocking drugs and deficient debrisoquine hydroxylation. *Lancet* 1:333, 1982.
8. Amery, A., DePlaen, J. F., Lijnen, P., et al. Relationship between blood

level of atenolol and pharmacologic effect. *Clin. Pharmacol. Ther.* 21:691, 1977.
9. Anchong, M. R., Piafsky, K. M., and Ogilvie, R. I. Duration of cardiac effects on timolol and propranolol. *Clin. Pharmacol. Ther.* 19:148, 1976.
10. Australian and Swedish Pindolol Study Group. The effect of pindolol on the two-year mortality after complicated myocardial infarction. *Eur. Heart J.* 4:367, 1983.
11. Basil, B., and Jordan, R. Pharmacological properties of diacetolol (M&B 16,942), a major metabolite of acebutolol. *Eur. J. Pharmacol.* 80:47, 1982.
12. Beller, G. A., Bittar, N., Coelho, J. B., et al. Double-blind, placebo-controlled trial of propranolol given once, twice and four times daily in stable angina pectoris: A multicenter study using serial exercise testing. *Am. J. Cardiol.* 54:37, 1984.
13. Belpaire, F. M., Bogaert, M. G., and Rosseneu, M. Binding of beta-adrenoceptor blocking drugs to human serum albumin, to alpha-1-acid glycoprotein and to human serum. *Eur. J. Clin. Pharmacol.* 22:253, 1982.
14. Benson, M. K., Berrill, W. T., Cruickshank, J. M., and Sterling, G. S. A comparison of four beta-adrenoceptor antagonists in patients with asthma. *Br. J. Clin. Pharmacol.* 5:415, 1978.
15. Bianchetti, G., Graziani, G., Brancaccio, D., et al. Pharmacokinetics and effects of propranolol in terminal uraemic patients and in patients undergoing regular dialysis treatment. *Clin. Pharmacokinet.* 1:373, 1976.
16. Boakes, A. J., and Prichard, B. N. C. The effect of AH 5158, pindolol, propranolol, d-propranolol on acute exercise tolerance in angina pectoris. *Br. J. Pharmacol.* 47:673P, 1973.
17. Bobik, A., Jennings, G. L., Ashley, P., and Korner, P. I. Timolol pharmacokinetics and effects on heart rate and blood pressure after acute and chronic administration. *Eur. J. Clin. Pharmacol.* 16:243, 1979.
18. Borg, K. O., Carlsson, E., Hoffmann, K. J., et al. Metabolism of metoprolol-(^{3}H) in man, the dog and the rat. *Acta Pharmacol. Toxicol.* 36(Suppl V):125, 1975.
19. Borgstrom, L., Johansson, C. G., Larsson, H., and Lenander, R. Pharmacokinetics of propranolol. *J. Pharmacokinet. Biopharm.* 9:419, 1981.
20. Boudoulas, H., Beaver, B. M., Kates, R. E., and Lewis, R. P. Pharmacodynamics of inotropic and chronotropic responses to oral therapy with propranolol: Studies in normal subjects and patients with angina. *Chest* 73:146, 1978.
21. Boudoulas, H., Dervenagas, S., Lewis, R. P., et al. Time course of the blockade effect of propranolol on sinus node and atrioventricular node. *J. Clin. Pharmacol.* 19:95, 1979.
22. Brandfonbrener, M., Landowne, M., and Shock, N. W. Changes in cardiac output with age. *Circulation* 12:557, 1955.
23. Cannon, R. E., Slavin, R. G., and Gonasun, L. M. The effect on asthma of a new beta blocker, pindolol. *Am. Heart J.* 104:438, 1982.
24. Castleden, C. M., and George, C. F. The effect of aging on the hepatic clearance of propranolol. *Br. J. Clin. Pharmacol.* 7:49, 1979.
25. Chidsey, C. A., Morselli, P., Bianchetti, G., et al. Studies of the absorption and removal of propranolol in hypertensive patients during therapy. *Circulation* 52:313, 1975.
26. Chidsey, C. A., Morselli, P., and Zanchetti, A. Blood levels and pharmacokinetics studies of propranolol in chronic therapy. *Clin. Res.* 22:100A, 1974.
27. Coelho, J. B., Dvornik, D., Mulland, J. F., et al. Dynamics of propranolol dosing schedules. *Clin. Pharmacol. Ther.* 34:440, 1983.

28. Conolly, M. E., Kersting, F., and Dollery, C. T. The clinical pharmacology of beta-adrenoceptor-blocking drugs. *Progr. Cardiovasc. Dis.* 19:203, 1976.
29. Cruickshank, J. M. The clinical importance of cardioselectivity and lipophilicity in beta blockers. *Am. Heart J.* 100:160, 1980.
30. Day, J. L., Simpson, N., Metcalfe, J., and Page, R. L. Metabolic consequences of atenolol and propranolol in treatment of essential hypertension. *Br. Med. J.* 1:77, 1979.
31. Decalmer, P. B. S., Chatterjee, S. S., Cruickshank, J. M., et al. Beta-blockers and asthma. *Br. Heart J.* 40:184, 1978.
32. Douglas-Jones, A. P., Baber, N. S., and Lee, A. Once daily propranolol in the treatment of mild to moderate hypertension: A dose range finding study. *Eur. J. Clin. Pharmacol.* 14:163, 1978.
33. Douglas-Jones, A. P., and Cruickshank, J. M. Once daily dosing with atenolol in patients with mild or moderate hypertension. *Br. Med. J.* 1:990, 1976.
34. Dreyfuss, J., Brannick, L. J., Vukovich, R. A., et al. Metabolic studies in patients with nadolol: Oral and intravenous administration. *J. Clin. Pharmacol.* 17:300, 1977.
35. Dubois, D., Petitcolas, J., Temperville, B., et al. Treatment of hypertension in pregnancy with beta-adrenoceptor antagonists. *Br. J. Clin. Pharmacol.* 13(Suppl):375, 1982.
36. Duff, H. J., Roden, D. M., Leif, B., et al. Electrophysiologic actions of high plasma concentrations of propranolol in human subjects. *J. Am. Coll. Cardiol.* 2:1134, 1983.
37. Duff, H. J., Wood, A. J. J., Dawson, A. K., et al. d-Propranolol: Nonadrenergically mediated electrophysiologic actions in man. *Circulation* 66(Suppl II):II-372, 1982.
38. du Souich, P., Caille, G., and Larochelle, P. Enhancement of nadolol elimination by activated charcoal and antibiotics. *Clin. Pharmacol. Ther.* 33:585, 1983.
39. Ellis, M. E., Sahay, J. N., Chatterjee, S. S., et al. Cardioselectivity of atenolol in asthmatic patients. *Eur. J. Clin. Pharmacol.* 21:173, 1981.
40. Esler, M., Zweifler, A., Randall, O., and De Quattro, V. Pathophysiologic and pharmacokinetic determinants of the antihypertensive response to propranolol. *Clin. Pharmacol. Ther.* 22:299, 1977.
41. European Infarction Study Group. European Infarction Study (E.I.S.): A secondary beta-blocker prevention trial after myocardial infarction. *Circulation* 68(Suppl III):III-294, 1983.
42. Evans, D. A. P., Mahgoub, A., Sloan, T. P., et al. A family and population study of genetic polymorphism of debrisoquine oxidation in a white British population. *J. Med. Genet.* 17:102, 1980.
43. Evans, G. H., and Shand, D. G. Disposition of propranolol: Drug accumulation and steady-state concentrations during chronic oral administration in man. *Clin. Pharmacol. Ther.* 14:487, 1973.
44. Evans, G. H., and Shand, D. G. Disposition of propranolol: Independent variation in steady-state circulating drug concentrations and half-life as a result of plasma drug binding in man. *Clin. Pharmacol. Ther.* 14:494, 1973.
45. Ferguson, R. K., Vlasses, P. H., Koplin, J. R., et al. Relationships among timolol doses, plasma concentrations and beta-adrenoceptor blocking activity. *Br. J. Clin. Pharmacol.* 14:719, 1982.
46. Flouvat, B., Decourt, S., Aubert, P., et al. Pharmacokinetics of atenolol in patients with terminal renal failure and influence of hemodialysis. *Br. J. Clin. Pharmacol.* 9:379, 1980.
47. Freestone, S., Silas, J. H., Lennard, M. S., and Ramsay, L. E. Comparison of two long-acting preparations of metoprolol with conventional metoprolol

and atenolol in healthy men during chronic dosing. *Br. J. Clin. Pharmacol.* 14:713, 1982.
48. Fremstad, D., Bergerud, K., Haffner, J. F. W., and Lunde, P. K. M. Increased plasma binding of quinidine after surgery. *Eur. J. Clin. Pharmacol.* 10:441, 1976.
49. Frishman, W. Clinical pharmacology of the new beta-adrenergic blocking drugs. Part 1. Pharmacodynamic and pharmacokinetic properties. *Am. Heart J.* 97:663, 1979.
50. Frishman, W., and Halprin, S. Clinical pharmacology of the new beta-adrenergic blocking drugs. Part 7. New horizons in beta-adrenoceptor blocking therapy: labetalol. *Am. Heart J.* 98:660, 1979.
51. Frishman, W., Smithen, C., Befler, B., et al. Non-invasive assessment of clinical response to oral propranolol. *Am. J. Cardiol.* 35:635, 1975.
52. Frishman, W., Stampfer, M., Strom, J., et al. Pindolol (LB-46) therapy for supraventricular arrhythmia: A viable alternative to propranolol in patients with bronchospasm. *Circulation* 56(Suppl III):III-180, 1977.
53. Frishman, W. H., Strom, J. A., Kirschner, M., et al. Labetalol therapy in patients with systemic hypertension and angina pectoris: Effects of combined alpha and beta adrenoceptor blockade. *Am. J. Cardiol.* 48:917, 1981.
54. Gabriel, R., Kaye, C. M., and Sankey, M. G. Preliminary observations on the excretion of acebutolol and its acetyl metabolite in the urine and faeces of man. *J. Pharm. Pharmacol.* 33:386, 1981.
55. Gaddie, J., and Skinner, C. Risk with beta-blocking in bronchial asthma. *Br. Med. J.* 1:749, 1972.
56. Galeazzi, R. L., Pirovino, M., and Weidmann, P. Constant kinetics and constant concentration-effect relationship during long-term beta-blockade with pindolol. *Clin. Pharmacol. Ther.* 33:733, 1983.
57. Gengo, F. M., Ermer, J. C., Carey, C., et al. The relationship between serum concentrations and central nervous system actions of metoprolol. *J. Neurol. Neurosurg. Psychiatry* 48:101, 1985.
58. George, C. F., and Gruchy, B. S. Elimination of drugs by active intestinal transport. *J. Pharm. Pharmacol.* 31:643, 1979.
59. Gomeni, R., Bianchetti, G., Sega, R., and Morselli, P. L. Pharmacokinetics of propranolol in normal healthy volunteers. *J. Pharmacokinet. Biopharm.* 5:183, 1977.
60. Gugler, R., Hobel, W., Bodem, G., and Dengler, H. J. The effect of pindolol on exercise-induced cardiac acceleration in relation to plasma levels in man. *Clin. Pharmacol. Ther.* 17:127, 1975.
61. Hager, W. D., Pieniaszek, H. J., Perrier, D., et al. Assessment of beta-blockade with propranolol. *Clin. Pharmacol. Ther.* 30:283, 1981.
62. Herrera, J., Vukovich, R. A., and Griffith, D. L. Elimination of nadolol by patients with renal impairment. *Br. J. Clin. Pharmacol.* 7:227S, 1979.
63. Hillis, L. D., and Braunwald, E. Coronary artery spasm. *N. Engl. J. Med.* 299:695, 1978.
64. Hoffmann, K. J., Regardh, C. G., Aurell, M., et al. The effect of impaired renal function on the plasma concentration and urinary excretion of metoprolol metabolites. *Clin. Pharmacokinet.* 5:181, 1980.
65. Ishizaki, T., Tawara, K., Oyama, Y., and Nakaya, H. Clinical pharmacologic observations on timolol. I. Disposition and effect in relation to plasma level in normal individuals. *J. Clin. Pharmacol.* 18:511, 1978.
66. Jackson, G., Schwartz, J., Kates, R. E., et al. Atenolol: Once-daily cardioselective beta blockade for angina pectoris. *Circulation* 61:555, 1980.
67. Johnsson, G., and Regardh, C. G. Clinical pharmacokinetics of beta-adrenoreceptor blocking drugs. *Clin. Pharmacokinet.* 1:233, 1976.
68. Johnsson, G., Regardh, C. G., and Solvell, L. Combined pharmacokinetic

and pharmacodynamic studies in man of the adrenergic beta-1-receptor antagonist metoprolol. *Acta Pharmacol. Toxicol.* 36(Suppl V):V-31, 1975.
69. Johnsson, G., Svedmyr, N., and Thiringer, G. Effects of intravenous propranolol and metoprolol and their interaction with isoprenaline on pulmonary function, heart rate and blood pressure in asthmatics. *Eur. J. Clin. Pharmacol.* 8:175, 1975.
70. Jordo, L., Attman, P. O., Aurell, M., et al. Pharmacokinetic and pharmacodynamic properties of metoprolol in patients with impaired renal function. *Clin. Pharmacokinet.* 5:169, 1980.
71. Joye, J. A., Lee, G., DeMaria, A. N., et al. Afterload advantage of cardioselective blockade by acebutolol versus propranolol: Hemodynamic assessment by cardiac catheterization in coronary patients. *Circulation* 58:11, 1978.
72. Kaye, C. M., and Oh, V. M. S. The biliary excretion of acebutolol in man. *J. Pharm. Pharmacol.* 28:449, 1976.
73. Kaye, C. M., Robinson, D. G., and Turner, P. The influence of urine pH on the renal excretion of practolol and propranolol. *Br. J. Pharmacol.* 49:155P, 1973.
74. Koch-Weser, J. Metoprolol. *N. Engl. J. Med.* 301:698, 1979.
75. Kornhauser, D. M., Wood, A. J. J., Vestal, R. E., et al. Biological determinants of propranolol disposition in man. *Clin. Pharmacol. Ther.* 23:165, 1978.
76. Kostis, J. B., Frishman, W., Hosler, M. H., et al. Treatment of angina pectoris with pindolol: The significance of intrinsic sympathomimetic activity of beta blockers. *Am. Heart J.* 104:496, 1982.
77. Kumana, C. R., Marlin, G. E., Kaye, C. M., and Smith, D. M. New approach to assessment of cardioselectivity of beta-blocking drugs. *Br. Med. J.* 4:444, 1974.
78. Lardoux, H., Gerard, J., Blazquez, G., and Flouvat, B. Which beta-blocker in pregnancy-induced hypertension? *Lancet* 2:1194, 1983.
79. Laverty, R., and Taylor, K. M. Propranolol uptake into the central nervous system and the effect on rat behaviour and amine metabolism. *J. Pharm. Pharmacol.* 20:605, 1968.
80. Lehtonen, A. The effect of acebutolol on plasma lipids, blood glucose and serum insulin levels. *Acta Med. Scand.* 216:57, 1984.
81. Lehtonen, A., Kanto, J., and Kleimola, T. Plasma concentrations of propranolol in patients with essential hypertension. *Eur. J. Clin. Pharmacol.* 11:155, 1977.
82. Lennard, M. S., Silas, J. H., Freestone, S., and Trevethick, J. Defective metabolism of metoprolol in poor hydroxylators of debrisoquine. *Br. J. Clin. Pharmacol.* 14:301, 1982.
83. Lennard, M. S., Silas, J. H., Freestone, S., et al. Oxidation phenotype—A major determinant of metoprolol metabolism and response. *N. Engl. J. Med.* 307:1558, 1982.
84. Lowenthal, D. T., Briggs, W. A., Gibson, T. P., et al. Pharmacokinetics of oral propranolol in chronic renal disease. *Clin. Pharmacol. Ther.* 16:761, 1974.
85. Lowenthal, D. T., Pitone, J. M., Affrime, M. B., et al. Timolol kinetics in chronic renal insufficiency. *Clin. Pharmacol. Ther.* 23:606, 1978.
86. Majid, P. A., Saxton, C., Stoker, J. B., and Taylor, S. H. Comparison of the hemodynamic effects of intravenous and oral therapy with propranolol and oxprenolol in hypertensive patients. *Cardiovasc. Res.* 6. VIth World Congress of Cardiology, London, 1970. P. 208.
87. Mason, J. W., Specter, M. J., Ingels, N. B., et al. Haemodynamic effects of acebutolol. *Br. Heart J.* 40:29, 1978.
88. Mason, W. D., Winer, N., Kochak, G., et al. Kinetics and absolute bioavailability of atenolol. *Clin. Pharmacol. Ther.* 25:408, 1979.

89. McAllister, R. G. Intravenous propranolol administration: A method for achieving and sustaining desired plasma levels. *Clin. Pharmacol. Ther.* 20:517, 1976.
90. McAinsh, J., Holmes, B. F., Smith, S., et al. Atenolol kinetics in renal failure. *Clin. Pharmacol. Ther.* 28:302, 1980.
91. McDevitt, D. G. Beta-adrenoceptor blocking drugs and partial agonist activity: Is it clinically relevant? *Drugs* 25:331, 1983.
92. McDevitt, D. G., Frisk-Holmberg, M., Hollifield, J. W., and Shand, D. G. Plasma binding and the affinity of propranolol for a beta receptor in man. *Clin. Pharmacol. Ther.* 20:152, 1976.
93. McDevitt, D. G., and Shand, D. G. Plasma concentrations and the time-course of beta-blockade due to propranolol. *Clin. Pharmacol. Ther.* 18:708, 1975.
94. McLean, A. J., Isbister, C., Bobik, A., and Dudley, F. J. Reduction of first pass hepatic clearance of propranolol by food. *Clin. Pharmacol. Ther.* 30:31, 1981.
95. McNeill, R. S. Effect of a beta-adrenergic-blocking agent, propranolol, on asthmatics. *Lancet* 2:1101, 1964.
96. McNeill, R. S., and Ingram, C. G. Effect of propranolol on ventilatory function. *Am. J. Cardiol.* 18:473, 1966.
97. Meffin, P. J., Winkle, R. A., Peters, F. A., and Harrison, D. C. Dose-dependent acebutolol disposition after oral administration. *Clin. Pharmacol. Ther.* 24:542, 1978.
98. Melander, A., Danielson, K., Schersten, B., and Wahlin, E. Enhancement of the bioavailability of propranolol and metoprolol by food. *Clin. Pharmacol. Ther.* 22:108, 1977.
99. Morganroth, J. Short-term evaluation of atenolol in hospitalized patients with chronic ventricular arrhythmias. *Drugs* 25(Suppl 2):181, 1983.
100. Morris, K. G., Higginbothan, M. B., Coleman, R. E., et al. Comparison of high-dose and medium-dose propranolol in the relief of exercise-induced myocardial ischemia. *Am. J. Cardiol.* 52:7, 1983.
101. Mudge, G. H., Grossman, W., Mills, R. M., et al. Reflex increase in coronary vascular resistance in patients with ischemic heart disease. *N. Engl. J. Med.* 295:1333, 1976.
102. Myers, M. G., Lewis, G. R. J., Steiner, J., and Dollery, C. T. Atenolol in essential hypertension. *Clin. Pharmacol. Ther.* 19:502, 1976.
103. Nies, A. S., Evans, G. H., and Shand, D. G. The hemodynamic effects of beta adrenergic blockade on the flow-dependent hepatic clearance of propranolol. *J. Pharmacol. Exp. Ther.* 184:716, 1973.
104. Ohlsson, O., and Lindell, S. E. The effects of pindolol and prazosin on hand blood flow in patients with cold extremities and on treatment with beta-blockers. *Acta Med. Scand.* 210:217, 1981.
105. Paterson, J. W., Conolly, M. E., Dollery, C. T., et al. The pharmacodynamics and metabolism of propranolol in man. *Pharmacologia Clinica* 2:127, 1970.
106. Piafsky, K. M. Disease-induced changes in plasma binding of basic drugs. *Clin. Pharmacokinet.* 5:246, 1980.
107. Piafsky, K. M., and Borga, O. Plasma protein binding of basic drugs. II. Importance of alpha-1-acid glycoprotein for interindividual variation. *Clin. Pharmacol. Ther.* 22:545, 1977.
108. Piafsky, K. M., Borga, O., Odar-Cederlof, I., et al. Increased plasma protein binding of propranolol and chlorpromazine mediated by disease-induced elevations of plasma alpha-1-acid glycoprotein. *N. Engl. J. Med.* 299:1435, 1978.
109. Pine, M., Favrot, L., Smith, S., et al. Correlation of plasma propranolol

concentration with therapeutic response in patients with angina pectoris. *Circulation.* 52:886, 1975.
110. Plotnick, G. D., Fisher, M. L., Wohl, B., et al. Improvement in depressed cardiac function in hypertensive patients during pindolol treatment. *Am J. Med.* 76:25, 1984.
111. Pratt, C. M., Yepsen, S. C., Bloom, M. G. K., et al. Evaluation of metoprolol in suppressing complex ventricular arrhythmias. *Am. J. Cardiol.* 52:73, 1983.
112. Raghuram, T. C., Koshakji, R. P., Wilkinson, G. R., and Wood, A. J. J. Polymorphic ability to metabolize propranolol alters 4-hydroxypropranolol levels but not beta blockade. *Clin. Pharmacol. Ther.* 36:51, 1984.
113. Raine, J. M., Palazzo, M. G., Kerr, J. H., and Sleight, P. Near-fatal bronchospasm after oral nadolol in a young asthmatic and response to ventilation with halothane. *Br. Med. J.* 282:548, 1981.
114. Reeves, P. R., McAinsh, J., McIntosh, D. A., and Winrow, M. J. Metabolism of atenolol in man. *Xenobiotica* 8:313, 1978.
115. Regardh, C. G., Borg, K. O., Johansson, R., et al. Pharmacokinetic studies on the selective beta-1-receptor antagonist metoprolol in man. *J. Pharmacokinet. Biopharm.* 2:347, 1974.
116. Regardh, C. G., and Johansson, G. Clinical pharmacokinetics of metoprolol. *Clin. Pharmacokinet.* 5:557, 1980.
117. Rosenthal, J., Kaiser, H., Raschig, A., and Welzer, D. Treatment of hypertension with a beta-adrenoceptor blocker: A multicentre trial with pindolol. *Br. J. Clin. Pract.* 33:165, 1979.
118. Roux, A., Aubert, P., Guedon, J., and Flouvat, B. Pharmacokinetics of acebutolol in patients with all grades of renal failure. *Eur. J. Clin. Pharmacol.* 17:339, 1980.
119. Rubin, P.C., Butters, L., Clark, D. M., et al. Placebo-controlled trial of atenolol in treatment of pregnancy-associated hypertension. *Lancet* 1:431, 1983.
120. Salem, S. A., and McDevitt, D. G. Central effects of beta-adrenoceptor antagonists. *Clin. Pharmacol. Ther.* 33:52, 1983.
121. Sankey, M. G., Gulaid, A., and Kaye, C. M. Preliminary study of the disposition in man of acebutolol and its metabolite, diacetolol, using a new stereoselective HPLC method. *J. Pharm. Pharmacol.* 36:276, 1984.
122. Schneck, D. W., and Pritchard, J. F. The inhibitory effect of propranolol pretreatment on its own metabolism in the rat. *J. Pharmacol. Exp. Ther.* 218:575, 1981.
123. Schneck, D. W., Pritchard, J. F., Gibson, T. P., et al. Effect of dose and uremia on plasma and urine profiles of propranolol metabolites. *Clin. Pharmacol. Ther.* 27:744, 1980.
124. Schneck, D. W., Pritchard, J. F., and Hayes, A. H. Measurement of propranolol, 4-hydroxypropranolol and propranolol glycol in human plasma. *Res. Commun. Chem. Pathol. Pharmacol.* 24:3, 1979.
125. Seiler, K. U., Schuster, K. J., Meyer, G. J., et al. The pharmacokinetics of metoprolol and its metabolites in dialysis patients. *Clin. Pharmacokinet.* 5:192, 1980.
126. Shand, D. G. Pharmacokinetic properties of the beta-adrenergic receptor blocking drugs. *Drugs* 7:39, 1974.
127. Shand, D. G., and Rangno, R. E. The disposition of propranolol. *Pharmacology* 7:159, 1972.
128. Simpson, W. T. Nature and incidence of unwanted effects with atenolol. *Postgrad. Med. J.* 53(Suppl 3):162, 1977.
129. Singh, B. N., Whitlock, R. M. L., Comber, R. H., et al. Effects of cardioselective beta adrenoceptor blockade on specific airways resistance in nor-

mal subjects and in patients with bronchial asthma. *Clin. Pharmacol. Ther.* 19:493, 1976.
130. Skinner, C., Gaddie, J., Palmer, K. N. V., and Kerridge, D. F. Comparison of effects of metoprolol and propranolol on asthmatic airway obstruction. *Br. Med. J.* 1:504, 1976.
131. Sotaniemi, E. A., Anttila, M., Pelkonen, R. O., et al. Plasma clearance of propranolol and sotalol and hepatic drug-metabolizing enzyme activity. *Clin. Pharmacol. Ther.* 26:153, 1979.
132. Steinberg, S. F., and Bilezikian, J. P. Total and free propranolol levels in sensitive and resistant patients. *Clin. Pharmacol. Ther.* 33:163, 1983.
133. Sum, C. Y., Yacobi, A., Kartzinel, R., et al. Kinetics of esmolol, an ultra-short-acting beta blocker, and of its major metabolite. *Clin. Pharmacol. Ther.* 34:427, 1983.
134. Sung, R. J., Blanski, L., Kirshenbaum, J., et al. Clinical experience with esmolol, a short-acting beta-adrenergic blocker in cardiac arrhythmias and myocardial ischemia. *J. Clin. Pharmacol.* 26(Suppl A):A15, 1986.
135. Svendsen, T. L. Central hemodynamics of beta-adrenoceptor blocking drugs: Beta-1 selectivity versus intrinsic sympathomimetic activity. *J. Cardiovasc. Pharmacol.* 5(Suppl):21, 1983.
136. Svensson, A., Gudbrandsson, T., Sivertsson, R., and Hansson, L. Metoprolol and pindolol in hypertension: Different effects on peripheral haemodynamics. *Clin. Sci.* 61:425S, 1981.
137. Svensson, C. K., Edwards, D. J., Mauriello, P. M., et al. Effect of food on hepatic blood flow: Implications in the "food effect" phenomenon. *Clin. Pharmacol. Ther.* 34:316, 1983.
138. Taylor, E. A., Jefferson, D., Carroll, J. D., and Turner, P. Cerebrospinal fluid concentrations of propranolol, pindolol and atenolol in man: Evidence for central actions of beta-adrenoceptor antagonists. *Br. J. Clin. Pharmacol.* 12:549, 1981.
139. Taylor, S. H., Silke, B., Ebbutt, A., et al. A long-term prevention study with oxprenolol in coronary heart disease. *N. Engl. J. Med.* 307:1293, 1982.
140. Thadani, U., and Parker, J. O. Propranolol in angina pectoris: Duration of improved exercise tolerance and circulatory effects after acute oral administration. *Am. J. Cardiol.* 44:118, 1979.
141. Thadani, U., and Parker, J. O. Propranolol in the treatment of angina pectoris: Comparison of duration of action in acute and sustained oral therapy. *Circulation* 59:571, 1979.
142. Thompson, F. D., Joekes, A. M., and Foulkes, D. M. Pharmacodynamics of propranolol in renal failure. *Br. Med. J.* 2:434, 1972.
143. Tocco, D. J., deLuna, F. A., and Duncan, A. E. W. Electron-capture GLC determination of timolol in human plasma and urine. *J. Pharm. Sci.* 64:1879, 1975.
144. Vermeij, P., el Sherbini-Schepers, M., and vanZwieten, P. A. The disposition of timolol in man. *J. Pharm. Pharmacol.* 30:53, 1978.
145. Vervloet, E., Pluym, B. F. M., Cilissen, J., et al. Propranolol serum levels during twenty-four hours. *Clin. Pharmacol. Ther.* 22:853, 1977.
146. Vestal, R. E., and Wood, A. J. J. Influence of age and smoking on drug kinetics in man: Studies using model compounds. *Clin. Pharmacokinet.* 5:309, 1980.
147. Vestal, R. E., Wood, A. J. J., Branch, R. A., et al. Effects of age and cigarette smoking on propranolol disposition. *Clin. Pharmacol. Ther.* 26:8, 1979.
148. Vestal, R. E., Wood, A. J. J., and Shand, D. G. Reduced beta-adrenoceptor sensitivity in the elderly. *Clin. Pharmacol. Ther.* 26:181, 1979.

149. von Bahr, C., Collste, P., Frisk-Holmberg, M., et al. Plasma levels and effects of metoprolol on blood pressure, adrenergic beta receptor blockade, and plasma renin activity in essential hypertension. *Clin. Pharmacol. Ther.* 20:130, 1976.
150. Vukovich, R., Dreyfuss, J., Brannick, L. J., et al. Pharmacologic and metabolic studies with a new beta-adrenergic blocking agent, nadolol. *Clin. Res.* 24:513A, 1976.
151. Walle, T., Conradi, E. C., Walle, U. K., et al. 4-hydroxypropranolol and its glucuronide after single and long-term doses of propranolol. *Clin. Pharmacol. Ther.* 27:22, 1980.
152. Walle, T., Conradi, E. C., Walle, U. K., and Gaffney, T. E. O-methylated catechol-like metabolites of propranolol in man. *Drug Metab. Dispos.* 6:481, 1978.
153. Walle, T., Conradi, E. C., Walle, U. K., et al. Steady-state kinetics of the active propranolol metabolite 4-hydroxypropranolol and its glucuronic acid conjugate in patients with hypertension and coronary artery disease. *Clin. Res.* 25:10A, 1977.
154. Walle, T., Conradi, E. C., Walle, U. K., and Gaffney, T. E. Steady-state plasma concentrations and urinary excretion of propranolol-o-glucuronide and propranolol in patients during chronic oral propranolol therapy. *Fed. Proc.* 35:665, 1976.
155. Walle, T., Conradi, E. C., Walle, U. K., et al. The predictable relationship between plasma levels and dose during chronic propranolol therapy. *Clin. Pharmacol. Ther.* 24:668, 1978.
156. Walle, T., Fagan, T. C., Walle, U. K., et al. Food-induced increase in propranolol bioavailability: Relationship to protein and effects on metabolites. *Clin. Pharmacol. Ther.* 30:790, 1981.
157. Walle, U. K., Walle, T., Bai, S. A., and Olanoff, L. S. Stereoselective binding of propranolol to human plasma, alpha-1-acid glycoprotein, and albumin. *Clin. Pharmacol. Ther.* 34:718, 1983.
158. Whitsett, T. L., Levin, D. C., and Manion, C. V. Comparison of the beta-1 and beta-2 adrenoceptor blocking properties of acebutolol and propranolol. *Chest* 82:668, 1982.
159. Wilson, T. W., Firor, W. B., Johnson, G. E., et al. Timolol and propranolol: Bioavailability, plasma concentrations, and beta blockade. *Clin. Pharmacol. Ther.* 32:676, 1982.
160. Winkle, R. A., Meffin, P. J., Ricks, W. B., and Harrison, D. C. Acebutolol metabolite plasma concentration during chronic oral therapy. *Br. J. Clin. Pharmacol.* 4:519, 1977.
161. Wollam, G. L., Cody, R. J., Tarazi, R. C., and Bravo, E. L. Acute hemodynamic effects and cardioselectivity of acebutolol, practolol and propranolol. *Clin. Pharmacol. Ther.* 25:813, 1979.
162. Woosley, R. L., Kornhauser, D., Smith, R., et al. Suppression of chronic ventricular arrhythmias with propranolol. *Circulation* 60:819, 1979.
163. Woosley, R. L., Shand, D., Kornhauser, D., et al. Relation of plasma concentration and dose of propranolol to its effect on resistant ventricular arrhythmias. *Clin. Res.* 25:262A, 1977.
164. Yusuf, S., Peto, R., Lewis, J., et al. Beta blockade during and after myocardial infarction: An overview of the randomized trials. *Progr. Cardiovasc. Dis.* 27:335, 1985.
165. Zacest, R., and Koch-Weser, J. Relation of propranolol plasma level to beta-blockade during oral therapy. *Pharmacology* 7:178, 1972.
166. Zaman, R., Wilkins, M. R., Kendall, M. J., and Jack, D. B. The effect of food and alcohol on the pharmacokinetics of acebutolol and its metabolite, diacetolol. *Biopharm. Drug Dispos.* 5:91, 1984.

CHAPTER 8

PHARMACOLOGY AND PHARMACOKINETICS OF CALCIUM ANTAGONISTS— INDIVIDUALIZED DOSING REGIMENS AND DRUG INTERACTIONS

LARRY M. LOPEZ
CARL J. PEPINE

The past 20 years have witnessed the movement of classic pharmacokinetics from the realm of the research scientist to that of the clinician. This movement out of the research laboratory has coincided with and resulted in the evolution of clinical pharmacokinetics. Classic pharmacokinetics refers to facts and inferences concerning liberation, absorption, distribution, metabolism, and elimination of drugs in patients. Clinical pharmacokinetics assesses the relationship of these facts and inferences to clinically important beneficial or adverse effects. Availability of this information is critical to development and optimal use of individualized dosing regimens in patients with various disorders and to the anticipation of beneficial or adverse effects of concomitant therapy with other agents.

Of growing importance are the classic and clinical pharmacokinetic characteristics of calcium channel antagonists. The importance of understanding pharmacokinetic characteristics of these agents lies not in any of their unusual chemical or physical properties but instead with the growing frequency with which these drugs are employed in practice. These agents were originally introduced as specific therapy for supraventricular tachycardia or management of ischemic heart disease. Now they are widely used for treatment of essential and emergent hypertension [16, 87, 106], migraine headaches [95], hypertrophic myocardial disease [102, 116], esophageal motor dysfunction, intermittent claudication, Raynaud's phenomenon, cerebrovascular spasm associated with subarachnoid bleeding, reversible airway obstruction, and pulmonary hypertension, among others [107]. Also, assay methodologies for each of these agents have progressed to the point where considerable pharmacokinetic and pharmacodynamic information is now available.

In this chapter we will review clinically relevant pharmacokinetic characteristics of calcium channel antagonists, effects of certain diseases on these characteristics, and resulting necessary dosing changes. Also, since calcium channel antagonists are frequently administered with other medications, their respective drug interaction profiles will be discussed from a pharmacokinetic point of view.

CLASSICAL AND CLINICAL PHARMACOKINETICS OF CALCIUM CHANNEL ANTAGONISTS

Classic Pharmacokinetics—Absorption

Classic pharmacokinetic parameters of currently available calcium channel antagonists are summarized in Table 8-1. Comparatively less is known about pharmacokinetic disposition of isradipine [2, 26, 151], nicardipine [20, 24, 25, 34, 44, 45, 54, 55, 62, 80, 118, 130, 133, 138], and nimodipine [9, 40, 66, 111] as compared with diltiazem, nifedipine, and verapamil [21, 49, 137]. Consequently, emphasis in this chapter will be placed primarily on discussion of these latter agents.

TABLE 8-1. *Pharmacokinetic Parameters of Calcium Channel Antagonists*

Parameter	Diltiazem	Nifedipine	Verapamil	Isradapine	Nicardipine	Nimodipine
T max (hr)[a]	1–4 6–11 (SR)[c]	0.5–4 6 (SR)	0.5–1 7–9 (SR)	1–3	0.5–2	0.7–1
Bioavailability (%)	24–74	43–65 29–85 (SR)	13–35	16–18	35	13
Protein Binding (%)	77–93	92–98	83–92	97	>98	95
Vd (L/kg)[b]	5.3 ± 1.7	0.8 ± 0.2	4.3	NR[d]	0.64	NR
Metabolism	deacetylation desacelylation	inactive acid, lactone	norverapamil plus 11 others	5 inactive metabolites	glucuronide conjugates	NR
Half-life (hr)	2–7	2–3 6 (SR)	2–7	5–11	0.75–2	8–9
Excretion (5) renal fecal	40 60	90 10	70 16	65 30	60 35	10 NR
Therapeutic Concentration (ng/ml)	40–200	20–100	80–300	NR	NR	NR

[a] Tmax = time to maximal concentration
[b] Vd = volume of distribution
[c] SR = sustained release
[d] Vd of isradipine is reportedly 60–161 L in healthy subjects and 250 L in the elderly

All of these agents are efficiently and extensively absorbed from oral dose forms and achieve maximal serum concentrations within 0.5 to 4 hours. While absorption is essentially complete for these drugs, bioavailability, the fraction of an administered dose which reaches systemic circulation, is incomplete and varies considerably. Since bioavailability measures amount of drug in systemic circulation after absorption, it is apparent that some of each dose of these agents is lost before it reaches systemic circulation. This loss of parent drug is due to presystemic elimination by the liver, sometimes referred to as first-pass effect. Presystemic elimination varies substantially among subjects and accounts, in part, for wide variation in dose required for desired effects in different individuals.

These tabulated absorption parameters are based primarily on results of studies using healthy, fasting individuals as study subjects. When nifedipine capsules are administered with food, peak nifedipine concentration is reduced by 68 percent (from a mean of 136 ng/ml to a mean of 43 ng/ml). Additionally, time to peak concentration and peak hemodynamic response are delayed by an average of 3 hours although duration of action may be correspondingly prolonged [42, 56]. Absorption of nicardipine is also diminished by 20 to 30 percent when taken with food while concentrations of isradipine are increased by 27 percent [90]. Delay and blunting of hemodynamic effects of nifedipine and effects on concentrations of nicardipine and isradipine by food suggest that these agents should be administered on an empty stomach to ensure maximal absorption and effects. These observations also suggest that dosing at mealtime may be useful for protecting a patient from excessive nifedipine-induced hypotension or other adverse effects. Similar studies evaluating effects of food on absorption of verapamil and diltiazem are needed. In the absence of definitive information, patients are best advised to take these medications in a consistent manner, preferably before meals on an empty stomach, to insure consistent drug absorption and effects.

Administration by a route other than oral may be an effective method for avoiding presystemic elimination. For example, use of 10 mg of verapamil intravenously yields plasma concentrations comparable to those observed after 80 mg given orally [91]. With nifedipine, however, administration of 10 mg by the sublingual route produces peak plasma concentrations considerably lower (42 ng/ml versus 100 ng/ml) and much later (74 minutes versus 40 minutes) than those found after an equivalent oral dose [4, 35]. Sublingual nifedipine is commonly thought to result in earlier and more intense effects than those observed after oral administration. Results of recent studies, however, indicated that buccal absorption of nifedipine is negligible.

Nifedipine, diltiazem, and verapamil are all now marketed as sustained-release preparations in addition to the standard immediate-release formulations. As expected, time to peak concentration after administration of any sustained-release formulation is delayed when compared with a corresponding immediate-release preparation. Both types of formulations are, however, comparable with respect to bioavailability. Also, food does not appear to influence absorption from these slow-release formulations. Indeed, administration of sustained-release nifedipine with food is preferred for optimal liberation and absorption.

Although not yet available for use in the United States, nifedipine is also marketed in Europe as a tablet formulation. Normally, pharmacokinetic characteristics of a drug should be unaffected by a variation in formulation. Such is not the case with nifedipine. Time to peak concentration after administration of a nifedipine tablet occurs much later than after the capsule (1.6 to 2.1 hours versus 0.5 to 0.6 hours) and elimination half-life is similarly prolonged (9.7 to 10.8 hours versus 1.5 to 3.4 hours) [11, 35, 144]. This apparent change in drug disposition associated with a different formulation is subject to question since there have been substantial problems with assay methodologies for nifedipine [61, 83, 85]. Nevertheless, these pharmacokinetic data imply that twice-daily dosing with the nifedipine tablet may be appropriate compared with the capsule which must be given more frequently.

Classic Pharmacokinetics— Distribution

The major determinants of distribution are molecular size, lipophilicity, extent of ionization at physiologic pH, and extent of protein binding [15]. Of these, only extent of protein binding would be affected by disease or other drugs. Extent of plasma protein binding for all of these compounds is similar (Table 8-1) and independent of concentration. Effects of other highly protein-bound drugs on extent of protein binding of calcium channel antagonists have been evaluated only with diltiazem and verapamil. Propranolol, warfarin, digoxin, phenylbutazone, hydrochlorothiazide, and salicylate failed to affect extent of diltiazem binding substantially [17]. On the other hand, binding of verapamil is significantly decreased by propranolol, diazepam, lidocaine, and disopyramide [93]. Also, norverapamil, the major active metabolite of verapamil, has also been shown to displace verapamil from its binding sites [158]. These in vitro studies have not yet been confirmed with in vivo investigations.

Interactions involving changes in plasma protein binding may be clinically important if the volume of distribution of the agent is small. Based on this proposition, occurrence of such an interaction appears most likely for nifedipine. Similar interactions involving the remainder of the calcium channel antagonists are likewise unlikely in view of their relatively large volumes of distribution. While extensively distributed to most tissues including the central nervous system, there is no evidence that these drugs accumulate in any tissue depot even with chronic dosing.

Classic Pharmacokinetics—Metabolism and Elimination

Clearance of these agents occurs largely through hepatic metabolism with subsequent renal elimination of a variety of metabolites (Table 8-1). Less than 5 percent of an oral dose of these drugs is eliminated by the kidney in an unchanged form. Nifedipine is metabolized primarily to a hydrocarboxylic acid and subsequently to a lactone, both of which are inactive [122]. Isradipine and nicardipine are similarly metabolized to inactive end products, while metabolic profile of nimodipine has not yet been reported. Verapamil, when given orally, forms at least 12 metabolites, two of which possess pharmacologic activity. One of the active metabolites is quickly deactivated by glucuronidation and another, norverapamil, retains approximately 20 percent of the activity of the parent compound [30, 98, 124]. Further, verapamil appears to undergo stereoselective metabolism with the l-isomer, the more active isomer, being eliminated faster than the d-isomer [31, 58]. Conventional drug assays are not presently able to detect metabolites of verapamil after intravenous administration of the drug. Diltiazem is also metabolized to multiple metabolites four of which are inactive and one, desacetyldiltiazem, which is active and possesses approximately 40 to 50 percent of the activity of the parent compound [74, 96, 118]. Contribution of active metabolites to overall effects of verapamil and diltiazem have yet to be determined.

An interesting aspect of elimination of verapamil and diltiazem is the effect of each drug on its own clearance. After multiple doses, half-life of verapamil increases from 3 to 7 hours up to 12 hours and its bioavailability increases twofold. This phenomenon has been observed to occur within a week of initiation of therapy with verapamil and apparently persists as long as the drug is taken [36, 127, 132, 146]. Similarly, during long-term oral dosing of diltiazem, accumulation of unchanged drug and the desacetyl metabolite has been observed [117, 124]. Bioavailability of diltiazem increases from 38 percent after the initial dose to 90 percent after multiple doses with minimal changes in elimination half-life. With chronic oral dosing it appears that presystemic elimination of verapamil and diltiazem is saturable, resulting in higher than expected concentrations of parent drug and metabolite. One implication from these changes is that twice-daily dosing of verapamil and diltiazem, instead of the currently recommended three to four daily doses, may be reasonable once steady-state has been reached. Clinical evaluation of these alternative dosing regimens is needed to verify these pharmacokinetic implications. Similar changes in disposition after multiple doses of other calcium channel antagonists has not been observed.

Clinical Pharmacokinetics

Establishment of pharmacokinetic parameters, per se, is only partially useful to the clinician. Association of these parameters, or drug concentration itself, to observed clinical effects allows the clinician to apply this information directly to patient care. Numerous investigations have attempted to correlate concentrations of nifedipine, verapamil, and diltiazem with hemodynamic, electrophysiologic, or clinical effects. Similar investigations are needed for isradipine, nicardipine, and nimodipine.

After one dose of verapamil by either the oral or intravenous route, hemodynamic and electrophysiologic effects have been directly related to its plasma concentration [31, 49, 75, 91, 120, 143]. Although not yet firmly established as a therapeutic range, after a single intravenous dose achievement of verapamil concentrations between 100 to 200 ng/ml is apparently associated with beneficial effects [50, 143]. Few studies have attempted to correlate verapamil concentrations with pharmacologic effects after chronic oral dosing. A therapeutic range of 100 to 400 ng/ml has been suggested for patients with hypertrophic obstructive cardiomyopathy [157]. Results of a study in such patients, however, were unable to confirm these recommendations [85]. A range of plasma concentrations from 150 to 500 ng/ml has been associated with an increased tolerance to exercise and reduced frequency of chest pain in patients with angina [6, 146]. Others, however, were unable to correlate clinical response to plasma concentrations in a group of similar patients [37, 160]. Further, it appears that effect of verapamil on P–R interval decreases or disappears during chronic dosing [112]. In studies evaluating plasma concentrations of verapamil and hypotensive effects, similar contradictions have been reported [131, 141]. Thus, routine monitoring of plasma verapamil concentrations is not helpful as a practical guide to therapy.

Attempts to identify a therapeutic range of plasma concentrations for nifedipine have encountered similar difficulties. Results of numerous studies have suggested that nifedipine concentration in plasma correlates with change in blood pressure and heart rate [7, 11, 47, 56, 70, 144, 149]. Also, a reduction in frequency of chest pain together with improved exercise tolerance has been reported in patients with nifedipine concentrations greater than 90 ng/ml [22]. Further, side effects from nifedipine may also be related to high peak concentrations [161]. Other studies, however, have failed to confirm any relationship between nifedipine concentrations and either hemodynamic or clinical effects [22, 84, 85, 113].

When diltiazem is administered in single intravenous or oral doses, systolic blood pressure and systemic vascular resistance decline in relation to plasma diltiazem concentrations. These effects are noted, however, only if diltiazem concentrations exceed 100 ng/ml [145]. In a study of diltiazem concentrations in patients with ischemic heart disease, plasma concentrations of 100 to 200 ng/ml were observed in responders. Lack of response in this patient group was generally associated with diltiazem concentrations below 100 ng/ml [96]. Failure to experience symptomatic improvement in another group of patients with angina was associated with diltiazem concentrations below 40 ng/ml [59]. In another study, administration of a slow intravenous infusion of diltiazem yielded concentrations greater than 700 ng/ml, but resulted in no significant changes in blood pressure or P–R interval. While the rate of administration of diltiazem may be an important determinant of its pharmacodynamic effects, there may also be a change in the concentration-effect relationship after intravenous dosing as compared with oral dosing [134].

In summary, hemodynamic, electrophysiologic, and clinical effects of all calcium channel antagonists are inconsistently associated with plasma concentrations. There are numerous potential reasons for these inconsistent findings. For example, nonlinear correlations have not been evaluated and hysteresis analysis has been employed infrequently [114]. Further, potential contributions of active metabolites of verapamil and diltiazem have been infrequently considered. Also, response to these agents may be complicated by variables such as endogenous sympathetic tone and ventricular function [152]. Clearly, routine monitoring of plasma concentrations of calcium channel antagonists is not yet a useful adjunct in the management of patients taking these medications. Existing pharmacokinetic and pharmacodynamic data may be useful, however, in developing individualized dosing guidelines for patients with other diseases in addition to heart disease.

INDIVIDUALIZED DOSING OF CALCIUM CHANNEL ANTAGONISTS

Calcium channel antagonists may be useful in some clinical situations where other cardiovascular drugs would be contraindicated or unsafe. For example, these drugs can be used to manage hypertension in patients with concurrent migraine headaches, bronchial asthma, angina, or diabetes mellitus. There are, however, a few clinical situations in which alteration of dosing regimens should be considered. Table 8-2 summarizes dosing adjustments recommended for diltiazem, nifedipine, and verapamil. Isradipine, nicardipine, and nimodipine are not included in the table since so little information is presently available concerning changes in their disposition by other diseases.

Liver Disease
Since all three calcium channel antagonists are cleared primarily by hepatic metabolism, it is reasonable to expect that liver disease would alter dosing requirements. Pharmacokinetic studies of some other drugs

TABLE 8-2. *Dose Alterations of Diltiazem, Nifedipine, and Verapamil*

	Diltiazem	Nifedipine	Verapamil
Liver Disease	No data available	Administer 50% of usual dose Prolong dose interval	Administer 50% of usual IV and 20% of usual oral doses Prolong dose interval
Geriatrics	Begin with low dose Increase dose interval	No data available	Begin with low dose Prolong dose interval
Renal Disease	No dose adjustment necessary	Initiate with lower dose (exaggerated hypotensive response)	Reduce dose by 50%

cleared by the liver have encountered considerable variability in changes of pharmacokinetic parameters in patients with liver disease [39, 105]. Indeed, some patients with relatively mild forms of liver disease, such as hepatitis, may not exhibit any changes in disposition of hepatically cleared drugs. Part of the problem in this regard relates to difficulty in defining liver disease from a pharmacokinetic point of view. For example, in patients with renal insufficiency or chronic renal failure, a change in clearance of creatinine can usually be correlated with changes in pharmacokinetic parameters of drugs eliminated renally. In patients with liver disease, there is no single test or combination of tests of liver function with which to correlate pharmacokinetic parameters of drugs cleared by the liver.

One manner of overcoming this difficulty has been to study drug disposition only in patients with biopsy-proven or characterized liver disease and compare pharmacokinetic parameters in these patients with those observed in normal subjects. When this design technique was employed with verapamil, considerable changes were noted in patients with severe liver disease [43, 136, 157]. Half-life and bioavailability were increased threefold to fourfold (2.9 to 3.7 hours versus 13.6 to 14.2 hours) and over twofold (22 percent versus 52 percent), respectively. Also, plasma protein binding of verapamil was reduced and volume of distribution was markedly increased (12.05 versus 6.76 L/kg) in concert with higher plasma concentrations and a reduction in time to peak concentrations in patients as compared with healthy subjects. Although considerable variability was observed as expected, these data suggest that 50 percent of the recommended intravenous dose and 20 percent of the recommended oral dose of verapamil should initially be given to patients with severe liver disease. In view of the prolonged elimination observed in these patients, an extension of dosing interval from 8 to 12 hours would also be reasonable.

When pharmacokinetic parameters and hemodynamic effects of nifedipine were compared in patients with hepatic cirrhosis and age-matched controls, similar observations were reported [72, 73]. Elimination half-life was prolonged by 268 percent (from 1.9 to 7 hours) and bioavailability was enhanced by 78 percent (51 percent versus 91 percent) in patients as compared with controls. Interestingly, maximal effects of nifedipine on heart rate and blood pressure were apparently unaffected by liver cirrhosis. This absence of hemodynamic effects in patients with liver disease suggests that a dosing alteration of nifedipine would be unnecessary. Since only a single dose of nifedipine was administered in these studies, such a conclusion may be premature. Unfortunately, similar investigations of nifedipine using a multiple-dose design have not yet been conducted. In view of the pronounced changes in pharmacokinetic disposition parameters observed in this study, a 50 percent reduction in total daily dose of nifedipine as well as prolongation in dosing interval would be reasonable in patients with severe liver disease.

Description of pharmacokinetic disposition of the newer compounds in patients with severe liver disease is limited to a single study involving isradipine [2]. After a single dose of isradipine, bioavailability and volume of distribution increased from 18 percent to 25 percent and 161 L to 247 L, respectively. Unfortunately, clinical consequences of these changes were not evaluated. Similar investigations of nicardipine, nimodipine, or diltiazem in patients with severe liver disease have not yet been reported. Based on accumulated experiences with nifedipine and verapamil, however, initial use of a 25 to 50 percent lower dose of these compounds seems reasonable.

Geriatrics

In addition to overt hepatic disease, a form of hepatic dysfunction may also be associated with aging. Metabolic functions such as oxidation and hepatic blood flow are known to decline with advancing age [41, 63]. These changes in hepatic function, while not pathological, may, nevertheless, result in changes of pharmacokinetic disposition of calcium channel antagonists which may necessitate dosing adjustments in order to prevent adverse effects [154].

Currently, little information is available concerning disposition of calcium channel antagonists in the elderly. Bioavailability of nifedipine is greater (61 percent versus 46 percent) and its elimination half-life is prolonged (6.7 versus 3.8 hours) in elderly subjects as compared with younger counterparts (48, 114). Rate of absorption of diltiazem is delayed, although bioavailability is unaffected in elderly subjects [96].

Also, when rate of elimination in a group of older patients was compared with that from a group of younger subjects, it was found that half-life was prolonged from 7 hours in the younger to 11 hours in the older group. Bioavailability of verapamil is quite variable in the elderly as compared with younger subjects. Reported mean values vary from 11 percent to 38 percent and in individuals range from 9 percent to 83 percent [124, 142, 157]. Volume of distribution is significantly diminished (1.99 versus 3.89 L/kg) while elimination half-life of verapamil appears to be unaffected by age. Preliminary observations from one study suggest that disposition of isradipine in the elderly is minimally affected [2, 23], while similar studies with nicardipine and nimodipine have yet to be reported. Recommendations concerning dosing changes based on these data must be withheld since these data were obtained from very few subjects and clinical consequences have been inconsistently evaluated. Considering the absence of information about nicardipine and nimodipine and the dearth of data from the remaining calcium channel antagonists in the elderly, the widely held axiom "start low, go slow" still applies when making dosing adjustments of these drugs in these patients.

Renal Disease

Usually, renal dysfunction does not markedly influence pharmacokinetic characteristics of drugs cleared by extra-renal processes. For example, disposition parameters of diltiazem and its primary metabolite, desacetyldiltiazem, are unaffected in patients with severely impaired renal function [108]. Use of oral nifedipine in similar patients results in significant increases in volume of distribution (1.47 versus 0.78 L/kg) and elimination half-life (230 versus 106 minutes) as compared with subjects with normal renal function, although extent of absorption declines approximately 20 percent [71]. Notably, these changes in nifedipine concentrations and disposition parameters in patients with renal disease are accompanied by an exaggerated decline in diastolic blood pressure [18, 71].

Initial evaluation of verapamil in patients with chronic renal failure yielded results similar to that reported with diltiazem [123]. Subsequently, it has been reported that renal clearance and total clearance of verapamil is reduced tenfold and twofold, respectively, in patients with advanced renal disease [142]. Thus, dose of verapamil should be reduced by 50 percent in patients with severe renal disease and a more modest reduction in dose should be considered for patients with less severe renal impairment, such as elderly patients. Neither disposition nor hemodynamic responses to nicardipine or nimodipine has been evaluated in patients with renal dysfunction. A marked increase in volume of distribution of isradipine (331 to 458 L versus 69 to 131 L) has been observed in patients with renal dysfunction, but clinical consequences of this finding, if any, are unknown at present [2].

In view of the absence of any effects on hemodynamic response as well as pharmacokinetic parameters, it appears, then, that use of diltiazem without altering its dose is reasonable in patients with renal dysfunction.

Summary

Few clinical situations are presently known which may require dosing modifications of calcium channel antagonists. Severe liver and renal dysfunction are the only diseases which presently require dose modifications or consideration of an alternative agent. Conspicuously absent from the previous discussion are effects of congestive heart failure on pharmacodynamic response and pharmacokinetic parameters of these drugs. Since clearance of these drugs is dependent upon hepatic blood flow, it is reasonable to expect higher concentrations, prolonged elimination, and impaired clearance of all three agents in relation to reduced hepatic flow associated with congestive heart failure. On the other hand, negative inotropic effects of these agents may be counterbalanced by sympathetic intervention secondary to calcium-channel-antagonist-induced vasodilation. Consequently, hepatic blood flow and concentrations of calcium channel antagonists would be unaffected. While dosing alterations of one or all of the currently available calcium channel antagonists may be necessary in the patient with impaired left ventricular function, precise recommendations await results of pharmacokinetic studies in such patients.

In addition to congestive heart failure, clinical pharmacokinetic characteristics of calcium channel antagonists have not been evaluated in pediatric patients. Verapamil has been advocated for use in these patients for treatment of supraventricular tachycardia by giving 0.1 mg/kg intravenously over 30 seconds and repeating the dose a maximum of two more times if hypotension does not intervene [107]. Resulting drug concentrations from this dosing regimen have not been reported and this dose regimen has not been fully evaluated.

Clearly, much about clinical pharmacokinetic profiles of calcium channel antagonists, especially effects of other diseases, awaits future investigations. An emerging area of more immediate interest, however, is that involving effects of other drugs on calcium channel antagonists, as well as effects of calcium channel antagonists on other agents.

DRUG INTERACTIONS OF CALCIUM CHANNEL ANTAGONISTS

Calcium channel antagonists are best utilized in patients with cardiovascular diseases, a group of patients in whom polypharmacy is not only likely but possibly desirable. Consequently, it is not surprising that

TABLE 8-3. *Selected Pharmacokinetic Drug Interactions of Calcium Channel Antagonists*

Drug	Effect	Recommendation
Digoxin	(with verapamil) 70% increase in digoxin concentration; (with diltiazem) 20%–30% increase in digoxin concentration	(with verapamil) reduce digoxin dose by 50% initially; monitor digoxin concentration and readjust accordingly (with diltiazem) reduce digoxin dose if digoxin concentration ≥1.5 ng/ml before diltiazem
Cimetidine	(with nifedipine) increased concentrations of nifedipine and exaggerated hypotensive response (with verapamil and diltiazem) probable increased concentrations of verapamil and diltiazem	reduce dose of calcium blocker by 50%; monitor for excessive blood pressure reduction; use sucralfate instead
Quinidine	(with nifedipine) reduced quinidine concentrations; increased nifedipine concentrations (with verapamil) increased quinidine concentrations	(with nifedipine) discontinue nifedipine and monitor for marked increase in quinidine concentrations

drug interactions occur involving these medications that, in some cases, have distinct clinical significance (Table 8-3).

Digoxin

Combination therapy of digoxin with some calcium channel antagonists may be useful in a variety of clinical situations. Digoxin and verapamil or diltiazem are useful for management of supraventricular tachycardia or atrial fibrillation. The combination of digoxin and nifedipine, nicardipine, or isradipine may be potentially beneficial in patients with congestive heart failure complicated by ischemic heart disease. Considerable data are now available concerning drug interactions between calcium blockers and digoxin (Table 8-3).

It is apparent that verapamil has the greatest effect on plasma digoxin concentrations. Initially reported to increase digoxin concentrations by 69 percent in 39 of 41 patients [68], subsequent investigations reported increases of digoxin concentrations from 60 percent to 77 percent. These pronounced changes in digoxin concentrations were accompanied primarily by a reduction in renal clearance and prolongation of half-life of the drug. Magnitude of the increase in digoxin concentration is apparently related to the total daily dose of verapamil [13, 14, 69]. Use of 240 mg/day of verapamil results in an increase in digoxin concentration greater than that reported with 160 mg/day. Daily doses of verapamil greater than 240 mg do not, however, further increase concentrations of digoxin. Interestingly, development of overt digoxin toxicity reportedly occurs in only 14 percent of patients [60].

Part of the explanation for this low frequency of adverse reactions with concurrent therapy may be due to the reversible nature of this interaction. After initiation of concomitant therapy, a new steady-state digoxin concentration is reached in approximately seven days [69, 104]. With continued dosing of both verapamil and digoxin for 6 weeks, however, digoxin concentrations return to baseline [104]. Thus, although a dose reduction of digoxin may be initially necessary, subsequent readjustment upward may also be required at a later time.

Effects of nifedipine, nicardipine, or isradipine on disposition of digoxin are considerably less profound. It was initially suggested that all patients receiving nifedipine along with digoxin should have their dose of digoxin reduced by 40 percent to 50 percent and be monitored for signs and symptoms of digoxin toxicity [10, 14]. These recommendations were based on a reported 45 percent increase in digoxin concentration after a single dose of nifedipine in healthy subjects [12, 14]. Subsequently, numerous single and multidose studies in patients and healthy subjects have failed to detect a significant pharmacokinetic interaction between nifedipine and digoxin or digitoxin [38, 52, 103, 128, 129, 162]. Although reasons for these conflicting results are not readily apparent, it is likely that most patients will not experience a clinically significant increase in digoxin concentrations when digoxin is concurrently used with nifedipine. Preliminary experience with isradipine or nicardipine given concomitantly with digoxin also suggest that concentrations of digoxin are minimally affected [27, 115].

Similarly, investigations into a diltiazem-digoxin interaction have revealed that diltiazem increases digoxin concentrations by an average of only 20 percent to 30 percent. Clearance and elimination half-life of digoxin are reduced by 24 percent to 26 percent and increased by 20 percent, respectively, without affecting protein binding or time to maximum digoxin concentration [76–79, 100, 110, 119, 125, 148, 159].

Thus, close monitoring of digoxin concentrations and one or more dose changes of digoxin may be necessary in patients receiving concurrent verapamil. In patients receiving concurrent nifedipine, isradipine, nicardipine, or diltiazem only minimal changes in digoxin concentration should be expected. Alteration of digoxin dosing regimen in these patients would be potentially necessary in those patients whose digoxin concentration was quite high before initiation of calcium channel antagonist therapy.

Cimetidine

From the earlier discussion of the effects of liver disease on disposition of calcium channel antagonists, it should follow that use of any other drug that affects hepatic function would result in similar changes. Such is the case with cimetidine, an agent widely and frequently used in the treatment of a variety of gastrointestinal disorders. Cimetidine has been shown to reduce hepatic blood flow and inhibit metabolic activity [33, 139], both of which may influence pharmacokinetic disposition and subsequent response.

Disparate results have been reported thus far with respect to effects of cimetidine on disposition of verapamil. Several investigators have failed to observe significant changes in pharmacokinetic characteristics of verapamil when coadministered with cimetidine [1, 156]. Others, however, have reported an increase in bioavailability along with a reduction in clearance of verapamil during cimetidine therapy [88, 135]. These contradictory findings are due mainly to two factors. First, effects of cimetidine on verapamil are subject to considerable interpatient variability. In one study, change in clearance of verapamil varied from +35 percent to −28 percent in study subjects. Second, all of these studies evaluated only a single dose of verapamil. Since administration of multiple doses of verapamil is known to result in drug accumulation, it is possible that chronic administration of both drugs would yield considerably different results. Although no important changes were detected in P–R interval in one such study, administration of cimetidine to patients taking verapamil may expose these patients to the risk of precipitating A–V block. Until this drug interaction is more thoroughly evaluated, cautious monitoring of these patients is advised together with a 50 percent reduction in dose of verapamil.

Both cimetidine and ranitidine appear to increase diltiazem concentrations, although only cimetidine produces increases which are significant [156]. Unfortunately, these observations also come from a study which employed a single-dose design and, consequently, effects of these H_2-receptor blockers on disposition of diltiazem are incompletely described. Initial dose of diltiazem should, nevertheless, be lowered by 50 percent in a manner similar to verapamil until this interaction is more completely characterized.

Evaluations of the effects of cimetidine on nifedipine disposition have yielded more consistent results. In one study, nifedipine and cimetidine were administered together for 7 days in order to more closely mimic actual use [64]. Bioavailability and clearance of nifedipine were increased by 80 percent and reduced by 40 percent, respectively. Additionally, when the drugs were administered together to a group of patients with hypertension, the combination was observed to exacerbate hypotensive adverse effects of nifedipine. In other studies [64, 65, 69] coadministration of ranitidine with nifedipine resulted in variable but significant increases in nifedipine concentrations accompanied by significant reductions in mean blood pressures. Concomitant use of cimetidine or other H_2-receptor antagonists and isradipine, nicardipine, or nimodipine have not yet been evaluated. From these data, it is apparent that if calcium blocker therapy is required for the patient with peptic ulcer disease, use of ranitidine instead of cimetidine, and perhaps sucralfate, would be less likely to cause adverse effects. Careful monitoring of blood pressure is still advisable, however, if either cimetidine or ranitidine is used along with any calcium channel antagonist.

Quinidine

A number of case reports have implicated nifedipine as a major influence on the pharmacokinetic characteristics of quinidine [8, 32, 46]. Although a pharmacodynamic interaction between quinidine and calcium channel antagonists is certainly possible, these case reports suggest that this interaction may be considerably more complex. In all these cases, marked decreases in quinidine concentrations associated with concurrent nifedipine therapy have been observed. Indeed, attempts to increase concentration by giving higher doses of quinidine have failed while nifedipine was coadministered. When nifedipine was discontinued, quinidine concentrations have increased an average of 116 percent. Only one study has attempted to evaluate this interaction in a systematic manner [97]. In this study, 12 patients receiving quinidine for management of ventricular or supraventricular arrhythmias were given nifedipine concurrently. Overall, no effect on disposition of quinidine was observed, although, in one patient, concentrations of quinidine declined by 41 percent. It appears, then, that clinically important effects of nifedipine on quinidine effects or concentrations occur in a minority of patients.

When effects of verapamil or diltiazem on disposition of quinidine were evaluated, markedly different observations were reported. Concomitant administration of verapamil and quinidine results in an increase in quinidine concentrations and elimination half-life [29, 82, 150]. Notably, no effect on disposition of either diltiazem or quinidine was observed in healthy volunteers [89]. Effects of quinidine on concentrations of verapamil have not been evaluated nor has the combination of diltiazem and quinidine been evaluated in patients. Reasons for these different effects on quinidine concentrations by nifedipine, verapamil, and diltiazem are not yet evident, but the implications of these interactions are considerable. The combination of nifedipine and quinidine should be used with caution due to the potential increase in quinidine concentrations when nifedipine is discontinued. Also, if adequate concentrations of quinidine cannot be achieved with usual dosing, concurrent calcium blocker therapy should be considered part of the etiology of this difficulty before more aggressive doses of quinidine are utilized.

Further, concurrent verapamil and quinidine should be used with caution because of the likelihood of verapamil-induced increased quinidine concentrations. Effects of concurrent therapy with other type I antiarrhythmic agents or diltiazem have yet to be assessed. Finally, since verapamil is known to affect concentrations of both quinidine and digoxin, the patient who requires treatment with all three agents should be monitored especially closely for changes in quinidine and digoxin concentrations.

Potential Interactions

A few reports suggest that verapamil and nifedipine are responsible for increases in phenytoin and theophylline concentrations [3, 19, 101]. Subsequent observations [53] of effects of nifedipine and diltiazem on theophylline concentrations have failed to confirm these initial observations. Also, bioavailability of verapamil was reportedly impaired by concurrent therapy with rifampin [109]. Full evaluation of these interactions has yet to be reported, however, and caution is advised when using calcium blockers with any of these agents.

One group of interactions with potential clinical importance involves concurrent use of beta blockers with calcium channel antagonists. This combination was originally thought to be beneficial since use of nifedipine, whose predominant action is vasodilation, was associated with reflex tachycardia. Administration of a beta blocker along with nifedipine was recommended to blunt this reflex increase in heart rate. This recommendation is still valid, and the combination of beta blocker with nifedipine is generally considered a beneficial interaction.

In contrast, dose-related negative inotropic and chronotropic effects appear to be much more likely and considerably more profound when verapamil is combined with a beta blocker. This interaction is believed to be due to overlapping effects of verapamil and beta blockers on left ventricular contractility as well as sinoatrial and atrioventricular nodal function. Patients thought to be at risk are those with preexisting left ventricular dysfunction, arrhythmias, aortic stenosis, and who use either high doses or the intravenous form of either agent. Preliminary results from one clinical investigation suggest that a similar interaction is possible when diltiazem is substituted for verapamil.

The pharmacokinetic aspects of these interactions have yet to be completely explored. One animal study has documented beta-blocker-induced reduction in hepatic blood that impaired clearance of verapamil and allowed accumulation of verapamil to toxic concentrations [51]. Also, marked increases in metoprolol concentrations have been observed when verapamil was concomitantly administered, while those of atenolol were unaffected [94, 147]. Both diltiazem and verapamil have been shown to increase concentrations of propranolol by approximately 25 percent and propranolol appears to effect similar changes in concentrations of diltiazem [60, 121]. Effects of concurrent beta-blocker therapy on concentrations of other calcium blockers have not yet been reported. Further, no correlation between changes in concentrations and subsequent hemodynamic alterations has yet been reported. Clearly, more work is needed to characterize fully these drug interactions, and it is apparent that the combination of any calcium channel antagonist with a beta blocker must be used with caution.

CONCLUSION

In summary, calcium channel antagonists are a chemically diverse group of cardiovascular agents with potentially wide applications. They share a number of pharmacokinetic characteristics including clearance by hepatic metabolism and short elimination half-life. Limited information is currently available in selected patients. Doses of all three drugs should be reduced in the elderly and dose of verapamil should be reduced in patients with advanced renal or hepatic dysfunction. Relatively few drug interactions have been fully evaluated thus far. Considering the potential of these agents for wide clinical use, however, it is reasonable to expect more to be characterized in the near future. Clinicians are well advised to monitor patients with multiple disease states taking multiple medications for adverse reactions or inadequate response to calcium channel antagonists.

REFERENCES

1. Abernethy, D. R., Schwartz, J. B., and Todd, E. L. Lack of interaction between verapamil and cimetidine. *Clin. Pharmacol. Ther.* 38:342, 1985.
2. Abernethy, D. R., and Schwartz, J. B. Pharmacokinetics of calcium antagonists under development. *Clin. Pharmacokin.* 15:1, 1988.
3. Ahmad S. Nifedipine-phenytoin interaction. *J. Am. Coll. Cardiol.* 3:1582, 1984.
4. Alessi, N. E., Walden, M. E., and Hseih, P. S. Nifedipine augments haloperidol in the treatment of Tourette syndrome (Letter). *Pediatr. Neurol.* 4:191, 1988.
5. Allen, G. S., et al. Cerebral arterial spasm—a controlled trial of nimodipine in patients with subarachnoid hemorrhage. *N. Engl. J. Med.* 308:619, 1983.
6. Anderson, P., et al. Plasma concentration response relationship of verapamil in the treatment of angina pectoris. *J. Cardiovasc. Pharmacol.* 4:609, 1982.
7. Aoki, K., et al. Acute and long-term hypotensive effects and plasma concentrations of nifedipine in patients with essential hypertension. *Eur. J. Clin. Pharmacol.* 23:197, 1982.
8. Appleby, D. H., and VanLith, R. M., Quinidine-nifedipine interaction. *Drug Intell. Clin. Pharm.* 19:829, 1985.
9. Auer, L. M., et al. Prevention of sympathetic vasospasm by topically applied nimodipine. *Acta. Neurochir.* 63:297, 1982.
10. Auricchio, R. J. Digoxin interactions with calcium channel blockers. *Drug Interactions Newsletter* 3:45, 1983.

11. Banzet, O., et al. Acute antihypertensive effect and pharmacokinetics of a tablet preparation of nifedipine. *Eur. J. Clin. Pharmacol.* 24:145, 1983.
12. Belz, G. G., et al. Effects of various calcium antagonists on blood level and renal clearance of digoxin. *Circulation* 64:24, 1981.
13. Belz, G. G., et al. Digoxin—antiarrhythmics: Pharmacodynamic and pharmacokinetic studies with quinidine, propafenon, and verapamil (Abstract). *Clin. Pharmacol. Ther.* 31:202, 1982.
14. Belz, G. G., et al. Interaction between digoxin and calcium antagonists and antiarrhythmic drugs. *Clin. Pharmacol. Ther.* 33:410, 1983.
15. Benet, L. Z., and Sheiner, L. B. Pharmacokinetics: The Dynamics of Drug Absorption, Distribution, and Elimination. In A. G. Gilman, L. S. Goodman, T. W. Roll, and F. Murad (eds.), *The Pharmacological Basis of Therapeutics* (7th ed.). New York: Macmillan, 1985.
16. Bertel, O., et al. Nifedipine in hypertensive emergencies. *Br. Med. J.* 1:1, 1983.
17. Bloedow, D. C., et al. Serum binding of diltiazem in humans. *J. Clin. Pharmacol.* 22:201, 1982.
18. Bogaert, M. G., et al. Plasma concentrations of nifedipine in patients with renal failure. *Arzneim. Forsch.* 34:307, 1984.
19. Burnakis, T. G., Seldon, M., and Czaplicki, A. D. Increased serum theophylline concentrations secondary to oral verapamil therapy. *Clin. Pharm.* 2:458, 1983.
20. Campbell, B. C., Kelman, A. W., and Hillis, W. S. Noninvasive assessment of the haemodynamic effects of nicardipine in normotensive subjects. *Br. J. Clin. Pharmacol* 20 (Suppl 1): 55s, 1985.
21. Chaffman, M., and Brogden, R. N. Diltiazem. A review of its pharmacological properties and therapeutic efficacy. *Drugs* 29:387, 1985.
22. Chaitman, B. R., et al. Improved exercise tolerance after propranolol, diltiazem, or nifedipine in angina pectoris: Comparison at 1, 3, and 8 hours and correlation with plasma drug concentration. *Am. J. Cardiol.* 53:19, 1984.
23. Chellingsworth, M. C., et al. Pharmacokinetics and pharmacodynamics of isradipine in young and elderly patients. *Am. J. Med.* 84:72, 1988.
24. Clair, F., et al. Hypotensive effect and pharmacokinetics of nicardipine in patients with severe renal failure. *Curr. Ther. Res.* 38:74, 1985.
25. Clarke, B., et al. Comparative calcium entry blocking properties of nicardipine, nifedipine, and PY 108068 on cardiac and vascular smooth muscle. *Br. J. Pharmacol.* 79 (Suppl):333P, 1983.
26. Clifton, G. D., et al. The pharmacokinetics of oral isradipine in normal volunteers. *J. Clin. Pharmacol.* 928:36, 1988.
27. Debruyne, D., et al. Nicardipine does not significantly affect serum digoxin concentrations at the steady-state of patients with congestive heart failure. *Int. J. Pharmacol.* 9:15, 1989.
28. Dow, R. J., and Graham, D. J. M. The effect of nicardipine hydrochloride, a calcium antagonist, on indices of hepatic microsomal enzyme activity in man. *Br. J. Clin. Pharmacol.* 18 (Suppl):296P, 1984.
29. Edwards, D. J., et al. The effect of coadministration of verapamil on the pharmacokinetics and metabolism of quinidine. *Clin. Pharmacol. Ther.* 41:68, 1987.
30. Eichelbaum, M., et al. The metabolism of ^{14}C-D,L-verapamil in man. *Drug Metab. Disp.* 7:145, 1979.
31. Eichelbaum, M., et al. Effects of verapamil in P-R intervals in relation to verapamil plasma levels following single intravenous and oral administration and during chronic treatment. *Klin. Wochenschr.* 58:919, 1980.

32. Farringer, V. A., et al. Nifedipine-induced alterations in serum quinidine concentrations. *Am. Heart J.* 108:1570, 1984.
33. Feely, J., Wilkinson, G. R., and Wood, A. Reduction of liver blood flow and propranolol metabolism by cimetidine. *N. Engl. J. Med.* 304:692, 1981.
34. Forette, F., et al. Effect of nicardipine in elderly hypertensive patients. *Br. J. Clin. Pharmacol.* 20 (Suppl):125s, 1985.
35. Foster, T. S., et al. Nifedipine kinetics and bioavailability after single intravenous and oral doses in normal subjects. *J. Clin. Pharmacol.* 25:161, 1983.
36. Freedman, S. B., et al. Verapamil kinetics in normal subjects and patients with coronary artery spasm. *Clin. Pharmacol. Ther.* 30:644, 1981.
37. Frishman, W., et al. Clinical relevance of verapamil plasma levels in stable angina pectoris. *Am. J. Cardiol.* 50:1180, 1982.
38. Garty, M., Shamer, E., and Rosenfeld, J. B. Nifedipine digoxin noninteraction. (Abstract No. H11) International Symposium on Calcium Entry Blockers and Tissue Protection, Rome 15–16, March 1984. P. 124.
39. Gengo, F. M., and Green, J. A. Beta-blockers. In W. E. Evans, J. J. Schentagg, and W. J. Jusko (eds.), *Applied Pharmacokinetics Principles of Therapeutic Drug Monitoring* (2d ed.). Spokane: Applied Therapeutics, 1986.
40. Gengo, F. M., et al. Nimodipine disposition and haemodynamic effects in patients with cirrhosis and age-matched controls. *Br. J. Clin. Pharmacol.* 23:47, 1987.
41. Geokas, M. C., and Haverback, B. J. The aging gastrointestinal tract. *Am. J. Surg.* 117:881, 1969.
42. George, C. F. Nifedipine: A calcium channel blocking drug. *Br. J. Clin. Pract.* 41:1059, 1987.
43. Giacomini, K. M., et al. Decreased binding of verapamil to plasma proteins in patients with liver disease. *J. Cardiovasc. Pharmacol.* 6:924, 1984.
44. Graham, D. J. M., et al. Pharmacokinetics of nicardipine following oral and intravenous administration in man. *Postgrad. Med. J.* 60:7, 1984.
45. Graham, D. J. M., et al. The metabolism and pharmacokinetics of nicardipine hydrochloride in man. *Br. J. Clin. Pharmacol.* 20 (Suppl):23s, 1985.
46. Green, J. A., et al. Nifedipine-quinidine interaction. *Clin. Pharm.* 2:461, 1983.
47. Gutierrez, L. M., et al. Pharmacokinetics and pharmacodynamics of nifedipine after chronic administration. *Clin. Pharmacol. Ther.* 35:245, 1984.
48. Gutierrez, L. M., et al. Pharmacokinetics and pharmacodynamics of nifedipine in patients at steady state. *J. Clin. Pharmacol.* 26:587, 1986.
49. Hamann, S. R., Blouin, R. A., and McAllister, R. G. Clinical pharmacokinetics of verapamil. *Clin. Pharmacokinet.* 9:26, 1984.
50. Hamann, S. R., Kaltenborn, K. E., and McAllister, R. G. Pharmacodynamic comparison of verapamil and nifedipine in anesthetized dogs. *J. Cardiovasc. Pharmacol.* 7:224, 1985.
51. Hamann, S. R., et al. Cardiovascular and pharmacokinetic consequences of combined administration of verapamil and propranolol in dogs. *Am. J. Cardiol.* 56:147, 1985.
52. Hansen, P. B., et al. Influence of atenolol and nifedipine on digoxin-induced inotropism in humans. *Br. J. Clin. Pharmacol.* 18:817, 1984.
53. Hendeles, L. H., and Christopher, M. A. Unpublished data, 1986.
54. Higuchi, S., and Shiobara, Y. Comparative pharmacokinetics of nicardipine hydrochloride, a new vasodilator in various species. *Xenobiotica* 10:447, 1980.
55. Higuchi, S., and Shiobara, Y. Metabolic fate of nicardipine hydrochloride, a new vasodilator, by various species in vitro. *Xenobiotica* 10:889, 1980.

56. Hirasawa, K., et al. Effect of food ingestion on nifedipine absorption and hemodynamic response. *Eur. J. Clin. Pharmacol.* 28:105, 1985.
57. Hongo, M., et al. Effects of nifedipine on esophageal motor function in humans: Correlation with plasma nifedipine concentration. *Gastroenterology* 86:8, 1984.
58. Horn, T. J., et al. The pharmacodynamic and pharmacokinetic differences of the D- and L-isomers of verapamil: Implications in the treatment of supraventricular tachycardia. *Am. Heart J.* 112:396, 1986.
59. Hosuda, S. Clinical Experience of Diltiazem. In R. J. Bing (ed.), *New Drug Therapy with a Calcium Antagonist*. Amsterdam: Excerpta Medica, 1978.
60. Hunt, B. A. Effects of calcium channel blockers on the pharmacokinetics of propranolol isomers. *Clin. Pharmacol. Ther.* 47:584, 1990.
61. Jakobsen, P., Lederballe-Pedersen, O., and Mikkelsen, E. Gas chromatographic determination of nifedipine and one of its metabolites using election capture detection. *J. Chromatogr.* 162:81, 1979.
62. Jamieson, M. J., et al. Nicardipine infusion: pharmacokinetics, haemodynamics and effects on the systolic time intervals. *Br. J. Clin. Pharmacol.* 19 (Suppl):536P, 1985.
63. Kato, R., and Takanaka, A. Metabolism of drugs in old rats. I. Activities of NADPH-linked electron transport and drug metabolizing enzyme systems in microsomes of old rats. *Jpn. J. Pharmacol.* 18:381, 1968.
64. Kirch, W., et al. Einflub von cimetidin und ranitidin auf pharmacokinetik und antihypertensiven effekt von nifedipin. *Deutsche Medizinische Wochenschrift* 108:1757, 1983.
65. Kirch, W., et al. Ranitidin-nifedipin interaktion. *Deutsche Medizinische Wochenschrift*; 109:1223, 1984.
66. Kirch, W., et al. Clinical pharmacokinetics of nimodipine in normal and impaired renal function. *Int. J. Clin. Pharm. Res.* 4:381, 1984.
67. Kirch, W., et al. Ranitidine increases bioavailability of nifedipine (abstract). *Clin. Pharmacol. Ther.* 37:204, 1985.
68. Klein, H. O., et al. Verapamil-digoxin interaction. *N. Engl. Med.* 303:160, 1980.
69. Klein, H. O., et al. The influence of verapamil on serum digoxin concentration. *Circulation* 65:998, 1982.
70. Kleinbloesen, C. H., et al. Nifedipine: Kinetics and dynamics in healthy subjects. *Clin. Pharmacol. Ther.* 35:742, 1984.
71. Kleinbloesen, C. H., et al. Nifedipine: Influence of renal function on pharmacokinetic/hemodynamic relationship. *Clin. Pharmacol. Ther.* 37:563, 1985.
72. Kleinbloesen, C. H., et al. Nifedipine: kinetics and hemodynamic effects in patients with liver cirrhosis after intravenous and oral administration. *Clin. Pharmacol. Ther.* 40:21, 1986.
73. Kleinbloesen, C. H., van Brummelen, and Breimer, D. D. Nifedipine: Relationship between pharmacokinetics and pharmacodynamics. *Clin. Pharmacokinet.* 12:12, 1987.
74. Kohno, K., et al. Pharmacokinetics and bioavailability of diltiazem (CRD-401) in dog. *Arzneim. Forsch.* 27:1424, 1977.
75. Koicke, Y., et al. Pharmacokinetics of verapamil in man. *Res. Commun. Chem. Pathol. Pharmacol.* 24:37, 1979.
76. Kuhlmann, J., and Marcin, S. Lack of significant effect of nifedipine and diltiazem on the pharmacokinetics of digitoxin. (Abstract No. 792). II. World Conference on Clinical Pharmacology and Therapeutics, Washington, D.C., (31 July–5 August 1983).
77. Kuhlmann, J., Marcin, J., and Frank, K. H. Effects of nifedipine and

diltiazem on the pharmacokinetics of digoxin. *Naunyn Schmiedebergs Arch. Pharmacol.* 324(Suppl):R81, 1983.
78. Kuhlmann, J., Marcin, S., and Frank, K. H. Pharmacokinetik und kardiale Wirksamkeit von β-acetyldigoxin und digitoxin unter uner Kombinationstherapie wit nifedipin. *Klin. Wochenshr.* 62:451, 1984.
79. Kuhlman, J. Effects of nifedipine and diltiazem on plasma levels and renal excretion of beta-acetyldigoxin. *Clin. Pharmacol. Ther.* 37:150, 1985.
80. Lagercrantz, C., et al. The efflux of spin label entrapped in human erythrocyte ghosts when suspended in hyperosmolar solutions: the effect of chlorpromazine, trifluoperazine, nicardipine and some other membrane active substances. *Biochem. Pharmacol.* 33:1851, 1984.
81. Lang, R., et al. Verapamil improves maximal exercise capacity in digitalized patients with chronic atrial fibrillation: A double-blind crossover study (Abstract). *Circulation* 64(Suppl IV): 296, 1981.
82. Lavoie, R., et al. The effect of verapamil on quinidine pharmacokinetics in man (Abstract). *Drug Intell. Clin. Pharm.* 20:457, 1986.
83. Lederballe-Pederson, O., and Mikkelsen, E. Acute and chronic effects of nifedipine in arterial hypertension. *Eur. J. Clin. Pharmacol.* 14:375, 1978.
84. Lederballe-Pedersen, O., et al. Effect of nifedipine on plasma renin, aldosterone, and catecholamines in arterial hypertension. *Eur. J. Clin. Pharmacol.* 15:235, 1979.
85. Lederballe-Pedersen, O., et al. Relationship between antihypertensive effect and steady state plasma concentration of nifedipine given alone or in combination with a beta-adrenoreceptor blocking agent. *Eur. J. Clin. Pharmacol.* 18:287, 1980.
86. Leon, M. B., et al. Clinical efficacy of verapamil alone and combined with propranolol in treating patients with chronic stable angina pectoris. *Am. J. Cardiol.* 48:131, 1981.
87. Lewis, G. R. C. Long-term results with verapamil in essential hypertension and its influence on serum lipids. *Am. J. Cardiol.* 57:35, 1986.
88. Loi, C.-M., et al. Effect of cimetidine on verapamil disposition. *Clin. Pharmacol.* 37:654, 1985.
89. Matera, M. G., et al. Quinidine-diltiazem: Pharmacokinetic interaction in humans. *Curr. Ther. Res.* 40:653, 1986.
90. Mazer, N., et al. Intragastric behavior and absorption kinetics of a normal and "floating" modified-release capsule of isradipine under fasted and fed conditions. *J. Pharm. Sci.* 77:647, 1988.
91. McAllister, R. G., and Kirsten, E. B. The pharmacology of verapamil. IV. Kinetic and dynamic effects after single intravenous and oral doses. *Clin. Pharmacol. Ther.* 31:418, 1982.
92. McAllister, R. G., Schloemer, G. L., and Hamann, S. R. Kinetics and dynamics of calcium entry antagonists in systemic hypertension. *Am. J. Cardiol.* 57:16D, 1986.
93. McGowan, F. X., et al. Verapamil plasma binding: Relationship to α-1-acid glycoprotein and drug efficacy. *Clin. Pharmacol. Ther.* 33:485, 1983.
94. McLean, A. J., et al. Clearance-based oral drug interction between verapamil and metoprolol and comparison with atenolol. *Am. J. Cardiol.* 55:1628, 1985.
95. Meyer, J. S., and Hardenberg, J. Clinical effectiveness of calcium entry blockers in prophylactic treatment of migraine and cluster headaches. *Headache* 23:266, 1983.
96. Morselli, P. L., et al. Pharmacokinetics and Metabolism of Diltiazem in Man (observations on healthy volunteers and angina pectoris patients). In

R. V. Bing (ed.), *New Drug Therapy With a Calcium Antagonist: Diltiazem.* Hakone symposium '78. Amsterdam: Excerpta Medica, 1979. P. 152.
97. Munger, M. A., et al. Elucidation of the nifedipine-quinidine interaction. *Clin. Pharmacol. Ther.* 45:411, 1989.
98. Neugebauer, G. Comparative cardiovascular actions of verapamil and its major metabolites in the anesthetized dog. *Cardiovasc. Res.* 12:247, 1978.
99. Oates, N. S., et al. Influence of quinidine on nifedipine plasma pharmacokinetics (abstract). *Br. J. Clin. Pharmacol.* 25:675P, 1988.
100. Oyama, Y., et al. Digoxin-diltiazem interaction. *Am. J. Cardiol.* 53:1480, 1984.
101. Parrillo, S. J., and Venditto, M. Elevated theophylline blood levels from institution of nifedipine therapy. *Ann. Emerg. Med.* 13:216, 1984.
102. Paulus, W. J., et al. Comparison of the effects of nitroprusside and nifedipine on diastolic properties in patients with hypertrophic cardiomyopathy: Altered left ventricular loading or improved muscle inactivation. *J.A.C.C.* 2:879, 1983.
103. Pedersen, K. E., et al. Effect of nifedipine on digoxin kinetics in healthy subjects. *Clin. Pharmacol. Ther.* 32:562, 1982.
104. Pedersen, K. E., et al. The long-term effect of verapamil on plasma digoxin concentration and renal digoxin clearance in healthy subjects. *Eur. J. Clin. Pharmacol.* 22:123, 1982.
105. Pieper, J. A., and Rodman, J. H. Lidocaine. In W. E. Evans, Schentag J. J., and Jusko, W. J. (eds.), *Applied Pharmacokinetics Principles of Therapeutic Drug Monitoring* (2d ed.). Spokane: Applied Therapeutics, 1986.
106. Pool, P. E., et al. Effects of diltiazem on serum lipids, exercise performance, and blood pressure: Randomized, double-blind, placebo-controlled evaluation for systemic hypertension. *Am. J. Cardiol.* 56:86h, 1985.
107. Porter, C. J., Garson, A., and Gilette, P. C. Verapamil: An effective calcium blocking agent for pediatric patients. *Pediatrics* 71:748, 1983.
108. Pozet, N., et al. Pharmacokinetics of diltiazem in severe renal failure. *Eur. J. Clin. Pharmacol.* 24:635, 1983.
109. Rahn, K. H., et al. Reduction of bioavailability of verapamil by rifampin. *N. Engl. J. Med.* 312:920, 1985.
110. Rameis, H., Magometschnigg, D., and Gonzinger, V. The diltiazem-digoxin interaction. *Clin. Pharmacol. Ther.* 36:183, 1984.
111. Ramsch, K. D., et al. Overview on pharmacokinetics of nimodipine in healthy volunteers and in patients with subarachnoid hemorrhage. *Neurochirurgia* 28:74, 1985.
112. Reddy, C. P., et al. Absence of specific electrocardiographic end points as indicators of drug effect during chronic oral verapamil therapy (Abstract). *Circulation* 64(Suppl IV):138, 1981.
113. Reves, J. G., Barker, S., and Smith, L. R. Significance of nifedipine plasma levels and hemodynamic changes during anesthesia induction. *Anesthesiology* 59:A41, 1983.
114. Robertson, D. R., et al. Age-related changes in the pharmacokinetics and pharmacodynamics of nifedipine. *Br. J. Clin. Pharmacol.* 25:297, 1988.
115. Rodin, S. M., et al. Comparative effects of verapamil and isradipine on steady-state digoxin kinetics. *Clin. Pharmacol. Ther.* 43:668, 1988.
116. Rosing, D. R., et al. Verapamil therapy: A new approach to the pharmacological treatment of hypertrophic-cardiomyopathy. I. Hemodynamic effects. *Circulation* 60:1021, 1979.
117. Rovei, V., et al. Pharmacokinetics and metabolism of diltiazem in man. *Acta. Cardiol.* 35:35, 1980.

118. Rush, W. R., et al. The metabolism of nicardipine hydrochloride in healthy male volunteers. *Xenobiotica* 16:341, 1986.
119. Sakai, M., et al. Comparison of the effects nifedipine and diltiazem have on serum digoxin concentrations. *Yakuri To Chiryo* 11(Suppl 1):318, 1983.
120. Sakurai, M., et al. Acute and chronic effects of verapamil in patients with paroxysmal supraventricular tachycardia. *Am. Heart J.* 105:619, 1983.
121. Schafer, H. G., et al. Pharmacokinetic interaction of diltiazem and propranolol enantiomers. *Pharm. Res.* 7:s-53, 1990.
122. Schlossman, K., Medenwald, H., and Rosenkranz, H. Investigations on the Metabolism and Protein Binding of Nifedipine. In W. Lockner, W. Braasch, G. Kroneberg (eds.), Second International Adolat symposium. New York: Springer-Verlag, 1975. P. 33.
123. Schols, M., et al. Studies on the disposition of verapamil in patients with renal failure. *Naunyn Schmiedeberg Arch. Pharmacol.* 322(Suppl):R130, 1983.
124. Schomerus, M., et al. Physiological disposition of verapamil in man. *Br. Med. J.* 10:605, 1976.
125. Schrager, B. R., et al. Diltiazem, digoxin interaction? *Circulation* 68(Suppl III):368, 1983.
126. Schwartz, J. B., et al. Acute and chronic pharmacodynamic interaction of verapamil and digoxin and digoxin in atrial fibrillation. *Circulation* 65:1163, 1982.
127. Schwartz, J. B., et al. Prolongation of verapamil elimination kinetics during chronic oral administration. *Am. Heart J.* 104:198, 1982.
128. Schwartz, J. B., and Miglione, P. J. Effect of nifedipine on serum digoxin concentration and renal digoxin clearance. *Clin. Pharmacol. Ther.* 36:19, 1984.
129. Schwartz, J. B., Raizner, A., and Akers, S. The effect of nifedipine on serum digoxin concentrations in patients. *Am. Heart J.* 107:669, 1984.
130. Seki, T., and Takenaka, T. Pharmacological evaluation of YC-93, a new vasodilator, in healthy volunteers. *Int. J. Clin. Pharmacol.* 15:267, 1977.
131. Semplicini, A., et al. Plasma levels of verapamil and its effects on blood pressure, body fluid volumes, and renal function in hypertensive patients. *Int. J. Clin. Pharmacol. Res.* 11:81, 1982.
132. Shand, D. G., et al. Reduced verapamil clearance during long-term oral administration. *Clin. Pharmacol. Ther.* 30:701, 1981.
133. Shibanuma, T., et al. Synthesis of metabolites of 2-(N-benzyl-N-methylamino methyl 2,6-dimethyl-4-[m-nitrophenyl]-1,4-dihydropyridine-3,5-dicarboxyl (nicardipine). *Chem. Pharm. Bull.* 28:2809, 1980.
134. Smith, M. S., et al. Pharmacokinetic and pharmacodynamic effects of diltiazem. *Am. J. Cardiol.* 51:1369, 1983.
135. Smith, M. S., et al. Influence of cimetidine on verapamil kinetics and dynamics. *J. Clin. Pharmacol. Ther.* 36:551, 1984.
136. Somogyi, A., et al. Pharmacokinetics, bioavailability, and ECG response of verapamil in patients with liver cirrhosis. *Br. J. Clin. Pharmacol.* 12:51, 1981.
137. Sorkin, E. M., et al. Nifedipine. A review of its pharmacodynamic and pharmacokinetic properties, and therapeutic efficacy, in ischemic heart disease, hypertension, and related cardiovascular disorders. *Drugs* 30:182, 1985.
138. Sorkin, E. M., and Clissold, S. P. Nicardipine: A review of its pharmacodynamic and pharmacokinetic properties, and therapeutic efficacy, in the treatment of angina pectoris, hypertension and related cardiovascular disorders. *Drugs* 33:296, 1987.
139. Speeg, K. V., et al. Inhibition of microsomal drug metabolism by histamine

H₂-receptor antagonist studied in vivo and in vitro in rodents. *Gastroenterology* 92:89, 1982.
140. Stern, Z., Zylber-Katz, E., and Levy, M. Nifedipine plasma concentration in patients treated for angina pectoris. *Int. J. Clin. Pharmacol. Ther. Toxicol.* 22:198, 1984.
141. Storstein, L., et al. Antihypertensive effect of verapamil in relation to plasma concentrations of verapamil and its active metabolite norverapamil. *Curr. Ther. Res.* 29:112, 1981.
142. Storstein, L., et al. Pharmacokinetics of calcium blockers in patients with renal insufficiency and in geriatric patients. *Acta. Med. Scand.* 681(Suppl):25, 1984.
143. Sung, R. J., Elser, B., and McAllister, R. G. Intravenous verapamil for termination of re-entrant supraventricular tachycardias. Intracardiac studies correlated with plasma concentrations. *Ann. Intern. Med.* 93:682, 1980.
144. Taburet, A. M., et al. Pharmacokinetic studies of nifedipine tablet. Correlation with antihypertensive effects. *Hypertension* 5(Suppl II):29, 1983.
145. Taeymans, Y., et al. Relationship between plasma diltiazem levels and its hemodynamic effects (Abstract). *Circulation* 66(Suppl II):81, 1982.
146. Tartaglione, T. A., et al. Pharmacokinetics of verapamil and norverapamil during long-term oral therapy. *Res. Commun. Chem. Pathol. Pharmacol.* 40:15, 1983.
147. Tateishi, T., et al. Effects of diltiazem on the pharmacokinetics of propranolol, metoprolol, and atenolol. *Eur. J. Clin. Pharmacol.* 36:67, 1989.
148. Thiercelin, J. F., et al. Interaction study between digoxin and calcium antagonists: Verapamil and diltiazem. Proceedings of the II World Conference on Clinical Pharmacology and Therapeutics, July 31–August 5:47, 1983.
149. Traube, M., et al. Correlation of plasma levels of nifedipine and cardiovascular effects after sublingual dosing in normal subjects. *J. Clin. Pharmacol.* 25:125, 1985.
150. Trohman, R. G., et al. Increased quinidine plasma concentrations during administration of verapamil: A new quinidine-verapamil interaction. *Am. J. Cardiol.* 57:706, 1986.
151. Tse, F. L. S., and Jaffe, J. M. Pharmacokinetics of PN 200–110 (isradipine) in normal volunteers. *J. Clin. Pharmacol.* 928:36, 1988.
152. Urthaler, F., and James, T. N. Experimental studies in the pathogenesis of asystole after verapamil in the dog. *Am. J. Cardiol.* 44:651, 1979.
153. van Harten, J., et al. Negligible sublingual absorption of nifedipine. *Lancet* 2:1363, 1987.
154. Vestal, R. E. Drug use in the elderly: A review of problems and special considerations. *Drugs* 16:358, 1978.
155. Wing, L. M. H., Miners, J. O., and Lillywhite, K. J. Verapamil disposition-effects of sulphipyrazone and cimetidine. *Br. J. Clin. Pharmacol.* 19:385, 1985.
156. Winship, L. C., et al. The effect of ranitidine and cimetidine on single-dose diltiazem pharmacokinetics. *Pharmacotherapy* 5:16, 1985.
157. Woodcock, B. G., et al. Verapamil disposition in liver disease and intensive care patients: Kinetics, clearance, and apparent blood flow relationships. *Clin. Pharmacol. Ther.* 29:27, 1981.
158. Yong, C. L., et al. Factors affecting the plasma protein binding of verapamil and norverapamil in man. *Res. Commun. Chem. Pathol. Pharmacol.* 30:329, 1980.
159. Yoshida, A., et al. Effects of diltiazem on plasma levels and urinary excretion of digoxin in healthy subjects. *Clin. Pharmacol. Ther.* 35:681, 1984.

160. Zanolla, L., et al. Long-term persistence of antianginal effect of oral verapamil in chronic stable angina. *J. Cardiovasc. Pharmacol.* 6:423, 1984.
161. Zylber-Katz, E., et al. Bioavailability of nifedipine. A comparison between two preparations. *Biopharm. Drug Disp.* 5:109, 1984.
162. Zylber-Katz, E., Koren, G., and Levy, M. Pharmacokinetic study of digoxin and nifedipine coadministration (Abstract). *Clin. Pharmacol. Ther.* 35:286, 1984.

CHAPTER 9

NITRATES IN TRANSIENT ISCHEMIC SYNDROMES

JONATHAN ABRAMS

Short- and long-acting nitrates are useful in the treatment of exertion- and emotion-induced angina, rest pain, as well as prophylaxis against chest pain attacks in stable and unstable anginal syndromes. While not every patient will respond favorably to nitrates, these drugs are usually effective; there is no convincing evidence that either of the other two antianginal classes of drugs are more effective as first-line agents for stable angina.

Nitrates are also used in patients with mixed angina, a syndrome that includes features of effort- or exertion-induced angina as well as episodes of unprovoked rest pain, suggesting an acute decrease in coronary blood supply. Because nitrates act on both the demand and supply side of the myocardial oxygen requirement equation (see Chapter 3), they should be effective in mixed angina. Unfortunately, there are no good studies available assessing the response of nitrates in this somewhat vaguely defined angina syndrome. Nitrates also appear to be useful in silent ischemia. While the data are limited, there is no reason to believe that these drugs should be any less potent than in the therapy of painful or symptomatic angina.

STABLE ANGINA PECTORIS

Mechanism of Action

As discussed in Chapter 3, there are a number of mechanisms through which nitrates may act to alleviate ischemia in stable angina pectoris (see Table 3-1). These compounds reduce myocardial oxygen demands at rest and during exercise through their vasodilatory effects on the veins and arteries. Most importantly, venodilation results in redistribution of the circulating blood volume with sequestration of blood away from the heart (Fig. 3-2), resulting in smaller cardiac chambers operating (Fig. 3-4) with lower filling pressures. In addition, the modest arterial dilating actions of these compounds result in a decrease in arterial conductance and systolic blood pressure, contributing to a decrease in left ventricular wall stress and an improvement in the myocardial oxygen demand-supply ratio. There is considerable evidence that nitrates act directly on the coronary circulation and improve nutrient flow to zones of myocardial ischemia. Thus, enhanced collateral flow, atherosclerotic stenosis dilation, enhancement of large coronary artery conductance, and reduction of left ventricular diastolic compressive pressure forces may all contribute to an improvement in coronary blood supply with restoration of adequate blood flow to ischemic endocardial zones. In individuals with coronary vasoconstriction or overt vasospasm, nitrates prevent or reverse transient decreases in coronary artery caliber.

The physiology of stable angina pectoris is reviewed in Chapter 1. Typical angina patients have large vessel coronary atherosclerosis with obstructive lesions in at least one major coronary artery. It is generally believed that for angina to occur a segment of the coronary artery must be narrowed to at least 50 to 70 percent of its diameter; often, more than one artery is involved in the process and most patients with angina have double- and triple-vessel disease. Many subjects will have multiple sites of significant narrowing. During physical activity or emotional stress, the diseased coronary circulation cannot augment its blood supply sufficiently to match the transient increase in myocardial energy requirements. This produces episodes of painful myocardial ischemia. Presumably, silent ischemia can be induced by the same mechanisms, although many episodes of painless ischemia are not accompanied by a detectable increase in blood pressure or heart rate.

Recent evidence indicates that residual smooth muscle within coronary atherosclerotic lesions is capable of vasomotion [8, 25]. This suggests another mechanism for the precipitation of angina and its relief by nitroglycerin. One study in effort angina demonstrated that during physical exertion the coronary atherosclerotic lesion may narrow further, increasing resistance across the stenosis and precipitating angina, whereas the normal response of an epicardial coronary artery is to vasodilate during exercise [25]. It has been shown that nitroglycerin can reverse or prevent this phenomena (Fig. 3-3) [25]. Whether or not exertion-related vasoconstriction at the site of coronary stenosis is a common event, it is clearly a potentially adverse phenomenon for patients with stable angina. In some individuals, physical exertion may induce vasoconstriction or overt spasm in epicardial coronary arteries that are not severely diseased [64]. Thus, exercise-related vasoconstriction within the atherosclerotic plaque or in more normal areas of the vessel provides another mechanism for nitrate action. It is likely that in many episodes of unstable angina, spontaneous reduction in coronary artery or atherosclerotic lesion caliber precipitates myocardial ischemia; nitrates should be effective in reversing this phenomenon.

Treatment of Acute Angina Attacks

Nitrates remain the mainstay for therapy of acute episodes of angina pectoris. Sublingual nitroglycerin (NTG) is the gold standard to which all other nitrates are compared. There are a variety of short-acting nitrates available (Table 9-1). Reichek has argued persuasively that many anginal episodes will improve spontaneously with cessation of the precipitating activity, even before sublingual nitroglycerin reaches its peak effect [45]. Nevertheless, there is little doubt that rapid-acting nitroglycerin preparations will attenuate and reverse most episodes of myocardial ischemia that last longer than 2 to 3 minutes, particularly if the cause of myocardial ischemia is not completely eliminated. This is true for patients who have reached a threshold "double product" during physical activity or when emotional stress is the driving force behind

TABLE 9-1. *Rapid-Acting Nitrate Formulations for Treatment or Prophylaxis of Acute Anginal Attacks*

Sublingual nitroglycerin
Sublingual isosorbide dinitrate
Chewable isosorbide dinitrate
Buccal or transmucosal nitroglycerin
Oral nitroglycerin spray
Oral isosorbide dinitrate spray (not available in United States)

the precipitation of angina. In the latter situation, coronary vasoconstriction is more likely to be present along with an increase in blood pressure; people cannot turn off their emotional state as readily as they can stop physical activity. Thus, emotion- or stress-related angina is likely to require nitroglycerin for relief.

HOW TO UTILIZE SHORT-ACTING NITRATES

Nitrate compounds are more effective when the patient remains in an upright position; this accentuates venous pooling and decreases blood pressure, leading to a further reduction in cardiac chamber size. Patients should be advised to take advantage of this effect, although there is a greater likelihood for adverse consequences related to symptomatic hypotension and reflex tachycardia following NTG administration when individuals are standing or sitting. Patients should be instructed to take a single dose of sublingual or oral spray NTG and then wait for 5 to 10 minutes to determine if there is an effect. Nitroglycerin tablets or spray begin to act within 2 minutes, with peak effects at 4 to 7 minutes (Fig. 9-1). The potential for significant hypotension is enhanced when several nitroglycerin tablets are taken in short succession; patients should be warned about the possibility of severe dizziness and even syncope when more than one dose is taken. As a general rule, no more than 3 to 4 doses of a short-acting nitrate should be administered over a period of 15 to 25 minutes. If chest pain continues or recurs the patient should immediately go to the nearest hospital emergency room for evaluation.

SUBLINGUAL NITROGLYCERIN

Sublingual tablets of NTG are extremely effective in alleviating anginal episodes. The amounts required range between 0.15 mg to 0.6 mg., with 0.4 mg (1/150 grain) or 0.6 mg (1/100 grain) as the most common dose employed. The small tablets are placed under the tongue where they rapidly dissolve; dry mouth, inadequate saliva production, or mucosal vasoconstriction can slow tablet dissolution.

Nitroglycerin tablets may have a variable nitroglycerin content, particularly when the medication is not fresh [15, 35]. Nitroglycerin is

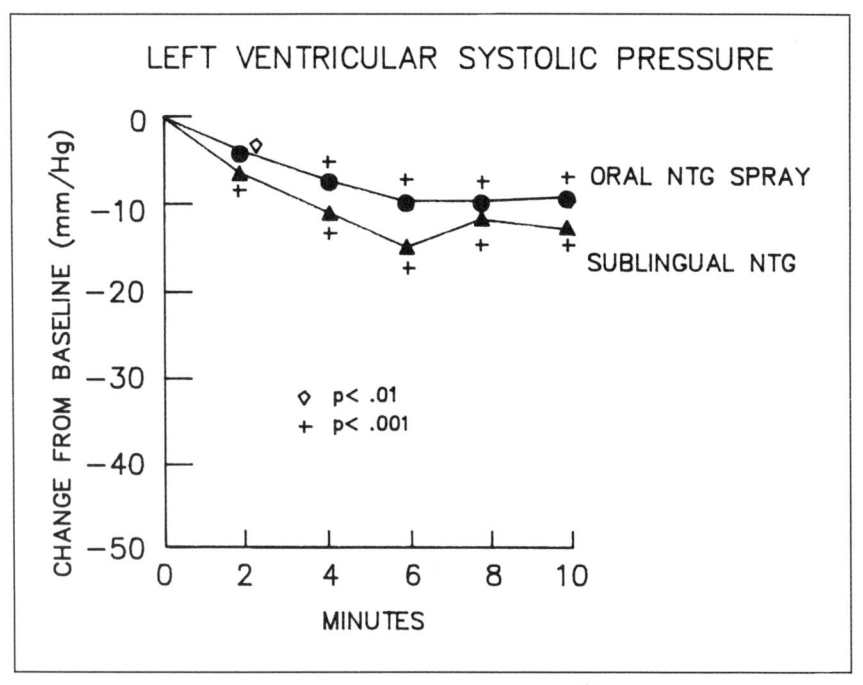

FIG. 9-1. Decrease in left ventricular systolic pressure following sublingual nitroglycerin and oral nitroglycerin spray. The data represent a group of 49 patients undergoing diagnostic cardiac catheterization given either oral nitroglycerin, 0.4 mg of oral nitroglycerin or 0.4 mg sublingual nitroglycerin. A rapid decrease in systolic pressure occurred in both groups. The peak fall in left ventricular systolic as well as diastolic pressure (not shown) occurred at 6 minutes for both preparations. (From Ref. 1, with permission.)

relatively volatile and disappears from the tablets over a period of weeks to months. The best way to maintain tablet potency is to keep the bulk of the prescription in the small brown bottles supplied by the manufacturer, with the cotton removed; the tablets should not be mixed with other pills and the bottle should be refrigerated. The patient keeps a supply of active tablets on his or her person at all times. Sublingual tablets should be renewed with a fresh supply no more than every 3 to 4 months to insure that full potency is maintained. New stabilized formulations of NTG have recently become available that should result in substantially longer tablet stability and may not require storage at cold temperature.

SUBLINGUAL ISOSORBIDE DINITRATE

Some physicians and patients prefer sublingual isosorbide dinitrate (ISDN), which has a slightly slower onset of action for antianginal attacks but has a more prolonged protective effect. Chewable ISDN tablets may also be used for acute episodes, but the onset of action is considerably slower compared to sublingual nitroglycerin.

BUCCAL NITROGLYCERIN

A relatively new formulation of NTG is the buccal or transmucosal tablet, comprised of NTG impregnated in a special methylcellulose matrix [2, 62]. The tablet is placed in the upper gum region in the buccal pouch behind the upper lip. A gel or seal quickly forms, allowing the tablet to adhere to the mucosal surface. Patients learn to eat and drink without difficulty. This formulation results in immediate release of NTG into the circulation; therapeutic plasma NTG levels are achieved within minutes, with peak NTG concentrations and onset of action equivalent to sublingual NTG. A unique aspect of buccal NTG is the sustained or continued release of NTG into the circulation over a period of hours in addition to its immediate action. As long as the tablet remains intact in the mouth it continues to provide therapeutic amounts of NTG for prevention of ischemic attacks. Once the tablet completely dissolves or is chewed, swallowed, or removed by the patient, NTG rapidly disappears from the plasma and the effects cease within 20 minutes.

The transmucosal formulation is effective both for acute treatment of antianginal attacks and as long-acting prophylactic therapy to prevent episodes of angina (Fig. 9-2). It is a particularly useful drug for people with infrequent angina or in those whom a certain type of activity or stressful situation is likely to induce chest pain. The patient can place the buccal tablet in the mouth and achieve immediate protection, which continues as long as the tablet remains in the buccal cavity.

The duration of activity of the buccal formulation ranges from 3 to 6 hours [2, 62]. Its pharmacokinetic profile is ideal to prevent tolerance (see Chapter 16), even when used on a tid basis (see Fig. 9-2) [41].

ORAL NITROGLYCERIN SPRAY

Oral spray formulations of NTG and ISDN have been used in Germany for some years. In 1986 an oral aerosolized spray of NTG was first marketed in America. This oil-based formulation consists of NTG contained in a special fluosol aerosol carrier. A single canister provides over 200 metered doses of 0.4 mg of NTG. The shelf life of this preparation is at least 2 years, a major advantage over sublingual NTG tablets. The oral spray is delivered directly into the mouth and acts as quickly as sublingual NTG. Abrams et al. compared the two formulations and demonstrated that the spray is almost as potent as an equivalent dose of NTG [1] (Fig. 9-1). This preparation has the advantage of being effective, easy to use, and cosmetically pleasing. It is comparable to sublingual NTG as an effective antianginal agent. Figure 9-3 shows data from a recent study comparing oral spray to sublingual NTG in patients with angina [42].

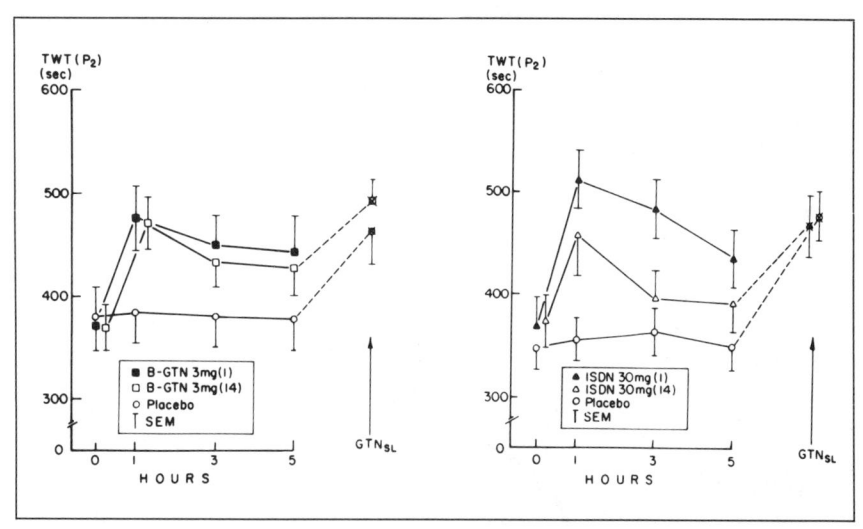

FIG. 9-2. Tolerance to oral isosorbide dinitrate but not to buccal nitroglycerin. In this placebo-controlled, crossover study, patients were treated with buccal nitroglycerin 3 mg. tid or placebo, and alternatively with ISDN 30 mg, qid or placebo. Exercise testing was carried out on day 1 as well as after two weeks of therapy [14]. Note that buccal nitroglycerin resulted in a sustained improvement in exercise performance compared to placebo at 1, 3, and 5 hours after dosing, which was not attenuated after two weeks of tid therapy. On the other hand, the initial day 1 effect of ISDN, resulting in improvement in exercise time up to 5 hours, was attenuated at 3 and 5 hours after two weeks of qid therapy. In both study arms, patients were tested with sublingual nitroglycerin after two weeks of therapy and showed continued responsiveness in spite of the development of tolerance to ISDN. TWT (P2) = treadmill walking time to angina of moderate severity. B-GTN = buccal nitroglycerin. (From Ref. 41, with permission.)

Table 9-2 lists the dosage recommendations, onset and duration of action of most of the available short-acting nitroglycerin formulations, as well as the common long-acting compounds.

USE OF SHORT-ACTING NITRATES AS PROPHYLAXIS AGAINST ANGINAL ATTACKS

Physicians often do not counsel their patients regarding the potential role of rapid-acting nitrate formulations for use immediately prior to activities likely to induce angina. Most individuals with chronic stable angina can predict situations when they are likely to have an episode of pain. This is true for recreational activity as well as employment-related tasks or emotionally stressful events. If a rapid-acting nitrate is taken within 5 minutes prior to the anticipated activity, there is a con-

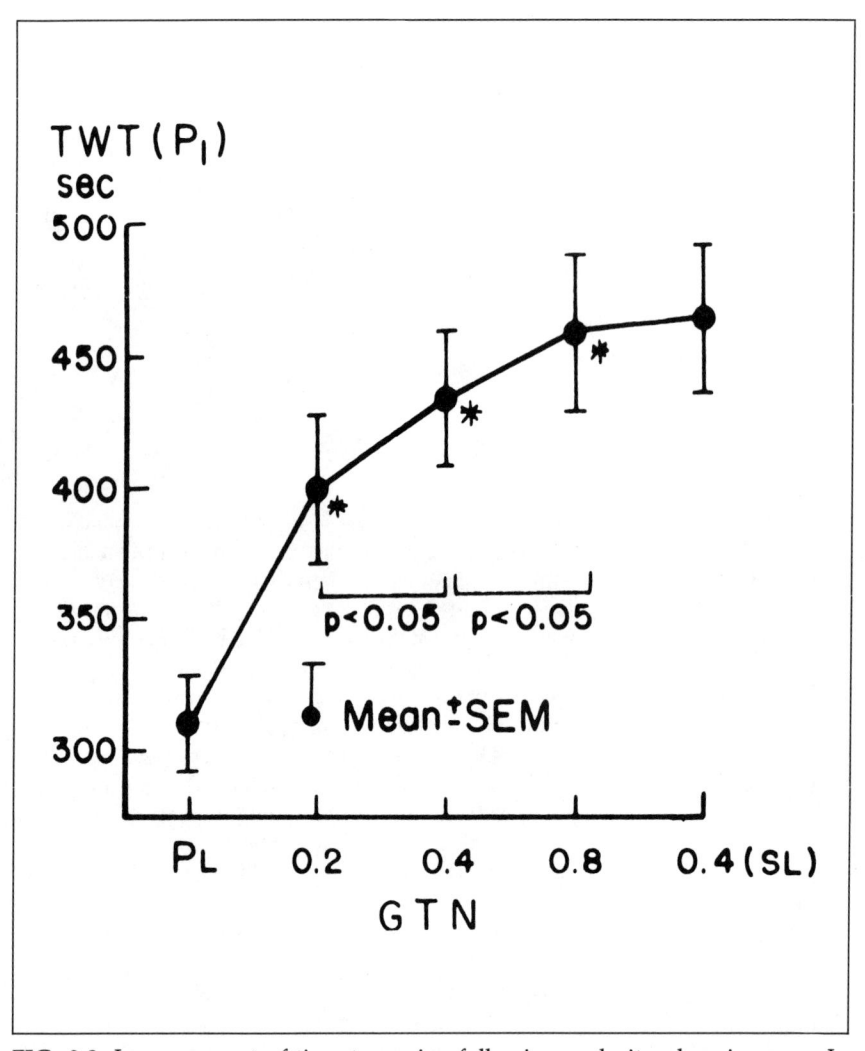

FIG. 9-3. Improvement of time to angina following oral nitroglycerin spray. In this protocol, patients were given placebo as well as three different doses of oral nitroglycerin spray (.2, .4, and .8 mg). Note the improvement of exercise performance for all three doses. A single dose of sublingual nitroglycerin of 0.4 mg was equivalent to the effect of 0.8 mg of oral spray. TWT (T1) = exercise time to the onset of angina. (From Ref. 42, with permission.)

TABLE 9-2. *Short- and Long-Acting Nitroglycerin and Isosorbide Dinitrate Formulations*

Medication	Recommended Dosage (mg)[a]	Onset of Action (minutes)	Peak Action (minutes)	Duration
Sublingual NTG	0.3–0.8	2–5	4–8	10–30 min
Sublingual ISDN	2.5–10	5–20	15–60	45–120 min[b]
Oral NTG spray	0.4	2–5	4–8	10–30 min
Buccal NTG	1–3	2–5	4–10	30–300 min
Oral ISDN	10–60	15–45	45–120	2–6 hr
Oral NTG	6.5–19.5	20–45	45–120	2–6 hr
NTG ointment (2%)	½–2 inches	15–60	30–120	3–8 hr
NTG discs (transdermal)	10–20 mg	30–60	60–180	Up to 24 hr[c]

NTG = nitroglycerin; ISDN = isosorbide.
[a]Higher doses of nitrates may be needed in congestive failure.
[b]Up to 3 to 4 hours in some studies.
[c]Clinical effects may not persist for 24 hours.

siderably decreased likelihood of angina, allowing the patient to proceed without fear of chest pain. This is also important for subjects who experience angina during sexual intercourse.

It is not uncommon for patients with chronic angina to experience chest pain following minimal activity in the early morning hours, perhaps due to a circadian increase in coronary vasomotor tone. The liberal use of prophylactic sublingual, buccal, or oral NTG spray can be beneficial in preventing these early morning anginal attacks.

FEAR OF NITROGLYCERIN

It is advisable to initiate new patients to rapid-acting NTG preparations by suggesting that they first use sublingual or spray NTG when they are not having angina. Subjects should be warned to sit or lie down immediately if marked dizziness or light-headedness appears. To obtain maximal benefits, patients should be advised to remain in an upright position when taking NTG, but it also must be explained that this may accentuate the side effects. Many patients are afraid to use sublingual NTG tablets because of headache or dizziness; if appropriate education is carried out prior to the initial use of NTG, patients are more likely to accept the adverse effects (if any) of the medication.

Dosage adjustment is often not considered by physicians. Patients who have limiting side effects with sublingual NTG tablets should try a smaller dose, utilizing a 0.15 or 0.3 mg tablet. It appears that the oral NTG spray produces less acute side effects than sublingual tablets [1].

A small dose of transmucosal NTG should be employed initially; thus one should start with 1 mg tablet and build up to 2 and 3 mg as tolerated. Remember that in congestive heart failure or in patients with significant left ventricular dysfunction, larger amounts of nitrate are usually required than in those with normal cardiac function, usually with fewer side effects.

TREATMENT OF CHRONIC STABLE ANGINA WITH LONG-ACTING NITRATES

Long-acting nitrates are a mainstay in the therapy of angina pectoris. For some patients monotherapy with a nitrate formulation is sufficient to maintain adequate control of the anginal syndrome. For many others, nitrates are used in conjunction with beta blockers or calcium channel antagonists. There is no evidence that any of the three classes of drugs is more efficacious than another with respect to anti-ischemic effects; it is therefore reasonable to consider nitrates as first-line therapy for patients being treated for angina. The rationale for this approach is the long safety record of these drugs, their low cost, lack of serious side effects, and the clear-cut benefit that nitrates provide in most patients with ischemic heart disease.

It is important for the physician to establish initially that a beneficial response occurs when patient takes sublingual NTG for an episode of angina. In those subjects in whom sublingual or oral spray NTG is promptly and predictably effective without marked adverse sequelae, it makes good sense to employ a long-acting nitrate for control of the anginal syndrome. Numerous studies have demonstrated the efficacy of long-acting nitrates in the treatment of stable angina [16–18, 21, 26, 27, 46, 52, 56, 58, 63].

One of the major advantages of organic nitrates is the remarkable diversity of formulations that is available to patients. Table 9-2 lists the nitrate compounds currently available for angina prophylaxis in the United States. Note that isosorbide-5 mononitrate (5-ISMN) is not included, as this formulation is still undergoing clinical testing; this compound is widely used in Europe and appears to be an effective drug when given two to three times a day [57, 61]. However, sustained acting formulations of 5-ISMN appear to produce tolerance [60].

Sustained release or retard forms of NTG and ISDN and its congeners are available. For the most part, such compounds should be avoided because of their increased propensity to induce nitrate tolerance (Chapter 16). Silber in Germany has successfully used a very large amount of sustained acting ISDN on a once daily basis [56]. This provides therapeutic ISDN and metabolite concentrations that decline during the last 8 to 10 hours of the day, resulting in low trough plasma ISDN and 5-ISMN concentrations that maintain vascular responsiveness compared to a more frequent dosing schedule [56]. Such an approach has not yet been used widely in the United States but is an interesting concept and deserves further study.

AVAILABLE FORMULATIONS

Oral Nitrates

The most commonly used long-acting nitrate is oral ISDN. There is much evidence documenting that this formulation is extremely effective in relieving angina pectoris [16, 21, 26, 41, 52, 56, 58]. It is likely that both the parent ISDN molecule as well as its major metabolite, 5-ISMN, are responsible for the clinical effects when a dose of oral ISDN is given [7]. Figure 9-4 demonstrates the plasma profile of ISDN and metabolites after ingestion of a single dose of ISDN. Note that 5-ISMN reaches a much higher plasma concentration and has a longer duration of action than the parent compound ISDN [7] (Chapter 6).

The lowest clinically effective dose of oral ISDN is 10 mg tid. However, this is not sufficient for most individuals with angina and one should aim for 30 to 40 mg per dose for effective antianginal prophylaxis. Some studies have used much higher individual doses (60 to 90 mg), but these amounts are difficult for most patients to tolerate and such a regimen should be reserved for truly refractory patients. Individuals with depressed left ventricular function or heart failure require larger amounts of nitrates. Parker et. al have demonstrated repeatedly that conventional four times daily ISDN administration predictably induces partial nitrate tolerance (Fig. 9-2) [41], whereas bid or tid dosing with oral ISDN maintains nitrate responsiveness in angina patients (Fig. 9-5) [39].

Oral nitroglycerin, usually in sustained release formulation, has been available for many years. There are relatively few studies documenting the efficacy of oral NTG [18, 63]. It appears that this drug is effective when enough oral NTG is given. There are no data comparing oral ISDN to oral NTG. The author recommends a minimum dose of 6.5 mg of NTG, preferably 9 to 13.5 mg per dose given tid or qid.

Topical Nitrates

NITROGLYCERIN OINTMENT

A topical formulation of 2% nitroglycerin has been available for many years [3]. This was initially used in Scandinavia for treatment of peripheral vascular disease and subsequently was employed in the United States in the 1950s for use in angina. Commercially available NTG ointment has a duration of action ranging from 4 to 8 hours after application. Several studies confirm clear-cut antianginal efficacy with acute dosing [17, 26]. There is some disagreement as to the size of the

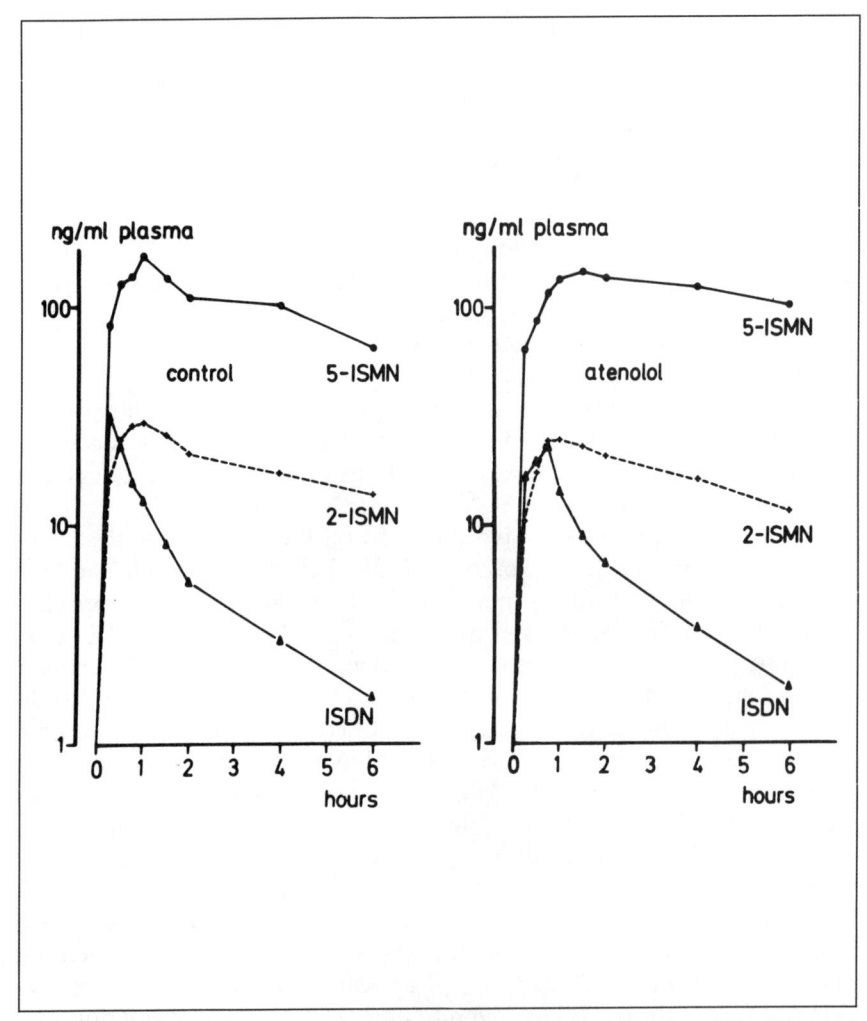

FIG. 9-4. Plasma concentrations of ISDN and its two metabolites following oral administration of a 40 mg dose. (Note that this is log scale.) Concentrations of 5-ISMN are substantially higher than those of the parent compound ISDN, and there is much longer duration of activity. Administration of the beta blocker atenolol does not affect the bioavailability or the pharmacokinetics of oral ISDN administration. (From Ref. 7, with permission.)

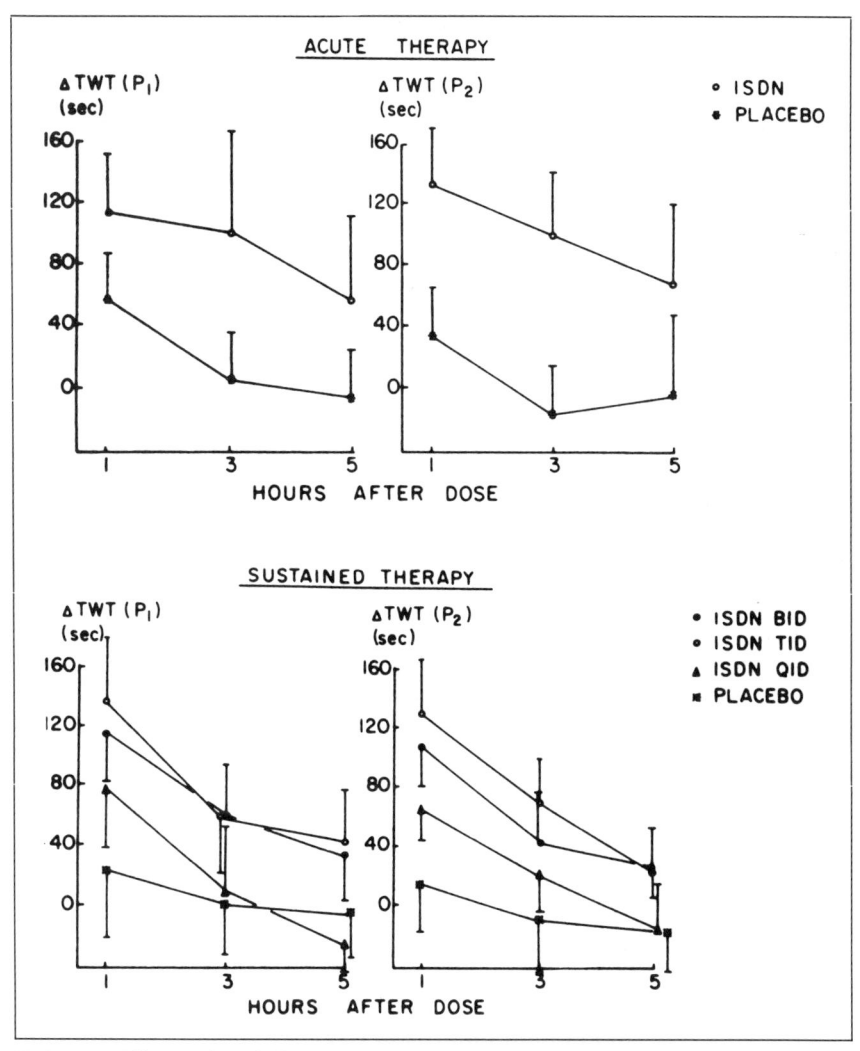

FIG. 9-5. Effects of oral ISDN given two, three, or four times daily. On the first day of the study protocol (acute therapy), there is a marked increase in treadmill walking time to the onset of angina (P1) and to angina of moderate intensity (P2) at 1, 3, and 5 hours after ISDN administration compared to placebo. Note the waning of effect at 5 hours. Ater one to two weeks of chronic therapy with oral ISDN in which the drug was given bid, tid, or qid, there is considerable attenuation of the duration of effect with tid and qid therapy at 3 and 5 hours. The peak effect is also blunted with qid therapy at one hour compared to the day 1 study. These data indicate that sustained dosing with oral ISDN 40 mg bid and tid does not result in significant nitrate tolerance, whereas qid dosing produces an attenuation of effect. (From Ref. 39, with permission.)

skin surface area over which the ointment should be administered. Some suggest a 3 times 3 cm area and others feel that a 6 times 6 inch area should be used. Plasma NTG concentrations are higher with a given dose with larger areas of application. It has been shown that although there may be minor differences in absorption between one skin site compared to another with respect to NTG plasma levels following ointment application, it makes no practical difference as to where the ointment is applied. The most common sites are the chest and arms.

The ointment must be taken off and reapplied several times daily. This is a messy formulation and the medication easily soils clothing. Thus, it is an awkward product for ambulatory subjects to use. Recently a self-contained adhesive unit has been marketed that allows for application of the NTG ointment with an adhesive-rimmed patch, providing a skin seal that prevents leakage of the ointment. This adhesive unit is effective and eliminates most of the application difficulties of the ointment. Nitroglycerin ointment is a particularly good formulation for hospitalized or house-bound subjects.

NITROGLYCERIN PATCHES OR DISCS

The innovative NTG discs or patches (transdermal NTG or TDNTG), marketed in 1982, have been remarkably successful. There are at least five different varieties currently available on the American market; all employ NTG imbedded in a matrix or reservoir system that provides continuous steady-state release of NTG across the dermal layer into the circulation. It is estimated that 0.4 to 0.6 mg per cm^2 of patch surface area reaches the systemic circulation. The patch is applied once daily; plasma concentrations are sustained for at least 24 hours, longer if the patch is not removed. This pharmacokinetic profile is different from any other nitrate formulation except continuous intravenous NTG administration. There are no peaks and valleys of NTG plasma or tissue levels. It is this feature that is particularly problematic with respect to long-term nitrate efficacy, as such a pharmacokinetic profile is most likely to induce tolerance (see Chapter 16).

The initial published reports concerning the NTG patches resulted in considerable controversy as to their effectiveness [40, 47, 53]. Most early studies employed small doses (5 to 10 mg per 24 hours), which result in low plasma NTG concentrations. The results of many such investigations were equivocal. However, with larger doses, utilizing a minimum of 10 to 30 mg per 24 hours, antianginal effects at 2 to 8 hours after administration are clearly seen [5, 34, 40, 47, 49, 59]. Some believe that the patches are not as potent as other nitrate formulations [44].

The major problem with NTG patches is the rapid induction of nitrate tolerance. Many studies in angina as well as congestive heart failure document an attenuation of NTG action within 12 to 18 hours after initial first-dose application [12, 24, 29, 32, 37, 40, 47, 54, 59]. While

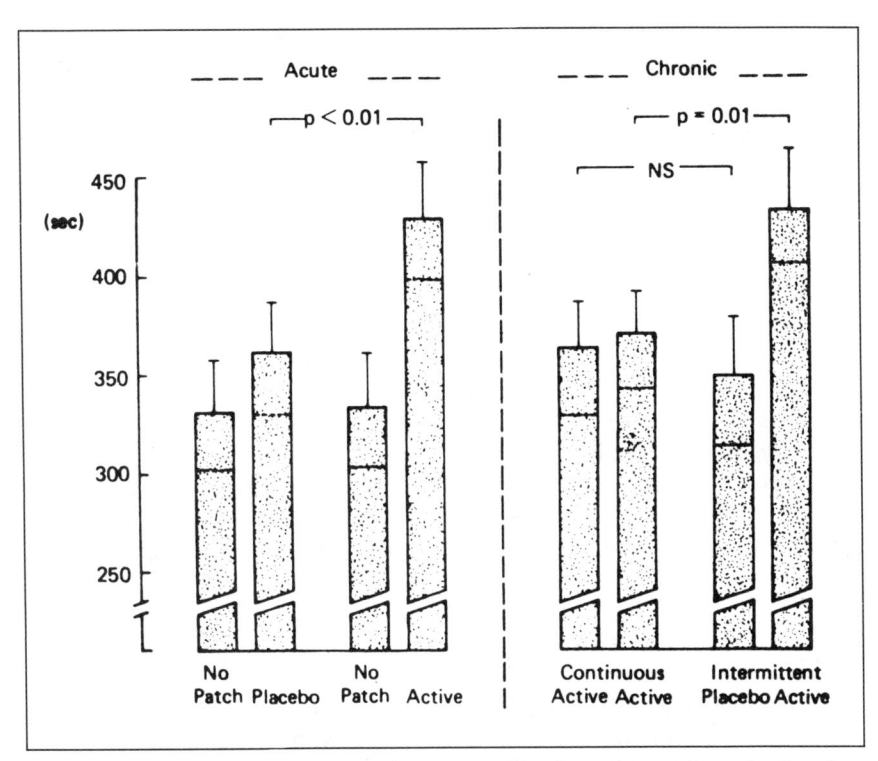

FIG. 9-6. Intermittent versus continuous application of transdermal nitroglycerin. This study in patients with angina demonstrates that intermittent application of the nitroglycerin patch with a 10-hour nitrate-free interval prevents the development of tolerance. Note that active patch administration on day 1 results in a substantial increase in exercise performance whereas placebo patch does not. After two weeks of patch administration, patients were again exercised. The intermittent group continued to show responsiveness to the nitroglycerin patch, whereas the continuous group showed complete loss of antianginal effect. This was a crossover study, with each patient serving as his/her own control. (From Ref. 12, with permission.)

some patients remain responsive to NTG at 24 hours, many others do not. Figure 15-5 shows treadmill test responses in angina patients after the first dose of TDNTG and following continuous therapy. With initial application antianginal effects were seen at 2 and 4 hours but not at 24 hours [40]. After daily application of TDNTG for 1 to 2 weeks there were no longer any antianginal effects at any test interval. Figure 9-6 displays data from one of the first studies that employed an on-off or intermittent NTG patch dosing strategy. In this protocol the patch was applied for 14 hours and then taken off for 10 hours [12]. Sustained antianginal effects were maintained during intermittent transdermal therapy with the patch for 2 weeks. Other small studies appear to confirm the efficacy of the on-off approach in angina as well as heart failure [32, 50, 54]. In 1989, the results of a large multicenter intermittent NTG patch trial in over 200 subjects with angina pectoris were published [20]. This placebo-controlled study was carried out for 1 month, employing a 12-hour patch on-off regimen. Continued responsiveness to administered NTG patch was observed for the 20, 30, and 40 cm^2 (10, 15, 20 mg/24 hour) doses using serial treadmill tests at 8 and 12 hours (see Fig. 15-7).

It is thus recommended that physicians instruct their patients to take the patches off at night to provide an 8 to 12 hour nitrate-free interval. It is critical to provide a lengthy nitrate-free interval of at least 8 hours. However, if a patient is using TDNTG continuously and is doing well clinically, there is no absolute need to alter the method of administration. If there is concern about nocturnal angina or silent ischemic events, the hours of patch on and patch off can be adjusted by the physician; additional antianginal therapy with a beta or calcium channel blocker may be advisable.

Buccal Nitroglycerin

As previously emphasized, this formulation is unique in that it provides both immediate action as well as sustained nitrate effects. Several studies in angina utilizing buccal or transmucosal NTG have documented excellent hemodynamic and anti-ischemic effects [2, 41, 62] (Fig. 9-2). The buccal tablet is well tolerated by most individuals. Patients learn not to dislodge the tablet with their tongues and also easily adapt to eat and drink without difficulty. Some individuals cannot tolerate the buccal formulation. The tablet slowly dissolves in the buccal cavity over 3 to 6 hours, continually releasing NTG into the circulation. The amount of saliva production as well as other factors affect the tablet half-life in the mouth. Subjects who dissolve the tablet within 1 to 2 hours are not good candidates for this formulation. In several clinical investigations comparing this formulation to other nitrate compounds, the appearance of nitrate tolerance with buccal NTG has yet to be demonstrated [36, 41, 48]. The unique pharmacokinetic profile with rapidly rising and falling NTG levels after dissolution mitigates against the development of tolerance by providing a nitrate-free interval as well as constantly changing plasma NTG concentrations (see Chapter 16).

Transmucosal nitroglycerin is available in 1, 2, and 3 mg strength tablets. It was initially marketed in 1982 in a larger tablet size, but the product was withdrawn from the market after poor sales. Buccal NTG has been reformulated in a smaller tablet. Proper use of this unusual product requires more time to educate patients and physicians than for other nitrates. Its unique profile with both rapid onset of action as well as sustained activity should be beneficial to many patients.

Dosing Guidelines for Chronic Angina Therapy

Table 9-2 displays the recommended maintenance dosage for the long-acting nitrates discussed in this chapter. There is a large variability in individual patient responsiveness to nitrates. Plasma nitrate concentrations are nonlinear and unpredictable after chronic oral or topical administration, thus making a fixed or standard dose difficult to recommend for most individuals. Patients with normal left ventricular function in general require less nitrate than those with congestive heart failure.

AVOIDANCE OF NITRATE TOLERANCE

Nitrate tolerance with long-acting nitrates is a real dilemma and is discussed further in Chapter 16. It is now recognized that some degree of tolerance or cross-tolerance among the nitrates can be commonly demonstrated in many patients who take long-acting nitrates over a period of weeks to months.

The pharmacokinetic profile most likely to induce tolerance is one that provides a relatively constant plasma nitrate concentration without a sufficiently long-nitrate-free interval. To preserve vascular responsiveness to nitrates, plasma nitrate levels should be allowed to fall to a nadir on a cyclic basis. The lowest plasma level required to avoid tolerance is not known and probably varies from formulation to formulation. Even shorter-acting nitrates given frequently or in large doses are more likely to induce tolerance when compared to smaller doses or less frequent dosing. An important study by Parker [39] indicated that oral ISDN 40 mg given qid readily induced tolerance as manifested by a shortening of nitrate effect and diminished peak action. However, when the same individuals received bid or tid therapy with oral ISDN, there was much less evidence for tolerance, suggesting that a less aggressive dosing regimen avoids attenuation of effect and preserves anti-ischemic actions (Fig. 9-5). Many other studies of similar design have reached the same conclusion [6, 13]. Table 9-3 outlines a rational approach to long-acting nitrate therapy that will help prevent tolerance development and allow for sustained nitrate effectiveness.

UNSTABLE ANGINA PECTORIS

The syndrome of unstable angina is defined in Chapter 1. Unstable angina generally implies (1) a history of stable angina that changes its character and becomes accelerated in nature or (2) new onset angina pectoris (usually defined as within 3 months) and (3) importantly, individuals with recent onset or prior angina who begin to have a more protracted duration of chest pain as well as pain at rest. Often, there is a decreased responsiveness to sublingual NTG.

TABLE 9-3. *Current Recommendations for Nitrate Therapy*

1. Begin with a small dose.
2. Establish a dose threshold that achieves the desired clinical effect.
3. Use the least amount of nitrate that provides continued symptomatic benefit.
4. Avoid use of sustained action or continuous delivery formulations; these preparations may more readily induce nitrate tolerance. If such regimens are employed, use with intermittent administration providing fluctuations in nitrate exposure.
5. Establish a dosing regimen that provides a nitrate-free interval of at least 8 hours.

The pathophysiology of unstable angina is multifactorial. While the distribution and severity of coronary atherosclerosis does not appear to be significantly different between stable and unstable angina patients, the precise pathogenesis of these two ischemic syndromes appears to differ in many patients, accounting in part for the poorer prognosis in unstable angina. Patients with unstable angina tend to have ulcerated atherosclerotic lesions, plaque fissuring, or underlying endothelial pathology that is associated with platelet aggregation and in situ acute thrombosis. A relatively rapid progression of coronary atherosclerosis has also been documented in some individuals with unstable angina. Increased coronary vasomotor tone or even overt coronary vasospasm has been implicated in this syndrome. It is widely believed that many to most episodes of unstable angina are precipitated by a primary decrease in regional coronary blood supply as opposed to a significant augmentation of myocardial oxygen demands necessitating an increase in coronary blood supply.

Whatever the mechanism, it is well established that unstable angina has a higher morbidity and mortality than stable angina. After clinical stabilization patients should be carefully stratified as to subsequent risk with conventional or radioisotope exercise testing and usually coronary arteriography to assess whether they will require aggressive interventions such as percutaneous angioplasty or coronary bypass surgery. The majority of patients will be treated with medical therapy, at least initially. Many will quiet down and convert to a stable angina pattern. Such individuals may be continued on medical therapy. A smaller but significant proportion of individuals continue to have symptoms or easily provokable ischemia necessitating early angioplasty or bypass surgery. Some progress to acute myocardial infarction within days to weeks of the onset of suggestions.

Nitrate Therapy in Unstable Angina

Unstable angina is a notoriously difficult syndrome to evaluate with rigorous clinial trials of therapy. There is no definite evidence that initial therapy with any one of the three classes of antianginal drugs is more effective than any other. A number of studies indicate that patients who are refractory to initial treatment with one drug who are then given an additional agent appear to respond to the second drug. As a practical matter, most individuals with unstable angina are hospitalized in coronary care units and treated with at least two different types of antianginal agents. The combination of a nitrate and a beta blocker is particularly efficacious: the mechanisms of ischemia relief are quite different, and some of the adverse consequences of each agent are neutralized by the use of the other drug (see Chapter 18).

There are a number of studies documenting that initial or combined treatment utilizing a nitrate is effective in the therapy of unstable angina [11, 13, 23 30]. The most persuasive data have come from protocols employing intravenous nitroglycerin or isosorbide dinitrate titrated to control chest pain. A recent study employed transmucosal NTG compared to intravenous ISDN and demonstrated marked anti-ischemic effects with the buccal preparation, with major improvement in ischemic left ventricular dysfunction after only 3 hours of high-dose transmucosal NTG therapy [31].

In my opinion, intravenous NTG is the initial drug of choice in the treatment of individuals with episodes of ischemic rest chest pain or those who are having frequent episodes of chest pain with little exertion. One must be prepared to use large amounts of intravenous NTG in poorly responsive patients, with meticulous monitoring of arterial pressure to avoid hypotension. Heart rate is a good indicator of the adequacy of central aortic pressure; if the heart rate increases during the nitrate infusion, one should decrease the infusion rate. High doses of intravenous nitroglycerin produce arterial vasodilation and may also have significant antiplatelet effects. One should initiate therapy with an infusion rate of 20 to 40 mcg/min, increasing the infusion rate by (10–20 mcg/min) every 10 to 30 minutes depending on the clinical response; the physician should also be prepared to use a dose of 200 to 300 mcg/minute in refractory patients. In in vitro experiments platelet antiaggregatory actions can be demonstrated with pharmocologic amounts of nitrate, but lower plasma concentrations of organic nitrate may have an important antiplatelet action in patients [19, 22].

One oft-cited study from Italy employed intravenous isosorbide dinitrate and demonstrated a reduction in both painful and painless episodes of resting ischemia [23]. Although this formulation is not yet available in the United States, its proponents believe it has a smoother action than intravenous NTG and may have other advantages [10]. Coronary thrombosis is often an underlying precipitant in unstable angina. Therapy of unstable angina should also include antiplatelet therapy, especially aspirin. When intravenous NTG is used initially, patients should be converted to topical or oral nitrate therapy within 36 to 48 hours after admission as the chest pain syndrome comes under control. There is increasing evidence that continuous infusion of intravenous NTG can induce tolerance [38, 65]. Therefore, it is important to try to decrease the total duration of NTG infusion while providing a dosing regimen that provides for a nitrate-free interval to maintain vascular responsiveness. This is not always clinically feasible; often one must continuously increase the dose of intravenous NTG while adding other antianginal drugs. One must be careful with the combination of intravenous NTG and high-dose calcium channel antagonists, as these drugs individually or in combination produce serious hypotension.

SILENT MYOCARDIAL ISCHEMIA

There is as yet little available data regarding the effectiveness of anginal therapy for silent ischemia. Assuming that the pathogenetic mechanisms responsible for silent ischemia are similar to those causing painful ischemic episodes, it stands to reason that an effective antianginal drug regimen should also reduce episodes of silent ischemia. Preliminary data with nitrates are promising. In 1977 Schang and Pepine gave patients repetitive doses of sublingual NTG and demonstrated a decrease in clinically silent abnormal ST segment shifts [51]. There are several studies that demonstrate improved resting left ventricular function after nitrates in patients with coronary disease [28, 33, 43]. Improvement in global as well as regional left ventricular function can often be documented in patients who are not having chest pain who are given nitroglycerin. The assumption is that the enhanced regional contraction may be related to relief of silent ischemia produced by the NTG [4, 9].

In addition, preliminary data indicate that painless ST abnormalities detected on ambulatory recordings can be improved with nitrate therapy [55]. It is likely that patients who demonstrate a decrease in painful ischemia (angina) during stress testing will also demonstrate a reduction in silent ischemic episodes with the same drug. In that the majority of episodes of ischemia in patients with angina appear to be painless and these silent attacks appear to be shorter than painful episodes, it is logical to conclude that these silent episodes will respond similarly to painful ischemic attacks with a given antianginal agent. Clearly, much more experience is necessary before definitive statements can be made in this regard.

MIXED ANGINA

The concept of mixed angina or angina with a variable exercise threshold implies a changing severity of coronary obstruction related to alterations in coronary vasomotion. The group at the National Institutes of Health have used the term *dynamic coronary obstruction* to stress the labile nature of ischemia in certain patients with coronary atherosclerosis. It is presumed there is large and/or small vessel vasoconstriction superimposed on underlying coronary atherosclerosis that can account for transient increases in resistance to coronary blood flow. Patients with mixed angina typically have effort-related angina that is variably exacerbated by increased myocardial oxygen demands, as well as attacks of chest pain that do not appear to be related to increased myocardial energy costs but are directly attributable to a putative decrease in coronary blood supply. The reason for the latter is not clear. Platelet factors, neurohormonal activity, and the autonomic nervous system may all be responsible for this phenomenon.

Recognition of Patients

Identification of patients with mixed angina is difficult, in that they do not meet standard criteria. A variable or changing angina threshold from day to day is one hallmark of this phenomenon. Individuals who have a prominent component of emotion- or cold-related angina may have transitory increases in coronary vasomotor tone and are more likely to have a mixed angina syndrome. Patients who have both exertion-related chest pain as well as rest pain on a chronic basis also fit into this category.

As we do not really understand the pathophysiologic mechanisms involved in mixed angina, it is difficult to demonstrate that one class of drug is more effective than another. Nitrates reduce myocardial work and improve blood supply by dilating the large epicardial arteries, coronary collaterals, as well as enlarging the stenotic site itself (at least in some patients); it therefore stands to reason that nitrate therapy should be effective in this poorly defined syndrome. Any clinical clue that suggests the occurrence of coronary vasoconstriction or fluctuations in coronary tone should prompt the physician to prescribe a nitrate or calcium channel antagonist (or both) in order to provide maximal coronary vasodilation, prevent vasoconstriction, and decrease myocardial oxygen consumption.

REFERENCES

1. Abrams, J., LeTourneau, J., and Junick, D. Hemodynamic effects of nitroglycerin spray. *Circulation* 76(Suppl IV):IV-126, 1987.
2. Abrams, J. New nitrate delivery systems. Buccal nitroglycerin. *Am. Heart J.* 105:848, 1983.
3. Abrams, J. Nitrate delivery systems in perspective: A decade of progress. *Am. J. Med.* 76(6A):38, 1984.
4. Abrams, J. Silent myocardial ischemia: Role of nitrate therapy. *Int. Med. for the Specialist* 9:51–69, 1988.

5. Abrams, J. The brief saga of transdermal nitroglycerin discs: Paradise Lost? *Am. J. Cardiol.* 54:220, 1985.
6. Abrams, J. Tolerance to organic nitrates. *Circulation* 74:1181, 1986.
7. Bogaert, M. G., and Rosseel, M. T. Fate of orally given isosorbide dinitrate in man: Factors of variability. *Z. Kardiol.* 72(Suppl 3):11, 1983.
8. Brown, G., Bolson, E., Petersen, R. B., et al. The mechanisms of nitroglycerin action. Stenosis vasodilatation as a major component of drug response. *Circulation* 65:1089, 1981.
9. Chatterjee, K. Role of nitrates in silent myocardial ischemia. *Am. J. Med.* 60:8H–25H, 1987.
10. Cintron, G. B., Glasser, S. P., Weston, B. A., et al. Effect of intravenous isosorbide dinitrate versus nitroglycerin on elevated pulmonary arterial wedge pressure during acute myocardial infarction. *Am. J. Cardiol.* 61:21–25, 1988.
11. Conti, R. Use of nitrates in unstable angina pectoris. *Am. J. Cardiol.* 60:31H, 1987.
12. Cowan, J. C., Bourke, J. P., Reid, D. S., and Julian, D. G. Prevention of tolerance to nitroglycerin patches by overnight removal. *Am. J. Cardiol.* 60:271, 1987.
13. Cowan, J. C. Nitrate tolerance. *Int. J. Cardiol.* 12:1, 1986.
14. Curfman, G. D., Heinsmer, J. A., Lozner, E. C., and Fung, H.-L. Intravenous nitroglycerin in the treatment of spontaneous angina pectoris: A prospective randomized trial. *Circulation* 67:276, 1983.
15. Curry, S. H., Mehta, K., Shavlik, T. A., and Felt, R. Survey of sublingual nitroglycerin-tablet potency under conditions of patient use. *Int. Med. for the Specialist* 8, 1987.
16. Danahy, D. T., and Aronow, W. S. Hemodynamics and antianginal effects of high dose oral isosorbide dinitrate after chronic use. *Circulation* 56:205, 1977.
17. Davidov, M. E., and Mroczek, W. J. The effect of nitroglycerin ointment on the exercise capacity in patients with angina pectoris. *Angiology* 27:205, 1976.
18. Davidov, M. E., and Mroczek, W. J. The effect of sustained-release nitroglycerin capsules on angina frequency and exercise capacity. *Angiology* 28:181–191, 1977.
19. DeCaterina, R., Giannessi, D., Crea, F., et al. Antiplatelet effects of isosorbide dinitrate in man. *Z. Kardiol.* 72 (Suppl 3):46, 1983.
20. DeMots, H., and Glasser, S. P. Intermittent transdermal nitroglycerin therapy in the treatment of chronic stable angina. *J.A.C.C.* 13:786–93, 1989.
21. DiBianco, R., Ronan, J. A., Donohue, D. J., and Lindgren, K. M. Effects of a new oral slow release form of isosorbide dinitrate on the hemodynamics and exercise capacity of patients with angina: A placebo controlled and double blind study. *Circulation* 66(Suppl II):II-381, 1982.
22. Diodati, J., Theroux, P., Latour, J.-G., et al. Nitroglycerin at therapeutic doses inhibits platelet aggregation in man (Abstract). *J.A.C.C.* 11:54A, 1988.
23. Distante, A., Maseri, A., Severi, S., et al. Management of vasospastic angina at rest with continuous infusion of isosorbide dinitrate. *Am. J. Cardiol.* 44:533, 1979.
24. Elkayam, U., Roth, A., Henriquez, B., et al. The hemodynamic and hormonal effects of high dose transdermal nitroglycerin in patients with chronic congestive heart failure. *Am. J. Cardiol.* 56:555, 1985.
25. Gage, J. E., Hess, O. M., Murakami, T., et al. Vasoconstriction of stenotic coronary arteries during dynamic exercise in patients with classic angina pectoris: Reversibility by nitroglycerin. *Circulation* 73:865, 1986.

26. Glancy, D. L., Richter, M. A., and Ellis, E. V. Effect of swallowed isosorbide dinitrate on blood pressure, heart rate, and exercise capacity in patients with coronary artery disease. *Am. J. Med.* 62:39, 1977.
27. Greengart, A., Lichstein, E., Hollander, G., et al. Efficacy of sustained-release buccal nitroglycerin in patients with angina pectoris. *Chest* 83:473, 1983.
28. Helfant, R. H., Pine, R., Meister, S. G., et al. Nitroglycerin to unmask reversible asynergy: Correlation with post-coronary bypass ventriculography. *Circulation* 50:108–14, 1974.
29. Jordan, R. A., Seth, L., Henry, D. A., et al. Dose requirements and hemodynamic effects of transdermal nitroglycerin compared to placebo in patients with congestive heart failure. *Circulation* 71:900–85, 1985.
30. Kaplan, K., Davison, R., Parker, M., et al. Intravenous nitroglycerin for the treatment of angina at rest unresponsive to standard nitrate therapy. *Am. J. Cardiol.* 51:694–98, 1983.
31. Lahiri, A., Bowles, M. J., Whittington, J. R., et al. A double blind trial of buccal nitroglycerin and intravenous isosorbide dinitrate in unstable angina (Abstract). Cardiovascular Pharmacology, International Symposium, Geneva, 1985. *Am. J. Cardiol.* 61:21, 1988.
32. Luke, R., Sharpe, N., and Coxon, R. Transdermal nitroglycerin in angina pectoris: Efficacy of intermittent application. *J.A.C.C.* 10:642, 1987.
33. McAnulty, J. H., Hattenhauer, M. T., Rosch, J., et al. Improvement in left ventricular wall motion following nitroglycerin. *Circulation* 51:140–46, 1975.
34. Muiesen, G., Agabita, I. R. E., Muiesen, L., et al. A multicenter trial of transdermal nitroglycerin in exercise-induced angina: Individual antianginal response after repeated administration. *Am. Heart J.* 112 (1):233, 1986.
35. O'Hanrahan, M., McGarry, K., Kelly, J. G., et al. Diminished activity of glyceryl trinitrate. *Brit. Med. J.* 284:1184–98, 1982.
36. Ohlmeier, H., Mertens, H. M., Mannbach, H., and Gleichmann, U. Tolerance and rebound phenomena in nitrate therapy. In J. N. Cohn and R. Rittinghausen (eds.), *Mononitrates*. Berlin: Springer-Verlag, 1985. Pp. 107–23.
37. Olivari, M. T., Carlyle, P. F., Levine, B., and Cohn, J. N. Hemodynamic and hormonal response to transdermal nitroglycerin in normal subjects and in patients with congestive heart failure. *J.A.C.C.* 2:872, 1983.
38. Packer, M., Lee, W. H., Kessler, P. D., et al. Prevention and reversal of nitrate tolerance in patients with congestive heart failure. *N. Engl. J. Med.* 317:799, 1987.
39. Parker, J. O., Farrell, B., Laney, K. A., and Moe, G. Effect of intervals between doses on the development of tolerance to isosorbide dinitrate. *N. Engl. J. Med.* 316:1440, 1987.
40. Parker, J. O., and Fung, H.-L. Transdermal nitroglycerin in angina pectoris. *Am. J. Cardiol.* 54:471, 1984.
41. Parker, J. O., VanKoughnett, K. A., and Farrell, B. Comparison of buccal nitroglycerin and oral isosorbide dinitrate for nitrate tolerance in stable angina pectoris. *Am. J. Cardiol.* 56:724, 1985.
42. Parker, J. O., VanKoughnett, K. A., and Farrell, B. Nitroglycerin lingual spray: Clinical efficacy and dose-response relation. *Am. J. Cardiol.* 57:1, 1986.
43. Pepine, C. J., Feldman, R. L., Ludbrook, P., et al. Left ventricular dyskinesia reversed by intravenous nitroglycerin: A manifestation of silent myocardial ischemia. *Am. J. Cardiol.* 58:38B–42B, 1986.

44. Reichek, N. Long-acting nitrates: Relative utility of nitroglycerin patches. *Am. J. Med.* 76(6A):63, 1984.
45. Reichek, N. Nitroglycerin in chronic stable angina pectoris. *Am. J. Cardiol.* 60:15H, 1987.
46. Reichek, N., Goldstein, R. E., Redwood, D. R., and Epstein, S. E. Sustained effects of nitroglycerin ointment in patients with angina pectoris. *Circulation* 50:348, 1974.
47. Reichek, N., Priest, C., Zimrin, D., et al. Antianginal effects of nitroglycerin patches. *Am. J. Cardiol.* 54:1, 1984.
48. Reichek, N., Priest, C., Zimrin, D., et al. Antianginal effect of nitroglycerin over 24 hours: Role of the method of administration. *Circulation* 70:II-190, 1984.
49. Scardi, S., Pivotti, F., Fonda, F., et al. Effect of a new transdermal therapeutic system containing nitroglycerin on exercise capacity in patients with angina pectoris. *Am. Heart J.* 110:546, 1985.
50. Schaer, D. H., Buff, L. A., and Katz, R. J. Sustained antianginal efficacy of transdermal nitroglycerin patches utilizing an overnight 10 hour nitrate-free interval. *Am. J. Cardiol.* 61:46, 1988.
51. Schang, S. J., and Pepine, C. J. Transient asymptomatic ST segment depression during daily activity. *Am. J. Cardiol.* 39:396–402, 1977.
52. Schneider, W. U., Bussman, W.-D., Stahl, B., and Kaltenbach, M. Dose-response relation of antianginal activity of isosorbide dinitrate. *Am. J. Cardiol.* 53:700, 1984.
53. Sharpe, D. N., and Coxon, R. Nitroglycerin in a transdermal therapeutic system in chronic heart failure. *J. Cardiovasc. Pharmacol.* 6:76–82, 1984.
54. Sharpe, N., Coxon, R., Webster, M., and Luke, R. Hemodynamic effects of intermittent transdermal nitroglycerin in chronic congestive heart failure. *Am. J. Cardiol.* 59:895, 1987.
55. Shell, W. E. Mechanisms and therapy of silent myocardial ischemia and the effect of transdermal nitroglycerin. *Am. J. Cardiol.* 56:231, 1985.
56. Silber, S., Krause, K. H., Garner, C., et al. Antiischemic effects of an 80 mg tablet of isosorbide dinitrate in sustained-release form before and after 2 weeks treatment with 80 mg once daily or twice daily. *Z. Kardiol.* 73(Suppl 3):211, 1983.
57. Tauchert, M., Jansen, W., Osterspey, A., et al. Dose dependence of tolerance during treatment with mononitrates. *Z. Kardiol.* 72(Suppl 3):218–28, 1983.
58. Thadani, U., Fung., H.-L., Darke, A. C., Parker, J. O. Oral isosorbide dinitrate in angina pectoris. Comparison of duration of action and dose response relationship during acute and sustained therapy. *Am. J. Cardiol.* 49:411, 1982.
59. Thadani, U., Hamilton, S. F., Olson, E., et al. Transdermal nitroglycerin patches in angina pectoris. *Ann. Int. Med.* 105:485, 1986.
60. Thadani, U., Hamilton, S., Teague, S., et al. Slow-release isosorbide-5-mononitrate for the treatment of angina pectoris: Duration of effects. In J. N. Cohn and R. Rittinghausen *Mononitrates*. Berlin: Springer-Verlag, 1985. Pp. 188–89.
61. Thadani, U., Prasad, R., Hamilton, S. F., et al. Isosorbide-5-mononitrate in angina pectoris: Plasma concentrations and duration of effects after acute therapy. *Clin. Pharmacol. Ther.* 42:58–65, 1987.
62. Transmucosal controlled-release nitroglycerin. *Med. Letter* 29:39, 1987.
63. Winsor, T., and Berger, H. Oral nitroglycerin as a prophylactic antianginal drug: Clinical, physiologic, and statistical evidence of efficacy based on a three-phase experimental design. *Am. Heart J.* 90:611, 1975.

64. Yasue, H., Omote, S., Takisawa, A., et al. Exertional angina pectoris caused by coronary arterial spasm: Effects of various drugs. *Am. J. Cardiol.* 43:647, 1979.
65. Zimrin, D., Reichek, N., Bogin, K. T., et al. Antianginal effects of nitroglycerin over 24 hours. *Circulation* 77:1376, 1988.

CHAPTER 10

BETA BLOCKERS IN TRANSIENT ISCHEMIC SYNDROMES

UDHO THADANI
VASU D. GOLI
EDWIN G. OLSON
STEPHEN F. HAMILTON

Since the introduction of the first beta blocker in 1958 by Powell and Slater [69], many similar agents have become available for clinical use. All have in common the property of blocking the beta receptors and thus competitively blocking the effects of sympathetic stimulation at rest and especially during exercise. In addition to the beta receptor blockade, many of the beta blockers possess ancillary pharmacologic properties like cardioselectivity, partial agonist or sympathomimetic activity, alpha blocking activity and quinidinelike activity. These ancillary properties are claimed by pharmaceutical companies to provide superiority of one beta blocker over another. The physician is faced with the difficult decision of deciding which beta blocker to use and the complexity of the situation is compounded by the number of beta blockers that have flooded the market in Europe and are expected to be released soon in the United States.

In this chapter, we will briefly discuss the rationale of use of beta blockers in various ischemic syndromes; the mechanism by which beta blockers favorably affect myocardial oxygen supply-demand ratio have been examined in detail in Chapter 4. Clinical trials with individual beta blockers, the comparative studies between different beta blockers, and clinical trials with nitrates and calcium channel antagonists, will be considered. The rationale of combination therapy will be reviewed and the relevance of ancillary pharmacologic properties of beta blockers in general and in special clinical situations will be analyzed.

BETA BLOCKERS IN STABLE ANGINA PECTORIS

Rationale of Beta Blocker Therapy in Stable Angina

Sympathetic stimulation induced by exercise augments myocardial oxygen demand by increasing the heart rate, systolic blood pressure, and myocardial contractility. In patients with obstructive coronary artery disease, the increase in myocardial oxygen demand during exercise cannot be compensated by a corresponding increment in coronary blood flow and when the myocardial oxygen demand outstrips the supply, myocardial ischemia develops and this often precipitates an attack of angina and associated electrocardiographic ST-T wave changes. Beta blocking agents attenuate the increase in heart rate, systolic blood pressure, and cardiac contractility during exercise and thereby reduce myocardial oxygen demand and have been shown to be effective in the treatment of patients with exertional angina pectoris [6, 70, 85, 93].

In this regard, it is well established that beta blocking agents are beneficial primarily by their ability to block competitively the beta-1-adrenergic receptors from the effects of sympathetic stimulation during exercise or emotional stress. Other ancillary properties like membrane stabilizing effect, intrinsic sympathomimetic activity, and beta-2- and alpha-receptor blockade are essentially irrelevant for the antianginal effects but are of importance in understanding the adverse effects observed during therapy with these agents.

Beta blockade, by reducing the heart rate, prolongs diastole and thereby increases the duration of coronary blood flow during diastole. In some patients, the beneficial effects of beta blockade may be offset by the increased wall tension due to ventricular dilation secondary to increase in ventricular fiber length and reduced contractility. Beta blockade also increases left ventricular end-diastolic pressure and hence has the potential of exacerbating occult heart failure and compromising subendocardial blood flow. In patients with normal left ventricular function, beta blockade has few detrimental effects and various beta blockers have been consistently shown to prolong exercise duration in patients with obstructive coronary artery disease when exercise is limited due to angina pectoris rather than breathlessness or fatigue.

Until recently it was felt that beta blockade might increase coronary vascular resistance and reduce coronary blood flow during exercise. Recent studies, however, suggest that beta blockade prevents either coronary collapse or an increase in coronary vascular tone during exercise and induces less ischemia [35]. Whether this effect is in response to lesser ischemia secondary to reduced myocardial oxygen demand due to beta blockade or improvement in collateral flow to the ischemic region remains unanswered at the present time.

Other minor mechanisms by which beta blocking agents might improve myocardial ischemia in stable angina are the ability to shift the oxyhemoglobin curve to the right [67] and to reduce platelet aggregation [32, 60].

Evaluation of Beta Blocking Drugs in Angina Pectoris

In order to evaluate the efficacy of beta blocking agents in angina pectoris, it is necessary to use the optimal dose. How to determine an optimal dose is, however, not always easy, although various methods outlined have been proposed [91]. The degree of beta blockade can be assessed by chronotropic response to isoproterenol before and after the administration of a beta blocking agent. Since the blockade can be reversed if enough agonist is given, there is never a maximum beta blockade [19, 36]. However, this method is of limited value in determining adequate beta blockade in patients who experience angina primarily during physical stress. Plasma drug concentrations are also of limited value despite a reasonable correlation between concentration and decrease in exercise heart rate [17, 20, 38, 51, 68, 78, 79]. The increase in exercise tolerance was poorly correlated with plasma concentration [94, 95]. However, plasma concentrations are useful for determining compliance and bioavailability of the drugs. The average plasma concentrations required to achieve maximal beta blockade after various drugs are shown in Table 10-1. Resting heart rate is not a good measure of optimal beta blockade because of the variability of resting heart rate, which is dependent on resting sympathetic tone. Also, the first dose produces the near maximum reduction in heart rate, while subsequent doses produce only slight additional effects (Fig. 10-1) [10,92]. Further, drugs with intrinsic sympathomimetic activity may not be able to produce desired reductions in resting heart rate. Resting heart rate, therefore, is a much better index of an initial dose rather than an optimal dose. Several other methods for evaluation of beta blockade offer significant advantages.

The frequency of anginal symptoms and nitroglycerin consumption is a good overall guide to therapy but has several limitations. Complicating this approach are the dynamic nature of angina, knowledge of frequent silent angina, and the occurrence of exercise-induced angina in patients without resting symptoms. The lack of spontaneous rest angina may reflect different mechanisms of ischemia in some patients and the fact that others have adjusted to low activity levels in order to avoid pain. Whether the adequacy of beta blockade can be assessed by the duration of ischemic events during a 24-hour ambulatory monitoring remains unexplored and must be considered experimental at this time. Silent ischemic episodes occur more frequently than symptomatic episodes in patients with stable angina pectoris [105], but in unselected patients with documented coronary artery disease, such episodes are encountered in less than 30 percent of the patients [100].

It is easy to assess maximum beta blockade during exercise testing. In normal subjects, maximal beta blockade leads to a 30 to 40 percent reduction in maximal heart rate [17, 20, 68, 90]. However, many patients with angina experience symptoms at relatively low or moderate levels of exercise. At these workloads, it is difficult to appreciate differences in heart rate for beta blockers, which may show a relatively flat dose-response curve (Fig. 10-1). The majority of patients who are on adequate beta blocker therapy have heart rates between 95 to 115 beats per minute during moderate physical exertion [17, 92, 94, 95]. If the heart rate is higher than 115 or 120 beats per minute, the degree of beta blockade is moderate [45]. This approach calls for multistage exercise testing but offers the advantage of assessment of any beta blocker regardless of ancillary pharmacologic properties. Unfortunately, some 20 to 30 percent of patients fail to respond to beta blocker therapy despite adequate reductions in exercise heart rates similar to responders [89, 92, 94, 95, 97]. However, in patients who respond to beta blockers, this exercise model has shown that when given in equipotent doses all beta blockers reduce exercise heart rates and systolic blood pressure to a similar extent [92, 94, 95]. The reduction of ST segment depression during exercise

TABLE 10-1. *Potency Ratio, Half-Lives, Optimal Plasma Concentration and Doses for Maximum Therapeutic Effects of Various Beta Blockers in Angina Pectoris*

Drug	Beta Blockade Potency Ratio	Plasma Half-Life (Hours)	Pharmaco-dynamic Half-Life (Hours)	Plasma Concentration		Total Daily Dose (mg)
Acebutolol	0.3	8	24	0.2–2	µg/ml	400–1800
Alprenolol	1	2–3		50–100	ng/ml	200– 800
Atenolol	1	5–9	24	0.2–0.5	µg/ml	100– 200
Labetalol	0.3	3–4	—	0.7–3	µg/ml	200–1200
Metoprolol	1	2–6	10–12	50–100	ng/ml	150– 400
Nadolol	1.5	14–24	39	50–100	ng/ml	80– 240
Oxprenolol	0.5–1	2–5	13	80–100	ng/ml	160– 320
Pindolol	6	3–4	8	5–15	ng/ml	10– 20
Practolol	0.3	6–8	12–24	1.5–5	µg/ml	400– 800
Propranolol	1	3.5–6	11	50–100	ng/ml	160– 320
Sotalol	0.3	5–13	24	0.5–4	µg/ml	240– 480
Timolol	6	3–4	15	5–10	ng/ml	15– 45
Tolamolol	1–2	2–3	10–12	—		200– 400

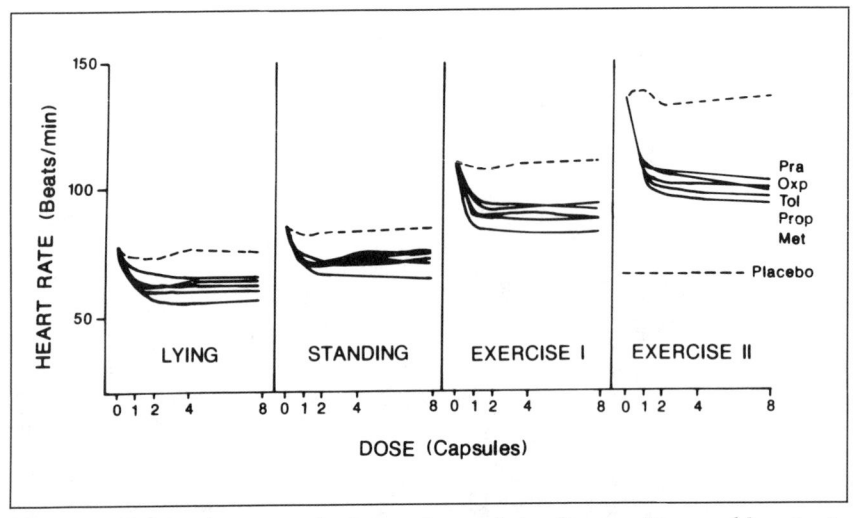

FIG. 10-1. Resting heart rate in the supine and standing position and heart rate during mild and moderate exercise before and after cumulative oral doses of beta blockers with different ancillary properties. The dose-response curves are relatively flat. (From Ref. 91, with permission.)

by beta blockers [89, 92, 94, 95, 97] is not sensitive enough to assess optimal beta blockade in patients. Similar reductions in ST segment depression have been observed in responders and nonresponders to beta blocker therapy [97], while other patients can increase exercise tolerance on beta blockade without a reduction in ST segment depression. Further, the degree of ST segment depression bears little relation to left ventricular dysfunction [53], and many patients have abnormal resting electrocardiograms that preclude ST segment analysis.

In conclusion, assessment of optimal beta blockade requires a comparison of the duration of exercise time to the onset of angina before and after various doses of beta blockers [89, 92, 94, 95, 97]. With this technique, one also evaluates the effects of therapy on heart rate and blood pressure, which are important determinants of myocardial oxygen demand, and of electrocardiographic ST segment depression. If a patient does not experience further improvement in exercise performance despite adequate suppression of heart rate and reduction in rate pressure product, there is little to be gained by increasing the doses.

Ideal Way to Assess Beta Blocker Therapy

The ideal way to determine optimal beta blockade would be to perform a baseline exercise test and to repeat the exercise test after increasing the doses until an adequate dose for a given patient is found. Individual dosing may be necessary in view of inter- and intraindividual variations in plasma concentrations and due to variable bioavailability of the drugs. This can be done in three ways: (1) Exercise tests can be repeated at hourly intervals after multiple cumulative oral doses. (2) The effect of a dose can be studied within 2 to 3 hours after oral ingestion and after doubling the dose on successive days. (3) One can double the doses at weekly intervals or monthly intervals and assess exercise performance before and after the morning dose of the medication. The first method has the advantage that it can be completed in 1 day. However, it does not allow adequate time between doses or equilibrium between tissue and plasma drug levels. The second approach is more reasonable but cumbersome. The third approach is more convenient for the patient but it may take several weeks before one can establish an optimal dose. Long-term studies will be needed to determine if these approaches reduce morbidity or mortality when compared to patients treated empirically.

Importance of Study Design in Evaluation of Beta Blockers in Angina Pectoris

In order to evaluate the effects of beta blockers in angina pectoris without bias, it is necessary that the active drug be compared to placebo in a double-blind fashion. Placebo alone has been shown to reduce angina frequency and improve exercise tolerance [41, 96]. The patients studied should have a stable pattern of angina that can be easily reproduced during mild to moderate exertion. It is essential to perform a symptom-limited exercise test on the bicycle or treadmill. Recently, there has been a trend to use placebo baseline as control followed by a period of active therapy, which is compared to an agent with proven efficacy. This approach, although not ideal, is better than open-label and uncontrolled study designs.

Since the response to beta blockers may vary from patient to patient, it is desirable to study the effects of the active drug at various dose levels and the placebo in a random-crossover design. An alternative is to study a larger number of patients in a parallel manner with each group assigned in a random manner to a given dose or drug.

In this chapter, we will only emphasize studies that have utilized double-blind protocols and were placebo-controlled. The acute, short- to medium-term, and long-term studies with beta blockers will be reviewed.

Acute Studies with Beta Blocking Drugs in Angina Pectoris

Acute studies with different beta blockers either used intravenously or orally (propranolol [70, 81, 97, 102], practolol [70, 102], sotalol [70], oxprenolol [70, 81, 97]) have shown that drugs with intrinsic sympathomimetic activity reduce heart rates to a smaller extent than drugs without this property. However, when used in equipotent doses, the degree of improvement in exercise tolerance is similar despite the differences in ancillary pharmacologic properties. Further, the majority of patients who respond to one drug also respond to other agents in this class.

The effects of cumulative doses of 40, 80, 160, and 320 mg propranolol; 40, 80, 160, and 320 mg oxprenolol; 100, 200, 400, and 800 mg practolol; 50, 100, 200, and 400 mg metoprolol; 50, 100, 200, and 400 mg tolamolol were studied in 12 patients with stable angina pectoris and compared to placebo [92]. All five drugs equally improved exercise tolerance, reduced ST segment depression, and attenuated rise in heart rate and systolic blood pressure. Near maximum improvement in exercise tolerance occurred after the cumulative oral dose had reached 160 mg for propranolol and oxprenolol, 200 mg for metoprolol and tolamolol, and 400 mg for practolol (Fig. 10-2). When these maximally effective doses were administered as single doses, increase in walking time before the development of angina and reduction in ST segment depression, heart rate, and blood pressure was apparent at 1 hour and the effects persisted for 8 hours—effects that markedly differed from response to placebo.

Limitations and Drawbacks of Acute Studies

Although acute studies clearly demonstrate the beneficial effects of beta blockers in patients with stable angina pectoris, they do not provide information regarding long-term effectiveness or late-occurring adverse effects. This was highlighted with practolol therapy, which produced serious oculocutaneous reactions only after prolonged use [4]. Therefore, it is necessary to evaluate the efficacy of beta blocking drugs in medium- to long-term studies.

Medium- to Long-Term Studies with Beta Blockers

For these studies, ideally one should have a run-in period of several weeks in order to assess the stability of the patient. A run-in period of 2 weeks is common and better than none. If a crossover design is used, the active treatment should be followed by an appropriate washout period in order to avoid carryover effects. It is preferable that each treatment should last for a period of a month or longer, although periods of only 1 or more weeks have been utilized. Using the randomized crossover design with adequate washout periods, it is difficult to evaluate multiple doses of a given drug. In recent years the emphasis has

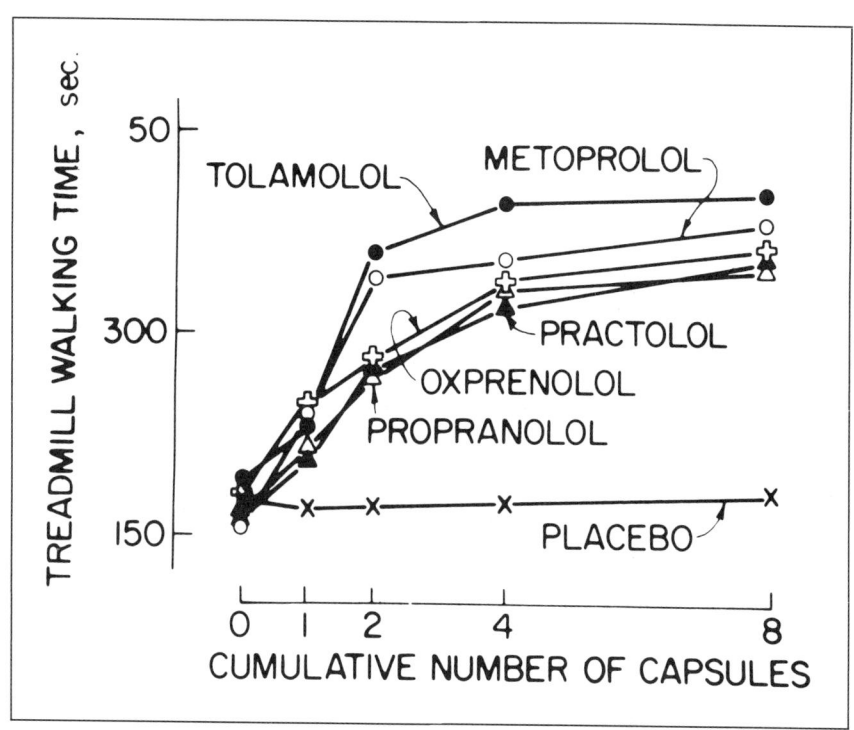

FIG. 10-2. Acute dose-response relation in angina pectoris (12 patients). Treadmill walking time before onset of angina increased significantly after all five drugs in comparison with placebo. Near maximum improvement was produced after four capsules when the cumulative oral dose was 160 mg for propranolol and oxprenolol, 200 mg for tolamolol and metoprolol, 400 mg for practolol, the contents of one capsule being either 40 mg of propranolol, 40 mg of oxprenolol, 100 mg of practolol, 50 mg of metoprolol or tolamolol, or placebo. (From Ref. 92, with permission.)

been on parallel design studies where effects of many doses or different drugs can be compared in similar cohort of patients. However, if one utilizes parallel design study, it is necessary to use patients with similar limitations of exercise tolerance in each of the study groups—otherwise, the results may be erroneous. Only double-blind studies with placebo control will be reviewed.

The medium- to long-term studies have the advantage that in addition to exercise testing one can also evaluate the effects of treatment on angina frequency and nitroglycerin consumption during daily activities. A drug that is truly antianginal should not only increase exercise capacity but should also reduce angina frequency. We will first review studies with individual drugs and then evaluate comparative studies with different beta blockers.

Studies of Individual Beta Blockers

Propranolol, metoprolol, atenolol, and nadolol are approved for use in angina pectoris in the United States. Both fixed and variable dosage trials of propranolol have been reported. The dosage has varied from 30 to 1380 mg per day, and the percentage of responders has varied from 52 to 100 percent [9]. Treadmill walking time to the onset of angina and to angina of moderate severity were significantly increased at 1, 8, and 12 hours postdose with both acute and sustained therapy (Fig. 10-3) [95]. On the basis of available data, the usual therapeutic dose of propranolol is 160 to 320 mg per day, which can be given twice rather than four times a day. A sustained release formulation of 160 mg of propranolol given daily was shown to be as effective as 40 mg given four times per day in nonplacebo randomized studies [39, 65].

Atenolol 100 and 200 mg once a day reduced angina frequency and nitroglycerin consumption and decreased mean heart rate throughout the dosing interval with preservation of diurnal variation in heart rate [47]. In a dose-response study, 25, 50, 100, and 200 mg of atenolol all increased exercise duration but near maximal improvement was seen after a dose of 100 mg [77]. Persistent beneficial increase in exercise duration has been reported for 1 year [77].

Metoprolol, in acute studies of 200 mg, increased exercise duration with persistence of effect for at least 8 hours [92]. From comparative studies an effective dose of metoprolol is between 120 and 240 mg per day. Therapy with 240 mg nadolol once a day has been shown to prolong exercise duration and reduce angina frequency over a 24-hour period [80]. Some studies have shown nadolol to be effective in doses as low as 180 mg per day [31].

Several beta blockers available in the United States have been studied but as yet do not have official indications for angina pectoris, including acebutolol, betaxolol, timolol, pindolol, labetalol, carteolol, and penbutolol. Acebutolol in doses of 600 to 1200 mg per day given in three divided doses has been found to be effective [23, 27]. While lower doses have been studied and found beneficial [86, 99], others have been unable to reproduce increases in exercise duration even at larger doses [56]. Timolol improved exercise tolerance after 10 to 30 mg administered three times a day [6, 7], but improvement at 3 hours postdose was greater compared to 12 hours postdose [6]. Carteolol in doses of 10 to 40 mg per day has been reported to reduce angina frequency [2].

In hypertensive patients with angina, labetalol can reduce angina frequency and improve exercise tolerance [33], though doses up to 1200 mg may be required. In normotensive angina patients, 200 to 300 mg twice daily can increase exercise tolerance and reduce ST segment evidence of spontaneous ischemia during 24-hour ambulatory monitoring [72].

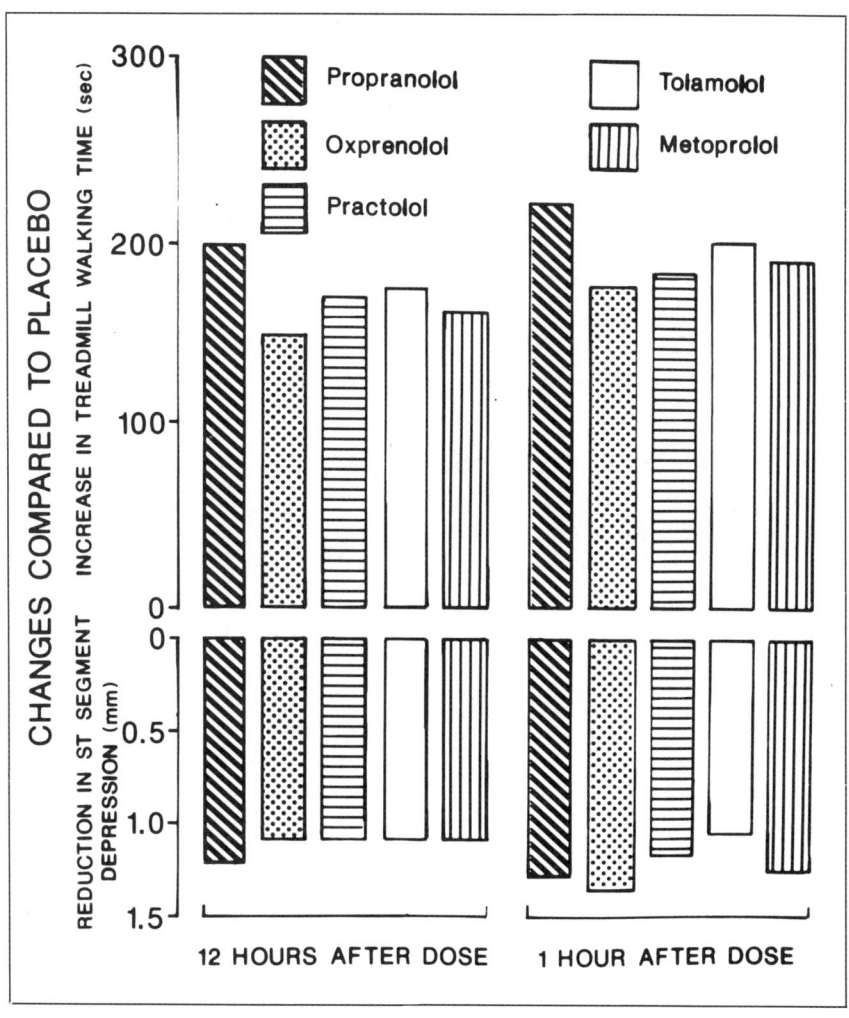

FIG. 10-3. Comparison of effects of five beta-adrenoceptor antagonists during sustained therapy (22 patients). Data represent mean values. Treadmill walking time prior to onset of angina increased significantly after treatment with each of the five drugs in comparison with treatment with placebo ($p < 0.001$) at 1 and 12 hours after propranolol, practolol, or metoprolol, and tolamolol. $p < 0.001$ at one hour and <0.01 at 12 hours after oxprenolol. ST segment was significantly reduced by all five drugs in comparison with placebo ($p < 0.001$). (From Ref. 93, with permission.)

Studies of pindolol report conflicting results. Some show the beneficial antianginal effects of 15 to 25 mg of pindolol per day [55] while others note a lack of effect at 15 to 30 mg per day [24, 40]. However, one report suggests that pindolol is as effective as propranolol [30].

Several beta blockers not marketed or not indicated for angina in the United States have been studied. These drugs include oxprenolol, sotalol [61, 83], bevantolol [25], celiprolol [12], carvedilol [8], and alprenolol [42]. Oxprenolol has been shown to be beneficial in both rapid release [89, 103] and slow release [59, 63] formulations. The beneficial effects of sotalol have been eclipsed by reports of Torsades de Pointes; the effects of 14 to 17 percent increases in exercise tolerance by alprenolol are relatively small compared to other agents in this class.

Comparative Studies of Beta Blockers with Different Ancillary Properties During Long-Term Therapy in Angina Pectoris

In order to make a meaningful comparison of various beta blockers in angina pectoris, it is essential that optimum doses for each drug should be utilized. However, many of these patients may not tolerate the maximum dose and this has compounded the results of some of the studies. Further, different exercise protocols have been utilized by different investigators, and it is not possible to compare the results of one study to another. Nonetheless, from the review of studies discussed below, the following conclusions can be made: (1) Comparative studies during sustained therapy with different beta blockers confirm previously reviewed intravenous and short-term oral studies, showing that all beta blockers irrespective of their ancillary pharmacologic properties are equally effective antianginal agents. (2) Drugs with intrinsic sympathomimetic activity reduce heart rate to a lesser extent than nonselective and cardioselective agents. (3) During exercise, all beta blockers reduce the rise in heart rate and systolic blood pressure and diminish the extent of electrocardiographic ST segment depression to a similar extent.

Sandler and Clayton compared the effects of practolol 200 to 600 mg twice a day and propranolol 80 mg four times a day with placebo in three 1-month treatment phases [76]. Both active drugs reduced angina frequency and improved exercise tolerance to a similar degree. Propranolol 160 mg per day and alprenolol 400 mg per day were found to be equally effective and both reduced angina frequency and improved exercise tolerance [48].

In 20 patients with angina pectoris, Sowton et al. gave 40 mg propranolol, 120 mg practolol, 100 mg alprenolol, 400 mg oxprenolol, and 5 mg pindolol for 2 weeks. All were effective; however, pindolol was less effective [84]. Jackson et al. compared the efficacy of propranolol 80 mg three times a day with tolamolol 100 and 200 mg as well as practolol 100 mg three times a day and placebo in 42 patients [44a]. Each treatment was prescribed for 4 weeks. Propranolol and tolamolol at both doses were superior to placebo ($p < 0.001$) while practolol was superior to placebo ($p < 0.05$). When active treatments were compared, the researchers were unable to identify any significant differences. Reported side effects were not different with any of the active preparations. Propranolol 80 to 640 mg and equipotent doses of practolol, tolamolol, and oxprenolol were found to be equally effective in a placebo-controlled study in 23 patients [93]. Each drug was prescribed twice a day for a period of 1 month. All drugs reduced anginal frequency and nitroglycerin consumption and improved exercise tolerance to a similar extent. At rest, heart rate reduction was more pronounced after metoprolol and propranolol than with the other three drugs. However, during exercise, all drugs attenuated the increase in heart rate and blood pressure to a similar degree in comparison to placebo.

Atenolol 25, 50, and 100 mg administered twice a day was as effective as propranolol 80 mg three times a day [46]. Improvement in exercise tolerance after 100 mg atenolol twice a day was similar to that after 320 mg of propranolol per day [46]. Metoprolol and nadolol have been reported to be equally efficacious to propranolol [18, 29, 34].

Comparing the long-acting beta blocker drugs and sustained release preparations, Jones and Mir reported that conventional propranolol, long-acting propranolol, sustained release oxprenolol, and nadolol all decreased angina frequency and nitroglycerin consumption while exercise duration was increased more after propranolol, long-acting propranolol, and nadolol than after sustained release oxprenolol [52].

Sustained release oxprenolol (160 mg) once a day has been reported to be equally effective to 40 mg three times a day of propranolol [63]. However, at 24 hours postdose, improvement in exercise tolerance after oxprenolol was less than that at 7.5 hours after oxprenolol and 4 and 12 hours after propranolol [63].

Pindolol 10 to 40 mg per day has been found to be equally effective in reducing angina frequency and improving exercise tolerance as propranolol 40 to 160 mg per day [30]. Labetalol and atenolol were equally effective [49]; so was celiprolol when compared to atenolol [48]. Similar results have been found comparing propranolol to sotalol [43], propranolol, metoprolol, and alprenolol [1, 3, 10], and acebutalol to propranolol [22].

Comparison of Beta Blocking Agents to Other Antianginal Drugs

NITRATES VERSUS BETA BLOCKERS
There are no good studies comparing the effects of beta blockers to long-term therapy with nitrates. Beta blockers do exert beneficial effects

during long-term therapy while tolerance develops rapidly during sustained therapy with nitrates.

BETA BLOCKERS VERSUS CALCIUM CHANNEL ANTAGONISTS
In 1973, Livesley et al. reported that therapy with fixed doses of 120 and 80 mg verapamil or 100 mg propranolol was superior to placebo and both agents reduced angina frequency and nitroglycerin consumption to a similar degree [57].

Acebutalol was found to be as effective as nifedipine [21], while verapamil 360 mg per day was found to be superior to metoprolol 40 mg per day, although both drugs reduced angina frequency and improved exercise capacity. Pindolol and nifedipine 10 mg three times a day were found to be equally effective [15].

Verapamil and propranolol have been shown to be equally effective [50], while propranolol was found to be superior to nifedipine in another study [88]. Similarly, propranolol and nifedipine have been reported to be equally effective [64]. From the published literature, one can conclude that beta blockers are equally effective to calcium channel antagonists when used as monotherapy in patients with angina pectoris and the choice of one drug over other is in part dependent on physician preference and in part due to other concomitant diseases present.

Combination of Beta Blocker and Nitrates in Angina Pectoris

Both beta blockers and nitrates reduce myocardial oxygen consumption, but in addition, nitrates also may increase the oxygen supply to the ischemic region. Beta blockade tends to increase the heart size, nitrates to decrease it. Beta blockade prevents nitrate-induced reflex tachycardia. Thus, there is a rationale basis for beta blockade and nitrate therapy in patients with angina pectoris. Patients already on beta blockers have been shown to increase exercise tolerance after sublingual nitroglycerin or sublingual isosorbide. In a recent acute study, combination of isosorbide dinitrate (mean dose 90 mg) and propranolol (mean dose 120 mg) was shown to be more effective than propranolol alone [62]. However, during long-term therapy, benefit of nitrate therapy in addition to beta blockade therapy has not been substantiated.

Combination of Beta Blocker and Calcium Channel Antagonists in Angina Pectoris

Combination therapy is often used in patients with angina, and beta blockade does block reflex tachycardia induced by nifedipine. However, the combination with diltiazem or verapamil, although used often without harm, should be used with caution as in sensitive patients extreme bradycardia and atrioventricular block or cardiac dilation may develop [64].

The combination therapy of propranolol and nifedipine has been reported to be superior to either drug alone [58, 62]. Similarly, combination of propranolol and diltiazem was superior to propranolol alone [87]. Atenolol plus nifedipine was also superior to either drug alone in another study [26].

Beta Blockers in Patients with Angina Pectoris and Concomitant Diseases

OBSTRUCTIVE AIRWAY DISEASE

Recently much discussion has centered around the possible therapeutic value of various ancillary pharmacologic properties of the beta receptor antagonists. On theoretical grounds, the cardioselective drugs like practolol, metoprolol, atenolol, and tolamolol may have an advantage over the noncardioselective drugs like propranolol, oxprenolol, and timolol in the treatment of patients with angina who also have evidence of obstructive airway disease. However, comparative studies in such patients are lacking, and it is not safe to assume that, in therapeutic doses, the cardioselective drugs will not have any deleterious effect on the respiratory function. Worsening of bronchospasm has been reported to occur with cardioselective drugs in patients with history of asthma or chronic bronchitis [101, 104].

INCIPIENT HEART FAILURE

It has been suggested that drugs with intrinsic sympathomimetic activity will precipitate heart failure less frequently than drugs without this property. However, no comparative studies are available to substantiate these claims. Moreover, heart failure has been reported following therapy with beta blockers, which also have intrinsic sympathomimetic activity [28].

DIABETES MELLITUS

Another area of concern has been in patients with angina pectoris who also have diabetes mellitus. Beta blockers are known to mask the symptom of hypoglycemia and it has been suggested that cardioselective agents are safer in this respect than nonselective drugs [54]. However, in practice serious problems during therapy with propranolol in patients with angina pectoris who also have diabetes have rarely been encountered. In diabetic patients, pretreatment with 40 mg propranolol or 50 mg metoprolol did not potentiate the effects of insulin [54]. However, blood glucose recovery was reduced significantly by propranolol but not metoprolol. Propranolol also caused more profound bradycardia and increased blood pressure during hypoglycemia.

Recommendations of Beta Blocker Therapy in Angina Pectoris

In an uncomplicated patient with angina pectoris with normal left ventricular function, beta blockers are very effective and reduce angina frequency and nitroglycerin consumption and increase exercise tolerance. In this regard, all beta blockers irrespective of ancillary pharmacologic properties are equally effective. In individual patients, the dose of a given beta blocker has to be titrated until a maximum benefit is obtained. Near maximum improvement usually is seen with propranolol 160 to 320 mg per day, atenolol 100 to 200 mg per day, metoprolol 200 mg per day, nadolol 160 to 240 mg per day, acebutolol 600 to 1200 mg per day, and labetalol 400 to 600 mg per day. Even the drugs with a shorter plasma half-life exert longer duration of effects, and drugs like propranolol and metoprolol, although recommended for use four times a day, have been used twice a day [93]. Long-acting drugs like atenolol, nadolol, and slow release formulations can be prescribed once a day.

In patients who have concomitant diseases in addition to angina pectoris, certain ancillary properties of beta blockers assume some importance. In patients with peripheral vascular disease, it is preferable to use cardioselective beta blockers. In patients with history of obstructive airway disease, it is better to avoid beta blockers, but if necessary one should either use cardioselective agents or drugs with intrinsic sympathomimetic activity in order to minimize the bronchospastic effects of beta blockade. Another alternative is concomitant therapy with a weak beta stimulant like albuteralol.

In patients with overt heart failure, beta blockers should be avoided when the patient has already been digitalized. In patients with incipient heart failure, even beta blockers with intrinsic sympathomimetic activity should be used with caution as overt heart failure may manifest itself.

In patients who have diabetes and angina pectoris, nonselective agents have been used without any problem, but on theoretical grounds, it is preferable to use a cardioselective agent.

If patients do not respond to one beta blocker, it is unlikely that they will respond to another. Change of one beta blocker to another is only indicated when central nervous system or other side effects develop. Patients who respond only partially to beta blocker therapy can be started on a combination of a beta blocker and a long-acting nitrate or a combination of a beta blocker and a calcium channel antagonist.

BETA BLOCKERS IN UNSTABLE ANGINA

The pathophysiological mechanisms responsible for unstable angina have been dealt with in detail in Chapter 1. A majority of the episodes of unstable angina are due to reversible myocardial ischemia secondary to a reduction in coronary blood flow either due to intermittent platelet occlusion or thrombus formation at the complicated plaque site or to a change in coronary artery tone. Some episodes are triggered by an increase in myocardial oxygen demand secondary to an increase in heart rate and/or blood pressure. Despite the emphasis on reduction in myocardial blood flow in patients with unstable angina, beta blockers are widely used in this group of patients.

Rationale of Beta Blocker Therapy in Unstable Angina

In a majority of patients with unstable angina, even when the initial episode is not due to an increase in myocardial oxygen demand, there is eventually an increase in heart rate and blood pressure due to an increase in sympathetic drive secondary to chest pain and myocardial ischemia [14, 75]. Beta blockade is likely to interrupt this sequence of changes and prevent development of symptoms and ischemia. Further, some beta blockers by reducing platelet aggregation may prevent reduction in coronary blood flow in the ischemic region.

Evaluation of Beta Blockers in Unstable Angina

Due to the waxing and waning of symptoms and electrocardiographic changes in unstable angina, it is necessary to evaluate a therapeutic agent against either placebo or proven therapy in a parallel fashion. Crossover studies may provide misleading information as the episodes of pain and ischemia may either resolve spontaneously or increase in frequency due to regression or progression of the thrombus at the complicated plaque site.

There is a paucity of double-blind studies evaluating beta blockers against placebo in unstable angina. In many of the studies, initial placebo period together with other concomitant therapy has been used as a baseline. These studies and one recently published controlled study will be evaluated.

Favorable clinical effects of therapy with beta blockers in unstable angina were reported in the early seventies. Guazzi et al. treated 36 patients with unstable angina, 21 of whom had ST segment depression and the remaining 15 patients had ST segment elevation in association with chest pain. The initial dose of propranolol was 20 mg four times a day and increased until symptom relief was observed or side effects developed [37]. Propranolol therapy abolished the symptoms in 80 percent of the patients in whom angina was associated with ST segment depression and in 73 percent of patients in whom angina was associated with ST segment elevation. Placebo therapy in the run-in period was ineffective in both groups.

In a randomized study comparing the effects of propranolol ($N = 50$)

and diltiazem ($N = 50$) in unstable angina, anginal episodes, morbidity, and mortality after a mean follow-up period of 5 months were similar with the two agents [98]. In a group of 70 patients with unstable angina, propranolol and diltiazem reduced the number of anginal episodes and ST segment changes to a similar degree [5].

On the other hand, in some reports beta blockade had either no beneficial effects or produced detrimental effects in patients with unstable angina. Capucci et al. in a double-blind, randomized crossover study compared placebo, propranolol (240 mg daily), or verapamil (480 mg daily) in 18 patients [13]. The mean frequency of anginal attacks was significantly lower after propranolol in comparison to first placebo period but verapamil was superior to propranolol. The findings of this study are of interest in that the number of episodes of chest pain decreased dramatically during the second placebo period.

Parodi et al. in a randomized, single-blind crossover trial compared antianginal effects of propranolol (300 mg daily) and verapamil (400 mg daily) in ten patients with unstable angina [66]. The number of ischemic episodes per 48 hours were: 25 ± 3 during placebo therapy, 23 ± 3 during propranolol therapy, and 5 ± 1 during verapamil therapy. Thus, only verapamil was shown to be effective.

These studies showing either a lack of or a beneficial effect of beta blocker therapy in unstable angina have serious limitations since placebo effects were not evaluated in the parallel manner that we feel is necessary for any meaningful conclusions. The Holland Interuniversity Nifedipine/Metoprolol Trial Research Group (HINT) compared the effects of placebo, nifedipine, metoprolol, and combination of metoprolol and nifedipine in 338 patients with unstable angina who had not received previous beta blocker therapy [73]. These patients were maintained on nitrate therapy. In addition, these workers also studied [73] patients who were already on beta blockers at time of admission; patients either continued to receive metoprolol plus placebo or metoprolol plus nifedipine. The main outcome event studied was recurrent ischemia or myocardial infarction within the first 48 hours of hospitalization. Trial medication effects were expressed as ratio of event rates relative to placebo. In patients not pretreated with a beta blocker, the event rate ratios with associated 90 percent confidence intervals were 1.15 (0.83, 1.64) for nifedipine, 0.76 (0.49, 1.16) for metoprolol, and 0.80 (0.53, 1.19) for metoprolol and nifedipine combined. In patients already on a beta blocker, the addition of nifedipine was beneficial.

The HINT study clearly documents the beneficial effect of metoprolol in patients with unstable angina. Fixed combination of metoprolol plus nifedipine provided no further benefit and nifedipine therapy alone was felt to be detrimental; the trial was terminated prematurely on that account. A combination of nifedipine and metoprolol was only effective when patients were already receiving beta blockers. Similar beneficial effects of propranolol plus nifedipine have been reported by other workers.

Recommendations for Beta Blocker Therapy in Unstable Angina

The pathogenic mechanisms underlying the development of unstable angina are complex and may vary from patient to patient. Only one large, randomized study has been performed, and it clearly shows the beneficial effects of beta blockers in unstable angina. Combination of beta blockers with nitrates or calcium channel antagonists has further advantage in that the latter agents may reduce vascular tone and prevent spasm, and this augments the beneficial effects of beta blocker therapy. Beta blockers are especially useful in patients with unstable angina who have heart rates about 70 beats per minute and/or associated hypertension. The doses of beta blockers used should be such that the resting heart rate stays below 80 beats per minute. In this regard, noncardioselective and cardioselective agents are preferable to agents with additional intrinsic sympathomimetic properties like pindolol as the latter may aggravate angina in the absence of high sympathetic drive at rest [71].

BETA BLOCKERS IN VARIANT ANGINA

Dynamic changes or frank coronary artery spasm is the main mechanism by which myocardial ischemia is produced in patients with variant angina. A majority of the patients have underlying fixed coronary artery disease, while a minority have angiographically normal coronary arteries. The main emphasis of treatment has been coronary vasodilator therapy with nitrates or calcium channel antagonists or the combination of the two. Despite the theoretical advantages of vasodilators, treatment with beta blockers has been used in patients with variant angina. Yasue et al. observed worsening of angina with propranolol in 13 patients with chest pain associated with ST segment elevation [106]. Robertson et al. [74] found that propranolol significantly prolonged the duration of ischemia during ambulatory electrocardiographic monitoring in patients with vasospastic angina. However, in their study, adverse effects of propranolol were observed in only a minority of the patients.

The adverse effects of beta blockade in variant angina have been explained by a change in the response of the smooth muscle cell to alpha-adrenergic stimulation caused by beta blockade. Whether beta blockers with additional alpha blocker properties will blunt this response is not known.

Whether beta blockade will aggravate chest pain or myocardial ischemia in the presence of concomitant therapy with nitrates and calcium channel antagonists also remains unknown. In patients who have significant frank coronary artery disease in addition to spasm, beta blockade may indeed be helpful in reducing myocardial ischemia and preventing coronary artery collapse during exercise [35].

Recommendations for Beta Blockers in Variant Angina

Beta blockers should not be used as initial therapy in patients with variant angina. They should be reserved for patients with variant angina who also have significant obstructive coronary artery disease and are symptomatic despite therapy with long-acting nitrates and calcium channel antagonists.

Beta Blockers for Mixed Angina Pectoris

Some patients with fixed coronary artery disease also experience rest pain due to a reduction in coronary artery flow. Whether the reduction in flow is due to frank spasm or intermittent platelet occlusion remains unknown. There are no studies with beta blockers or other therapeutic agents in this syndrome. On theoretical grounds, combination therapy with a beta blocker and nitrates or calcium channel antagonists is justified.

Beta Blockers for Silent Myocardial Ischemia

Silent myocardial ischemia occurs more frequently than manifest ischemia. During ambulatory monitoring it is detected by electrocardiographic ST segment and T wave changes. However, many patients with coronary artery disease also have electrocardiographic ST-T changes, depression of left ventricular function, or abnormal thallium perfusion scans during exercise in absence of symptoms. The latter manifestations are no doubt due to increase in myocardial oxygen demand induced by increased sympathetic discharge during exercise. In this group of patients, there is a clear role of therapy with beta blockers and an increase in exercise duration associated with a significant reduction in ST segment depression has been reported [16].

Silent myocardial ischemia detected during ambulatory electrocardiographic monitoring and in patients with unstable angina pectoris is believed to be due to a primary reduction in myocardial oxygen supply secondary to a reduction in coronary blood flow. How this reduction in flow is brought about is not known.

Both changes in coronary vasoconstriction and intermittent platelet occlusion have been proposed in the pathogenesis of silent myocardial ischemia. Therefore, many authorities advocate treatment with calcium channel antagonists or nitrates for silent myocardial ischemia. Recent careful studies, however, suggest that silent myocardial ischemia has definite diurnal variation with increased frequency between 6:00 A.M. and 12:00 noon [11, 82]. Many of the episodes are preceded by and associated with some increase in heart rate (10 to 12 beats per minute) and minor alterations in blood pressure [11, 82]. These changes in heart rate are less pronounced than those observed during exercise testing, which also produces ischemia in these patients [11, 82].

Despite the claims that silent myocardial ischemia is induced by a primary reduction in myocardial blood flow, recent placebo-controlled studies have shown that propranolol, metoprolol, and labetalol all significantly reduce silent myocardial ischemia; this is brought about by reduction in heart rate and possibly myocardial contractility [44].

In patients with unstable angina, silent ischemia occurs frequently and can probably be explained on the basis of intermittent platelet or thrombotic occlusion, which has been documented angiographically. In this group of patients, the main emphasis of treatment should be antiplatelet agents or antithrombotic agents. There are no controlled studies evaluating the effects of beta blockade in this group of patients.

Recent studies, however, suggest that beta blocker therapy is very effective in patients with unstable angina; the effects of such therapy on episodes of silent ischemia are now being explored.

Recommendations of Beta Blocker Therapy for Silent Myocardial Ischemia

Beta blockers are very effective in reducing silent myocardial ischemia in patients with fixed coronary artery disease and such treatment is recommended routinely in this group of patients. The role of beta blockers in patients with unstable angina who also manifest silent ischemia is unknown at the present time, but there are no contraindications for the use of beta blockers in this group of patients.

REFERENCES

1. Adolfsson, L., and Sonnhag, C. Hemodynamic effects of two cardioselective beta-adrenoceptive antagonists, metoprolol and H87/07, in coronary insufficiency. *Scand. J. Clin. Lab. Invest.* 36:755, 1976.
2. Alcocer, L., Aspe, J., Arce, E., and Vieyra, J. The effect of carteolol, a new beta-blocker, on angina pectoris. *Curr. Ther. Res.* 31:67, 1982.
3. Alderman, E. L., Coltart, D. J., Wettach, G. E., and Harrison, D. C. Coronary artery syndromes after sudden propranolol withdrawal. *Ann. Intern. Med.* 81:625, 1974.
4. Amos, H. E., Brigden, W. D., and McKerron, R. A. Untoward effects associated with practolol: Demonstration of antibody binding to epithelial tissue. *Br. Med. J.* 1:598, 1975.
5. Andre-Fouet, X., Usdin, J. P., Gayet, C., et al. Comparison of short-term efficacy of diltiazem and propranolol in unstable angina at rest: A randomized trial in 70 patients. *Eur. Heart J.* 4:691, 1983.
6. Aronow, W. S., Plasencia, G., Wong, R., and Landa, D. Exercise duration to angina at two and twelve hours after timolol. *Clin. Pharmacol. Ther.* 29:155, 1981.

7. Aronow, W. S., Turbow, M., Van Camp, S., et al. The effect of timolol vs placebo on angina pectoris. *Circulation* 61:66, 1980.
8. Astrom, H., and Jonsson, B. Haemodynamic effects of different beta blockers in angina pectoris. *Scot. Med. J.* 22:64, 1977.
9. Boakes, A. J., and Prichard, B. N. C. The effect of AH 5158, pindolol, propranolol, and D-propranolol on acute exercise tolerance in angina pectoris. *Br. J. Pharmacol.* 47:673P, 1973.
10. Borer, J. S., Comerford, M. B., and Sowton, E. Assessment of metoprolol, a cardioselective beta-blocking agent, during chronic therapy in patients with angina pectoris. *J. Intern. Med. Res.* 4:15, 1976.
11. Campbell, S., Barry, J., Rebecca, G. S., et al. Active transient myocardial ischemia during daily life in asymptomatic patients with positive exercise tests and coronary artery disease. *Am. J. Cardiol.* 57:1010, 1986.
12. Capone, P., and Mayol, R. Celiprolol in the treatment of exercise induced angina pectoris. *J. Cardiovasc. Pharmacol.* 8(Suppl 4):S135, 1986.
13. Capucci, A., Brachetti, D., Carini, G. C., et al. Propranolol versus verapamil in patients with unstable angina. *Amsterdam Excerpta Medica* 198:1981.
14. Chierchia, S., Brunelli, C., Simonetti, I., Lazzari, M., and Maseri, A. Sequence of events in angina at rest: Primary reduction in coronary flow. *Circulation* 61:759, 1980.
15. Cocco, G., Strozzi, C., Chu, D., et al. Therapeutic effects of pindolol and nifedipine in patients with stable angina pectoris and asymptomatic resting ischemia. *Eur. J. Cardiol.* 10:59, 1979.
16. Cohn, P. F. Influence of beta blockers on exercise-induced silent myocardial ischemia. In P. F. Cohn (ed.) *Silent Myocardial Ischemia*. New York: Marcel Dekker, 1986.
17. Coltart, D. J., and Shand, D. G. Plasma propranolol levels in the quantitative assessment of beta-adrenergic blockade in man. *Br. Med. J.* 3:731, 1970.
18. Comerford, M. B., and Besterman, E. M. M. An eighteen months' study of the clinical response to metoprolol, a selective beta-one receptor blocking agent, in patients with angina pectoris. *Postgrad. Med. J.* 52:481, 1976.
19. Conolly, M. E., Kersting, F., and Dollery, C. T. The clinical pharmacology of beta-adrenoceptor-blocking drugs. *Progr. Cardiovasc. Dis.* 19:203, 1976.
20. Davidson, C., Thadani, U., Taylor, S. H., et al. Pharmacological studies with slow-release formulations of oxprenolol in man. *Eur. J. Clin. Pharmacol.* 10:189, 1976.
21. DePonti, C., DeBiase, A. M., Pirelli, S., et al. Effects of nifedipine, acebutolol and their association on exercise tolerance in patients with coronary artery disease. *Am. J. Cardiol.* 49:1259, 1982.
22. DiBianco, R., Singh, S. N., Shah, P. M., et al. Comparison of the antianginal efficacy of acebutolol and propranolol: A multicenter, randomized, double-blind, placebo-controlled study. *Circulation* 65:1119, 1982.
23. DiBianco, R., Singh, S., Singh, J. B., et al. Effects of acebutolol on chronic stable angina pectoris: A placebo-controlled, double-blind, randomized crossover study. *Circulation* 62:1179, 1980.
24. Dwyer, E. M., Jr., Pepe, A. J., and Pinkernell, B. H. Effects of beta-adrenergic blockade with pindolol versus placebo in coronary patients with stable angina pectoris. *Am. Heart J.* 103:830, 1982.
25. Farnham, D. J. Effectiveness of bevantolol in the treatment of angina—A placebo-controlled study. *Angiology* 37:226, 1896.
26. Findlay, I. N., MacLeod, K., Ford, M., et al. Treatment of angina pectoris with nifedipine and atenolol: Efficacy and effect on cardiac function. *Br. Heart J.* 55:240, 1986.

27. Fiserova, J., Hlavacek, K., Vavra, M., et al. Acebutolol (sectral) in angina pectoris treatment. *Acta Universitatis Carolinae Medica* 25:335, 1979.
28. Forrest, W. A. A monitored release study: A clinical trial of oxprenolol in general practice. *Practitioner* 208:412, 1972.
29. Frick, M. H., and Luurila, O. Double-blind titrated-dose comparison of metoprolol and propranolol in the treatment of angina pectoris. *Ann. Clin. Res.* 8:385, 1976.
30. Frishman, W., Kostis, J., Strom, J., et al. Clinical pharmacology of the new beta-adrenergic blocking drugs. Part 6. A comparison of pindolol and propranolol in treatment of patients with angina pectoris: The role of intrinsic sympathomimetic activity. *Am. Heart J.* 98:526, 1979.
31. Frishman, W. H. Nadolol: A new beta-adrenoceptor antagonist. *N. Engl. J. Med.* 305:678, 1981.
32. Frishman, W. H., Christodoulou, J., Weksler, B., et al. Abrupt propranolol withdrawal in angina pectoris: Effects on platelet aggregation and exercise tolerance. *Am. Heart J.* 95:169, 1978.
33. Frishman, W. H., Strom, J. A., Kirschner, M., et al. Labetalol therapy in patients with systemic hypertension and angina pectoris: Effects of combined alpha and beta adrenoceptor blockade. *Am. J. Cardiol.* 48:917, 1981.
34. Furberg, B., Dahlqvist, A., Raak, A., and Wrege, U. Comparison of the new beta-adrenoceptor antagonist, nadolol, and propranolol in the treatment of angina pectoris. *Curr. Med. Res. Opin.* 5:388, 1978.
35. Gaglione, A., Hess, O. M., Corin, W. J., et al. Is there coronary vasoconstriction after introcoronary beta-adrenergic blockade in patients with coronary artery disease? *J. Am. Coll. Cardiol.* 10:299, 1987.
36. George, C. F., Conolly, M. E., Fenyvesi, F., et al. Intravenously administered isoproterenol sulfate dose-response curves in man. *Arch. Intern. Med.* 130:361, 1972.
37. Guazzi, M., Fiorentini, C., Polese, A., et al. Treatment of spontaneous angina pectoris with beta blocking agents: A clinical, electrocardiographic, and haemodynamic appraisal. *Br. Heart J.* 37:1235, 1975.
38. Gugler, R., Krist, R., Raczinski, H., et al. Comparative pharmacodynamics and plasma levels of beta-adrenoceptor blocking drugs. *Br. J. Clin. Pharmacol.* 10:337, 1980.
39. Halkin, H., Vered, I., Saginer, A., and Rabinowitz, R. Once-daily administration of sustained release propranolol capsules in the treatment of angina pectoris. *Due J. Clin. Pharmacol.* 16:387, 1979.
40. Harston, W. E., and Friesinger, G. C. Randomized double-blind study of pindolol in patients with stable angina pectoris. *Am. Heart J.* 104:504, 1982.
41. Hartman, K. E., Nordstrom, L. A., and Gobel, F. L. The effect of placebo therapy on exercise response and nitroglycerin consumption in patients with angina pectoris (Abstract). *Circulation* 50(Suppl III):III-115, 1974.
42. Hickie, J. B. Alprenolol ("aptin") in angina pectoris: A double-blind multicentre trial. *Med. J. Australia* 2:268, 1970.
43. Horn, M. E., and Prichard, B. N. C. Variable dose comparative trial of propranolol and sotalol in angina pectoris. *Br. Heart J.* 35:555, 1973.
44. Imperi, G. A., Lambert, C. R., Coy, K., et al. Effects of titrated beta blockade (metoprolol) on silent myocardial ischemia in ambulatory patients with coronary artery disease. *Am. J. Cardiol.* 60:519, 1987.
44a. Jackson, G., Atkinson, L., and Oram, S. Double-blind comparison of tolamolol, propranolol, practolol, and placebo in the treatment of angina pectoris. *Br. Med. J.* 1:708, 1975.
45. Jackson, G., Atkinson, L., and Oram, S. Reassessment of failed beta-

blocker treatment in angina pectoris by peak-exercise heart rate measurements. *Br. Med. J.* 3:616, 1975.
46. Jackson, G., Harry, J. D., Robinson, C., et al. Comparison of atenolol with propranolol in the treatment of angina pectoris with special reference to once daily administration of atenolol. *Br. Heart J.* 40:998, 1978.
47. Jackson, G., Schwartz, J., Kates, R. E., et al. Atenolol: Once-daily cardioselective beta blockade for angina pectoris. *Circulation* 61:555, 1980.
48. Jackson, N. C., Lee, P. S., and Taylor, S. H. A single-blind randomized comparison of the 24-h antianginal efficacy of celiprolol versus atenolol. *J. Cardiovasc. Pharmacol.* 8(Suppl 4):S145, 1986.
49. Jee, L. D., and Opie, L. H. Double-blind trial comparing labetalol with atenolol in the treatment of systemic hypertension with angina pectoris. *Am. J. Cardiol.* 56:551, 1985.
50. Johnson, S. M., Mauritson, D. R., Corbett, J. R., et al. Double-blind, randomized, placebo-controlled comparison of propranolol and verapamil in the treatment of patients with stable angina pectoris. *Am. J. Med.* 71:443, 1981.
51. Johnsson, G., Regardh, C. G., and Solvell, L. Combined pharmacokinetic and pharmacodynamic studies in man of the adrenergic beta$_1$-receptor antagonist metoprolol. *Acta Pharmacol. Toxicol.* 36(Suppl V):V-31, 1975.
52. Jones, G. R., and Mir, M. A. Comparison of antianginal efficacy of one conventional and three long acting beta-adrenoreceptor blocking agents in stable angina pectoris. *Br. Heart J.* 46:503, 1981.
53. Kronenberg, M. W., Born, M. L., Pederson, R. W., and Friesinger, G. C. The degree of ST-segment depression is unrelated to left ventricular performance on exercise (Abstract). *J. Am. Coll. Cardiol.* 1:650, 1983.
54. Lager, I., Blohme, G., and Smith, U. Effect of cardioselective and nonselective beta-blockade on the hypoglycaemic response in insulin-dependent diabetics. *Lancet* 1:458, 1979.
55. Leary, W. P., and Asmal, A. C. Treatment of coexistent angina pectoris and hypertension with pindolol. *S. Afr. Med. J.* 49:11, 1975.
56. Lee, G., DeMaria, A. N., Favrot, L., et al. Efficacy of acebutolol in chronic stable angina using single-blind and randomized double-blind protocol. *J. Clin. Pharmacol.* 22:371, 1982.
57. Livesley, B., Catley, P. F., Campbell, R. C., and Oram, S. Double-blind evaluation of verapamil, propranolol, and isosorbide dinitrate against placebo in the treatment of angina pectoris. *Br. Med. J.* 1:375, 1973.
58. Lynch, P., Dargie, H., Krikler, S., and Krikler, D. Objective assessment of antianginal treatment: A double-blind comparison of propranolol, nifedipine, and their combination. *Br. Med. J.* 281:184, 1980.
59. Majid, P. A., de Feijter, P. J., Wardeh, R., et al. Comparison of clinical effects of propranolol (inderal) with once daily slow-release oxprenolol (slow trasicor) in angina pectoris. *J. Int. Med. Res.* 7:194, 1979.
60. Mehta, J., Mehta, P., and Pepine, C. J. Differences in platelet aggregation in coronary artery sinus and aortic blood in patients with coronary artery disease: Effect of propranolol. *Clin. Cardiol.* 1:96, 1978.
61. Milei, J., and Fortunato, M. R. A new beta adrenergic blocking agent, sotalol, in the treatment of angina pectoris: A double blind-crossed treatment study. *Rev. Bras. de Pesquisas Med. e Biol.* 8:279, 1975.
62. Morse, J. R., and Nesto, R. W. Double-blind crossover comparison of the antianginal effects of nifedipine and isosorbide dinitrate in patients with exertional angina receiving propranolol. *J. Am. Coll. Cardiol.* 6:1395, 1985.
63. Olowoyeye, J. O., Thadani, U., and Parker, J. O. Slow release oxprenolol

in angina pectoris: Study comparing oxprenolol, once daily, with propranolol, four times daily. *Am. J. Cardiol.* 47:1123, 1981.
64. Opie, L. H., Sonnenblick, E. H., Kaplan, N. M., and Thadani, U. Beta-blocking agents. In L. H. Opie (ed.), *Drugs for the Heart.* Orlando: Grune & Stratton, 1984. P. 1.
65. Parker, J. O., Porter, A., and Parker, J. D. Propranolol in angina pectoris: Comparison of long-acting and standard-formulation propranolol. *Circulation* 65:1351, 1982.
66. Parodi, O., Simonetti, I., and Michelassi, C. Comparison of verapamil and propranolol therapy for angina pectoris at rest: A randomized, multiple-crossover, controlled trial in the coronary care unit. *Am. J. Cardiol.* 57:899, 1986.
67. Pendleton, R. G., Newman, D. J., Sherman, S. S., et al. Effect of propranolol upon the hemoglobin-oxygen dissociation curve. *J. Pharmacol. Exp. Ther.* 180:647, 1972.
68. Pine, M., Favrot, L., Smith, S., et al. Correlation of plasma propranolol concentration with therapeutic response in patients with angina pectoris. *Circulation* 52:886, 1975.
69. Powell, C. E., and Slater, I. H. Blocking of inhibitory adrenergic receptors by a dichloro analog of isoproterenol. *J. Pharmacol. Exp. Ther.* 122:480, 1958.
70. Prichard, B. N. C., Aellig, W. H., and Richardson, G. A. The action of intravenous oxprenolol, practolol, propranolol and sotalol on acute exercise tolerance in angina pectoris: The effect on heart rate and the electrocardiogram. *Postgrad. Med. J.* 46(Suppl):77, 1970.
71. Quyyumi, A. A., Efthimiou, J., Quyyumi, A., et al. Nocturnal angina: Precipitating factors in patients with coronary artery disease and those with variant angina. *Br. Heart J.* 56:346, 1986.
72. Quyyumi, A. A., Wright, C., Mockus, L., et al. Effects of combined alpha and beta adrenoceptor blockade in patients with angina pectoris: A double blind study comparing labetalol with placebo. *Br. Heart J.* 53:47, 1985.
73. Report of the Holland Interuniversity Nifedipine/Metoprolol Trial (HINT) Research Group. Early treatment of unstable angina in the coronary care unit: A randomised, double-blind, placebo controlled comparison of recurrent ischaemia in patients treated with nifedipine and metoprolol or both. *Br. Heart J.* 56:400, 1986.
74. Robertson, R. M., Wood, A. J. J., Vaughn, W. K., and Robertson, D. Exacerbation of vasotonic angina pectoris by propranolol. *Circulation* 65:281, 1982.
75. Roughgarden, J. W. Circulatory changes associated with spontaneous angina pectoris. *Am. J. Med.* 41:947, 1966.
76. Sandler, G., and Clayton, G. A. Clinical evaluation of practolol, a new cardioselective beta-blocking agent in angina pectoris. *Br. Med. J.* 2:399, 1970.
77. Schwartz, J. B., Jackson, G., Kates, R. E., and Harrison, D. C. Long-term benefit of cardioselective beta blockade with once-daily atenolol therapy in angina pectoris. *Am. Heart J.* 101:380, 1981.
78. Shand, D. G., Nuckolls, E. M., and Oates, J. A. Plasma propranolol levels in adults: With observations in four children. *Clin. Pharmacol. Ther.* 11:112, 1970.
79. Shanks, R. G., Carruthers, S. G., Kelly, J. G., and McDevitt, D. G. Correlation of reduction of exercise heart rate with blood levels of atenolol after oral and intravenous administration. *Postgrad. Med. J.* 53(Suppl 3):70, 1977.
80. Shapiro, W., Park, J., DiBianco, R., et al. Comparison of nadolol, a new

long-acting beta-receptor blocking agent, and placebo in the treatment of stable angina pectoris. *Chest* 80:425, 1981.
81. Sharma, B., Meeran, M. K., Galvin, M. C., et al. Comparison of adrenergic beta-blocking drugs in angina pectoris. *Br. Med. J.* 3:152, 1971.
82. Shea, M. J., Deanfield, J. E., Wilson, R., et al. Transient ischemia in angina pectoris: Frequent silent events with everyday activities. *Am. J. Cardiol.* 56:34E, 1985.
83. Slome, R. Sotalol in angina pectoris: A double-blind study. *S. Afr. Med. J.* 50:469, 1976.
84. Sowton, E., Das Gupta, D. S., and Baker, I. Comparative effects of beta adrenergic blocking drugs. *Thorax* 30:9, 1975.
85. Srivastava, S. C., Dewar, H. A., and Newell, D. J. Double-blind trial of propranolol (inderal) in angina of effort. *Br. Med. J.* 2:724, 1964.
86. Steele, P., and Gold, F. Favorable effect of acebutolol on exercise performance and angina in men with coronary artery disease. *Chest* 82:40, 1982.
87. Strauss, W. E., and Parisi, A. F. Superiority of combined diltiazem and propranolol therapy for angina pectoris. *Circulation* 71:951, 1985.
88. Subramanian, B., Bowles, M. J., Davies, A. B., and Raftery, E. B. Combined therapy with verapamil and propranolol in chronic stable angina. *Am. J. Cardiol.* 49:125, 1982.
89. Taylor, S. H., and Thadani, U. Oxprenolol in angina pectoris. *Br. J. Pharmacol.* 58:412P, 1976.
90. Taylor, S. H., Thadani, U., Davidson, C., et al. A comparative study of the activity of beta-adrenoceptor antagonists in man. *Int. J. Clin. Pharmacol. Biopharm.* 12I-II:305, 1975.
91. Thadani, U. Assessment of optimal beta blockade in treating patients with angina pectoris. *Acta Medica Scand.* 694(Suppl):178, 1984.
92. Thadani, U., Davidson, C., Chir, B., et al. Comparison of the immediate effects of five beta-adrenoreceptor-blocking drugs with different ancillary properties in angina pectoris. *N. Engl. J. Med.* 300:750, 1979.
93. Thadani, U., Davidson, C., Singleton, W., and Taylor, S. H. Comparison of five beta-adrenoreceptor antagonists with different ancillary properties during sustained twice daily therapy in angina pectoris. *Am. J. Med.* 68:243, 1980.
94. Thadani, U., and Parker, J. O. Propranolol in angina pectoris: Duration of improved exercise tolerance and circulatory effects after acute oral administration. *Am. J. Cardiol.* 44:118, 1979.
95. Thadani, U., and Parker, J. O. Propranolol in the treatment of angina pectoris: Comparison of duration of action in acute and sustained oral therapy. *Circulation* 59:571, 1979.
96. Thadani, U., Shapiro, W., and DiBianco, R. Effect of long term placebo therapy on angina frequency and exercise tolerance in patients with stable angina pectoris. *Circulation* 70(Suppl II):II-44, 1984.
97. Thadani, U., Sharma, B., Meeran, M. K., et al. Comparison of adrenergic beta-receptor antagonists in angina pectoris. *Br. Med. J.* 1:138, 1973.
98. Theroux, P., Taeymans, Y., Morissette, D., et al. A randomized study comparing propranolol and diltiazem in the treatment of unstable angina. *J. Am. Coll. Cardiol.* 5:717, 1985.
99. Tremblay, G., Biron, P., Caille, G., et al. Double-blind crossover trial of single- versus twice-daily doses of acebutolol in angina. *Curr. Ther. Res.* 29:644, 1981.
100. Vaghaiwalla, F., Mody, K., Nademanee, V., et al. Prognostic significance of silent myocardial ischemia in chronic stable angina based on correlation with coronary angiography (Abstract). *Circulation* 76(Suppl IV):IV-78, 1987.

101. Waal-Manning, H. J., and Simpson, F. O. Practolol treatment in asthmatics. *Lancet* 2:1264, 1971.
102. Wilson, A. G., Brooke, O. G., Lloyd, H. J., and Robinson, B. F. Mechanism of action of beta-adrenergic receptor blocking agents in angina pectoris: Comparison of action of propranolol with dexpropranolol and practolol. *Br. Med. J.* 4:399, 1969.
103. Wilson, D. F., Watson, O. F., Peel, J. S., and Turner, A. S. Trasicor in angina pectoris: A double-blind trial. *Br. Med. J.* 2:155, 1969.
104. Wiseman, R. A. Practolol—accumulated data on unwanted effects. *Postgrad. Med. J.* 47(Suppl):68, 1971.
105. Wolf, E., Tzivoni, D., and Stern, S. Comparison of exercise tests and 24-hour ambulatory electrocardiographic monitoring in detection of ST-T changes. *Br. Heart J.* 36:90, 1974.
106. Yasue, H., Omote, S., Takizawa, A., et al. Pathogenesis and treatment of angina pectoris at rest as seen from its response to various drugs. *Jpn. Circ. J.* 42:1, 1978.

CHAPTER 11

CALCIUM ANTAGONISTS IN TRANSIENT MYOCARDIAL ISCHEMIC SYNDROMES AND SYSTEMIC HYPERTENSION

DEBORAH A. JALOWIEC
CARL J. PEPINE

The major use of calcium channel antagonists to date has been in patients with ischemic syndromes who have coronary artery disease. These uses, as well as their application in patients with hypertension, are discussed in detail in the following chapter.

REST ANGINA

Spasm of major epicardial coronary arteries is a likely etiology for transient ischemia in most patients with recurrent rest angina associated with ST segment elevation. Rationale for use of calcium channel antagonists in patients with coronary artery spasm derives from the dependence of coronary artery vasculature smooth muscle on transmembrane calcium ion flux for maintenance of vessel tone [103]. Spontaneous phasic contractions of the large coronary arteries may contribute to spasm. Blockade of these oscillations is possible by calcium channel antagonists [96]. All three first-generation calcium-blocking agents have been shown to afford excellent short-term efficacy for rest angina in controlled trials. A 50 to 90 percent reduction in frequency of angina and consumption of nitroglycerin has been reported [1, 21, 48, 76]. Long-term efficacy studies have substantiated the short-term results and further demonstrated a paucity of adverse effects [1, 21, 48, 77, 86]. Since the first-generation calcium channel antagonists are different compounds with different properties in addition to their calcium antagonizing effects at the smooth muscle membrane, it is appropriate to consider them separately.

Diltiazem

Initial evidence for effectiveness of diltiazem in controlling rest angina came from an uncontrolled trial in Japan, which reported 90.8 percent efficacy [51]. In a controlled study by Pepine and colleagues [76], a very favorable short-term response in 12 patients with variant angina was found. Subsequently, Feldman and coworkers [21] described an open label long-term follow-up of these patients. Responses during short-term trial accurately predicted long-term response, with 42 percent of patients remaining asymptomatic and an additional 33 percent obtaining a good (less than 50 percent decrease in angina frequency) or partial response. Thus, 75 percent of patients had favorable responses, and important adverse effects attributable to diltiazem were not detected. The dose was limited to 240 mg daily.

During a mean of 17.5 months of follow-up with diltiazem therapy for coronary artery spasm, others also demonstrated a marked reduction in frequency of angina (mean 21.5 attacks per week decreased to 1.3 attacks per week). Thirty-one percent of the 36 patients were pain free taking 240 mg/day, with 23 percent of remaining patients becoming pain free taking 360 mg/day. Seventy-three percent of the remaining patients achieved a 70 percent or greater reduction in frequency of angina at this higher dose. Again, important adverse effects were uncommon, with 17 percent of the patients developing mild pedal edema during long-term therapy [86].

Nifedipine

The beneficial effects of nifedipine in variant angina appear to arise from prevention of coronary spasm rather than dilation of the large coronary arteries [22]. In an uncontrolled trial of 127 patients with variant angina, nifedipine significantly reduced the mean weekly rate of anginal attacks to 16 from 22. Sixty-three percent of patients achieved complete control of angina and 87 percent had at least a 50 percent reduction in the frequency of angina. In another uncontrolled study of 716 patients with refractory angina, complete prevention of angina with nifedipine was most frequent in patients with documented vasospasm (42 percent of patients in this group), intermediate in those with evidence of both classical exertional angina as well as superimposed vasospasm (20 percent), and least frequent in patients with classic exertional angina alone (3 percent) [91]. Overall, a total of 83 percent of the patients experienced reduction in angina episodes to at least 50 percent of the baseline frequency. These studies however, actually represented results obtained with nifedipine and other antianginal agents, usually nitrates.

A controlled study of 19 patients with coronary artery spasm compared the effectiveness of monotherapy nifedipine with isosorbide dinitrate [40]. The mean frequency of angina was less during both nifedipine (0.69 episodes/day) and isosorbide dinitrate (0.77 episodes/day) therapy than during the lead-in (pretherapy) phase (1.71 episodes/day). Consumption of nitroglycerin decreased from 1.86 tablets/day to 0.89 tablets/day with nifedipine and to 0.63 tablets/day with isosorbide nitrate. Some patients responded better to nifedipine while others had greater symptomatic improvement with isosorbide dinitrate. Prediction of this response, however, was not possible with usual clinical criteria.

Verapamil

Verapamil also does not cause major dilation of epicardial coronary arteries in the doses usually found to be clinically useful. Verapamil, like the other first-generation calcium channel antagonists, prevents constriction of coronary segments induced by alpha-adrenergic and seratonergic coronary receptor stimulation [4]. Verapamil will almost completely abolish the constriction of coronary arteries after ergonovine.

In a 9-month randomized double-blind study of 16 patients with variant angina, there was a decrease in both the frequency of angina (12.6 episodes/week with placebo to 1.7 episodes/week with verapamil) and in consumption of nitroglycerin (14.4 tablets/week with placebo to 2.1 tablets/week with verapamil) [48]. Additionally, significant reductions in hospitalizations and episodes of transient ST segment deviation recorded during ambulatory electrocardiographic (ECG) monitoring were observed during therapy with verapamil. No important side effects were observed. In a short-term trial of verapamil in 15 coronary care unit patients with continued rest angina after 24 hours of treatment with placebo, 12 of 13 patients obtained a prompt and marked reduction in both chest pain frequency and nitroglycerin consumption [60]. In our studies, after 1 year follow-up of 16 patients with rest angina, 56 percent had a greater than 50 percent decrease in angina frequency compared to placebo [77]. Sixty-nine percent of these patients, however, developed drug-related side effects. The most frequent side effects were either constipation or abdominal distention. Prolongation of A–V conduction was less frequent.

Comparison Studies

In a 1-year comparative evaluation of the three currently used calcium channel antagonists, angina frequency, adverse effects, and occurrence of coronary events, (e.g., sudden death, infarction, hospitalization for rest angina control and coronary artery bypass surgery) were evaluated [77]. Sixty percent of the 45 patients in the study had angiographically important coronary artery disease, while 78 percent had coronary spasm either documented during catheterization or suspected from recurrent ST segment elevation with angina. Age, frequency of angina, duration of symptoms, and ejection fractions were similar in all three therapeutic groups. The presence and extent of coronary artery disease, however, was greatest in the verapamil group (14 of 16 patients) in comparison with the nifedipine group (only 8 of 16 patients) and the diltiazem group (only 5 of 13 patients). Sixty-four percent of the patients had a 50 percent decrease in angina without a coronary event through the initial year of therapy (9 of the 16 who were receiving verapamil, 11 of the 16 who were receiving nifedipine, and 9 of the 13 who were receiving diltiazem). Forty-four percent of these patients (20 patients), however, required additional antianginal therapy (7 of the 16 in the verapamil group, 9 of the 16 in the nifedipine group, and 4 of the 13 in the diltiazem group). Although all 45 patients were responders in short-term controlled trials, coronary events occurred in 13 patients (29 percent) (7 of 16 taking verapamil, 4 of 16 taking nifedipine, and 2 of 13 taking diltiazem). Frequency of side effects ranged from none in the diltiazem group to 11 patients in the verapamil group, with the nifedipine group in the middle with 6 patients experiencing side effects. Additionally, it was noted that 1-year response to calcium channel antagonists in patients with coronary artery disease was not significantly different from the response in those without coronary artery disease. It was evident that in the majority of patients (71 percent) the initial symptom response was sustained without events during the first year of therapy with calcium channel antagonists.

TABLE 11-1. *Physiologic Factors Important in Effort Angina Modified by Calcium Antagonists*

Definite	Probable
Increased blood pressure (N ≫ V > D)*	Inappropriate arteriolar constriction (N)
Increased heart rate (D > V)	Reduced ventricular compliance (V > D > N)
Increased contractility (V > D > N)	
Increased heart size (N)	Reduced diastolic pressure-time (D > N)

*D = Diltiazem; N = Nifedipine; V = Verapamil.

EXERTIONAL ANGINA

Patients with multivessel atherosclerotic obstruction experience effort angina primarily due to increased myocardial oxygen demand. Short- and long-term efficacy has been demonstrated for all three first-generation calcium channel antagonists in patients with exertional angina. The mechanism responsible for this beneficial effect is probably reduction in hemodynamic determinants of myocardial oxygen demand during exercise. The major hemodynamic determinants of myocardial oxygen supply are heart rate, systolic wall stress (which is determined by systolic blood pressure and ventricular size), and contractility. All these agents decrease blood pressure during exercise. There are several differential effects of these calcium channel antagonists in exercise-induced angina worthy of mention. Nifedipine produces a marked reduction in blood pressure during exercise but does not suppress heart rate augmentation. Diltiazem and verapamil, on the other hand, produce much less diminution in exercise blood pressure but also suppress exercise-associated increases in heart rate. While all will decrease the rate–blood pressure product at various levels of exercise, the mechanisms are different (Table 11-1).

Diltiazem

Acute hemodynamic and ECG effects were evaluated after a single 120 mg oral dose of diltiazem in patients with exercise-induced angina [44]. Frequency of pain during exercise testing was reduced and exercise duration was increased after administration of diltiazem. A significant reduction in arterial and pulmonary artery wedge pressures and exercise heart rate was also demonstrated. Additionally, in patients with marked left ventricular dysfunction on exercise, a significant improvement in cardiac output during exercise was observed, reflecting prevention of exercise-induced, ischemia-related left ventricular dysfunction. In a similar study of the effects of single-dose diltiazem in exercise, Wagniart and colleagues demonstrated a significant increase in exercise tolerance and time to onset of important ST segment depression in patients with fixed coronary artery stenosis [97]. This response was associated with a decrease in heart rate, systolic pressure, and rate-pressure product at submaximal exercise but not at peak exercise when compared with placebo. Several studies of long-term efficacy of diltiazem in chronic stable angina that evaluated exercise performance have substantiated persistent improvement. Improvement in exercise end points including time to onset of angina, significant ST segment depression, and termination of exercise during treadmill exercise testing were shown to be maximal at 3 months with a continued effect seen during exercise testing at 12 to 16 months [79].

In two multicenter trials of patients with effort angina, diltiazem was demonstrated to decrease significantly the frequency of angina and nitroglycerin consumption, with a greater total exercise duration after 10 weeks of therapy [92]. A significant dose-related response was observed, with 240 mg/day being the most effective dosage in increasing total duration of exercise, time to onset of angina, and time to onset of significant ST depression [43]. The ability of diltiazem to reduce myocardial oxygen demand at submaximal exercise is represented by the observed significant reduction in submaximal rate-pressure product.

Nifedipine

Evidence suggests that nifedipine improves exercise tolerance in patients with stable effort angina by reducing myocardial oxygen requirements for a given workload largely through reduction of systolic blood pressure during exercise. A 40 percent reduction in weekly angina episodes associated with a significant increase in exercise time to onset of angina was demonstrated in an early study by Moskowitz [62]. This was associated with a decrease in heart rate–pressure product at various workloads. An exercise tolerance increase of 20 percent associated with a 22 mmHg decrease in systolic blood pressure during exercise was shown by Ekelund and Oro [16]. A further increase in average exercise time by 40 percent from baseline was observed after addition of beta blockers to nifedipine, secondary to further decreases in exercise systolic blood pressure and heart rate.

While it has been suggested that nifedipine acts as a direct coronary arterial dilator, several coronary hemodynamic and metabolic studies during pacing-induced angina have failed to show an increase in coronary blood flow or myocardial oxygen consumption [18, 39]. Recent work with intracoronary and intravenous nifedipine has shown a significant increase in coronary blood flow as well as reduction in systemic vascular resistance, but the relevance of these parenteral doses to usual oral therapy remains to be proven [94].

Verapamil

The major mechanism responsible for improvement in exercise tolerance with verapamil is reduction in both heart rate and blood pressure. Depression of myocardial contractility probably further decreases myocardial oxygen requirements and contributes to this drug's antianginal effect. Studies as early as 1966 demonstrated beneficial effects of verapamil in patients with exertional angina [67]. Reduction in heart rate and blood pressure associated with an increase in exercise duration and reduction in anginal attacks per week after administration of verapamil has been shown in subsequent studies [31, 56]. When compared with propranolol, verapamil was found by some to be more effective in increasing total exercise time.

In addition their beneficial actions on the major determinants of oxygen consumption (i.e., heart rate, blood pressure, and contractility), these agents may possess other cardioprotective effects. Several studies have proposed that these drugs may decrease atherogenesis by preventing progressive arterial calcium overload [27, 70, 83]. The calcium channel antagonists also have inhibitory effects on platelet aggregation [7] and do not appear to affect adversely serum lipoproteins [80].

SILENT MYOCARDIAL ISCHEMIA

Clinically unrecognized or *silent myocardial ischemia* (asymptomatic and painless) are terms used to describe a syndrome characterized by objective evidence for myocardial ischemia in the absence of angina or equivalent symptoms. Exercise stress testing and ambulatory electrocardiographic monitoring are the most frequently used methods of detection. Studies utilizing these methods have demonstrated that silent episodes represent 75 to 84 percent of the total ischemic episodes occurring during daily life in many patients with effort angina [11, 84, 87]. These episodes occurred at heart rates significantly lower than those observed at onset of angina during exercise testing and with ordinary daily activities including mental stress, cold, and cigarette smoking [11]. Additionally, it has been suggested that patients with silent ischemia may have a higher coronary-related mortality and frequency of cardiac events during long-term follow-up [90, 98].

It has been proposed that both an increase in myocardial oxygen demand and a reduction in coronary blood flow may be important factors in the pathogenesis of silent ischemia. There are data to suggest that nifedipine [8, 68, 81], verapamil [48, 71, 93, 99], nicardipine [34], and diltiazem [20, 30] are effective therapies in relieving episodes of silent ischemia.

One study compared nifedipine to pindolol in 12 patients with stable angina and silent ischemia documented by ambulatory electrocardiographic monitoring [8]. After 30 days of therapy, four of seven patients receiving nifedipine had improvement in ischemia, whereas only one of five of the pindolol-treated patients improved. Another study demonstrated improvement in both silent and painful episodes recorded during ambulatory monitoring with propranolol and nifedipine. The combination of the two drugs was significantly superior to either drug alone [68]. When specifically applied to patients with variant angina, total abolition of ischemic attacks in 11 of 13 patients with evidence of silent ST segment ECG changes was demonstrated by Prevatali and coworkers [81].

Verapamil has been shown to be effective therapy in silent ischemia when compared with placebo and beta blockers. In a study combining verapamil with propranolol, a reduction in the number of ST segment depression episodes and maximum depth of ST segment depression compared with placebo was demonstrated [93]. Winniford and colleagues [99] showed that verapamil and nifedipine each significantly reduced the number of both silent and painful ST segment shifts on ambulatory ECG monitoring in patients with variant angina. Johnson and coworkers [48] treated 16 patients with variant angina with verapamil and demonstrated a decrease in ischemic episodes from 33.1 ± 39.3 (12.2 ± 28.4 symptomatic) per week with placebo to 7.7 ± 11.7 (1.6 ± 3.0 symptomatic) per week with verapamil. Parodi and coworkers [71] treated coronary care unit patients with unstable angina and asymptomatic ST segment shifts with verapamil and found a significant decrease in both symptomatic and asymptomatic episodes.

Gelman and colleagues [34] used the investigational calcium channel antagonist nicardipine to treat 17 patients with coronary artery spasm and silent ischemic episodes. Using a placebo-controlled, double-blind crossover design, they demonstrated a significant decrease in total silent episodes of ischemic ST segment shifts. Most recently diltiazem has been shown by Frishman and coworkers to be effective for silent ischemia while nifedipine was not [20, 30].

In general, calcium channel antagonists have been shown to be beneficial in the treatment of silent myocardial ischemia in anginal patients. It is yet to be determined which of the calcium channel antagonists is most effective in treatment of this entity.

EXPERIMENTAL CALCIUM CHANNEL ANTAGONISTS

Nicardipine dihydropyrine, a second-generation calcium channel antagonist similar in chemical structure to nifedipine, is currently used in Japan for treatment of ischemic heart disease, cerebral vascular insufficiency, and hypertension. It differs from other calcium channel antagonists in that it is a potent vasodilator with slightly greater selectivity for the coronary bed than the systemic bed [54]. Its anti-ischemic effects have been evaluated in patients with either chronic stable effort angina or angina at rest with favorable results. Systemic and hemodynamic effects after a 2 mg intravenous bolus followed by continuous intravenous infusion of nicardipine titrated to maintain a 10 to 20 min mmHg decrease in systolic blood pressure include an increase in heart rate, cardiac output, and stroke volume with a decrease in systemic vascular resistance. Coronary blood flow increased while coronary resistance decreased. The left ventricular end-diastolic pressure was unchanged. Nicardipine was demonstrated to produce a coronary resistance change 1.24 times the resistance for the systemic vascular bed [54].

Myocardial ischemia during intravenous nicardipine administration has been reported by Lambert and colleagues [55]. Angina associated with ECG ST segment changes and an elevation in left ventricular end-diastolic pressure was produced in a patient with severe coronary artery disease. This occurred following a 2 mg bolus and during continuous intravenous infusion at 50 µg per minute of nicardipine. The presumed etiology included production of an area of ischemia due to failure of collateral flow to augment in proportion to the demands of the reflex tachycardia, increased myocardial contraction state, and increased myocardial oxygen consumption.

The reflex increase in heart rate seen with intravenous administration is not seen with long-term oral use; this has been attributed to a resetting of the baroreceptors [102]. Numerous placebo-controlled, double-blind studies with oral nicardipine for treatment of effort angina [15, 35, 50, 85] demonstrated an increase in total exercise duration during exercise stress testing (average 20 percent), an increase in time to onset of 1 mm ST segment depression (average 29 percent), a decrease in angina frequency (50 percent average), and a decrease in nitroglycerin consumption (average 41 percent).

When used to treat patients with angina at rest due to coronary artery spasm, nicardipine was demonstrated to decrease significantly angina frequency, daily nitroglycerin consumption, and episodes of ischemic-type ST segment shifts during ambulatory ECG monitoring when compared with placebo. These results were shown in a number of patients who had previous unsatisfactory results with long-acting nitrates or other calcium channel antagonists [74]. Predominant side effects reported during therapy with nicardipine have included light-headedness, flushing, headache, increased angina, and skin rash. No significant ECG abnormalities or change in clinical, hematologic, chemical, or urinary testing were seen when nicardipine and placebo periods were compared [75].

Several other second-generation dihydropyridines (i.e., insoldipine, inmoldipine) are under clinical investigation.

Bepridil

Bepridil hydrochloride is a novel calcium channel antagonist [53] with a half-life of 42 hours and ventricular antiarrhythmic properties. It is also a potent coronary vasodilator [9] and has been used in patients with ischemic heart disease [13, 38, 66]. In addition to its vasodilatory properties, bepridil has electrophysiologic effects consisting of a decreased phase zero depolarization with prolongation of the action potential duration and blunting of the action potential height [100]. Its effects on the resting ECG include a decreased sinus rate, increased Q-T and QTc intervals, and production T wave changes [41]. These properties make it a potential antiarrhythmic agent as well [10, 49, 57].

When evaluated for its anti-ischemic potential in chronic stable angina and ST segment depression during exercise stress testing, bepridil significantly increased total exercise time, time to onset of angina, time to 1 mm ST segment depression, time to 2 mm ST segment depression, and total work achieved compared with placebo [37, 38]. Studies thus far suggest that bepridil is an effective drug for prevention of exercise-induced myocardial ischemia. Its long half-life and electrophysiologic properties make it a potentially beneficial drug in a select subset of patients.

HYPERTENSION

The sensitivity of arterial vasculature to the inhibitory effects of the calcium channel antagonists has been shown to be even greater than that of the myocardium [23-26, 28, 36]. Although widely used in Europe for many years as antihypertensive agents, calcium channel antagonists have only recently received approval for this indication in the United States. The basic mode of action of this class of drugs—as potent smooth muscle relaxation promoters resulting in vasodilation with lowering of blood pressure and reduction of vascular resistance—has prompted investigation into their use as first step monotherapeutic agents for mild to moderate hypertension. In addition, these agents have been extensively used as both anti-ischemic and antihypertensive agents in patients with angina and high blood pressure.

Some of the first studies of the antihypertensive and hemodynamic effects of calcium channel antagonists came from Italy. Oliveri and colleagues [69] noted a reduction in arterial pressure with nifedipine without a resultant increased heart rate and a slight increase in cardiac output, indicating a decrease in peripheral vascular resistance. This response was not accompanied by an increase in intravascular volume, and the glomerular filtration rate was preserved. Verapamil was compared to nifedipine in a study by Muiesan and colleagues [64] revealing significant blood pressure lowering without orthostatic hypotension or resultant tachycardia and no change in plasma volume. Numerous subsequent investigators have supported these early findings. Fleckenstein and coworkers [27], using spontaneously hypertensive rats as a model for essential hypertension, demonstrated a dramatic fall in blood pressure using verapamil, nifedipine, and other 1,4 dihydropyridine derivatives (Fig. 11-1). Direct observation of the acute spasmolytic effects of calcium channel antagonists in the retinal artery was made. They additionally suggested an anticalcinotic action of diltiazem on the coronary, aorta, cerebral, mesenteric, and renal arterial walls. These findings suggested a vascular protective action, which could be beneficial in certain patients with chronic arterial diseases such as hypertension and atherosclerosis.

Reflex Actions

Favorable antihypertensive effects were shown by Frohlich and coworkers [33] in hypertensive rats and human patients with essential hypertension using diltiazem and nifedipine. They noted a small initial reflex increase in heart rate with diltiazem, which resolved after 4 weeks of chronic therapy despite even further reduction of peripheral vascular resistance. Absence of reflex tachycardia has been a favorable attribute noted by other investigators in sharp contrast to the reflex stimulation of the sympathomimetic and renin angiotension system caused by other vasodilators, an important limiting factor in their use as monotherapeutic agents. Of the three currently used agents, nifedipine has been established as having the greatest reflex sympathetic response [2, 47, 65, 73, 89]. Diltiazem and verapamil, on the other hand, are associated with a decrease in heart rate owing to their slowing of the sinoatrial node activity and weak alpha-adrenergic blocking actions [29, 61, 80].

Renal Actions

Calcium channel antagonists exert their antihypertensive action without causing sodium and water retention. Diltiazem and nifedipine have been shown to increase urine volume and sodium excretion in a dose-related manner [65]. This effect does not appear to be clinically significant in long-term use [3]. The natriuretic effects of diltiazem appear to be complex. Renal blood flow and glomerular filtration rate were observed to increase markedly after infusion of diltiazem into the renal artery; however, maintenance of constant renal blood flow and glomerular filtration rate using an aortic clamp still produced a significant increase in sodium excretion. Inhibition of sodium reabsorption along the distal nephron tubule has been proposed as the natriuretic mechanism of diltiazem (Fig. 11-2) [3]. Verapamil has also been suggested to have a direct action on the renal tubules without affecting the glomerular filtration rate [14, 59]. Calcium channel antagonists effectively lower blood pressure while preserving renal perfusion and function.

Renin-Angiotension-Aldosterone-Effects

During chronic use, none of the calcium channel antagonists produced a clinically significant effect on any component of the renin angiotension

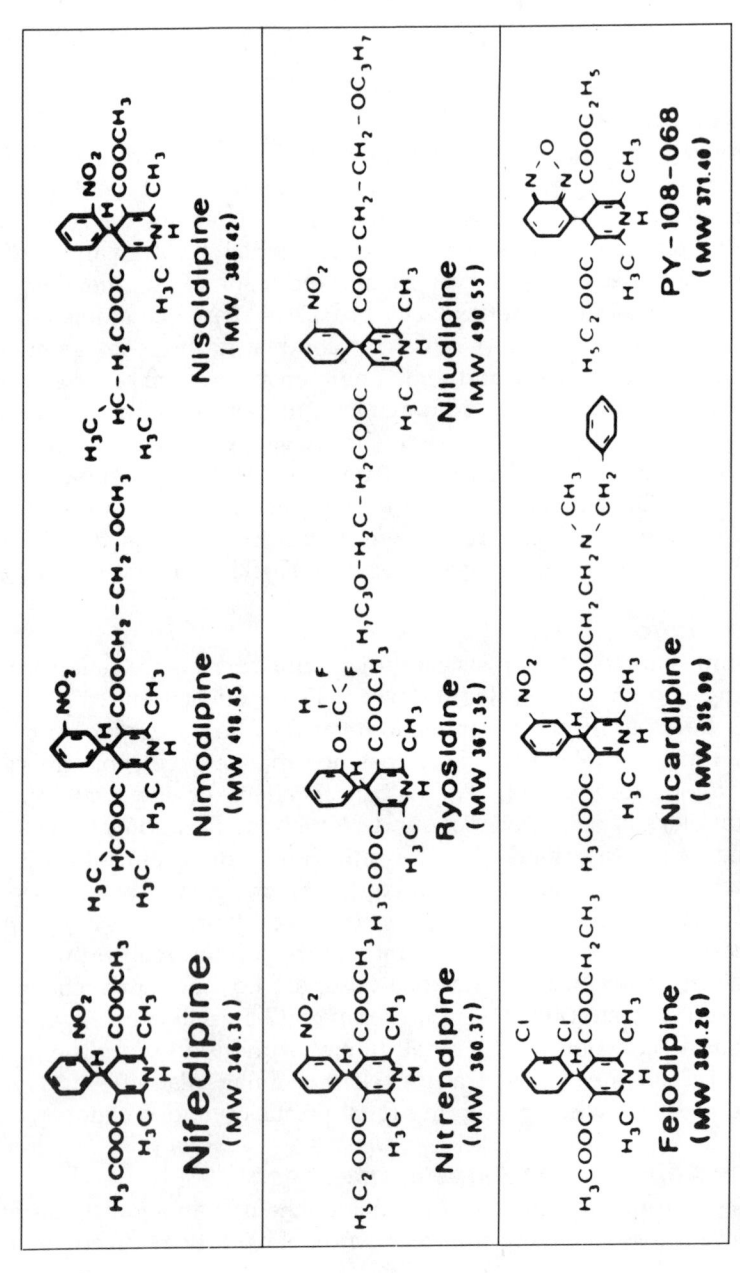

FIG. 11-1. Highly specific 1,4 dihydropyridine calcium channel antagonists derived from the prototypical substance nifedipine. (From Ref. 27, with permission.)

	V	$U_{Na}V$	U_KV	PV/ECF	WT
Effects of Calcium Entry Blockers on Salt and Water Excretion and Body Fluid Composition					
Short-term					
Diltiazem	↑	↑	No Δ	...	...
Nifedipine	↑	↑	No Δ	...	...
Verapamil	No Δ	No Δ	No Δ	...	...
Nitrendipine	...	...	...	...	...
Long-term					
Diltiazem	No Δ	No Δ	No Δ	No Δ	No Δ
Nifedipine	No Δ	No Δ	No Δ	No Δ	No Δ
Verapamil	No Δ	No Δ	No Δ	No Δ	No Δ
Nitrendipine	No Δ	No Δ	No Δ	...	...

PV/ECF = plasma volume/extracellular fluid volume; U_KV = urinary potassium excretion; $U_{Na}V$ = urinary sodium excretion; V = urinary flow rate; WT = weight.

FIG. 11-2. Effects of calcium entry blockers on salt and water excretion and body fluid composition. Abbreviations: PV/ECF = plasma volume/extracellular fluid volume; U_KV = urinary potassium excretion; $U_{Na}V$ = urinary sodium excretion; V = urinary flow rate; WT = weight. (From Ref. 3, with permission.)

aldosterone system [3]. Nifedipine, given sublingually or orally in doses of 10 to 30 mg to normotensive and hypertensive subjects, significantly increased plasma renin activity and angiotension concentration. However, the renin and aldosterone systems do not appear activated with long-term oral therapy [42, 72]. Verapamil and nifedipine, in particular, have been proposed as being selectively beneficial in low renin volume–dependent hypertensive states [5, 6, 19]. Clinically, these drugs have been shown to be efficacious in both older patients and blacks, many of whom have low plasma renin activity [6, 52].

Effects on Atherogenic Risk Factor
Calcium channel antagonists appear to have a favorable or neutral effect on plasma lipids and uric acid with long-term use. While verapamil has been shown not to change significantly serum cholesterol, triglycerides, and HDL levels after three months [58], diltiazem was associated with a statistically significant increase in HDL cholesterol [80]. It is evident that the adverse effects on atherogenic lipid fractions seen with beta blocker and diuretic use are not seen with calcium channel antagonists.

While earlier studies suggested that verapamil inhibits insulin release from pancreatic beta cells [12], a recent study indicates that both oral and intravenous therapy may improve oral glucose tolerance in patients with type II diabetes [82]. There was no detectable effect on insulin release. Verapamil did not appear to affect glibenclamide therapy. The potential beneficial effect on glucose was suggested to result from verapamil's effect on the liver with decreased hepatic glucose output secondary to inhibitory influences on gluconeogenic and glycogenolytic enzymes. Similarly, diltiazem has been shown not to influence plasma glucose and insulin, although specific studies in diabetics have not been reported [78, 80]. In contrast, some adverse effects with nifedipine have been reported, yet other studies have been unable to support these findings [78].

Comparison Studies

Comparative studies involving beta-adrenergic blockers and calcium channel antagonists have substantiated similar antihypertensive responses in patients with mild to moderate hypertension. Verapamil was the first calcium channel antagonist used in hypertension, and numerous trials comparing verapamil and beta blockers have been published. When tested against propranolol, verapamil in the twice daily and three times daily doses produced a uniform and comparable reduction in blood pressure throughout a 24-hour interval [88], with comparable effects demonstrated during exercise [45, 46]. Investigations of diltiazem with propranolol [101] and metoprolol [95] also revealed comparable antihypertensive effects. Frishman and colleagues [31] have compared verapamil and propranolol in patients with angina and hypertension using a double-blind, placebo-controlled protocol. Both verapamil and propranolol were similarly effective in controlling hypertension and angina during exercise. Nifedipine, when compared with metoprolol, decreased supine, systemic, and diastolic pressures similarly, with metoprolol once again showing a greater decrease in exercise systemic pressure. This latter effect is most likely due to blunting of the stroke volume response to exercise by the beta blockers [17].

When combined, calcium channel antagonists and beta blockers appear to produce additive antihypertensive responses. While the antihypertensive effects of the two classes of drugs are similar, patients with airway constriction, peripheral vascular disease, insulin-dependent diabetes mellitus, or left ventricular dysfunction may derive greater overall benefits from calcium channel antagonists compared with beta blockers.

Diltiazem has been shown to have equivalent antihypertensive efficacy as a monotherapeutic agent when compared with hydrochlorothiazide. A preliminary report of a large multicenter study, using sustained release diltiazem and twice daily hydrochlorthiazide, showed attainment of goal blood pressure in 42 and 45 percent of patients, respectively, which was sustained for the trial period of 6 months [32].

Diltiazem has also been shown to be as effective as hydrochlorothiazide in black hypertensive patients [63]. Additive effects were seen when the two classes of drugs were combined.

CALCIUM CHANNEL ANTAGONISTS FOR COMBINED ANGINA PECTORIS AND SYSTEMIC HYPERTENSION

Many patients have systemic hypertension complicated by coronary artery disease. As the calcium channel antagonists have been demonstrated to be effective therapy in each of these disorders separately, it is a natural progression that they join the ranks of beta-adrenergic blocking drugs as effective single therapeutic agents for patients with coexisting disorders.

The rationale for utilizing these agents in treatment of combined disease stems from their favorable effect on factors that influence myocardial demands combined with their vasodilatory effect on systemic and coronary arteries. Calcium channel antagonists reduce the heart rate–blood pressure product at rest and during submaximal exercise; diltiazem and nifedipine decrease arterial blood pressure during exercise while verapamil and diltiazem decrease heart rate during exercise.

Frishman and colleagues [28] compared nifedipine and diltiazem in a double-blind, placebo-controlled crossover study in patients with stable angina pectoris and mild to moderate hypertension. Compared with placebo, anginal frequency and nitroglycerin consumption were significantly reduced with both diltiazem and nifedipine, and exercise tolerance was increased. A reduction of standing systolic and diastolic blood pressure, as well as a decrease in exercise diastolic blood pressure, was noted equally with diltiazem and nifedipine. Nifedipine produced a small and insignificant increase in resting heart rate compared with placebo, whereas the resting heart rate with diltiazem was 11 beats per minute lower than that with nifedipine.

Frishman and coworkers [31] also compared the calcium channel antagonists with beta blockers for use in hypertensive patients with angina pectoris. Verapamil and propranolol were compared in 11 patients with mild to moderate hypertension and chronic stable angina. A reduction in anginal attacks per week was demonstrated with both drugs with no difference between verapamil and propranolol in the magnitude of reduction. Increases in total exercise time and calculated workload were produced with both drugs when compared with placebo. Verapamil was significantly more effective in improving exercise time when compared with propranolol. Systolic and diastolic blood pressure were reduced similarly by both drugs. Resting and exercise heart rate were likewise reduced by both drugs with a more marked reduction in both categories with propranolol.

CONCLUSIONS

Calcium channel antagonists are established antianginal agents and clearly effective antihypertensive agents. Several studies have demonstrated their beneficial effects in patients with coexisting disease. The favorable safety profile of calcium channel antagonists when compared with other commonly used agents adds to their potentially useful role for therapy in patients with hypertension and ischemic heart disease.

REFERENCES

1. Antman, E. M., et al. Nifedipine therapy for coronary artery spasm. *N. Engl. J. Med.* 302:1269, 1980.
2. Aoki, K., et al. Antihypertensive effect of cardiovascular Ca^{2+} antagonist in hypertensive patients in the absence and presence of beta-adrenergic blockade. *Am. Heart J.* 96:218, 1978.
3. Bauer, J. H., Sunderrajan, S., and Reams, G. Effects of calcium entry blockers on renin-angiotensin-aldosterone system, renal function and hemodynamics, salt and water excretion and body fluid composition. *Am. J. Cardiol.* 56:62H, 1985.
4. Brown, B. G. Response of normal and diseased epicardial coronary arteries to vasoactive drugs: Quantitative arteriographic studies. *Am. J. Cardiol.* 56:23E, 1985.
5. Buhler, F., et al. Renin profiling to select antihypertensive baseline drugs. *Am. J. Med.* 77:36A, 1984.
6. Buhler, F. R., et al. Greater antihypertensive efficacy of the calcium channel inhibitor verapamil in older and low renin patients. *Clin. Sci.* 82:439S, 1982.
7. Burns, E. R., and Frishman, W. H. The antiplatelet effects of calcium channel blockers add to their antianginal properties. *Int. J. Cardiol.* 4:372, 1983.
8. Cocco, G., et al. Therapeutic effects of pindolol and nifedipine in patients with stable angina pectoris and symptomatic resting ischemia. *Eur. J. Cardiol.* 10:59, 1979.
9. Cosnier, D., et al. Cardiovascular pharmacology of bepridil (1{3-isobutoxy-2(benzylphenyl) amino} propyl pyrolidine hydrochloride) a new potential antianginal compound. *Arch. Int. Pharmacodyn.* 225:133, 1977.
10. Davy, J. M., et al. Bepridil, a new calcium antagonist for the treatment of ventricular tachycardia (Abstract). *Circulation* 68:III-310, 1983.
11. Deanfield, J. E., and Selwyn, A. P. Characteristics and causes of transient myocardial ischemia during daily life. *Am. J. Med.* 80:18, 1986.
12. Devis, G., et al. Calcium antagonists and islet function. I. Inhibition of insulin release by verapamil. *Diabetes* 24:547, 1975.
13. DiBianco, R., et al. Bepridil for chronic stable angina pectoris: Results of a prospective multi-center, placebo-controlled, dose-ranging study in 77 patients. *Am. J. Cardiol.* 53:35, 1984.
14. Dietz, J. R., et al. Effects of intrarenal infusion of calcium entry blockers in anesthetized dogs. *Hypertension* 5:482, 1983.
15. DiPasquale, G., et al. Comparative efficacy of nicardipine, a new calcium antagonist, versus nifedipine in stable effort angina. *Int. J. Cardiol.* 6:673, 1984.
16. Ekelund, L. G., and Oro, L. Antianginal efficiency of nifedipine with and

without a beta-blocker, studied with exercise test. A double-blind randomized subacute study. *Clin. Cardiol.* 2:203, 1979.
17. Ekelund, L., Ekelund, C., and Rossner, S. Antihypertensive effects at rest and during exercise of a calcium blocker, nifedipine, alone and in combination with metoprolol. *Acta Med. Scand.* 212:71, 1982.
18. Emanuelsson, H., and Holmberg, S. Mechanisms of angina relief after nifedipine: A hemodynamic and myocardial metabolic study. *Circulation* 68:124, 1983.
19. Erne, P., et al. Factors influencing the hypertensive effects of calcium antagonists. *Hypertension* 5:II-97, 1983.
20. Fazzini, P. F., Multino, D., and Zambaldi, G. Diltiazem in spontaneous angina: Double-blind cross-over study with Holter. *G. Ital. Cardiol.* 15:1085, 1985.
21. Feldman, R. L., et al. Short- and long-term responses to diltiazem in patients with variant angina. *Am. J. Cardiol.* 49:554, 1982.
22. Feldman, R. L., et al. Analysis of coronary responses to nifedipine alone and in combination with intracoronary nitroglycerin. *Am. Heart J.* 105:651, 1983.
23. Fleckenstein, A. Specific pharmacology of calcium in myocardium, cardiac pacemakers and vascular smooth muscle. *Ann. Rev. Pharmacol. Toxicol.* 17:119, 1977.
24. Fleckenstein, A. Calcium antagonism in heart and smooth muscle-experimental factors and therapeutic prospects. Monograph. New York: Wiley, 1983.
25. Fleckenstein, A., et al. The basic Ca antagonist actions of nifedipine on cardiac energy metabolism and vascular smooth muscle tone. In K. Hoshimoto, E. Kimara, and T. Kobayashi (eds.), *New Therapy of Ischemic Heart Disease, First International Adalat Symposium, Tokyo, 1973.* Tokyo: University of Tokyo Press, 1975. Pp. 31–44.
26. Fleckenstein, A., et al. Interactions of vasoactive ions and drugs with calcium-dependent excitation contraction coupling of vascular smooth muscle. In E. Carafoli, F. Clemeti, W. Drabikowski, and A. Magreth (eds.), *Calcium Transport in Contraction and Secretion, Proceedings of an International Symposium in Bressanone, Italy, May 1975.* Amsterdam: North Holland Publishing, 1975. Pp. 555–66.
27. Fleckenstein, A., et al. Experimental basis of the long-term therapy of arterial hypertension with calcium antagonists. *Am. J. Cardiol.* 56:3H, 1985.
28. Fleckenstein-Grun, G., and Fleckenstein, A. Calcium antagonism, a basic principle in vasodilatation. In A. Zanchetti and D. M. Krikler (eds.), *Calcium Antagonism in Cardiovascular Therapy: Experience with Verapamil, International Symposium, Florence, Italy, October, 1980.* Amsterdam: Excerpta Medica, 1981. Pp. 30–48.
29. Frishman, W. H., et al. Comparison of diltiazem and nifedipine for both angina pectoris and systemic hypertension. *Am. J. Cardiol.* 56:41H, 1985.
30. Frishman, W., et al. Effects of diltiazem, nifedipine, and their combination on transient ST-segment deviations on the ambulatory ECG in patients with stable angina pectoris (Abstract). *J. Am. Coll. Cardiol.* 9:177A, 1987.
31. Frishman, W. H., et al. Calcium-channel blockers for combined angina pectoris and systemic hypertension. *Am. J. Cardiol.* 57:22D, 1986.
32. Frishman, W. H., et al. Diuretics versus calcium-channel blockers in systemic hypertension: A preliminary multicenter experience with hydrochlorothiazide and sustained-release diltiazem. *Am. J. Cardiol.* 56:92H, 1985.
33. Frolich, E. D. Hemodynamic effects of calcium entry-blocking agents in normal and hypertensive rats and man. *Am. J. Cardiol.* 56:21H, 1985.

34. Gelman, J. S., et al. Nicardipine for angina pectoris at rest and coronary arterial spasm. *Am. J. Cardiol.* 56:232, 1985.
35. Gheorghiade, M., et al. Short- and long-term treatment of stable effort angina with nicardipine, a new calcium channel blocker: A double-blind, placebo-controlled, randomized repeat cross-over study. *Br. J. Clin. Pharmacol.* 20:195S, 1985.
36. Grun, G., and Fleckenstein, A. Excitation-contraction uncoupling of vasculature smooth musculature as fundamental effect in coronary dilatation produced by 4-(2^1-nitrophenyl)-2,6-dimethyl-1,4 dihydropyridine-3,5 dicarbonic acid dimethyl ester (Bay a 1040, nifedipin). *Arzneimittelforsch* 22:334, 1972.
37. Hill, J. A., et al. Effects of bepridil on exercise tolerance in chronic stable angina: A double-blind, randomized, placebo-controlled, crossover trial. *Am. J. Cardiol.* 53:679, 1984.
38. Hill, J. A., et al. Effects of bepridil in patients with chronic stable angina: Results of a multicenter trial. *Circulation* 71:98, 1985.
39. Hill, J. A., et al. Nifedipine improves collateral coronary flow in man at rest but not during pacing. *Clin. Res.* 31:2, 1983.
40. Hill, J. A., et al. Randomized double-blind comparison of nifedipine and isosorbide dinitrate in patients with coronary arterial spasm. *Am. J. Cardiol.* 49:431, 1982.
41. Hill, J. A., and Pepine, C. J. Effects of bepridil on the resting electrocardiogram. *Int. J. Cardiol.* 6:319, 1984.
42. Hiramatsu, K., et al. Acute effects of the calcium antagonist, nifedipine, on blood pressure, pulse rate, and the renin-angiotension-aldosterone system in patients with essential hypertension. *Am. Heart J.* 104:1346, 1982.
43. Hossack, K. F., et al. Efficacy of diltiazem in angina on effort: A multicenter trial. *Am. J. Cardiol.* 49:567, 1982.
44. Hossack, K. F., et al. Divergent effects of diltiazem in patients with exertional angina. *Am. J. Cardiol.* 49:538, 1982.
45. Hornung, R. S., et al. Twice-daily verapamil for hypertension: A comparison with propranolol. *Am. J. Cardiol.* 57:93D, 1986.
46. Hornung, R., et al. Propranolol versus verapamil for the treatment of essential hypertension. *Am. Heart J.* 108:554, 1984.
47. Husted, S. E., et al. Long-term therapy of arterial hypertension with nifedipine given alone or in combination with beta-adrenoceptor blocking agents. *Eur. J. Clin. Pharmacol.* 22:101, 1982.
48. Johnson, S. M., et al. A controlled trial of verapamil for Prinzmetal's variant angina. *N. Engl. J. Med.* 15:862, 1981.
49. Kane, K. A., and Winslow, E. Antidysrhythmic and electrophysiological effects of a new antianginal agent, bepridil. *J. Cardiovasc. Pharmacol.* 2:193, 1980.
50. Khurmi, N. S., et al. Short- and long-term efficacy of nicardipine, assessed by placebo-controlled single- and double-blind crossover trials in patients with chronic stable angina. *J. Am. Coll. Cardiol.* 4:908, 1984.
51. Kimura, E., and Ishida, H. Treatment of variant angina with drugs: a survey of 11 cardiology institutes in Japan. *Circulation* 63:844, 1981.
52. Kiowski, W., et al. Age, race, blood pressure and renin: Predictors for antihypertensive treatment with calcium antagonists. *Am. J. Cardiol.* 56:81H, 1985.
53. Labrid, C., et al. Some membrane interactions with bepridil, a new antianginal agent. *J. Pharmacol. Exp. Ther.* 211:546, 1979.
54. Lambert, C. R., et al. Coronary and systemic hemodynamic effects of nicardipine. *Am. J. Cardiol.* 55:652, 1985.

55. Lambert, C. R., et al. Myocardial ischemia during intravenous nicardipine administration. *Am. J. Cardiol.* 55:844, 1985.
56. Leon, M. G., et al. Clinical efficacy of verapamil alone and combined with propranolol in treating patients with chronic stable angina pectoris. *Am. J. Cardiol.* 48:131, 1981.
57. Levy, S., et al. Treatment of recurrent ventricular tachycardias with bepridil, a slow and fast channel blocking agent (Abstract). *Circulation* 68:III-272, 1983.
58. Lewis, G. R. J. Long term results with verapamil in essential hypertension and its influence on serum lipids. *Am. J. Cardiol.* 57:35D, 1986.
59. McCrorey, H. L., et al. Effects of verapamil, an inhibitor of calcium transport across plasma membrane on renal hemodynamics and electrolyte excretion in dogs (Abstract). *Clin. Res.* 27:424A, 1979.
60. Mehta, J., et al. Short-term efficacy of oral verapamil in rest angina: A double-blind placebo controlled trial in CCU patients. *Am. J. Med.* 71:977, 1981.
61. Millard, R. W., et al. Differential cardiovascular effects of calcium channel blocking agents: Potential mechanisms. *Am. J. Cardiol.* 49:499, 1982.
62. Moskowitz, R. M., et al. Nifedipine therapy for stable angina pectoris. *Am. J. Cardiol.* 44:81, 1979.
63. Moser, M., Lunn, J., and Materson, B. J. Comparative effects of diltiazem and hydrochlorthiazide in blacks with systemic hypertension. *Am. J. Cardiol.* 56:101H, 1985.
64. Muiesan, G., et al. Antihypertensive and humoral effects of verapamil and nifedipine in essential hypertension. *J. Cardiovasc. Pharmacol.* 4:S325, 1982.
65. Nagao, T., et al. Calcium entry blockers: Antihypertensive and natriutetic effects in experimental animals. *Am. J. Cardiol.* 56:56H, 1985.
66. Narahara, K. A., et al. Evaluation of bepridil, a new antianginal agent: Clinical and hemodynamic alterations during treatment of stable angina pectoris. *Am. J. Cardiol.* 53:29, 1984.
67. Newmann, M., and Luisada, A. A. Double-blind evaluation of orally administered iproveratril in patients wtih angina pectoris. *Am. J. Med. Sci.* 251:552, 1966.
68. Oakley, G. D. G., et al. Objective assessment of treatment in severe angina. *Br. Med. J.* 1:1540, 1979.
69. Oliveri, M., et al. Treatment of hypertension with nifedipine, a calcium antagonist agent. *Circulation* 59:1056, 1979.
70. Parmley, W. W., Blumlein, S., and Sievers, B. S. Modification of experimental atherosclerosis by calcium channel blockers. *Am. J. Cardiol.* 55:165B, 1985.
71. Parodi, O., Maseri, A., and Simonetti, I. Management of unstable angina at rest by verapamil. *Br. Heart J.* 41:167, 1979.
72. Pedersen, O. L., et al. Effects of nifedipine on plasma renin, aldosterone and catecholamines in arterial hypertension. *Eur. J. Clin. Pharmacol.* 15:235, 1979.
73. Pederson, O. L., et al. Relationship between antihypertensive effects and steady state plasma concentration of nifedipine given alone or in combination with a beta-adrenoreceptor blocking agent. *Eur. J. Clin. Pharmacol.* 18:287, 1980.
74. Pepine, C. J., and Gelman, J. S. Prevention of vasospastic angina with nicardipine. *Br. J. Clin. Pharmac.* 20:187S, 1985.
75. Pepine, C. J., and Lambert, C. R. Usefulness of nicardipine for angina pectoris. *Am. J. Cardiol.* 59:13J, 1987.

76. Pepine, C. J., et al. Effect of diltiazem in patients with variant angina: A randomized double-blind trial. *Am. Heart J.* 101:719, 1981.
77. Pepine, C. J., et al. Clinical outcome after treatment of rest angina with calcium blockers: Comparative experience during the initial year of therapy with diltiazem, nifedipine and verapamil. *Am. Heart J.* 106:1341, 1983.
78. Piepho, R. W. Individualization of calcium entry-blocker dosage for systemic hypertension. *Am. J. Cardiol.* 56:105H, 1985.
79. Pool, P. E., and Seagren, S. C. Long-term efficacy of diltiazem in chronic stable angina associated with atherosclerosis: Effect on treadmill exercise. *Am. J. Cardiol.* 49:573, 1982.
80. Pool, P. E., Seagren, S. C., and Salel, A. F. Effects of diltiazem on serum lipids, exercise performance and blood pressure: Randomized, double-blind, placebo-controlled evaluation for systemic hypertension. *Am. J. Cardiol.* 56:86H, 1985.
81. Previtali, M., et al. Treatment of angina at rest with nifedipine: A short-term controlled study. *Am. J. Cardiol.* 45:825, 1980.
82. Rojdmark, S., and Andersson, D. E. H. Influence of verapamil on human glucose tolerance. *Am. J. Cardiol.* 57:39D, 1986.
83. Rouleau, J. L., et al. Verapamil suppresses atherosclerosis in cholesterol-fed rabbits. *J. Am. Coll. Cardiol.* 1:1453, 1983.
84. Schang, S. J., and Pepine, C. J. Transient asymptomatic ST segment depression during daily activity. *Am. J. Cardiol.* 39:396, 1977.
85. Scheidt, S., et al. Nicardipine for stable angina pectoris. *Br. J. Clin. Pharmacol.* 20:178S, 1985.
86. Schroeder, J. S., et al. Diltiazem for long-term therapy of coronary arterial spasm. *Am. J. Cardiol.* 49:533, 1982.
87. Selwyn, A. P., et al. Myocardial ischemia in patients with frequent angina pectoris. *Br. Med. J.* 2:1594, 1978.
88. Singh, B. N., et al. Calcium antagonists and beta blockers in the control of mild to moderate systemic hypertension, with particular reference to verapamil and propranolol. *Am. J. Cardiol.* 57:990, 1986.
89. Spinach, C., Ockens, S., and Frishman, W. H. Calcium antagonists: Clinical use in the treatment of systemic hypertension. *Drugs* 25:154, 1983.
90. Stern, S., and Tzivoni, D. Early detection of silent ischemic heart disease by 24-hour electrocardiographic monitoring of active subjects. *Br. Heart J.* 36:481, 1974.
91. Stone, P. H., et al. Efficacy of nifedipine therapy in patients with refractory angina pectoris: Significance of the presence of coronary vasospasm. *Am. Heart J.* 106:644, 1983.
92. Strauss, W. E., et al. Safety and efficacy of diltiazem hydrochloride for the treatment of stable angina pectoris: Report of a cooperative clinical trial. *Am. J. Cardiol.* 49:560, 1982.
93. Subramanian, B., et al. Combined therapy with verapamil and propranolol in chronic stable angina. *Am. J. Cardiol.* 49:125, 1982.
94. Terris, S., et al. Direct cardiac and peripheral vascular effects of intracoronary and intravenous nifedipine. *Am. J. Cardiol.* 58:25, 1986.
95. Trimarco, B., et al. Diltiazem in the treatment of mild or moderate essential hypertension. Comparison with metoprolol in a crossover double-blind trial. *J. Clin. Pharmacol.* 24:218, 1984.
96. Van Breeman, C., et al. Selectivity of calcium antagonistic action in vascular smooth muscle. *Am. J. Cardiol.* 49:507, 1982.
97. Wagniart, P., et al. Increased exercise tolerance and reduced electrocardiographic ischemia with diltiazem in patients with stable angina pectoris. *Circulation* 66:23, 1982.

98. Weiner, D., et al. Significance of silent myocardial ischemia during exercise testing in coronary artery disease. *Am. J. Cardiol.* 59:725, 1987.
99. Winniford, M. D., et al. Verapamil therapy for Prinzmetal's variant angina: Comparison with placebo and nifedipine. *Am. J. Cardiol.* 50:913, 1982.
100. Winslow, E., and Kane, K. A. Supraventricular antidysrhythmic and electrophysiological effects of bepridil, a new antianginal agent. *J. Cardiovasc. Pharmacol.* 3:655, 1981.
101. Yamakado, T., et al. Effects of diltiazem on cardiovascular responses during exercise in systemic hypertension and comparison with propranolol. *Am. J. Cardiol.* 52:1023, 1983.
102. Young, M. A., Watson, R. D., and Littler, W. A. Baroreflex setting and sensitivity after acute and chronic nicardipine therapy. *Clin. Sci.* 66:233, 1984.
103. Zelis, R., and Flaim, S. F. Calcium influx blockers and vascular smooth muscle: Do we really understand the mechanisms? *Ann. Intern. Med.* 94:124, 1981.

CHAPTER 12

THE ROLE OF NITRATES IN ACUTE MYOCARDIAL INFARCTION AND POST-INFARCTION

JOHN T. FLAHERTY

Friedberg's textbook of cardiology as recently as 1966 warned that nitroglycerin was contraindicated in patients with acute myocardial infarction [14]. While carefully monitoring ST segment changes cardiologists at the Johns Hopkins Hospital began studying the short-term hemodynamic and anti-ischemic effects of intravenous nitroglycerin in patients with acute myocardial infarction more than 15 years ago [5, 6, 9, 10]. More recently they conducted a randomized, placebo-controlled trial of intravenous nitroglycerin administered for 48 hours with the goals of reducing infarct size and improving clinical outcomes [12].

On October 1, 1981, nitroglycerin for intravenous infusion was released for general clinical use by the Federal Food and Drug Administration. The approved indications included: (1) unstable angina, (2) left ventricular failure complicating acute myocardial infarction, (3) perioperative hypertension, and (4) controlled hypotension during noncardiac surgery.

The following discussion will review (1) short-term hemodynamic responses in patients with acute myocardial infarction, (2) results of our placebo-controlled trial of longer term infusion of intravenous nitroglycerin in patients with acute myocardial infarction, (3) results of other clinical studies utilizing intravenous nitroglycerin in an attempt to reduce infarct size, (4) comparative hemodynamic and intercoronary collateral flow effects of nitroglycerin and nitroprusside, (5) results of two placebo-controlled clinical trials of nitroprusside in acute myocardial infarction, and (6) effects on infarct expansion and ventricular remodeling. Finally, recommendations for the use of intravenous nitroglycerin in patients with acute myocardial infarction will be presented.

SHORT-TERM HEMODYNAMIC RESPONSES OF PATIENTS WITH ACUTE MYOCARDIAL INFARCTION

As early as 1972 cardiologists at the Johns Hopkins Hospital began administering intravenous nitroglycerin to patients with acute myocardial infarction with the goal of reducing regional myocardial ischemia and, when possible, improving left ventricular hemodynamics. In order to be sure that by lowering coronary perfusion pressure regional ischemia was not being made worse, ST segments were monitored using precordial ST segment mapping. In the first 12 patients only small mean blood pressure lowerings were induced (7 mm Hg). In all cases a reduction in the sum of the ST segment voltages was documented [9].

Following this initial experience, higher infusion rates of nitroglycerin were employed, which resulted in greater reductions in mean arterial pressure (15–30 mm Hg) [10]. Again beneficial anti-ischemic effects were found in all patients irrespective of the presence or absence of left ventricular failure. By employing Swan-Ganz thermodilution catheters

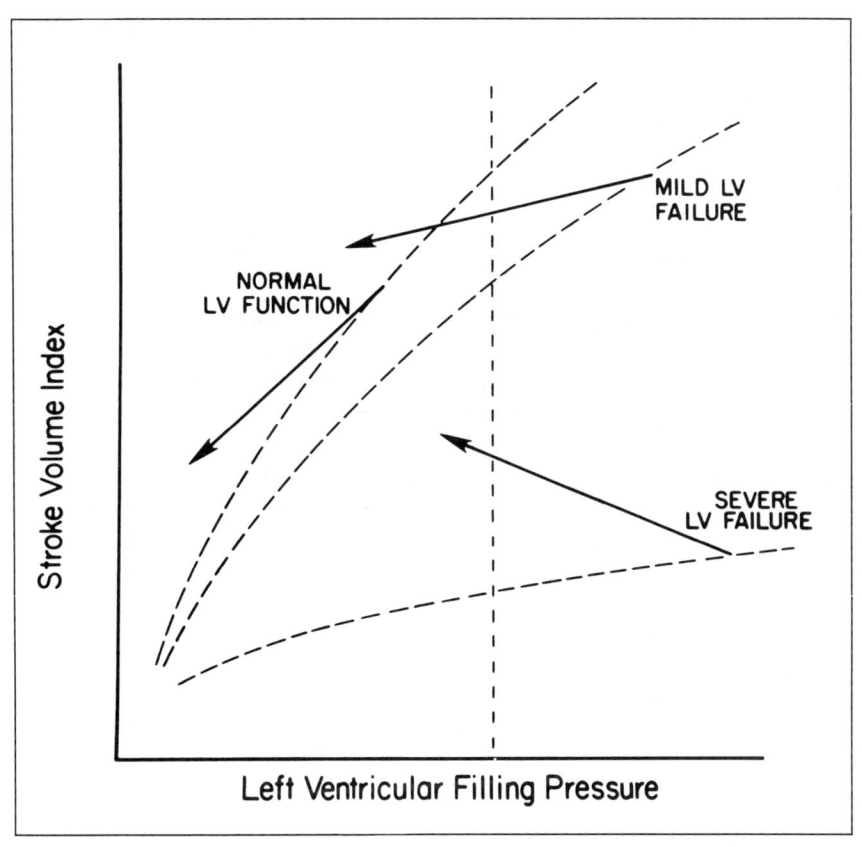

FIG. 12-1. Hemodynamic effects of intravenous nitroglycerin in the presence and absence of left ventricular (LV) failure. Stroke volume index is plotted versus LV filling pressure. The responses obtained with intravenous nitroglycerin in individual hemodynamic subgroups are indicated by arrows. A family of hypothetic Starling ventricular function curves is indicated by dashed curves with diminished contractility expressed by downward and rightward displacement. The vertical dashed line indicates an upper limit of normal LV filling pressure.

in all these patients, nitroglycerin was shown to act principally as a venodilator at lower infusion rates, lowering left ventricular filling pressure 10 mm Hg (45 percent) while causing minimal (7 percent) lowering of mean arterial pressure. In contrast, at higher infusion rates, more balanced venous and arterial dilating effects were observed. A similar lowering of left ventricular filling pressure (52 percent) was associated with a greater lowering of mean arterial pressure (20 percent). Effects on left ventricular hemodynamics varied with the degree of left ventricular failure (Fig. 12-1). Patients without left ventricular failure demonstrated a decrease in stroke volume and a decrease in the left ventricular filling pressure, evidence of a predominant preload lowering or diuretic-like effect induced by venodilation. Patients with mild left ventricular failure as evidenced by elevated left ventricular filling pressure and more normal stroke volume demonstrated a similar lowering of left ventricular filling pressure but with maintenance of stroke volume, suggesting that nitroglycerin was inducing, in addition to preload, a degree of afterload lowering as well. Patients evidencing the most severe degree of left ventricular failure demonstrated the most beneficial hemodynamic effects. In these patients left ventricular filling pressure was again lowered but, in addition, stroke volume was increased, compatible with balanced venous and arterial dilating effects. Similar differential effects on hemodynamics have been reported for nitroprusside. This differential effect of vasodilators on stroke volume for a given lowering of peripheral vascular resistance could be the result of inappropriate elevation in arterial impedance in patients with heart failure, due at least in part to increased sympathetic stimulation and/or circulating catecholamines in patients with moderate or severe left ventricular failure (Fig. 12-2). In the studies conducted at Johns Hopkins, while the hemodynamic response to intravenous nitroglycerin varied with the hemodynamic subgroup, patients in all hemodynamic subgroups demonstrated a beneficial anti-ischemic effect, as evidenced by a reduction in the sum of precordial ST segment voltages.

In summary, short-term administration of intravenous nitroglycerin to patients with acute myocardial infarction resulted in improvement of electrocardiographic evidence of regional ischemia in all hemodynamic subgroups. Patients with the most severe degree of left ventricular failure obtained the most beneficial hemodynamic effect, demonstrating both a reduction in pulmonary venous congestion as well as an improvement in forward cardiac output. Slow upward titration of the infusion rate allowed these beneficial anti-ischemic and hemodynamic effects to be obtained without excessive lowering of blood pressure and without reflex tachycardia. In fact, the mean heart rate during intravenous nitroglycerin infusion was lower than control in all hemodynamic subgroups, most notably in those subgroups of patients with evidence of left ventricular failure.

Two additional short-term clinical studies were conducted in an effort to determine whether or not the anti-ischemic effects could be augmented by the addition of phenylephrine, which by maintaining coronary perfusion pressure might augment the anti-ischemic effects of nitroglycerin alone, or propranolol, which by adding negative inotropic and negative chronotropic effects might augment the anti-ischemic effects of nitroglycerin by further reducing myocardial oxygen demand. The addition of phenylephrine not only increased arterial

12. THE ROLE OF NITRATES IN ACUTE MYOCARDIAL INFARCTION   313

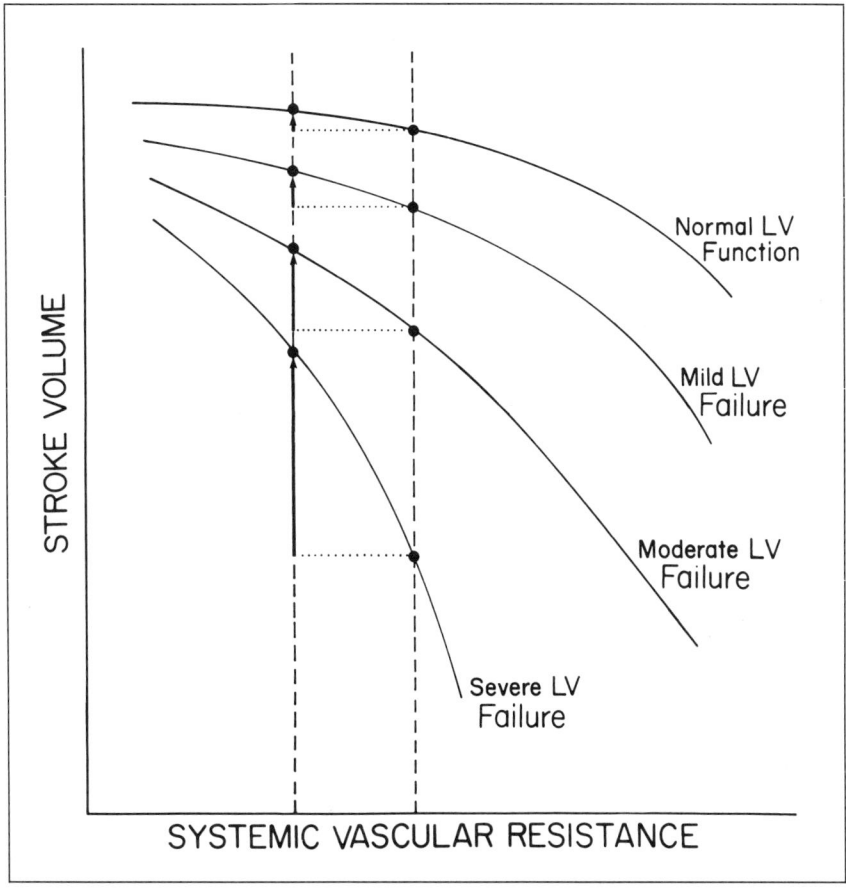

FIG. 12-2. Differential effects of afterload reduction on stroke volume according to hemodynamic subgroup. Curves shown are for patients with normal left ventricular (LV) function as well as for patients with mild, moderate, and severe LV failure. Vertical dashed lines indicate pretreatment (right) and posttreatment (left) levels of systemic vascular resistance (SVR). Vertical arrows indicate the magnitude of the increase in stroke volume index that would be expected from this reduction in SVR for each hemodynamic subgroup.

pressure but also increased left ventricular filling pressure, thereby reversing the beneficial anti-ischemic effects obtained with nitroglycerin alone [5]. Addition of propranolol also resulted in a reversal of the left ventricular filling pressure lowering obtained with nitroglycerin alone. Further, when the nitroglycerin infusion was discontinued, left ventricular filling pressures rose above control levels, especially in patients with significant left ventricular dysfunction [6].

CLINICAL TRIAL OF LONGER-TERM INFUSION OF NITROGLYCERIN IN PATIENTS WITH ACUTE MYOCARDIAL INFARCTION

Based on the positive results of our initial short-term studies, a randomized prospective trial of long-term infusion of nitroglycerin in patients with acute myocardial infarction was undertaken [12]. Patients received 48 hours of either intravenous nitroglycerin or placebo, followed by application of nitroglycerin or placebo ointment for an additional 72 hours. Included in this study were patients with chest pain and electrocardiographic changes suggestive of acute myocardial infarction, presenting less than 12 hours after the onset of symptoms. Excluded were patients with systolic blood pressure less than 95 mm Hg, heart rate less than 55 beats/min, or age greater than 75 years. Also excluded were patients with significant arterial hypertension, from whom intravenous vasodilator therapy could not ethically be withheld, patients unable or unwilling to give informed consent, or patients with severe life-threatening disease of other organ systems.

Initiation of the study drug infusion was preceded by obtaining a thallium-201 perfusion scan and a technetium 99m labeled gated blood-pool scan. A computer-assisted scoring technique was used to obtain a thallium defect score that quantified the extent and severity of the myocardial perfusion defect(s). The thallium defect score provided an estimate of the total area at risk, including both infarcted and reversibly ischemic myocardium. The gated blood-pool scan defined pretreatment left ventricular function. In a few patients two-dimensional echocardiography was employed instead to assess pretreatment left ventricular function.

Infusion of intravenous nitroglycerin was begun at 5 to 10 mcg/min, and the infusion rate increased stepwise until a 10 percent lowering of mean arterial pressure was obtained. Blood pressure was monitored noninvasively with an ultrasonic blood pressure cuff. Once this end point had been reached, the final infusion rate was continued for 48 hours, unless side effects or hemodynamic instability required reduction or discontinuation of the infusion. The mean infusion rate required to obtain the 10 percent mean blood pressure lowering was 90 mcg/min. After 48 hours the nitroglycerin infusion was discontinued; patients were treated with 1 inch of nitroglycerin ointment every 4 hours, with the dosage increased in a stepwise fashion, in an attempt to maintain the arterial pressure previously obtained with intravenous therapy. Control patients received placebo ointment. Seven to 14 days later a repeat thallium-201 myocardial perfusion scan and a gated blood-pool scan or a two-dimension echocardiogram were obtained. Comparison of paired measurements of pre- and posttreatment myocardial perfusion and left ventricular function in nitroglycerin and placebo-treated patients allowed separation of the effects of nitroglycerin from the spontaneous changes occurring with time.

Fifty-six patients were randomized to nitroglycerin, and forty-eight were randomized to placebo. No significant differences in admission clinical, laboratory, or scintigraphic parameters were found between the groups randomized to nitroglycerin or placebo. Patients were also divided to early- and late-treatment subgroups, according to the time interval between the onset of symptoms and the initiation of treatment. Patients treated less than 10 hours from the onset of symptoms were considered to have had early treatment, and those treated 10 hours or more after symptom onset, late treatment. This arbitrary cutoff at 10 hours divided the 56 nitroglycerin-treated patients into two equal subgroups. Coincidentally, the mean time interval from onset of chest pain to initiation of therapy for the entire population of 104 patients was also 10 hours.

Three-month mortality was lower in the early nitroglycerin treatment subgroup (14 percent) when compared with the other three treatment subgroups (21–28 percent). Because of the relatively small size of the study population this difference approached but did not reach statistical significance. When the clinical outcomes of in-hospital death, infarct extension, or the new development of congestive heart failure were examined separately, differences clearly favored early nitroglycerin treatment but again were not quite statistically significant. However, when the incidence of any one of these three unfavorable outcomes was combined, a highly significant reduction was noted with early nitroglycerin treatment ($p < .003$).

The change in ejection fraction between day 1 and days 7 to 14 was also strikingly better with early nitroglycerin therapy (Fig. 12-3). Patients with an abnormal ejection fraction on admission who received early treatment with nitroglycerin demonstrated an 11 percent improvement in left ventricular ejection fraction. In contrast, patients with an initially abnormal ejection fraction in the other three treatment subgroups demonstrated no significant changes ($p = 0.058$). Subgroups of patients with initially normal ejection fractions (greater than 50 percent) all demonstrated decreases in ejection fraction between day 1 and days 7 to 14 irrespective of therapy. It seems likely that the pretreatment ejection fractions were artificially augmented by the high circulating catecholamine levels associated with an acute myocardial infarction. Seven to 14 days later, in the absence of chest pain and associated sympathetic/catecholamine stimulation, a lower overall ejection fraction might be expected.

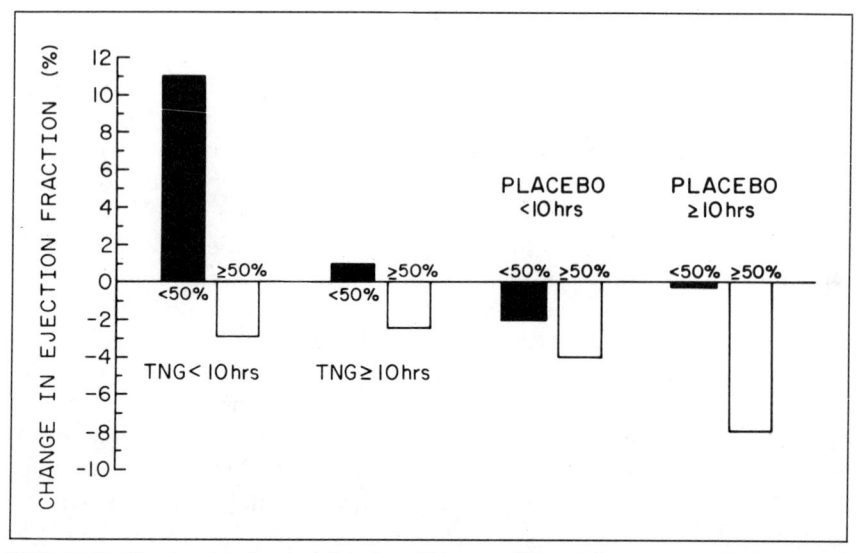

FIG. 12-3. Change in ejection fraction (%) according to treatment subgroup and initial ejection fraction. Ejection fraction defined as abnormal (< 50%) or normal (≥ 50%). Treatment subgroups were defined as early (< 10 hours) or late (≥ 10 hours) relative to time of symptom onset for nitroglycerin (TNG) and placebo-treated patients.

FINDINGS OF OTHER CLINICAL TRIALS OF INTRAVENOUS NITROGLYCERIN IN ACUTE MYOCARDIAL INFARCTION

In addition to the study at Johns Hopkins, several other studies have been published that employed long-term infusion of nitroglycerin in an attempt to reduce infarct size (Table 12-1). Bussman et al. studied 31 patients with acute myocardial infarction who received intravenous nitroglycerin for 48 hours and 29 control patients who did not receive nitroglycerin [1]. They included only patients with pulmonary artery diastolic or pulmonary capillary wedge pressures of 12 mm Hg or more. To be included, patients had to have a transmural infarction as evidenced by ST segment elevations and, subsequently, the development of pathologic Q waves and a rise in creatine kinase blood levels. Treatment was instituted a mean of 10 hours after the onset of symptoms of acute infarction. Nitroglycerin was titrated to lower the pulmonary artery diastolic pressure an unspecified amount, but excessive lowering of arterial pressure was specifically avoided. Nitroglycerin infusion rates of 12 to 100 mcg/min were employed (mean 47 mcg/min).

Creatine kinase (CK) infarct size was found to be 23 percent lower for nitroglycerin-treated versus control patients ($p < .05$). Similarly,

TABLE 12-1. *Clinical Trials of Intravenous Nitroglycerin (NTG) in Acute Myocardial Infarction*

Authors	Patients (N)	Inclusion Criteria	Mean Time from Symptom Onset to Rx[b] (hrs)	IV NTG Mean Dose	Duration	Titration End-Point	Outcome
Bussman et al. [1]	60	Only transmural infarcts with LVFP[a] >12 mm Hg	10	47 µg/min	48 hours	↓ LVFP	↓ CK[c] infarct size
Jaffe et al. [16]	85	All infarcts	6	54 µg/min	24 hours	↓ SAP 10%	↓ CK infarct size 37% but in inferior transmural infarcts only
Derrida et al. [7]	24	All infarcts	10	51 µg/min	1–7 days	↓ SAP 20 mm Hg	↓ In-hospital mortality–from 23% to 5% and precordial R waves better preserved in anterior infarcts

↓ = decrease.
[a]LVFP = left ventricular filling pressure.
[b]Rx = treatment.
[c]CK = creatine kinase.

infarct size calculated from serum levels of the myocardial specific (MB) isoenzyme of creatine kinase, peak total CK level, and peak MB isoenzyme blood levels were also lower with nitroglycerin compared with control treatment.

The routine use of Swan-Ganz catheters allowed for serial measurements of the hemodynamic effects of nitroglycerin during the 48-hour infusion and also for documenting spontaneous hemodynamic changes in control patients. Pulmonary artery diastolic pressure decreased from 19 ± 4 to 11 ± 3 mm Hg ($p < .005$ versus control patients) and cardiac output increased from 5.1 ± 1.2 to 5.5 ± 1.4 L/min ($p < .025$ versus control patients) after 48 hours of nitroglycerin infusion. Heart rate increased only slightly, from 88 ± 19 to 93 ± 16 beats/min (not significant versus control patients). Mean arterial pressure decreased from 108 ± 19 to 93 ± 13 mm Hg (not significant versus control patients).

Jaffe et al. reported a randomized prospective study of 85 patients receiving 24-hour infusion of nitroglycerin or placebo beginning a mean of 6 hours after the onset of symptoms of acute infarction [16]. Nitroglycerin infusion was titrated to lower systolic blood pressure by 10 percent, unless heart rate increased by 20 beats/min or a maximum dose of 200 mcg/min was reached. The mean infusion rate required was 54 mcg/min. Creatine kinase infarct size was 37 percent lower with nitroglycerin treatment only in the subgroup of patients with inferior transmural infarctions ($p < .05$). In contrast, patients with anterior transmural infarctions did not show evidence of benefit. Patients with subendocardial infarctions demonstrated an intermediate response.

In another randomized prospective study, Derrida et al. reported a reduction in in-hospital mortality from 23 to 5 percent in 74 patients with acute myocardial infarction, comparing nitroglycerin-treated with untreated controls ($p < .05$) [7]. Nitroglycerin was titrated to lower systolic arterial pressure 20 mm Hg, with the infusion maintained for 1 to 7 days. The mean nitroglycerin infusion rate was 51 mcg/min, and the mean time interval between the onset of symptoms and the initiation of therapy was 10 hours. Precordial mapping studies in the subgroup of 46 patients with anterior transmural infarctions revealed better preservation of R waves in the subset of precordial leads initially demonstrating ST segment elevation of greater than 1.5 mm and a persistent R wave ($p < .05$).

Based on the premise that the published clinical trials of intravenous nitroglycerin in acute myocardial infarction had been unable to detect a moderate reduction in mortality due to relatively small sample sizes, Yusuf and Collins pooled mortality data from seven randomized, placebo-controlled studies [27]. In only two of the seven trials did the reduction in mortality achieve statistical significance. In contrast, the pooled data for all seven studies, which included more than 1000 patients, revealed a 30 percent reduction in mortality [74/522 (14 percent)

TABLE 12-2. *Comparison of Intravenous Nitroglycerin with Nitroprusside in Acute Myocaridal Infarction*

	Nitroglycerin	Nitroprusside
Chiarello et al. [3]		
Patients with anterior transmural myocardial infarction	↓ ST elevations ↓ ST elevations and ↑ MBF[a]	↑ ST elevations
Open-chest anesthetized dog model with acute coronary ligation	↓ ST elevations and ↑ MBF[a]	↑ ST elevations and ↓ MBF*
Mann et al. [22]		
Patients with angiographically visible intercoronary channels	↑ MBF	↓ MFB

↓ = decrease; ↑ = increase.
*MBF = myocardial blood flow.

among intravenous nitroglycerin-treated patients versus 107/507 (21 percent) among control patients, $p < .001$].

MECHANISM OF NITROGLYCERIN'S REDUCTION OF INFARCT SIZE ASSESSED IN A CANINE MODEL

That intravenous nitroglycerin might be reducing infarct size by effects on collateral flow was suggested by the results of a placebo-controlled study performed by Jugdutt et al. using an unanesthetized canine model of acute myocardial infarction [17]. Nitroglycerin was infused for 6 hours beginning 3 minutes after coronary artery ligation. The titration end point of a 10 percent lowering of mean arterial pressure was identical to that employed in our clinical trial. Jugdutt et al. demonstrated a 50 percent increase in intercoronary collateral blood flow and a 47 to 50 percent reduction in infarct size with nitroglycerin therapy.

COMPARISON OF THE EFFECTS OF NITROGLYCERIN AND NITROPRUSSIDE ON REGIONAL MYOCARDIAL BLOOD FLOW

Several studies have compared the hemodynamic and anti-ischemic effects of nitroglycerin and nitroprusside (Table 12-2). Chiarello et al. reported a study in which ten patients with acute anterior transmural myocardial infarction received sodium nitroprusside at an infusion rate sufficient to lower mean arterial pressure by 25 mm Hg [3]. During nitroprusside infusion all ten patients showed an increase or worsening of their precordial ST segment elevations, suggesting a worsening rather than an improvement in the severity of their regional myocardial ischemia. After stopping the nitroprusside infusion, five of these patients were given sublingual nitroglycerin at a dose that lowered mean arterial pressure 14 mm Hg. All five patients demonstrated a decrease or an improvement in their precordial ST segment elevations, suggesting an improvement in regional ischemia with nitroglycerin. In order to define the mechanisms responsible for the apparent opposite effects of nitroglycerin and nitroprusside on the severity of regional ischemia, these same investigators carried out an analogous study in an open-chest canine model. Following ligation of the left anterior descending coronary artery, nitroprusside was infused at a rate sufficient to lower mean arterial pressure 20 mm Hg. After the nitroprusside infusion had been discontinued, nitroglycerin was infused at a rate sufficient to lower mean arterial pressure by an equal amount. Utilizing the radioactive microsphere technique these investigators found that myocardial blood flow distal to the ligated left anterior descending coronary artery decreased and epicardial ST segment voltages increased or worsened during nitroprusside infusion. In contrast, during nitroglycerin infusion, myocardial blood flow increased and epicardial ST segments decreased, suggesting an improvement in the severity of ischemia in the region of myocardium supplied by the occluded left anterior descending coronary artery. Since the coronary artery remained ligated, the improvement in regional ischemia observed with nitroglycerin must be due to an increase in intercoronary collateral blood flow. During nitroprusside infusion, in contrast, intercoronary collateral flow to the ischemic zone actually decreased, as flow to the nonischemic zone increased, evidencing a coronary steal.

In the cardiac catheterization laboratory, Mann et al. used the xenon washout technique to study the effects of nitroglycerin and nitroprusside on regional myocardial blood flow [21]. In a subgroup of patients with fixed coronary artery disease and angiographically visible intercoronary collaterals, myocardial blood flow distal to a severe coronary artery stenosis was found to increase with nitroglycerin and to decrease with nitroprusside. Cappuro et al., using an open-chest anesthesetized dog model with well-developed collateral vessels induced by previous implantation of an ameroid constrictor, demonstrated greater sensitivity of intercoronary collateral channels to the vasodilating effects of nitroglycerin than nitroprusside [2]. Finally, Marcho and Vatner demonstrated in a conscious, previously instrumented dog model that, compared to nitroprusside, nitroglycerin induces relatively less dilation of the small resistance vessels and greater dilation of the large (conductance) coronary vessels, which include intercoronary collateral channels [23].

COMPARISON OF BLOOD PRESSURE LOWERING EFFECTS OF NITROGLYCERIN AND NITROPRUSSIDE

Based on previous observations in patients with acute myocardial infarction that significant lowering of arterial pressure could be obtained with intravenous nitroglycerin, the Johns Hopkins cardiologists designed a crossover study to test the arterial vasodilating potency of nitroglycerin and sodium nitroprusside in patients developing acute hypertension during the first 5 hours following coronary artery bypass surgery [11]. Seventeen patients were studied using a randomized crossover protocol. The infusion rate of nitroglycerin and nitroprusside was increased stepwise until the mean arterial pressure was lowered 20 mm Hg or more. Nitroglycerin and nitroprusside resulted in equal lowering of mean arterial pressure at comparable infusion rates in 14 of 17 patients. In the remaining three patients, which we termed nitroglycerin resistant, infusion rates in excess of 1000 mcg/min were employed with variable success in an attempt to match the blood pressure lowering obtained with nitroprusside.

Analysis of the hemodynamic effects revealed that equal lowerings of mean arterial pressure and systemic vascular resistance were obtained with nitroglycerin and nitroprusside. Neither drug resulted in a significant increase in heart rate nor a significant decrease in pulmonary capillary wedge pressure. The latter finding was likely the result of simultaneous volume administration in these early postoperative patients with active surgical bleeding. Measurements of pulmonary and tissue gas exchange in eight of the 17 patients revealed a significantly greater increase in alveolar-arterial (A-a) oxygen gradient observed with nitroprusside than the increase with nitroglycerin. Likewise, calculated intrapulmonary shunting, which decreased with nitroglycerin, in contrast, increased with nitroprusside.

In summary, it would appear that nitroglycerin is equally effective as nitroprusside for lowering blood pressure in acutely hypertensive patients. For the minority in whom nitroglycerin resistance is observed, nitroprusside would appear to remain the drug of choice. Intravenous nitroglycerin is frequently used in the perioperative setting concomitantly with nitroprusside, with nitroprusside used for coarse-tuning and the nitroglycerin used for fine-tuning. Patients initially receiving the combination of nitroglycerin and nitroprusside are most often switched to nitroglycerin alone when the vasodilator requirement and/or the stimuli to vasoconstriction (e.g., hypothermia) diminish.

TABLE 12-3. *Clinical Trials of Intravenous Nitroprusside (NP) in Acute Myocardial Infarction*

Clinical Trial	Early Treatment Group	Late Treatment Group
Cohn et al. [4] 812 patients, mean time of Rx 17 hours after onset of symptoms. Only transmural infarcts and LVFP[a] >12 mm Hg	↑ Mortality (13 wks) 24% for NP vs. 13% for placebo	↓ Mortality (13 wks) 14% for NP vs. 22% for placebo
Durrer et al. [8] 328 patients, mean time of Rx 5 hours after onset of symptoms. All infarcts. (Patients with hypertension on admission were not excluded.)	↓ Mortality (4 wks) 6% for NP vs. 12% for placebo ↓ Peak MB-CK[b] blood levels (anterior infarcts only)	

↑ = increase.
↓ = decrease.
[a]LVFP = left ventricular filling pressure.
[b]MB − CK = MB isoenzyme of creatine kinase.
[c]Rx = treatment.

CLINICAL TRIALS OF NITROPRUSSIDE IN ACUTE MYOCARDIAL INFARCTION

In two published randomized prospective placebo-controlled trials nitroprusside or placebo was administered to patients with acute myocardial infarction in an attempt to reduce infarct size and/or improve short-term mortality (Table 12-3). In a large multicenter Veterans Administration Cooperative Trial nitroprusside was titrated to reach one of four end points: (1) a reduction of left ventricular filling pressure to less than 60 percent of control, (2) a lowering of systolic arterial pressure to 20 percent of the control pressure plus 76 mm Hg, (3) the development of significant side effects, or (4) a maximum infusion rate of 200 mcg/minute [4]. Included were 812 patients with onset of chest pain less than 24 hours prior to admission and transmural infarction as evidenced by ST segment elevations and subsequent development of pathologic Q waves or a new conduction defect (Table 12-3). Approximately 67 percent of patients had anterior wall infarctions. A left ventricular filling pressure of greater than or equal to 12 mm Hg was also required. Excluded were patients with (1) normal left ventricular filling pressures, (2) cardiogenic shock, (3) hypertension requiring vasodilator therapy, (4) severe bronchopulmonary disease or other serious illnesses, or (5) a systolic blood pressure of less than 100 mm Hg.

Patients received either 48-hour infusion of sodium nitroprusside or placebo. The mean time interval between the onset of symptoms and initiation of therapy was 17 hours. Three-week mortality was 10.4 percent among the total population of placebo-treated patients compared with 11.5 percent among all nitroprusside-treated patients (NS). Likewise, after 13 weeks of follow-up, mortality rates were 19 percent in placebo-treated and 17 percent in nitroprusside-treated patients (NS). No significant differences were noted in the peak MB isoenzyme of creatine kinase blood levels. However, with early treatment defined as treatment initiated less than 9 hours after the onset of chest pain, mortality rate after 13 weeks of follow-up was higher, 24 percent in those treated early with nitroprusside compared to only 13 percent in those treated early with placebo ($p < 0.025$) (Table 12-3). In contrast, in those patients treated late, 13-week mortality was found to be lower (14 percent with nitroprusside versus 22 percent with placebo, $p < 0.04$).

While several explanations were offered for the apparent opposite effects of nitroprusside with early versus late treatment, one was particularly plausible. First, a spontaneous decline in left ventricular filling pressure has been documented to occur during the early hours of an acute myocardial infarction. Thus, many patients included in the early treatment subgroup might have been excluded from the study had their filling pressure been measured later. The early treatment subgroups would therefore contain more patients without significant left ventricular dysfunction. By lowering coronary perfusion pressure and dilating small resistance vessels in nonischemic myocardium more than intercoronary collateral channels (i.e., inducing a coronary steal), nitroprusside might have made regional ischemia worse. Such a deleterious effect might have been magnified in patients with low left ventricular filling pressures, in whom the reduction in myocardial oxygen demand by reduction of diastolic wall tension would have been minimal. In contrast, patients treated later with persistently elevated left ventricular filling pressures could obtain a greater reduction in myocardial oxygen demand and a greater improvement in subendocardial perfusion, perhaps counteracting any deleterious effects on collateral flow.

In a second randomized clinical trial, Durrer et al. administered nitroprusside or placebo for 24 hours to 328 patients with acute myocardial infarction [8] (Table 12-3). Nitroprusside was titrated to lower systolic blood pressure to 100 mm Hg or to reach a maximum infusion rate of 500 mcg/min. Inclusion criteria were chest pain lasting 1 or more hours and electrocardiographic changes consisting of ST segment elevation or depression or T wave inversion, thereby including subendocardial as well as transmural infarctions. Approximately 50 percent of the infarctions were anterior. Swan-Ganz catheters were not routinely placed. Exclusion criteria were (1) cardiogenic shock, (2) pulmonary edema, (3) hypotension as defined by systolic blood pressure less than 95 mm Hg,

(4) heart rate greater than 120 beats/min, and (5) patients in whom infarction was unlikely or in whom the time of onset of symptoms was uncertain.

The mean interval between the onset of symptoms and the initiation of therapy was 5 hours. Durrer et al. [8] found a significant reduction in mortality after 23 days of follow-up comparing nitroprusside (6 percent) and placebo-treated patients (12 percent) (Table 12-3). Eighteen patients died in the placebo group compared with only five in the nitroprusside-treated group ($p < 0.05$). Of the 18 deaths in the placebo group, seven occurred within 24 hours and the remaining 11 within the first week. In contrast, of the five deaths in the nitroprusside treatment group, there were no deaths during the first 24 hours, with all five deaths occurring later in the first week. It was noteworthy that the cause of death in nine of the 18 placebo patients was rupture of the left ventricular free wall, a papillary muscle, or the interventricular septum. This relatively high (7 percent) incidence of myocardial rupture of one form or another in a population of patients that included both subendocardial and transmural infarctions and normal as well as abnormal left ventricular filling pressures seems unusually large. Since initially hypertensive patients appeared not to be excluded, it is possible that some of these patients suffering myocardial rupture had been significantly hypertensive on admission and that their hypertension had remained untreated if they were randomized to receive placebo treatment. The beneficial effect found for nitroprusside could therefore be reflecting the ability of a vasodilator to reduce elevated blood pressures during the early hours of acute infarction and thereby prevent subsequent myocardial rupture. These investigators were also able to demonstrate a reduction in peak blood levels of the MB isoenzymes of creatine kinase only in patients with anterior infarction (Table 12-3) and a reduction in the incidence of congestive heart failure during the in-hospital period in all nitroprusside-treated patients.

In any event, the results of these two studies raise several questions regarding the advisability of nitroprusside treatment in patients with acute myocardial infarction and, compared to the uniformly beneficial results of the nitroglycerin studies, would appear to favor the use of intravenous nitroglycerin over nitroprusside in this clinical setting.

EFFECTS ON INFARCT EXPANSION AND LEFT VENTRICULAR REMODELING

Interest in the issue of ventricular remodeling following myocardial infarction has been generated by the results of several experimental animal model studies [18, 24] and a randomized, placebo-controlled clinical study, which showed that administration of an afterload lowering agent, such as the angiotensin-converting enzyme inhibitor captopril, to patients with anterior transmural myocardial infarctions limits left ventricular dilation during a 1-year follow-up [25]. Left ventricular remodeling can be the result of stretching and thinning of the infarct segment, which has been termed infarct expansion and, in addition, stretching of remote noninfarcted myocardium, which is presumably trying to utilize the Starling mechanism to compensate for the loss of contractility in infarcted segments. A recent study by Jugdutt and Warnica reported the beneficial effects of acute administration of intravenous nitroglycerin on left ventricular ejection fraction, left ventricular asynergy, and derived indices of infarct expansion and thinning [19]. These authors randomized 310 patients to intravenous nitroglycerin infusion for an average of 39 hours or routine therapy (controls). Serial two-dimensional echocardiography was employed to assess the incidence and severity of infarct expansion. Not only was infarct expansion, assessed 10 days after admission, reduced, but in addition, creatine kinase infarct size and 3-month mortality were also significantly decreased. Tymchak et al. have also recently reported the results of a smaller randomized clinical trial where they compared reperfusion with intracoronary streptokinase or coronary angioplasty in combination with intravenous nitroglycerin, with intravenous nitroglycerin alone for 45 hours, and with saline infusion in controls [26]. The extent of left ventricular asynergy and the evidence of infarct expansion were reduced significantly by both reperfusion plus intravenous nitroglycerin and with intravenous nitroglycerin alone. Michorowski et al. have also reported the beneficial effects of prolonged nitroglycerin therapy on left ventricular function and indices of infarct expansion in a randomized, placebo-controlled clinical trial [23]. Patients received intravenous nitroglycerin infusion for 48 hours and then were randomized to receive either buccal nitroglycerin 1 to 3 mg three times a day, with an 8 hour overnight nitrate-free interval, or placebo. Nitroglycerin-treated patients demonstrated a significant reduction in indices of infarct expansion assessed 12 weeks after study entry and 6 weeks after discontinuing the therapy. These exciting new results would suggest that prolonged (6 week) nitroglycerin therapy is able to exert beneficial effects on both infarct expansion and subsequent left ventricular remodeling.

A randomized clinical trial performed at the Johns Hopkins Hospital compared intravenous nitroglycerin infusion plus intra-aortic balloon counterpulsation therapy for 4 to 5 days with routine medical management in a group of patients with large transmural myocardial infarctions, as judged by their admission thallium defect score [13]. This study, carried out in patients without overt clinical evidence of left ventricular decompensation, revealed that even this combined aggressive approach to lowering left ventricular afterload was not sufficient to reduce infarct expansion in these patients with large risk regions but was able to reduce the degree of stretching or remodeling of the contralateral wall; this was assessed by two-dimensional echocardiography 7 to 14 days after initiation of afterload lowering therapy but at least two days after the therapy had been discontinued. Those patients with smaller and thus lower risk thallium perfusion defects were entered into a second randomized, placebo-controlled trial of the calcium channel antagonist nifedipine [15]. The results of this trial showed significant beneficial effects on infarct segment length, suggesting that with smaller risk regions afterload lowering with nifedipine, like nitroglycerin or captopril, can prevent or minimize infarct expansion.

In summary, initiation of intravenous nitroglycerin infusion at the time of admission followed by chronic therapy with a long-acting nitrate preparation for the next 6 weeks would appear to have long-term beneficial effects on left ventricular remodeling, which are similar to those obtained with the angiotensin converting enzyme (ACE) inhibitors. The need for a nitrate-free interval to avoid the development of nitrate tolerance or hemodynamic attenuation in this setting has not been documented. However, since the majority of clinical studies demonstrate loss of arterial blood pressure lowering effects with chronic continuous administration of long-acting nitrates, it might seem prudent to utilize a nitrate-free interval in this particular clinical setting, where afterload lowering is the primary goal. Of interest, the results of a recent study by Kelly et al. suggest that measuring the brachial artery pressure might not be an adequate assessment of the afterload lowering effects of nitroglycerin [20]. These authors were able to show in some patients large reductions in central aortic systolic pressure in the absence of a significant lowering of brachial arterial pressure. The authors reason that nitroglycerin's effect on pulse wave transmission does not alter the peak systolic in the brachial artery but does reduce the aortic peak systolic pressure, which is the sum of a primary systolic pressure wave and a secondary reflected wave.

CURRENT RECOMMENDATIONS FOR USE OF NITRATES IN PATIENTS WITH ACUTE MYOCARDIAL INFARCTION

The author recommends the administration of intravenous thrombolytic therapy (tissue plasminogen activator or streptokinase) to patients reaching the emergency room within 4 hours of symptom onset. These patients will initially have intravenous nitroglycerin titrated to lower mean or systolic arterial pressure 10 percent, with the infusion then maintained for up to 48 hours. Patients seen more than 4 hours after symptom onset but with evidence of viable myocardium (e.g., persistent R waves in those EKG leads demonstrating ST elevation) may also receive intravenous nitroglycerin and thrombolytic therapy. Results of the large number of clinical trials of intravenous nitroglycerin in acute myocardial infarction would support the routine use of intravenous nitroglycerin for patients seen 4 to 12 hours after onset of symptoms or for patients seen earlier in whom thrombolytic therapy cannot be utilized. Intravenous nitroglycerin is also useful for the treatment of acute congestive heart failure and/or hypertension complicating acute myocardial infarction as well as for the treatment of postinfarction unstable angina. Definitive therapy consisting of percutaneous transluminal angioplasty or, on occasion, early bypass surgery is frequently employed after successful thrombolytic therapy. It is likely that this combined treatment will result in optimal salvage of ischemic myocardium as well as improved long-term prognosis.

REFERENCES

1. Bussman, W. D., Passek, D., Seidel, W., et al. Reduction of CK and CK-MB indexes of infarct size by intravenous nitroglycerin. *Circulation* 63:615, 1981.
2. Cappuro, N. L., Kent, K. M., and Epstein, S. E. Comparison of nitroglycerin, nitroprusside and phenolamine induced changes in coronary collateral function in dogs. *J. Clin. Invest.* 60:295, 1977.
3. Chiarello, M., Gold, H. K., Leinbach, R. C., et al. Comparison between the effects of nitroprusside and nitroglycerin on ischemic injury during acute myocardial infarction. *Circulation* 54:766, 1976.
4. Cohn, J. N., Franciosa, J. A., Francis, G. S., et al. Effect of short-term infusion of sodium nitroprusside on mortality rate in acute myocardial infarction complicated by left ventricular failure. *N. Engl. J. Med.* 306:1129, 1982.
5. Come, P. C., Flaherty, J. T., Baird, M. G., et al. Reversal by phenylephrine of the beneficial effects of intravenous nitroglycerin in patients with acute myocardial infarction. *N. Engl. J. Med.* 293:1003, 1975.
6. Come, P. C., Flaherty, J. T., Becker, L. C., et al. Combined administration of nitroglycerin and propranolol to patients with acute myocardial infarction. *Chest* 80:416, 1981.
7. Derrida, J. R., Sal, R., and Chiche, P. Effects of prolonged nitroglycerin infusion in patients with acute myocardial infarction (Abstract). *Am. J. Cardiol.* 41:407, 1978.
8. Durrer, J. D., Lie, K. L., Van Capell, F. J. T., et al. Effect of sodium nitroprusside on mortality in acute myocardial infarction. *N. Engl. J. Med.* 306:1121, 1982.
9. Flaherty, J. T., Reid, P. R., Kelly, D. T., et al. Intravenous nitroglycerin in acute myocardial infarction. *Circulation* 51:132, 1975.
10. Flaherty, J. T., Come, P. C., Baird, M. G., et al. Effects of intravenous nitroglycerin on left ventricular function and ST segment changes in acute myocardial infarction. *Br. Heart J.* 38:612, 1976.
11. Flaherty, J. T., Magee, P. A., Gardner, T. J., et al. Comparison of intravenous nitroglycerin and sodium nitroprusside for the treatment of acute hypertension developing after coronary artery bypass surgery. *Circulation* 65:1172, 1981.
12. Flaherty, J. T., Becker, L. C., Bulkley, B. H., et al. A randomized prospective trial of intravenous nitroglycerin in patients with acute myocardial infarction. *Circulation* 68:576, 1983.

13. Flaherty, J. T., Becker, L. C., Weiss, J. L., et al. Results of a randomized prospective trial of intraaortic balloon counterpulsation and intravenous nitroglycerin in patients with acute myocardial infarction. *J.A.C.C.* 56:434–46, 1985.
14. Friedberg, C. K. *Diseases of the Heart* (3rd ed.). Philadelphia: W. B. Saunders, 1966. P. 193.
15. Gottlieb, S. O., Becker, L. C., Weiss, J. L., et al. Nifedipine in acute myocardial infarction: An assessment of infarct size, left ventricular function and infarct expansion: A double-blind, randomized placebo-controlled trial. *Br. Heart J.* 59:411–18, 1988.
16. Jaffe, A. S., Geltman, E. M., Tiefenbrunn, A. J., et al. Relation of the extent of inferior myocardial infarction with intravenous nitroglycerin: A randomized prospective study. *Br. Heart J.* 49:452, 1983.
17. Jugdutt, B. I., Becker, L. C., Hutchins, G. M., et al. Effect of intravenous nitroglycerin on collateral blood flow and infarct size in the conscious dog. *Circulation* 63:17, 1981.
18. Jugdutt, B. I., Michorowski, B. L., and O'Kelly, B. F. Pharmacologic modification of left ventricular remodeling after myocardial infarction in the dog (Abstract). *J.A.C.C.* 11:252A, 1988.
19. Jugdutt, B. I., and Warnica, J. W. Intravenous nitroglycerin therapy to limit myocardial infarct size, expansion, and complications. *Circulation* 78:906–19, 1988.
20. Kelly, R., Gibbs, H., Morgan, J., et al. Brachial artery pressure measurements underestimate beneficial effects of nitroglycerin on left ventricular afterload (Abstract). *J.A.C.C.* 13:231A, 1989.
21. Mann, T., Cohn, P. F., Holman, B. L., et al. Effect of nitroprusside on regional myocardial blood flow in coronary disease: Results in 25 patients and comparison with nitroglycerin. *Circulation* 57:732, 1978.
22. Marcho, P., and Vatner, S. F. Effects of nitroglycerin and nitroprusside in large and small coronary vessels in conscious dogs. *Circulation* 64:1101, 1981.
23. Michorowski, B. L., Tymchak, W. T., and Jugdutt, B. I. Improved left ventricular function and topography by prolonged nitroglycerin therapy after acute myocardial infarction (Abstract). *Circulation* 76(Suppl IV):IV-128, 1987.
24. Pfeffer, J. M., Pfeffer, M. A., and Braunwald, E. Influence of chronic captopril therapy on the infarcted left ventricle of the rat. *Circ. Res.* 57:84–95, 1985.
25. Pfeffer, M. A., Lamas, G. A., Vaughan, D. E., et al. Effect of captopril on progressive ventricular dilatation after anterior myocardial infarction. *N. Engl. J. Med* 319:80–86, 1988.
26. Tymchak, W. J., Michorowski, B. L., Burton, J. R., et al. Preservation of left ventricular and topography with combined reperfusion and intravenous nitroglycerin in acute myocardial infarction (Abstract). *J.A.C.C.* 11:90A, 1988.
27. Yusuf, S., and Collins, R. IV nitroglycerin and nitroprusside therapy in acute myocardial infarction reduces mortality: Evidence from randomized controlled trials (Abstract). *Circulation* 72:III-224, 1985.

CHAPTER 13

THE ROLE OF BETA BLOCKERS IN ACUTE MYOCARDIAL INFARCTION AND POST-INFARCTION

VASU D. GOLI
EDWIN G. OLSON
STEPHEN F. HAMILTON
UDHO THADANI

Coronary artery disease is still the major cause of death in the Western world and most patients succumb to myocardial infarction. Efforts to prevent the occurrence of myocardial infarction (primary prevention) have centered around alterations in life-style, but the difficulties in conducting such trials have been enormous and to date the success of such an approach has not been effectively documented. In patients with increased cholesterol LDL levels, lipid-lowering agents have reduced cardiovascular mortality in two large studies. The problem of preventing death following a recent myocardial infarction (secondary prevention) is more amenable to study. Over the past 25 years several studies have been undertaken to evaluate drug efficacy in secondary intervention of myocardial infarction. The medications tested include lipid-lowering agents, traditional antiarrhythmic agents, anticoagulants, antiplatelet drugs, nitrates, beta blockers, calcium channel antagonists, and thrombolytic agents. In this chapter we will discuss the rationale of beta blocker therapy in primary and secondary interventions of myocardial infarction, review the published trials, and suggest guidelines for beta blocker therapy in post-myocardial infarction patients.

ADRENERGIC ACTIVITY AND ACUTE MYOCARDIAL INFARCTION

In patients with an acute myocardial infarction, the presence of severe pain, tissue injury, and circulatory disturbances provides an important physiologic stimulus for endogenous catecholamine release. Further, physiologic stresses and reflexes originating in the border zone of infarcting tissue may also trigger an increase in plasma and local catecholamine concentration [54]. This increase in sympathetic tone may play an important supportive role in maintaining contractile function in ischemic areas of the myocardium, as well as enhancing the function of residual nonischemic areas. However, the positive inotropic and chronotropic effects of catecholamines may lead to increased myocardial oxygen consumption [64]. Further detrimental effects of increasing necrosis in ischemic areas may provoke further catecholamine release [31], leading to a vicious cycle that could include extension of infarction and serious arrhythmias.

RATIONALE FOR BETA BLOCKER THERAPY IN MYOCARDIAL INFARCTION

Beta blockers have been considered useful in patients with an acute myocardial infarction, and these agents prevent the undesirable consequences of increased sympathoadrenal discharge and, hence, arrhythmogenesis and infarct extension [51]. Beta blockers do not directly affect the progression of coronary atheroma, but by reducing myocardial oxygen requirement [19] these agents may enable the cardiac muscle to tolerate, for a while, what could otherwise be an inadequate supply of oxygen. Beta-adrenergic blockade may also increase coronary perfusion by slowing the heart rate and lengthening cardiac diastole. In experimental studies, beta blockade improves distribution of blood flow in the ischemic myocardium, as well as utilization of myocardial substrates [41]. Beta blockers are also effective antiarrhythmic agents [18, 28], and some are known to inhibit platelet aggregation and improve oxygen hemoglobin dissociation curve [20, 50]. By blocking the effects of catecholamines, beta blockade reduces free fatty acid levels and shifts the myocardial metabolism from fatty acids to glucose and decreases oxygen demand by this mechanism as well. In isolated perfused hearts this results in decreased lactate production, enzyme leakage, and preservation of mitochondria [38, 42]. In the ischemic heart, beta blockade can also reduce local catecholamine levels [37] and produce a favorable redistribution of blood flow with greater diversion to the subendocardial regions where ischemia is particularly severe [43, 63].

INFARCT PREVENTION

Acute Intervention Studies with Beta Blockers in Patients with Threatened Myocardial Infarction

When severe myocardial ischemia, rather than necrosis, is the cause of prolonged chest pain, beta blockers are recommended along with nitrates and calcium channel antagonists. Yusuf and colleagues [68] reported that fewer patients with preinfarction angina went on to develop frank infarctions when intravenous and oral atenolol, rather than placebo, was administered. The potentially protective properties of propranolol [13, 16], metoprolol [49], and atenolol [15, 68] for prolonged myocardial ischemia in the absence of infarction have also been reported by several groups. In a randomized, double-blind study of 68 patients with unstable angina, the propranolol-treated patients experienced fewer coronary events than placebo-treated patients [13]. In patients admitted to coronary care units because of prolonged chest pain, mitral regurgitation developed less frequently in patients treated with propranolol [13]. Thus, from these limited studies, it appears that early beta blocker administration in patients with unstable angina may offer some protective effect.

BETA BLOCKERS IN POST-INFARCTION PERIOD

Acute Intervention (Short-Term) Beta Blocker Trials in Survivors of Myocardial Infarction

Snow's initial uncontrolled study [53], involving less than 100 patients and showing a substantial reduction in mortality after oral beta blockade in the early phases of a myocardial infarction, was not confirmed by several subsequent randomized studies of oral and intravenous short-term beta blockade [2, 5, 6, 9, 10, 32, 44, 55, 62]. However, other end points in these studies (infarction size reduction, occurrence of arrhythmias, and effect on chest pain and serum enzymes) were utilized and are suggestive of beneficial effects. The effects of beta blocker therapy on these end points are discussed below.

Effects on Infarct Size

Readily available measurements most directly related to infarct size are electrocardiographic quantification of Q wave development, loss of R wave, and serologic estimation of the quantity of creatine kinase released from necrotic myocardium [25, 26]. Indirect techniques such as enzyme release or electrocardiographic changes, however, have their limitations [47]. Evidence from more than one such technique may be necessary before it can be concluded that infarct size is truly reduced.

Early intravenous therapy with beta blockers has a moderate influence on enzyme release, but no such effects occur when treatment is delayed until 12 hours after the onset of pain [52]. Typical reduction in cumulative enzyme release appears to be around 20 percent for patients who are entered within the first 2 hours of onset of chest pain (Fig. 13-1). Such benefit has been shown with a variety of beta blockers with different ancillary properties, for example, atenolol [68], propranolol [40], metoprolol [56], sotalol [33], timolol [61], and perhaps alprenolol [30].

There is also evidence that beta blockade lessens the size of infarct by electrocardiographic criteria. Electrocardiographic evidence that is more directly suggestive of limitation of infarct size is provided by the highly significant ($p < 0.001$) preservation of R waves with atenolol [68] and significant reduction of Q waves with propranolol [40] and timolol [61]. These findings show that beta-1 blockade is responsible for reducing the infarct size; ancillary properties (e.g., cardioselectivity, membrane stabilizing action) are irrelevant in this regard.

The beneficial effects of beta blockers on the electrocardiogram, together with reduction in enzyme levels, suggest that a true reduction in infarct size can be produced by early use of intravenous beta blockers following an acute myocardial infarction.

Effects on Chest Pain

Three separate studies have reported relief or lessening of chest pain in patients with acute myocardial infarction following treatment with propranolol [21], metoprolol [16], and atenolol [45]. The results of the MIAMI Trial [56] and those studies that preceded it (Goteberg trial [27]) indicate that the early use of metoprolol in acute myocardial infarction prevents chest pain in many patients and significantly reduces the intensity in those patients who experience chest pain. Narcotic anal-

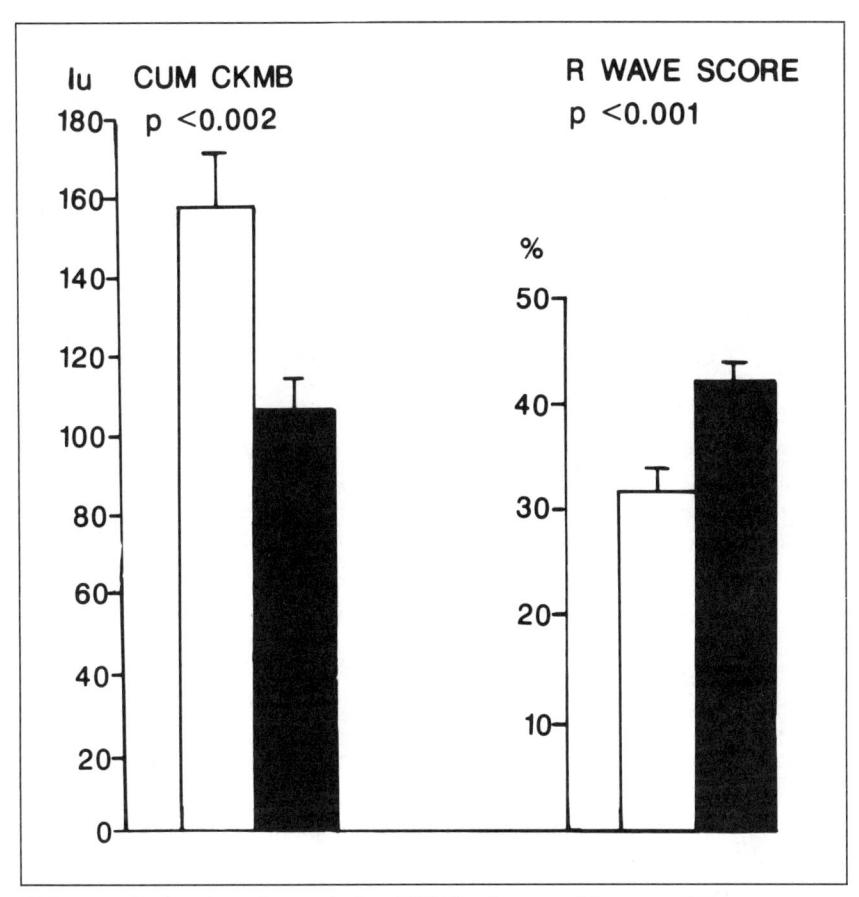

FIG. 13-1. Reduction of cumulative CKMB release and improved R wave scores after intravenous atenolol (solid bars) compared to placebo (open bars) in acute myocardial infarction. (From Ref. 68, with permission.)

gesics were used in 49 percent of the placebo-treated patients versus 44 percent of metoprolol-treated patients ($p < 0.001$); similarly, there was a slight trend toward lower usage of nitrates and calcium channel antagonists in the metoprolol group. The chest pain reduction by beta blockers was most pronounced in those patients with increased heart rate and systolic blood pressure, reflecting beneficial effects of beta blockade in the presence of increased sympathetic activity.

Effects on Arrhythmias

Two randomized studies have been reported that involved analysis of continuous Holter monitoring to assess the effect of intravenous beta blockers on arrhythmias during the early phase of myocardial infarction [48, 49]. In the study by Rossi and colleagues [48], 182 patients were studied for a period of about 24 hours early in their clinical course. Intravenous atenolol was given at a mean of 5 hours after the onset of chest pain [48]. There was a threefold ($p < 0.001$) reduction both in the frequency of isolated premature ventricular contractions and the percentage of "R on T" premature beats. The atenolol study [68] also revealed a promising reduction in nonfatal cardiac arrest, from 4 percent in control patients (9/233) to 1 percent in atenolol-treated patients (4/244). Ryden and colleagues [49] reported significant reduction in ventricular fibrillation and lidocaine use during the hospital phase of myocardial infarction in patients treated with intravenous metoprolol followed by oral therapy (6/697 patients) compared to the control group (17/698) (Fig. 13-2). Similar findings were reported after propranolol by Norris and colleagues [39]. A study of atenolol with other principal end points mentioned, incidentally, a reduction in atrial fibrillation [68].

Thus, the antiarrhythmic effects of beta blockers with different ancillary properties are similar and appear to be related to their common beta-adrenergic blocking properties [20].

EFFECTS ON SHORT-TERM MORTALITY

Intravenous Beta Blockers

The TIMI II Trial was designed to study invasive and conservative strategies of catheterization and angioplasty in 3262 patients with evolving myocardial infarction [60]. All patients received tissue plasminogen activator heparin and aspirin within 4 hours of symptom onset. A subgroup of 1390 patients were considered eligible for treatment with beta blockers and received either intravenous metoprolol followed by oral metoprolol or only oral metoprolol, which was deferred until day 6 of hospitalization. There was similar total mortality for the two beta blocker groups for the first 6 and 42 days of therapy. However, further subgroup analysis did expose some benefit of early beta blocker therapy. There was a significant reduction in death and reinfarction (5 percent versus 12.1 percent) within the first 42 days in the 181 patients receiving IV metoprolol within 2 hours of symptom onset as compared to 190 similar patients in whom metoprolol was deferred during the first 6 days of treatment. This difference was not apparent in a similar cohort of patients who received IV metoprolol between 2 and 4 hours of symptoms. In patients considered to be at "low risk" there were no deaths in those receiving IV metoprolol compared to 7 deaths in 246 (2.8 percent) similar patients who deferred beta blocker therapy. No similar benefit could be demonstrated in patients considered "now low risk." While these results are encouraging, the discovery of beneficial effects upon subgroup analysis when overall analysis did not identify a difference inspires some skepticism.

In the Goteborg Intravenous Metoprolol Trial [27], 3-month mortality

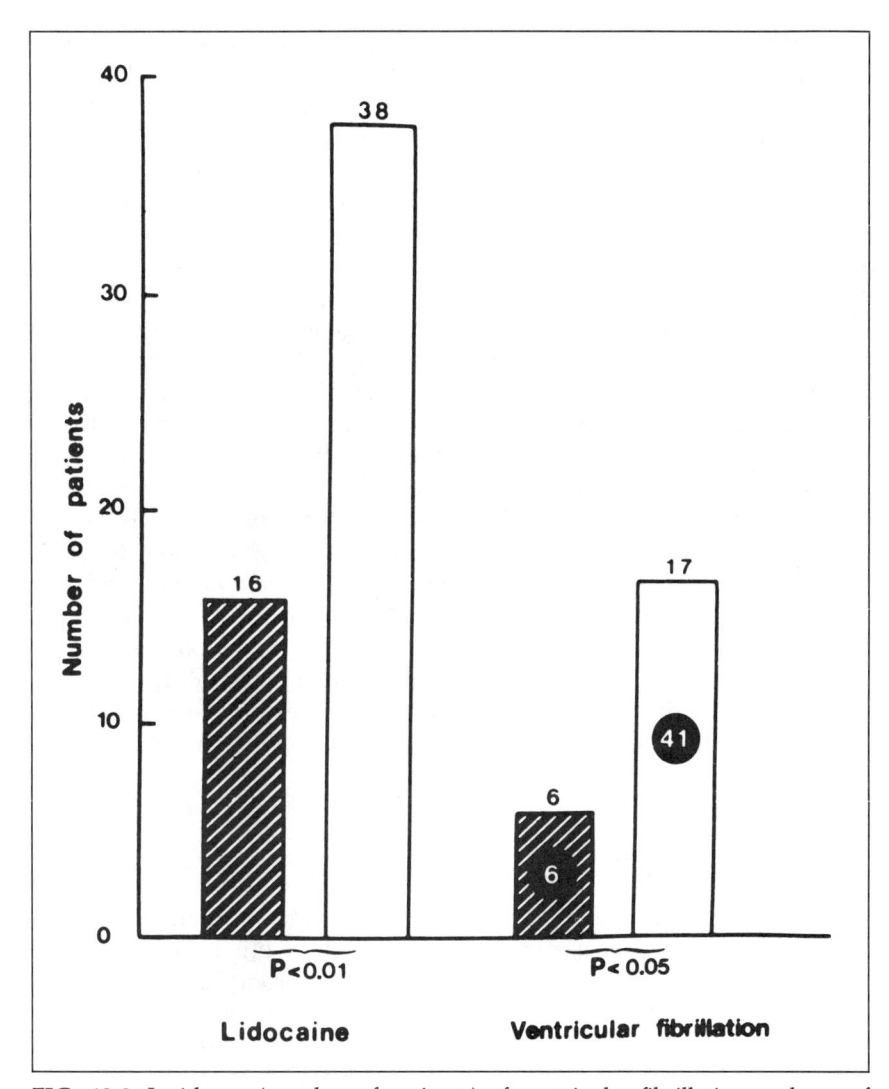

FIG. 13-2. Incidence (number of patients) of ventricular fibrillation and use of lidocaine during metoprolol (hatched bars) or placebo (open bars) therapy. The number of separate attacks of ventricular fibrillations is given in the circles within the bars. (From Ref. 49, with permission.)

was reduced in the metoprolol-treated group. There were 62 deaths (8.90 percent) in the placebo group of 697 patients and 40 deaths (5.73 percent) in the metoprolol group of 698 patients ($p < 0.05$). In the MIAMI Trial [56], the cumulative mortality for the total period of 15 days was 4.9 percent in the placebo group and 4.3 percent in the metoprolol-treated group, a difference that was not statistically significant. When a retrospective subgroup analysis was performed by risk stratification, a reduction in mortality was reported in high-risk groups treated with metoprolol (6.0 percent) compared to placebo (8.5 percent). The high-risk group was characterized by age above 60 years, presence of diabetes, sinus tachycardia at entry, signs of mild congestive heart failure, and usage of diuretics and digitalis glycosides. Yusuf's group [67], in their recent review on this subject, analyzed the pooled data from 28 studies. Overall results were not at all impressive: mortality of 3.6 percent for the control group versus 3.4 percent for the active treatment group. However, calculating the confidence interval, the differences in the two groups from pooled data suggested that the data were compatible with a 20 percent reduction in the odds of death being produced by beta blocker treatment [67]. However, in reality, one has to treat 500 myocardial infarction patients with intravenous beta blockade to save one life, which is not a cost-effective proposal. Estimates of mortality reduction with active beta blocker treatment for individual long-term studies and calculated 95 percent confidence intervals are given in Figure 13-3.

Oral Beta Blockade

Snow's initial report [53] of a substantial reduction in mortality using oral beta blockade in a small series of patients in comparison to nonrandomized controls has not been confirmed by other studies. Yusuf and colleagues [67] analyzed the pooled data from 22 such studies; again, overall results were not impressive. The mortality was 8.7 percent (165/1900 patients) in the treated group versus 9.6 percent (165/1711 patients) in the control group. This difference in mortality was not statistically significant.

One can conclude that during the acute phase of a myocardial infarction, intravenous and oral beta blocker therapy does reduce infarct size and arrhythmias, but there is no demonstrable reduction in early mortality.

Late Intervention Beta Blocker Trials in Survivors of Myocardial Infarction

Following discharge from the hospital, survivors of an acute myocardial infarction remain in an unstable state [11]. For patients under the age of 70 years, there is a 10 percent mortality during the first posthospital year and a 4 percent annual mortality rate subsequently. The mortality

13. THE ROLE OF BETA BLOCKERS IN ACUTE MYOCARDIAL INFARCTION

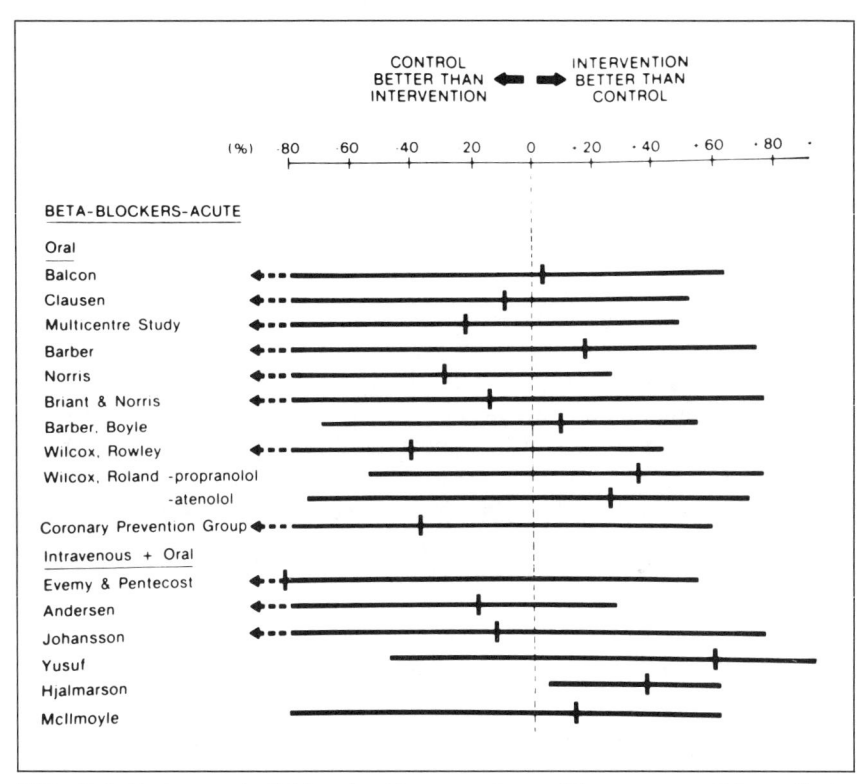

FIG. 13-3. Estimates (solid bars) with approximate 95 percent confidence limits of the relative differences in total mortality between control and intervention groups in 11 beta blocker trials in the acute phase of myocardial infarction. (From Ref. 35, with permission.)

rate is highest in the first 3 months after hospital discharge, with a progressive decline thereafter [34]. Many of these deaths are sudden, the primary mechanism being ventricular fibrillation. Arrhythmic deaths are about one half of total deaths throughout the postinfarction period.

The risk factors that are operative during the postinfarction period include residual myocardial ischemia, cardiac arrhythmias, and mechanical left ventricular dysfunction [57]. The degree of sympathetic drive influences the incidence of arrhythmias [23] and the work done by the ventricles. Denervation of the heart by stellate ganglionectomy has been shown to reduce arrhythmias and improve survival after coronary ligation in animals. Thus, beta blockers appear attractive and logical to modify the natural history of the postmyocardial infarction period by preventing the undesirable consequences of reinfarction and sudden cardiac death.

Limitations of Long-Term Trials

Before reviewing the results of long-term trials, it is worthwhile to note some of the inherent limitations of these studies. The published results of long-term postinfarction beta blocker trials are difficult to compare because they were derived from studies using different protocol designs, different study patient populations, different types and dosages of several beta blockers, different times when beta blockers were started after the documentation of the infarct (times ranging from a few hours to a few weeks), and variable clinical follow-up ranging from 3 weeks to 7 years. In analyzing and comparing the findings of beta blocker secondary prevention trials, there are certain prerequisites that should be met. First, the trial must be placebo-controlled and double-blind. It has been estimated that for a properly designed, placebo-controlled, double-blind, randomized trial, one needs to follow 2000 patients to demonstrate conclusively that an intervention caused a 30 percent reduction in death over a 2-year period [22]. Second, the study end points should be properly defined at the onset of the trial and findings should be analyzed on an intention to treat basis.

EFFECTS ON MORTALITY

Inconclusive Studies

Keeping in mind all the above limitations, it is not surprising that some studies have been inconclusive while others have shown a substantial decrease in mortality with beta blockers in postmyocardial infarction patients.

Several studies with inconclusive results include: The Coronary Prevention Research Study of oxprenolol (1981) [12], the Australian-Swedish Pindolol Study (1983) [4], the European Infarction Study with oxprenolol (1984) [14], Reynolds and Whitlock with alprenolol (1972) [46], Barber et al. with practolol (1975) [6], Wilcox et al. with propranolol and atenolol (1980) [65], and a multicenter trial of propranolol [7].

Conclusive Studies

The first of the conclusive studies on the beneficial effect of beta blockers on postmyocardial infarction was reported by Wilhelmsson and colleagues in 1974 [66]. In this study, 230 postinfarct patients with ages ranging from 57 to 67 years were stratified to four risk groups and were treated with either 400 mg of alprenolol daily or placebo. Treatment was started 2 to 4 weeks postinfarct and patients were followed for 2 years. Overall, there were 11 deaths in the placebo group and three in the treated group, a difference not statistically significant. However, there was a reduction in the mortality in the highest risk group.

The multicenter international trial [1] utilized practolol at a fixed dose of 200 mg twice a day; 3038 patients were given either practolol or placebo 4 weeks postmyocardial infarction and followed for 1 year. There was a reduction in mortality of 38 percent ($p = 0.05$). A trend toward reduction in nonfatal reinfarction was also observed but was not statistically significant. Subgroup analysis showed a mortality reduction only in patients with an anterior myocardial infarction. This is the only trial of a beta blocker with intrinsic sympathomimetic activity to show conclusive beneficial effects.

Anderson and colleagues in 1979 [3] treated patients with definite or suspected myocardial infarction following admission to the coronary care unit with either 5 or 10 mg intravenous alprenolol or placebo. Those treated with intravenous alprenolol were continued on oral alprenolol 200 mg twice daily. During the year of follow-up, mortality was significantly reduced only in patients 65 years of age or younger.

Another trial that addressed the question of whether early initiation of treatment with an intravenous beta blocker had any advantage over delayed treatment was reported by Hjalmarson [27]. A total of 1395 patients with definitive or suspected myocardial infarction were randomized to receive either intravenous metoprolol 15 mg followed by 100 mg orally twice daily for 90 days or placebo. Mortality was 8.9 percent in placebo versus 5.7 percent in the metoprolol group at 3 months, a reduction of 36 percent, which was highly significant.

The first large-scale postmyocardial infarction trial of the use of beta blockers was the Norwegian Multicenter Timolol Study in 1981 [24]. More than 3600 patients were stratified into three risk groups: those with reinfarction at entry, high risk, and low risk. Treatment was started 7 to 28 days postinfarct in 1884 patients, with 945 taking 10 mg timolol twice daily and 939 patients taking placebo. Patients were followed for 12 to 33 months. The cumulative reinfarction rate was 20.1 percent in the placebo group and 14.4 percent in the timolol group. The cumulative sudden death rate was 13.9 percent in the placebo group and 7.7 percent in the timolol group, a reduction of 44.6 percent. Recently, the same group reported their extended follow-up of participating patients for up to 72 months. The mortality curves of the two groups continued to rise in parallel with cumulative mortality rates of 32.3 percent in placebo group versus 26.4 percent in the timolol group ($p = 0.0028$) (Fig. 13-4). The authors concluded that the previously observed beneficial effect of beta blocker therapy was maintained for at least 6 years after infarction [58].

Another large multicenter study was the Beta Blocker Heart Attack Trial [8] where 3837 patients who had experienced at least one myocardial infarction were treated either with propranolol (180 to 240 mg daily) or placebo. Treatment was started 5 to 21 days after an acute myocardial infarction. During the average of 25 months follow-up period, there was 7.2 percent mortality in the propranolol group versus 9.8 percent

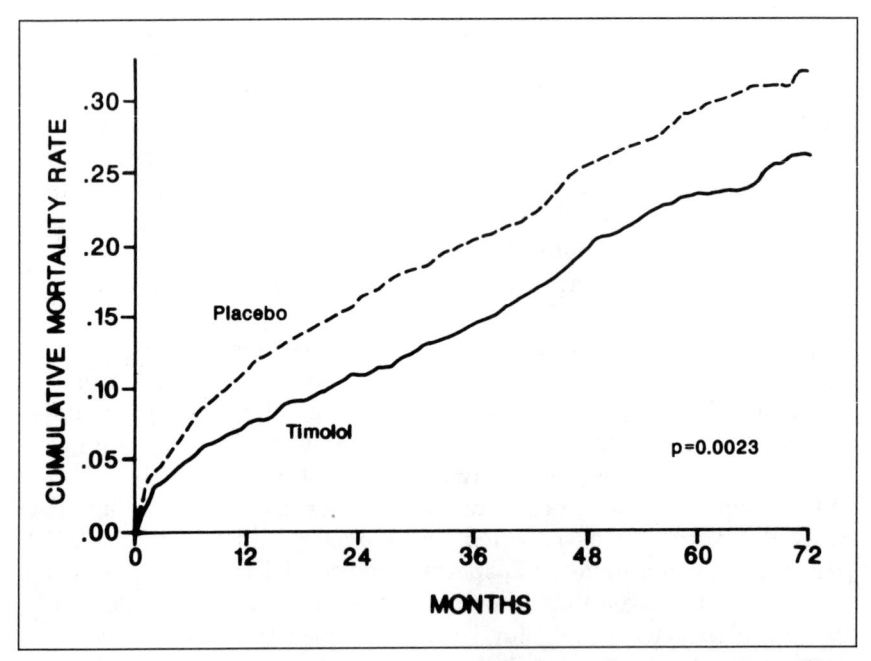

FIG. 13-4. Life-table cumulated mortality rates from all causes among all patients randomly assigned to treatment with either placebo or timolol. (From Ref. 58, with permission.)

in the placebo group, a mortality reduction of 28 percent (Fig. 13-5). There was a greater reduction in mortality in patients above 65 years compared to those under 65 years of age.

In a preliminary report of a Norwegian Multicenter Trial in 1981 [18] involving 560 patients treated 4 to 5 days postmyocardial infarction with either propranolol 40 mg 4 times a day or placebo, there was a significant (32 percent) reduction in 1 year total mortality in the propranolol-treated group.

Julian and colleagues in 1982 [29], in a large multicenter study, reported a reduction in total mortality of only 18 percent in patients treated with 320 mg sotalol a day and followed for 1 year. However, the reinfarction rate was 41 percent lower in the sotalol than in the placebo-treated group.

Yusuf and colleagues [67], in a recent review on the topic, analyzed the pooled data from the 16 randomized trials involving 18,000 patients. In the beta blocker treated group, the risk of death was reduced to 8 percent from 10 percent in the placebo-treated group, a reduction of 20 percent (Fig. 13-6). The individual data from different trials are shown in Figure 13-7 [36].

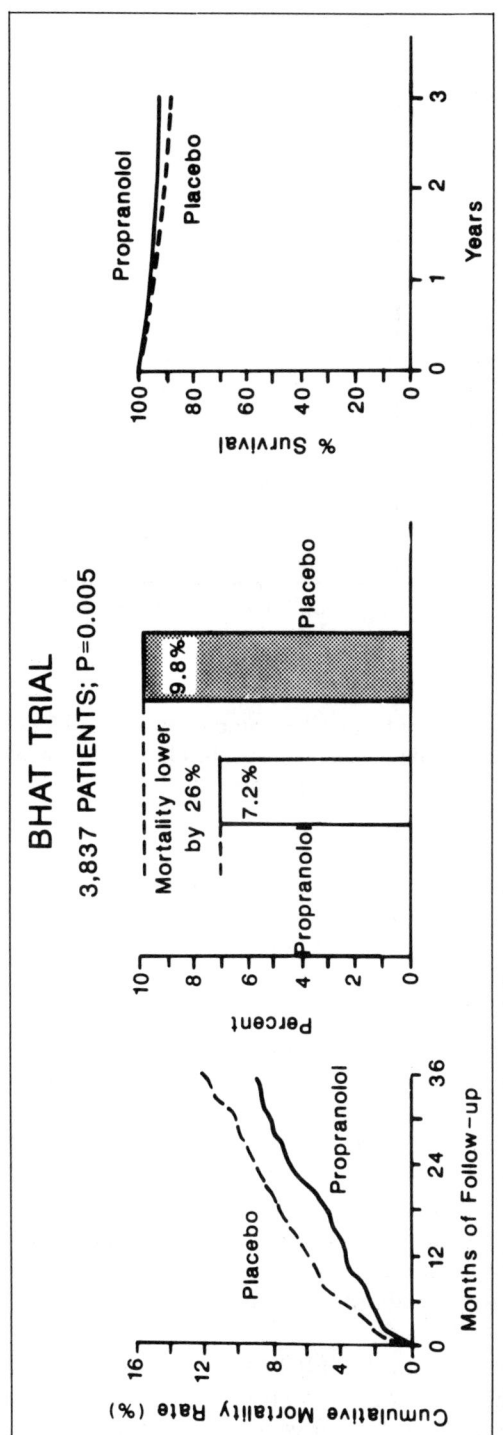

FIG. 13-5. Mortality and survival rates following therapy with propranolol or placebo following acute myocardial infarction. (From Ref. 8, with permission.)

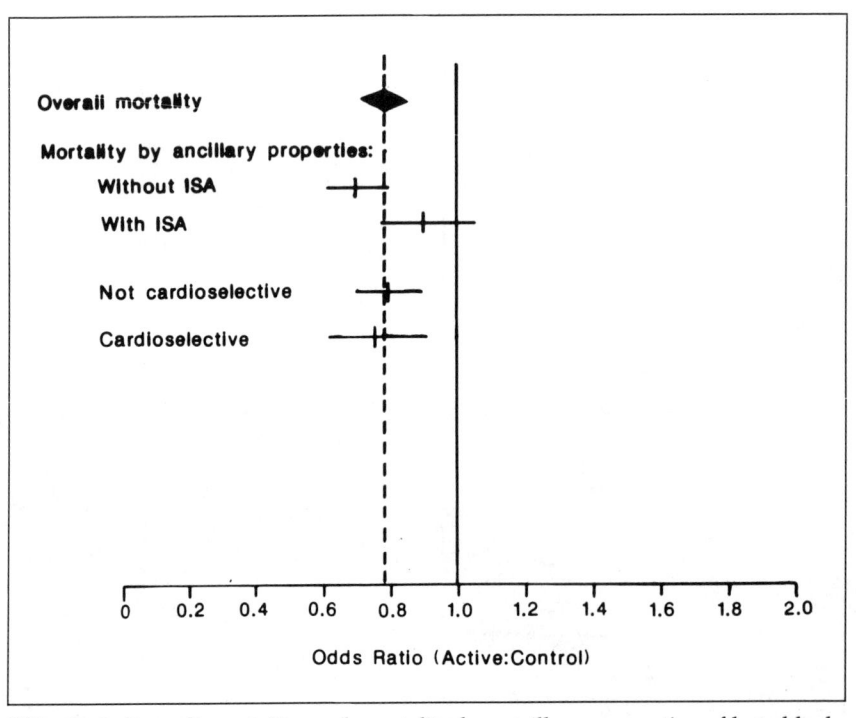

FIG. 13-6. Overall mortality and mortality by ancillary properties of beta blockers in long-term beta-blocker trials. Odds ratios (active: control) together with 95 percent confidence ranges. (From Ref. 67, with permission.)

Effects of Reinfarction

The frequency of nonfatal reinfarction was not well documented in many of the reported trials. In the Goteborg Metoprolol Trial [27], there was a 35 percent reduction in the incidence of fatal and nonfatal reinfarction during a 4 to 90 day period. In the Norwegian Multicenter Study Group Trial [59] using timolol, there was reduction of 28 percent in the incidence of nonfatal reinfarction ($p < 0.0006$). In the study reported by Julian et al. [29] using sotalol, there was a 41 percent reduction in reinfarction rate in the treated group. However, in the Beta Blocker Heart Attack Trial [8], which consisted of 3837 participants, there was only a 16 percent reduction in reinfarction rate, a difference that did not reach statistical significance. Combining the information from various trials suggests that treatment with long-term beta blockade reduces the odds of reinfarction by about one-fourth ($p < 0.001$) [67] (Fig. 13-8).

The most recent data comes from the TIMI II Trial, which has shown, during the first 6 days of hospitalization, a significant reduction in nonfatal reinfarction (16 versus 31) and other ischemic events (107 ver-

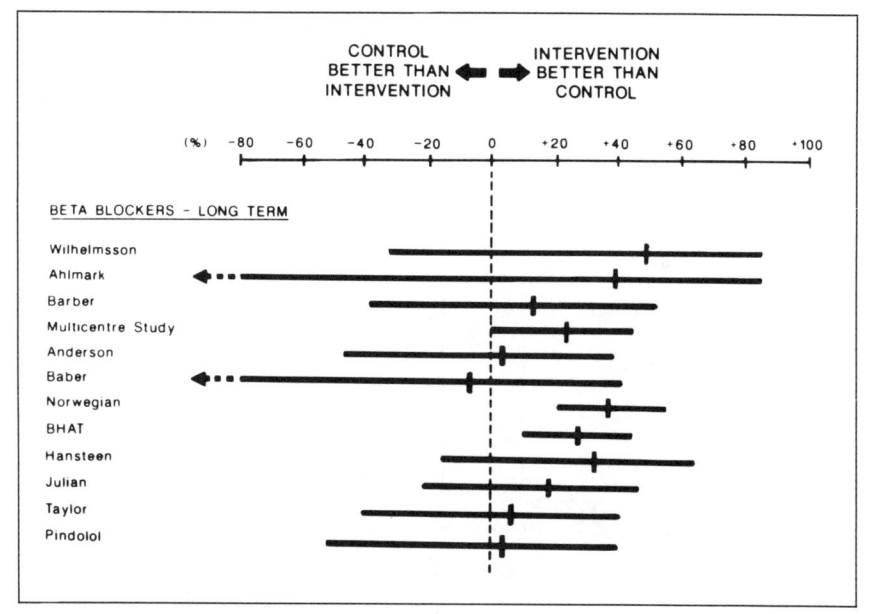

FIG. 13-7. Estimates (solid bars) with approximate 95 percent confidence limits of the relative differences in total mortality between control and intervention groups in 13 long-term trials of beta blockers after myocardial infarction. (From Refs. 36 and 67, with permission.)

sus 147) in patients treated with IV metoprolol within 4 hours of symptom onset compared to those patients who deferred beta blocker therapy [60].

Effects on Sudden Death

In an attempt to elucidate the mechanisms by which beta blockers may prevent death, most of the long-term trials have classified death into sudden (presumably arrhythmic or cardiac rupture) and nonsudden (presumably nonarrhythmic and including a few noncardiovascular deaths), based on the time of death from the onset of chest pain. The definition of precisely what counted as sudden varied from instantaneous in one study to within 24 hours of symptoms in another. In the Norwegian Timolol Study [59], sudden cardiac death accounted for approximately two-thirds of the total deaths. The sudden death rate at 33 months of follow-up was 13.9 percent in placebo versus 7.7 percent in the timolol group, an impressive reduction of 44.6 percent ($p = 0.0001$).

In the Beta Blocker Heart Attack Trial Study [8], sudden cardiac death among the propranolol-treated group was 3.3 percent versus 4.6 percent in the placebo group, a 28 percent reduction ($p < 0.05$). In a Multicenter

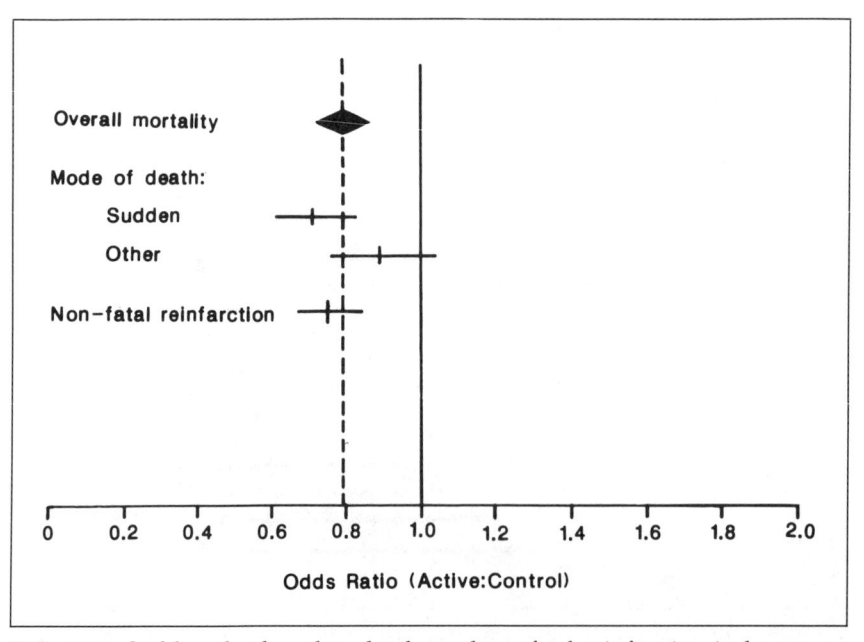

FIG. 13-8. Sudden death, other death, and nonfatal reinfarction in long-term beta blocker trials that reported these end points separately: Odds ratios (active:control), together with approximate 95 percent confidence ranges. (Reproduced from Ref. 67, with permission.)

International Study using propranolol [1], there were 73 sudden cardiac deaths in the placebo group versus 47 in the treated group (significant at $p < 0.01$), a net reduction of 30.9 percent.

Overall, the pooled data show a highly significant reduction ($p < 0.00001$) of about 30 percent in the odds of sudden death, with 95 percent confidence and limits of about 20 percent to 40 percent in those treated with beta blockers [67].

INDIVIDUAL STUDIES WITH DIFFERENT BETA BLOCKERS

Propranolol

Propranolol is a nonselective beta blocking agent with membrane stabilizing properties and no intrinsic sympathomimetic action. In the European Multicenter Trial, Barber and colleagues [7] compared placebo to oral propranolol in 720 patients who were enrolled 2 to 14 days postmyocardial infarction. At 3 months, there was no difference in mortality between the placebo and propranolol (120 mg daily) group, nor was there any difference in nonfatal reinfarction. In the Beta Blocker Heart Attack Trial [8], 3837 patients were randomized to either propranolol (180 to 240 mg daily) or placebo 5 to 21 days following myocardial infarction. At 25 months follow-up, there was a 26 percent reduction in total mortality, 28 percent reduction in sudden cardiac death, and 16 percent reduction in reinfarction in propranolol-treated patients. Incidence of ventricular arrhythmias at 6 weeks postinfarct was reduced in the propranolol group compared to placebo.

In the Norwegian Multicenter Trial [24], Hansteen and colleagues randomized 3795 patients 4 to 6 days following myocardial infarction to either propranolol (40 mg 4 times a day) or placebo. In a preliminary report, there was a 32 percent reduction in mortality at 1 year follow-up. Currently, propranolol (180 to 240 mg/day) is approved for postmyocardial infarction secondary prevention.

Metoprolol
Metoprolol is a cardioselective beta-1 selective agent with no membrane stabilizing or partial agonist activity. In the placebo-controlled Goteborg study, Hjalmarson [27] treated 1395 patients with either 15 mg intravenous metoprolol followed by 100 mg oral metoprolol twice daily or placebo for 3 months. Overall, mortality was reduced by 36 percent at 3 months. Further, there was a reduction in frequency of ventricular fibrillation and lactic dehydrogenase (LDH) isoenzymes in patients treated within 12 hours of infarction. About 19 percent of patients in both treatment and placebo groups were withdrawn because of side effects. Hypotension (less than 90 mmHg) and bradycardia (less than 40 bpm) were the most common causes of withdrawal in the metoprolol-treated groups. In the MIAMI Trial [56], a reduction in infarct size was reported but the reduction in mortality of 13 percent at 15 days was not statistically significant. Metoprolol is not currently approved for postmyocardial infarction secondary prevention in the United States.

Timolol
Timolol is a nonselective beta blocker with no membrane stabilizing or partial agonist activity and was the first beta blocker approved by the United States Food and Drug Administration for postmyocardial infarction secondary prophylaxis. In the Norwegian Multicenter Timolol Study [61], 1884 patients were randomized to either timolol at a fixed dose (10 mg twice daily) or placebo at 7 to 28 days postinfarct. At a 3-year follow-up [61], mortality decreased by 36 percent, sudden death incidence decreased by 44.6 percent, and nonfatal reinfarction was reduced by 20.1 percent in the timolol-treated group. At long-term follow-up at 6 years [58], the cumulative mortality was 32.3 percent in the placebo and 26.4 percent in the timolol-treated group.

Atenolol
Atenolol is a cardioselective agent with no membrane stabilizing or partial agonist action. Wilcox and colleagues [65] randomized 388 pa-

tients to oral atenolol (50 mg twice daily), propranolol (40 mg 3 times daily), or placebo. There was no difference in mortality between placebo and active treatment groups at 1 year.

In an acute intervention trial with intravenous and oral atenolol, there was a favorable trend in the atenolol-treated group on in-hospital mortality, a reduction in ventricular arrhythmias, and a reduction in creatine kinase myocardial (CK-MB) isoenzyme levels compared to placebo treatment [68].

Alprenolol

Alprenolol is a nonselective beta blocker with membrane stabilizing and a partial agonist activity. In a small study on 87 patients by Reynolds and Whitlock [46], there was no difference in mortality at the 1-year follow-up between alprenolol (450 mg/day) and placebo-treated groups. Wilhelmsson [66] treated 230 patients with either alprenolol (400 mg a day) or placebo at 5 to 8 weeks postmyocardial infarction and reported a 50 percent reduction in mortality at 2 years.

In an early intervention study, Anderson and colleagues [3] randomly treated elderly myocardial infarction patients with either intravenous alprenolol (5 to 10 mg) or placebo, followed by corresponding oral treatment. At 1-year follow-up, mortality was reduced significantly only in patients less than 65 years of age.

Sotalol

Sotalol is a nonselective beta blocker without membrane stabilizing or partial agonist action but unlike other beta blocking agents, sotalol prolongs the action potential duration. Julian and colleagues [29] treated patients with either sotalol (320 mg/day) or placebo and reported a nonsignificant reduction in mortality of 18 percent, and a significant reduction of 41 percent reinfarction rate at 1-year follow-up in the sotalol group.

Pindolol

Pindolol is a nonselective beta blocker with partial agonist activity and no membrane stabilizing action. In a study conducted by a Swedish-Australian group [4], pindolol (10 mg daily) was compared to placebo in high-risk patients with electrical mechanical complication postmyocardial infarction. Patients were entered 1 to 21 days postinfarct and followed for 2 years. There were no significant differences in mortality, sudden death, or reinfarction rates between pindolol and the placebo group.

Oxprenolol

Oxprenolol is a nonselective agent with partial agonist action and without membrane stabilizing activity. In the European Infarction Study [14] and the Coronary Prevention Research Study using oxprenolol [12], there was no significant difference in mortality and reinfarction rates between the oxprenolol- and placebo-treated group.

Issues Regarding the Use of Beta Blockers in Postinfarct Patients

There are considerable data indicating that long-term treatment of postmyocardial infarction patients with beta blockers significantly reduces subsequent mortality and reinfarction, yet the postmyocardial infarction usage of beta blockers remains erratic both in the United States and abroad. There is no consensus on numbers of relevant issues and the clinician is faced with practical decisions regarding each individual patient. Since the subsequent outcome of patients following myocardial infarction varies widely, one has to consider several issues before prescribing long-term beta blocker therapy to every patient. Factors influencing these decisions are discussed below.

SITE AND NATURE OF INFARCTION

In the Multicenter International Practolol Trial [1], beneficial effects were seen primarily in those with an anterior wall myocardial infarction. In the Beta Blocker Heart Attack Propranolol Trial [8] and the Norwegian Timolol Study [61], a reduction in mortality was reported regardless of the site of infarct only in patients who had transmural myocardial infarctions. The timolol trial also showed a substantial reduction in mortality in the subgroups of patients with nontransmural myocardial infarction. A similar reduction was not seen in the Beta Blocker Heart Attack Trial Study. While there is less than complete evidence to support a definitive statement, it would be reasonable to recommend beta blocker therapy to otherwise appropriate patients regardless of the site and type of infarction.

TIME OF INITIATION OF THERAPY

One can divide myocardial infarction into three separate periods: (1) initial few hours while the infarct is still evolving, the aim of treatment being to limit infarct size and reduce morbidity and mortality, (2) subsequent few days when the process of infarction is complete but the patient is still not yet considered to be in a stable condition; and (3) the subsequent weeks, months, or years.

In some of the early intervention trials using intravenous and oral beta blockers, reduction in mortality was not the primary aim and the trials were often of inadequate size to evaluate mortality as an end point. Further, even in the Goteborg Trial [27] where treatment was initiated early by intravenous route, the mean entry time was 11.3 hours, too late to influence the evolution of infarction in many patients.

Although there are some data to support limitation of infarct size by very early beta blockade, none of the trials has demonstrated a significant reduction in mortality conclusively.

The large clinical trials documenting a reduction in mortality have used protocol designs, starting beta blockade as early as 4 days [24] to as late as 28 days [41]. In the Practolol Multicenter Trial [1], patients who were entered earlier had the highest mortality, which was reduced by practolol. A similar finding was reported in the Propranolol Multicenter Study [8]. In the latter study, patients started on beta blocker therapy 5 to 9 days or 10 to 21 days after myocardial infarction had a mortality reduction of 36 percent and 18 percent, respectively. The mortality in the placebo-treated group was similar whether the placebo was started on days 5 to 9 (9.9 percent) or 10 to 21 days (9.7 percent) postinfarct.

No conclusive data are available regarding the effect of beta blocker therapy on survival, initiated months to years after an acute myocardial infarction. Retrospective subgroup analysis from a placebo versus oxprenolol trial [57] suggested beneficial effects on survival if treatment was started within 4 months of the infarction. When beta blocker therapy was delayed for longer than 4 months no benefits were seen.

The available data suggest that one should initiate beta blockade therapy between 5 days after a myocardial infarction and prior to hospital discharge. Although the preliminary results of large studies with intravenous beta blockade at the onset of chest pain are encouraging, routine use cannot be recommended to reduce mortality at the present time [27]. The TIMI II Trial was encouraging in reducing mortality in a highly select group of patients who receive IV metoprolol within 2 hours of symptom onset [60].

DURATION OF THERAPY

At present, there is no consensus as to how long the treatment with beta blockers in a postmyocardial infarction patient should continue. Neither are there adequate data regarding the outcome when such therapy is discontinued. However, the accrued benefit at 1 year is well documented. In the Beta Blocker Heart Attack Trial [8], the timolol [41], practolol [1], sotalol [29], and the Norwegian Propranolol Trials [24], the follow-up of all patients was virtually complete to 1 year and the mortality reduction at 1 year ranged from 18 percent to 39 percent, with an average reduction of 25 percent [67].

In the Beta Blocker Heart Attack Trial [8], the timolol [41], and the practolol trials [1], a subgroup of patients was followed for 3 years. The survival curves for the drug and placebo were different at 3 years, suggesting a beneficial effect for up to 3 years of continued beta blocker therapy.

In the Norwegian Multicenter Study [58], the mortality curves of the timolol- and placebo-treated groups continued to rise in parallel for up to 6 years of follow-up. Cumulative mortality rates were 32.3 percent in placebo and 26.4 percent in the timolol group ($p = 0.0028$), suggesting that the early beneficial effect of therapy was maintained for up to 6 years (Fig. 13-4). Based on available data, beta blocker therapy, once begun, should be continued for at least 3 years or longer.

CHOICE OF BETA BLOCKER

Trials with seven different beta blockers reveal similar favorable mortality trends. One could conclude that the benefit is conferred by the drug class rather than by a specific beta blocker. In general, beta blockers without intrinsic sympathomimetic activity or partial agonist activity have shown a greater benefit than beta blockers with this ancillary property as reviewed by Yusuf and colleagues (Fig. 13-6). The only exception is the result of beneficial effects of practolol [1] in a large multicenter study. However, it should be noted that with the exception of the practolol trial, the sample size used for drugs with partial agonist activity using oxprenolol and pindolol has been relatively small [4, 14, 57]. In the United States, only timolol and propranolol are officially approved for use as secondary intervention in postmyocardial infarction, and it seems prudent to use agents with proven benefits.

OPTIMAL DOSAGE REGIMEN

In most of the long-term studies, with the exception of the Beta Blocker Heart Attack Trial [8], fixed empiric doses of beta blockers have been employed. None have reported whether an adequate beta blockade was achieved during the long-term therapy. In the Beta Blocker Heart Attack Study [8], attempts were made to adjust dosage on the basis of plasma propranolol concentrations, which is not practical in routine clinical practice.

The fixed dose regimen used in secondary prevention trials was 200 mg per day for metoprolol [27], 20 mg per day for timolol [61], and 160 to 240 mg per day for propranolol [8, 24]. It is not known whether the fixed empiric dose regimen is superior to a variable dose schedule defined on the basis of adequate beta blockade. Until further studies address this question, the fixed dosages outlined for different drugs used in the major studies should be utilized.

SAFETY PROFILE OF DIFFERENT BETA BLOCKERS

Severe side effects from beta blockers in postmyocardial infarction patients who were considered suitable for such therapy have been infrequent. Compared to placebo, there has been a higher incidence of heart failure, bradycardia, hypotension, bronchospasm, fatigue, and mental depression. In this regard, various beta blockers studied appear to have similar safety profiles [17]. Practolol was an exception and, due to oculocutaneous reactions, was withdrawn from clinical use [1]. Therefore, close monitoring of patients for adverse effects is required regardless of which drug is used.

CHOICE OF PATIENTS TO RECEIVE TREATMENT WITH BETA BLOCKERS

Recent studies show that patients with preserved left ventricular function following a myocardial infarction have very low mortality in subsequent years of follow-up compared to those showing an impairment of global left ventricular function. There is a serious question whether low-risk postinfarct patients (those with a recent myocardial infarction but normal left ventricular function, no PVC's, and normal submaximal exercise tolerance test who have a 1-year postmyocardial infarction mortality of 2 percent) should be treated with beta blockers; this is a hotly debated issue. The patients who benefit most are those who are also at a greater risk of experiencing adverse effects from beta blocker therapy. In patients with very low ejection fraction, signs of heart failure, or chronic obstructive lung disease, beta blocker therapy should be used with caution. In the other 30 percent to 40 percent of postinfarct patients in whom beta blocker therapy is not contraindicated and who are considered to be a higher risk (those with impaired left ventricular function, frequent PVC's, evidence of myocardial ischemia during exercise testing), beta blocker therapy is strongly recommended. Clinical experience has shown that beta blockers are often well tolerated in patients with global ejection fraction of 35 percent or greater. In such patients, beta blocker therapy is recommended irrespective of the site or size of infarct or the age of the patient, provided there are no other contraindications to beta blocker therapy. However, based on the demonstration of the trend toward reduction in mortality even in the low-risk group from major studies [8, 67], therapy can be justified even in this group.

CONCLUSIONS

Long-term beta blocker therapy for up to 3 years (and perhaps as long as 6 years) following an acute myocardial infarction is of proven benefit, especially in high-risk patients. When all patients are considered, the rate of mortality is reduced by about 25 percent and there is an added benefit of reduction in reinfarction and arrhythmia rates. In this regard, all beta blockers are effective. Data from trials with small sample size suggest that beta blockers with partial agonist activity may confer less benefit. Only fixed dosing regimens proven effective in large multicenter studies should be used. Very early use of beta blockade following myocardial infarction can limit the infarct size, but available data for the effects of such treatment on mortality are limited and not compelling. Preliminary results from a larger international study are encouraging [27]. The TIMI II Trial has shown that a significant reduction in death and reinfarction can be achieved in a small subgroup of patients treated with intravenous metoprolol within 2 hours of symptom onset [60]. However, no overall effect on mortality was seen in the study.

The adverse effects of beta blocker therapy in postmyocardial infarction patients are infrequent provided patients are carefully selected. Once the patient tolerates the first few doses of beta blocker, adverse effects during long-term therapy are uncommon. However, one should carefully monitor for worsening of heart failure, hypotension, or excessive bradycardia during beta blocker therapy. Severe adverse reactions necessitate discontinuation of beta blocker therapy, but substitution of one beta blocker for another is justified when adverse effects are of a minor nature.

REFERENCES

1. A Multicentre International Study. Improvement in prognosis of myocardial infarction by long-term beta-adrenoreceptor blockade using practolol. *Br. Med. J.* 3:735, 1975.
2. A Multicentre Trial. Propranolol in acute myocardial infarctions. *Lancet* 2:1435, 1966.
3. Anderson, M. P., Bechsgaard, P., Frederiksen, J., et al. Effect of alprenolol on mortality among patients with definite or suspected acute myocardial infarction: Preliminary results. *Lancet* 2:865, 1979.
4. Australian and Swedish Pindolol Study Group. The effect of pindolol on the two year mortality after complicated myocardial infarction. *Eur. Heart J.* 4:367, 1983.
5. Balcon, R., Jewitt, D. E., Davies, J. P. H., and Oram, S. A controlled trial of propranolol in acute myocardial infarction. *Lancet* 2:917, 1966.
6. Barber, J. M., Boyle, D. M. C., Chaturvedi, N. C., et al. Practolol in acute myocardial infarction. *Acta Med. Scand.* 574(Suppl):213, 1975.
7. Barber, J. M., Murphy, F. M., and Merrett, J. D. Clinical trial of propranolol in acute myocardial infarction. *Ulster Med. J.* 36:127, 1967.
8. Beta-Blocker Heart Attack Trial Research Group. A randomized trial of propranolol in patients with acute myocardial infarction. I. Mortality results. *Circulation* 72:449, 1985.
9. Briant, R. B., and Norris, R. M. Alprenolol in acute myocardial infarction: Double-blind trial. *N.Z. Med. J.* 71:135, 1970.
10. Clausen, J., Felsby, M., Jorgensen, F., et al. Absence of prophylactic effect of propranolol in myocardial infarction. *Lancet* 2:920, 1966.
11. Coronary Drug Project Research Group. Factors influencing long-term prognosis after recovery from myocardial infarction—three-year findings of the coronary drug project. *J. Chronic. Dis.* 27:267, 1974.
12. Coronary Prevention Research Group. An early intervention secondary prevention study with oxprenolol following myocardial infarction. *Eur. Heart J.* 2:389, 1981.
13. Davies, R. O., Mizgala, H. F., Tinmouth, A. L., et al. Prospective controlled trial of long-term propranolol on acute coronary events in patients with unstable coronary artery disease (Abstract). *Clin. Pharmacol. Ther.* 17:232, 1975.
14. The European Infarction Study Group. European infarction study (E.1.5).

A secondary prevention study with slow release oxprenolol after myocardial infarction: Morbidity and mortality. *Eur. Heart J.* 5:189, 1984.
15. First International Study of Infarct Survival Collaborative Group. Randomized trial of intravenous atenolol among 16,027 cases of suspected acute myocardial infarction: ISIA-1. *Lancet* 2:57, 1986.
16. Fox, K. M., Chopra, M. P., Portal, R. W., and Aber, C. P. Long-term beta blockade: possible protection from myocardial infarction. *Br. Med. J.* 1:117, 1975.
17. Friedman, L. M. How do the various beta blockers compare in type, frequency and severity of their adverse effects? *Circulation* 67(Suppl I):I-89, 1983.
18. Frishman, W., and Silverman, R. Clinical pharmacology of the new beta-adrenergic blocking drugs. Part 2. Physiologic and metabolic effects. *Am. Heart J.* 97:797, 1979.
19. Frishman, W. H. Multifactorial actions of beta-adrenergic blocking drugs in ischemic heart diesease: Current concepts. *Circulation* 67(Suppl I):I-11, 1983.
20. Frishman, W. H., and Weksler, B. B. Effects of beta-adrenoceptor blocking drugs on platelet function in normal subjects and patients with angina pectoris. In H. Roskamm and K. H. Graefe (eds.), Advances in Beta-Blocker Therapy: Proceedings of an International Symposium. Amsterdam: Excerpta Medica, 1980. P. 165.
21. Gold, H. K., Leenbach, R. C., and Moroko, P. R. Propranolol-induced reduction of signs of ischemic injury during acute myocardial infarction. *Am. J. Cardiol.* 38:689, 1976.
22. Hampton, J. R. Use of beta blockers for the reduction of mortality after myocardial infarction. *Eur. Heart J.* 2:259, 1981.
23. Han, J. Mechanisms of ventricular arrhythmias associated with myocardial infarction. *Am. J. Cardiol.* 24:800, 1969.
24. Hansteen, V., Moinichen, E., Lorentsen, E., et al. One year's treatment with propranolol after myocardial infarction: Preliminary reports of Norwegian Multicentre Trial. *Br. Med. J.* 284:155, 1982.
25. Hillis, L. D., and Braunwald, E. Myocardial ischemia (First of three parts). *N. Engl. J. Med.* 296:971, 1977.
26. Hillis, L. D., and Braunwald, E. Myocardial ischemia (Second of three parts). *N. Engl. J. Med.* 296:1034, 1977.
27. Hjalmarson, A. Goteborg metoprolol trial in acute myocardial infarction. *Am. J. Cardiol.* 53(Suppl):1D, 1984.
28. Hoffman, B. F., and Singer, D. H. Appraisal of the effects of catecholamines on cardiac electrical activity. *Ann. N.Y. Acad. Sci.* 139:914, 1967.
29. Julian, D. G., Prescott, R. J., Jackson, F. S., and Szekely, P. Controlled trial of sotalol for one year after myocardial infarction. *Lancet* 1:1142, 1982.
30. Jurgensen, H. J., Frederiksen, J., Hansen, D. A., and Pedersen-Bjergaard, O. Limitation of myocardial infarct size in patients less than 66 years treated with alprenolol. *Br. Heart J.* 45:583, 1981.
31. Kirk, E. S., and Sonnenblick, E. H. Newer concepts in the pathophysiology of ischemic heart disease. *Am. Heart J.* 103:756, 1982.
32. Ledwich, J. R. A trial of propranolol in myocardial infarction. *Can. Med. Assoc. J.* 98:988, 1968.
33. Lloyd, E. A., Gordon, G. D., Mabin, T. A., et al. Intravenous sotalol in acute myocardial infarction (Abstract). *Circulation* 66(Suppl II):II-3, 1982.
34. May, G. S., Eberlein, K. A., Furberg, C. D., et al. Secondary prevention after myocardial infarction: A review of long-term trials. *Prog. Cardiovasc. Dis.* 24:331, 1982.

35. May, G. S. A review of acute-phase beta-blocker trials in patients with myocardial infarction. *Circulation* 67(Suppl I):I-21, 1983.
36. May, G. S. A review of long-term beta-blocker trials in survivors of myocardial infarction. *Circulation* 67(Suppl I):I-46, 1983.
37. Mueller, H. S., and Ayres, S. M. Propranolol decreases sympathetic nervous activity reflected by plasma catecholamines during evolution of myocardial infarction in man. *J. Clin. Invest.* 65:338, 1980.
38. Naylor, W., Yepez, C. E., Fassold, E., and Ferrari, R. Prolonged protective effect of propranolol on hypoxic heart muscle. *Am. J. Cardiol.* 42:217, 1978.
39. Norris, R. M., Barnaby, P. F., Brown, M. A., et al. Prevention of ventricular fibrillation during acute myocardial infarction by intravenous propranolol. *Lancet* 2:883, 1984.
40. Norris, R. M., Clarke, E. D., Sammel, N. L., et al. Protective effect of propranolol in threatened myocardial infarction. *Lancet* 2:907, 1978.
41. Opie, L. H. Myocardial infarction size. Part 2. Comparison of anti-infarct effects of beta-blockade, glucose-insulin-potassium, nitrates, and hyluronidose. *Am. Heart J.* 100:531, 1980.
42. Opie, L. H., and Thomas, M. Propranolol and experimental myocardial infarction: Substrate effects. *Postgrad. Med. J.* 52(Suppl 4):124, 1976.
43. Pitt, B., and Craven, P. Effect of propranolol on regional myocardial blood flow in acute ischemia. *Cardiovasc. Res.* 4:176, 1970.
44. Pitt, B., Weiss, J. I., Schulze, R. A., et al. Reduction of myocardial infarct extension in man by propranolol (Abstract). *Circulation* 53(Suppl II):II-29, 1976.
45. Ramsdale, D. R., Faragher, E. B., Bennett, D. H., et al. Ischemic pain relief in patients with acute myocardial infarction by intravenous atenolol. *Am. Heart J.* 103:459, 1982.
46. Reynolds, J. L., and Whitlock, R. M. L. Effects of a beta-adrenergic receptor blocker in myocardial infarction treated for one year from onset. *Br. Heart J.* 34:252, 1972.
47. Roe, C. R., Cobb, F. R., and Starmer, C. F. Relationship between enzymatic and histologic estimates of the extent of myocardial infarction in conscious dogs with permanent coronary occlusion. *Circulation* 55:438, 1977.
48. Rossi, P. R., Yusuf, S., Ramsdale, D., et al. Reduction of ventricular arrhythmias by early intravenous atenolol in suspected myocardial infarction. *Br. Med. J.* 286:506, 1983.
49. Ryden, L., Ariniego, R., Arnman, K., et al. A double-blind trial of metoprolol in acute myocardial infarction: Effects on ventricular tachyarrhythmias. *N. Engl. J. Med.* 308:614, 1983.
50. Schrumpf, J. D., Sheps, D. S., Wolfson, S., et al. Altered hemoglobin-oxygen affinity with long-term propranolol therapy in patients with coronary artery disease. *Am. J. Cardiol.* 40:76, 1977.
51. Singh, B. N. Beta-adrenoceptor blocking drugs and acute myocardial infarction. *Drugs* 15:218, 1978.
52. Sleight, P., Yusuf, S., Ramsdale, D., et al. Early intravenous beta-blockade in myocardial infarction. *Br. J. Clin. Pharmacol.* 14(Suppl I):I-375, 1982.
53. Snow, P. J. D. Effect of propranolol in myocardial infarction. *Lancet* 2:551, 1965.
54. Stascewska-Barczak, J. Reflex stimulation of catecholamine secretion during the acute state of myocardial infarction in the dog. *Clin. Sci.* 41:419, 1971.
55. Taylor, S. H., Silke, B., Ebbutt, A., et al. A long-term prevention study with oxprenolol in coronary heart disease. *N. Engl. J. Med.* 307:1293, 1982.
56. The MIAMI Trial Research Group. Metoprolol in acute myocardial infarction

(MIAMI). A randomized placebo-controlled international trial. *Eur. Heart J.* 6:199, 1985.
57. The Multicenter Postinfarction Research Group. Risk stratification and survival after myocardial infarction. *N. Engl. J. Med.* 309:331, 1983.
58. The Norwegian Multicenter Group. Six-year follow-up of the Norwegian Multicenter Study of timolol after acute myocardial infarction. *N. Engl. J. Med.* 313:1055, 1985.
59. The Norwegian Multicenter Study Group. Timolol-induced reduction in mortality and reinfarction in patients surviving acute myocardial infarction. *N. Engl. J. Med.* 304:801, 1981.
60. The TIMI Study Group. Comparison of invasive and conservative strategies after treatment with intravenous tissue plasminogen activator in acute myocardial infarction. Results of the Thrombolysis in Myocardial Infarction (TIMI) Phase II Trial. *N. Engl. J. Med.* 320:618–27, 1989.
61. Timolol-International Collaborative Study Group. Reduction of infarct size with the early use of timolol in acute myocardial infarction. *N. Engl. J. Med.* 310:9, 1984.
62. Tonkin, A. M., Joel, S. E., Reynolds, J. L., et al. Beta-blockade in acute myocardial infarction. Inability of relatively late administration to influence infarct size and arrhythmias. *Med. J. Aust.* 2:145, 1981.
63. Vatner, S. F., Baig, H., Manders, T., et al. Effects of propranolol on regional myocardial function, electrograms, and blood flow in conscious dogs with myocardial ischemia. *J. Clin. Invest.* 60:353, 1977.
64. Vatner, S. F., McRitchie, R. J., Maroko, P. R., et al. Effects of catecholamines, exercise, and nitroglycerin on the normal and ischemic myocardiums in conscious dogs. *J. Clin. Invest.* 54:563, 1974.
65. Wilcox, R. G., Roland, J. M., Banks, D. C., et al. Randomized trial comparing propranolol with atenolol in immediate treatment of suspected myocardial infarction. *Br. Med. J.* 280:885, 1980.
66. Wilhelmsson, C., Vedin, J. A., Wilhelmsen, L., et al. Reduction of sudden deaths after myocardial infarction by treatment with alprenolol. *Lancet* 2:1157, 1974.
67. Yusuf, S., Peto, R., Lewis, J., et al. Beta blockade during and after myocardial infarction: An overview of the randomized trials. *Prog. Cardiovasc. Dis.* 27:335, 1985.
68. Yusuf, S., Sleight, P., Rossi, P., et al. Reduction in infarct size, arrhythmias and chest pain by early intravenous beta blockade in suspected acute myocardial infarction. *Circulation* 67(Suppl I):I-32, 1983.

CHAPTER 14

THE ROLE OF CALCIUM ANTAGONISTS IN ACUTE MYOCARDIAL INFARCTION AND POST-INFARCTION

CHARLES R. LAMBERT
CARL J. PEPINE

In recent years considerable interest has arisen regarding treatment of the patient suffering an acute myocardial infarction with calcium channel antagonists. This interest is based on experimental evidence suggesting beneficial effects of calcium channel antagonist treatment with respect to salvage of ischemic myocardium or limitation of infarct size in acute animal studies. In this chapter we will review the theoretical basis for and experimental evidence in favor of using calcium channel antagonists for treatment of the patient with acute myocardial infarction and consider the major clinical trials published to date in this area.

EXPERIMENTAL EVIDENCE SUPPORTING THE USE OF CALCIUM CHANNEL ANTAGONISTS IN ACUTE MYOCARDIAL INFARCTION

There are a number of theoretical reasons suggesting possible benefit from calcium channel antagonists in the setting of acute myocardial infarction. These include prevention of vasospasm, improvement of regional blood flow either directly or through collaterals, and relative improvement in myocardial oxygen demand through direct depression of myocardial contractile state, heart rate, and systemic blood pressure. In addition to these hemodynamic and direct myocardial effects, calcium channel antagonists may alter the kinetics of intracellular calcium channel accumulation, which is felt to be instrumental in causing ischemia-mediated cell death [19]. This mode of cell injury is manifested by cell swelling, accumulation of intracellular cytoplasmic calcium, formation of myofibrillar contraction bands, and massive mitochondrial accumulation of calcium with deposition of calcium pyrophosphate [15, 24]. Calcium channel antagonists might also help prevent ischemic cell injury by modulating accelerated ATP utilization or activation of phospholipases [14]. These possible mechanisms of ischemic myocardial salvage have led to a plethora of experimental studies concerning calcium channel antagonists and acute myocardial ischemia. These studies have been performed in a variety of experimental models with coronary reflow after occlusion, no reflow, varying periods and degrees of coronary occlusion, varying routes and relative times of drug administration, and varying methods for assessment of ischemic injury. We will not attempt to recapitulate all the literature in this area but will discuss some representative studies that are germane to the clinical setting of acute myocardial infarction. In this light, we will not consider the widely accepted beneficial effects of calcium channel antagonists on myocardial function during relatively brief periods of myocardial ischemia. Instead we will concentrate on investigations designed to assess the effects of calcium channel antagonists on limitation of infarct size with more prolonged periods of coronary occlusion. In general, this latter situation more closely parallels the pathophysiology of acute myocardial infarction in humans.

In 1978, Henry and coinvestigators [13] reported results of a study in 24 conscious dogs instrumented for hemodynamic measurements and with left anterior descending coronary artery occluders in place. After initial measurements, coronary occlusion was performed and nifedipine was administered as a 5 µg/kg bolus followed by a 24-hour infusion (IV) titrated by systemic arterial pressure. At the end of the infusion the animals were sacrificed and infarct area measured. Nifedipine was found to (1) increase coronary collateral blood flow during occlusion, (2) reduce creatine kinase depletion, and (3) reduce infarct size. The magnitude of the infarct limitation in the treated group compared to the control group was on the order of 1.5 to 3 times by both creatine kinase and morphometric estimates. The mechanism for the observed effects was felt to be related to the measured increase in collateral flow produced by nifedipine.

DeBoer and coworkers [6] reported results of a study in 25 anesthetized dogs with acute left anterior descending coronary artery occlusion. Verapamil was administered intravenously after 1 hour of occlusion as a loading dose of 0.2 mg/kg followed by an infusion of 0.6 mg/kg/hr. After 8 hours the animals were sacrificed and infarct size was determined as a percentage of the area at risk (ischemic area) measured by microsphere deposition. The verapamil-treated animals infarcted 70.5 percent of the ischemic area while the control animals infarcted 92 percent of the ischemic area ($p < 0.01$). Thus, a second study showed a beneficial effect of acute calcium channel antagonist administration in the setting of experimental myocardial infarction. A similar beneficial effect was demonstrated in rats for diltiazem by Zamanis and coworkers [29]. In this study diltiazem was administered at either 30 or 100 mg/kg/min by infusion given 20 minutes before and 1 hour after left coronary artery ligation. Planimetry of infarcted regions demonstrated complex topology, control infarct size of around 40 percent and a treated group infarct size of 22 to 25 percent when expressed as a percentage of ventricular mass.

Yellon and coworkers [28] studied the effects of verapamil on infarct size in 25 anesthetized greyhounds. Infarction was produced by embolization of a 2.5 mm plastic bead and verapamil was administered as a bolus of 0.2 mg/kg followed by an infusion of 0.005 mg/kg. Drug administration was initiated within 5 minutes of coronary embolization. After 24 hours, infarct size was determined by tetrazolium staining and the area at risk for infarction was measured by autoradiography. In the control group 62 percent of the area of risk was infarcted while in the verapamil group this percentage was reduced to 18 ($p < 0.001$).

In contrast to the studies cited above, Geary and coworkers [9] reported the effects of nifedipine on infarct size in eight baboons with acute left anterior descending coronary artery (LAD) occlusion followed by reperfusion. Nifedipine was administered as a 5 µg/kg bolus followed by an infusion of 30 µg/kg/hr begun 1 hour before a 2-hour LAD occlusion. Nifedipine administration was discontinued 2 hours after reperfusion. In the control animals 50 percent of the LAD perfusion bed was infarcted, and this figure was not statistically different (41.7 percent) in the nifedipine-treated group. Similar results were recently published for the NIH Cooperative Study in Animal Models for Protecting Ischemic Myocardium [22]. This study was designed to assess animal models for quantification of limitation in infarct size and included data for both conscious and anesthetized canine experiments. Administration of verapamil as a 0.03 mg/kg/min acute dose followed by 0.01 mg/kg/min for 6 hours did not have any effect on infarct size in this study.

In order to define more accurately the time related effects of verapamil on limitation of infarct size, Reimer and Jennings studied dogs with a variable period of circumflex coronary artery (Cx) occlusion followed by reperfusion [21]. One group of animals underwent a 40-minute period of Cx occlusion with or without verapamil pretreatment. After 4 days of recovery, untreated animals sustained subendocardial infarcts sized at 34 percent of the risk area while verapamil-treated animals sustained subendocardial infarcts involving only 8 percent of the risk area. In order to determine whether this protective effect was seen with longer periods of ischemia, a similar experiment was performed with 3 hours of coronary occlusion. Control dogs in this experiment sustained infarctions that involved 60 percent of the area at risk. Treatment with verapamil beginning 15 minutes after coronary occlusion and throughout the remaining 3-hour period did not limit infarct size. Verapamil did not alter collateral blood flow in this study.

Studies of a newer dihydropyridine calcium channel antagonist, nicardipine, have been reported for a 6-hour left anterior descending coronary occlusion model in baboons [1]. Dosing by intravenous pretreatment, post-ligation treatment, or 6-month oral pretreatment all limited infarct size significantly (22 percent, 21 percent, and 20 percent, respectively). In contrast, comparative studies using intravenous nifedipine or verapamil in the same model showed no beneficial effect. Nicardipine has also been studied in a canine model of myocardial infarction [7]. Significant myocardial salvage was observed with pretreatment (15 minutes before occlusion) and early postocclusion treatment (15 minute delay) but not when nicardipine administration was delayed 3 hours.

Although the studies mentioned above represent only a sampling of those reported in this area, they illustrate several pertinent points regarding the experimental evidence for use of calcium channel antagonists in acute myocardial infarction. First, such studies yield highly variable results. With the same drug, one study may demonstrate a salutary effect while another fails to do so. Possible reasons for such discrepancies are many and include species variability, interanimal variation in collateral development, uncontrolled hemodynamic effects, dose, time of administration relative to coronary occlusion, presence or absence of reperfusion, and inaccuracies in determination of the area at risk for infarction. All studies demonstrating limitation of infarct size by administration of calcium channel antagonists during the first 6 hours of ischemia have been noted to lack adequate control of one or more variables determining infarct size [21]. It is also interesting to note that in the NIH-sponsored study cited above, multivariate analysis showed that with a sample size of 15 dogs, an intervention limiting infarct size by 10 to 13 percent of the area at risk would be detected (using excellent experimental methodology and technique) only 50 percent of the time. With all these considerations, variability in results of such studies is not surprising. Despite these problems, a general theme that is present throughout most animal work in this area is that calcium channel antagonist administration, in order to be effective, must be administered early in the course of acute experimental myocardial infarction. This point becomes crucial in considering results of clinical trials.

RESULTS OF CLINICAL TRIALS

Multiple clinical trials have been done, based upon beneficial effects seen in animal studies of calcium channel antagonists in acute myocardial infarction. An early randomized, double-blind, placebo-controlled trial (NAMIS) of nifedipine therapy in acute myocardial infarction was done in 1982 and published in 1984 [17]. A total of 3143 patients were screened for the study who presented with ischemic pain of more than 45 minutes in duration. From this group, 105 patients with threatened myocardial infarction and 66 patients with acute myocardial infarction were randomized. Patients received either nifedipine 20 mg orally every 4 hours for 14 days or placebo plus standard care. Infarct size was determined by measurement of creatine kinase myocardial isoenzyme (CK-MB). The mean delay between onset of pain and beginning therapy was 4.6 hours. For the group of patients with threatened myocardial infarction, progression to documented myocardial infarction was not altered by treatment with nifedipine. In both placebo and treatment groups 75 percent of patients progressed to infarct. In addition, infarct size, in those patients who progressed, was identical in both placebo and nifedipine groups. Overall 6-month mortality for the 171 randomized patients was 8.5 percent for the placebo group and 10.1 percent for the nifedipine treatment group (not statistically different). However, 2-week mortality was significantly higher (7.9 percent) for the nifedipine group when compared to the placebo group (0 percent). Thus, in this trial with small patient numbers, treatment with nifedipine had no beneficial effect on any indicator related to myocardial infarction and may have had a deleterious effect with respect to early mortality.

Results of the Norwegian Nifedipine Multicenter Trial were also published in 1984 [25]. In this double-blind study 227 patients with suspected acute myocardial infarction were randomized within 12 hours of the onset of symptoms. A total of 885 patients were screened and inclusion criteria were based on chest pain characteristics and electrocardiographic changes. A similar number of patients evolved a documented myocardial infarction for both the treatment ($N = 74$) and placebo ($N = 83$) groups. Nifedipine was administered 10 mg orally five times a day for the first 2 days followed by 10 mg four times a day for 6 weeks. Just as for the study noted above, infarct size was estimated by the CK-MB method. Both the nifedipine and placebo groups had identical infarct size indices. Six-week mortality was also identical in each group (ten patients). Thus, a second clinical trial failed to demonstrate a beneficial effect of nifedipine therapy in acute myocardial infarction, although patient numbers in this study were also small.

The TRENT study [27] included 4491 patients with suspected acute myocardial infarction who were randomized to receive nifedipine 40 mg/day or placebo. One-month mortality was 10.2 percent in the nifedipine group and 9.2 percent in the placebo group; the study was terminated early due to this lack of effect.

An interesting study using nifedipine in concert with thrombolytic therapy for acute myocardial infarction was recently described by Erbel and coworkers [8]. A total of 149 patients entered a double-blind, placebo-controlled trial in which they received sublingual nifedipine or placebo in the emergency room and either nifedipine or placebo given intracoronary after reperfusion followed by a maintenance dose. Treatment was started in both groups in less than 3 hours from the onset of symptoms. A variety of indicators supported the conclusion that even very early administration of nifedipine combined with reperfusion and intracoronary administration does not enhance the salvage of myocardium in the clinical setting of acute infarction.

The Belfast trial [26] randomized patients with suspected myocardial infarction within 6 hours of the onset of symptoms to nifedipine (10 mg sublingual every 4 hours for 24 hours then orally for the next 24 hours) or placebo. Nifedipine had no effect on enzymatically estimated infarct size, incidence of ventricular arrhythmias, or in-hospital mortality.

A trial performed by Johns Hopkins investigators [11] randomized 132 patients with acute myocardial infarction within 12 hours of symptom onset to nifedipine (120 mg/day) or placebo. The nifedipine group did not achieve any benefit with respect to infarct size or left ventricular function; however, there was less infarct expansion in that group (7 percent) compared to placebo (47 percent).

In contrast to the studies outlined above, Bussman and coworkers reported a 30 percent reduction in infarct size in a small prospective study using verapamil in acute myocardial infarction [2]. Verapamil was administered intravenously at 5 to 10 mg/hr for 2 days beginning at a mean of 8 hours following the onset of symptoms. Crea and coworkers also reported the results of a small trial using intravenous verapamil in patients with acute myocardial infarction [3]. Reinfarction rate, creatine kinase release, and postinfarction angina all failed to respond favorably to verapamil treatment.

Unlike the small studies noted above, the Danish Verapamil Infarction Trial (DAVIT I) randomized a large number of patients ($N = 1436$); however, the primary goal of that trial was to assess the effects of the drug on reinfarction [4]. Patients were randomized to placebo or verapamil given as an initial intravenous bolus followed by 360 mg per day orally. Of the total study population, approximately 100 patients received treatment within 6 hours of the onset of symptoms. Verapamil had no effect on infarct size in this group, and the rate of reinfarction did not differ between the treatment and placebo groups as a whole. Treatment and follow-up continued for 6 months and, again, no influence of therapy on survival was seen. Another recent trial assessing the effects of calcium channel antagonist therapy in acute myocardial infarction was designed to study patients with non-Q wave infarctions who are known to have a particularly high incidence of reinfarction [10]. Diltiazem was selected for the study drug because of its relatively high safety profile, the observation that it does not increase heart rate, and some evidence suggesting preferential effects on coronary versus peripheral blood flow. Several end points other than reinfarction were monitored in these patients. These included postinfarction angina, refractory angina, and short-term (14 day) mortality. A total of 1600 patients were screened for the study and 576 were enrolled. These patients were similar with respect to 36 baseline characteristics in both treatment and placebo groups. Diltiazem was administered 90 mg orally every 6 hours to 287 patients and the remainder received placebo. Treatment was instituted 24 to 72 hours after the onset of infarction and continued for 14 days. Reinfarction was defined as an abnormal additional rise in CK-MB in plasma. Of the 576 patients enrolled, 42 developed reinfarction. Nine percent of patients in the placebo group and 5 percent of those in the diltiazem group sustained reinfarction. Expressed another way, treatment was associated with a 51.2 percent reduction in cumulative life table incidence, although the confidence limits for this figure are wide. Diltiazem therapy also decreased the frequency of refractory postinfarction angina by 50 percent. Mortality was 3.1 percent in the placebo group and 3.8 percent in the treatment group (not significantly different). Overall, 95 percent confidence limits indicate a significant beneficial effect of diltiazem therapy in this group of patients with respect to reinfarction alone as well as reinfarction and postinfarction angina. Thus, for the first time, calcium channel antagonist therapy was shown to be effective in the setting of acute myocardial infarction, albeit in the special case of reinfarction in the non-Q wave setting.

Further results from the Multicenter Diltiazem Postinfarction Trial Research Group have recently been published [18]. Patients with previous myocardial infarction were randomized to receive diltiazem (240 mg/day, $N = 1234$) or placebo ($N = 1232$) and followed for a mean period of 25 months. Total and cumulative mortality was identical in the two groups. Recurrent cardiac events (recurrent infarction or cardiac death) were less (11 percent) in the diltiazem group; however, significant interaction between diltiazem treatment and pulmonary congestion on chest x-ray was observed. Thus, while diltiazem therapy was associated with a lower number of cardiac events in the absence of pulmonary congestion, an increased cardiac event rate was observed in treated patients with pulmonary congestion or, similarly, with left ventricular ejection fraction less than 40 percent.

Several trials, some of which have been previously mentioned, have been designed to assess the efficacy of calcium channel antagonists in secondary prevention after acute myocardial infarction. The SPRINT Trial (Secondary Prevention Reinfarction Nifedipine Trial) had as a basic objective evaluation of nifedipine titrated to a dose of 60 mg/day as secondary prevention in patients with acute infarction and high-risk indicators [20]. A total of 828 patients were included in the trial study group and no difference was observed in mortality (9.3 percent for both groups) or nonfatal myocardial infarction (5.0 percent versus 3.5 percent) for the nifedipine versus placebo groups, respectively. However, in the group of 1373 randomized patients, mortality was 15.8 percent in the nifedipine group compared to 12.6 percent in the placebo group. This difference was due to excess 6-day mortality in the nifedipine group during the titration period: 7.0 percent mortality was seen in the nifedipine group and 4.2 percent in those on placebo. When this trend was observed, the study was discontinued. Retrospective analysis showed that most of the excess mortality occurred in patients with admission blood pressures of less than 100 mm Hg.

The Holland Interuniversity Nifedipine/Metoprolol Trial (HINT) compared nifedipine, metoprolol, and the combination of the incidence of recurrent ischemia and infarction in patients with unstable angina [23]. The trial showed that patients not on beta blockers had a beneficial response to metoprolol and that the combination of metoprolol and nifedipine offered nothing further. Therapy with nifedipine alone appeared detrimental; however, addition of nifedipine to metoprolol when patients became unstable appeared beneficial.

Recently the Danish Verapamil Infarction Trial II results were reported [5]. The objective of DAVIT II was to assess the effect of therapy with verapamil beginning on the second week after an acute myocardial infarction and continued for 12 to 18 months on mortality and major events. A total of 878 patients were randomized to receive either verapamil 360 mg/day or placebo. Eighteen-month total mortality rates were 11.1 and 13.8 percent ($p = 0.11$) while major event rates were 18 and 22 percent ($p = 0.03$) in verapamil and placebo groups, respectively. Mortality (7.7 versus 11.8 percent) and major event rates (14.6 versus 19.7 percent) for patients without heart failure in the coronary care unit were significantly reduced in the verapamil group. In patients with heart failure no benefit of verapamil treatment was seen on mortality or major event rate; however, no detrimental effects were observed. Thus, verapamil was shown to be beneficial in secondary prevention of death and major cardiac events after acute myocardial infarction in patients without heart failure.

CONCLUSIONS

Theoretical evidence abounds at the molecular and cellular level suggesting a possible beneficial effect of calcium channel antagonists in ischemic myocardial injury. Indeed, ample evidence exists in animal models for such a salutary effect in the setting of acute reversible ischemia. When one moves to animal models of acute myocardial infarction due to prolonged coronary occlusion, variable results are obtained. Some studies demonstrate a benefit of calcium channel antagonist therapy in limiting infarct size and others do not. Although many variables enter into interpretation of these discrepancies, early administration of the calcium channel antagonist appears to be the most important issue if a beneficial effect is to be observed.

The one study [10, 18] showing acute benefit of calcium channel antagonist therapy in myocardial infarction does so in a select group of patients who have already sustained a non-Q wave infarct and who are at risk for extension or reinfarction. Considering the need for early administration of drug demonstrated in animal studies, the salutary effects seen in the reinfarction scenario might be anticipated since these patients are essentially pretreated with regard to secondary events. This contrasts with most acute trials, which, by necessity, treat patients after the fact (acute transmural myocardial infarction) by varying periods of time. Since it is unlikely that patients will ever present within 30 minutes or an hour of the actual onset of infarction (not of symptoms), it appears doubtful that relatively late treatment with calcium channel antagonists will ever show an effect in terms of limiting infarct size. This view is supported by the fact that such a demonstration is far from universally present even in the controlled setting of the animal laboratory.

Although secondary prevention trials have been largely negative, most of these have utilized nifedipine. The DAVIT II trial shows convincing evidence for benefit from verapamil therapy in this regard in patients without heart failure.

Recently Held and coworkers examined the effects of calcium channel antagonists on initial infarction, reinfarction, and mortality in 24 trials, retrospectively [12]. Patients in these trials had unstable angina, acute myocardial infarction, or were followed postinfarction on long-term therapy. Results are summarized in Tables 14-1 and 14-2 and show that calcium channel antagonists that do not slow heart rate do not prevent myocardial events in such patients as evidenced by odds ratios of 1.19 [95% (10.92–1.53) and 1.16 (0.99–1.35)], and 1.05 for reinfarction and death. Thus, retrospective analysis does not seem to support the prophylactic use of calcium channel antagonists to prevent these end points in patients with acute ischemic syndromes. It should be noted, however, that such analyses are heavily weighted by the preponderance of investigations utilizing nifedipine. There is clear and emerging evidence showing beneficial effects of compounds other than nifedipine [5, 10] that slow the heart rate where the odds ratios were 0.79 (0.67–0.94, $p < 0.01$) and 0.95 (0.82–1.09) for reinfarction and death. Clearly all calcium channel antagonists are not created equal [16].

Theoretical, experimental, and clinical considerations regarding calcium channel antagonists and acute myocardial infarction are summarized in, and the results of some major clinical trials are given in, Tables 14-1 and 14-2. Clearly, before firm recommendations regarding calcium channel antagonist therapy for salvage of ischemic myocardium or prevention of events after acute myocardial infarction can be made, more clinical trials must be done. Indications for calcium channel antagonist therapy in the various chronic or unstable ischemic syndromes and for dysrhythmias are covered elsewhere in this volume. Clearly the effects, in terms of reduction of reinfarction and death, are not as significant as that seen with beta blockers and aspirin. But in the post-infarction patient in whom a beta blocker is contraindicated, it seems appropriate to consider a heart-rate-slowing calcium channel antagonist.

TABLE 14-1. *Updates on Trials of the Effect of Dihydropyridine Calcium Blockers on Mortality and Subsequent Infarction*

	Active (Number of Events/Number of Patients)	Control	Odds Ratio	(95% CI)
Mortality				
Held et al (1989) (overview)	365/4731	330/4733	1.13	(0.97–1.32)
Waters et al (1990)	2/192	3/191	0.66	(0.06–1.9)
Lichtien et al (1990)	12/214	2/211	4.4	(1.5–12.6)
Total	379/5137 (7.4%)	335/5135* (6.5%)	1.16	(0.99–1.35)
	$2 = 1.86; p = 0.07$			
Reinfarction				
Held et al (1989) (overview)	124/3646	111/3680	1.14	(0.68–1.92)
Waters et al (1990)	14/192	8/191	1.77	(0.75–1.43)
Lichtien et al (1990)	?/214	?/211	—	
Total	138/3838 (3.5%) +?/214	119/3871* (3.1%) +?/211	1.19	(0.92–1.53)
	$p = $ not significant			

*If death and reinfarction reported in the trials are largely independent of each other, then the data on both the end points can be combined. In this case, the excess in death or reinfarction, or both, has a $Z = 2.29$, which has a nominal p value of <0.02. CI = confidence interval.

TABLE 14-2. *Update on Trials of Calcium Channel Antagonists That Slow Heart Rate (Verapamil, Diltiazem)*

	Active (Number of Events/Number of Patients)	Control	Odds Ratio	(95% CI)
Mortality				
Verapamil				
Held et al (1989) (overview)	149/1766	147/1752	1.01	(0.79–1.28)
DAVIT-II (1990)	95/878	119/897	0.79	(0.06–1.05)
Subtotal (verapamil)	244/2644	266/2649	0.91	(0.76–1.1)
Diltiazem				
Held et al (1989)	180/1574	181/1577	0.99	(0.80–1.24)
Total	424/4218 (10.0%)	447/4226 (10.6%)	0.95	(0.82–1.09)
Reinfarction				
Verapamil				
Held et al (1989) (overview)	54/1728	64/1727	0.83	(0.57–1.21)
DAVIT-II (1990)	84/878	107/897	0.78	(0.58–1.05)
Subtotal (verapamil)	138/2606	171/2624	0.80	(0.63–1.01)
Diltiazem				
Held et al (1989)	113/1557	142/1560	0.79	(0.61–1.02)
Total	251/4163 (6.0%)	313/4184 (7.5%)	0.79	(0.67–0.94)*

*$Z = 2.61$; $p < 0.01$.
DAVIT-II = the second Danish Verapamil Infarction Trial; other abbreviations as in Table 14-1.

REFERENCES

1. Alps, B. J., Calder, C., and Wilson A. The beneficial effect of nicardipine compared with nifedipine and verapamil in limiting myocardial infarct size in baboons. *Arzneim.-Forsch. Drug Res.* 33:868, 1983.
2. Bussman, W., Seher, W., and Gruengras, M. Reduction of creatine kinase and creatine kinase-MB indexes of infarct size by intravenous verapamil. *Am. J. Cardiol.* 54:1224, 1984.
3. Crea, F., et al. Effects of verapamil in preventing postinfarction angina and reinfarction. *Am. J. Cardiol.* 55:900, 1985.
4. Danish Study Group on Verapamil in Myocardial Infarction. Verapamil in acute myocardial infarction. *Eur. Heart J.* 5:516, 1984.
5. The Danish Study Group on Verapamil in Myocardial Infarction. Effect of verapamil on mortality and major events after acute myocardial infarction (the Danish verapamil infarction trial II). *Am. J. Cardiol.* 66:779, 1990.
6. DeBoer, L. W. V., et al. Autoradiographic method for measuring the ischemic myocardium at risk: Effects of verapamil on infarct size after experimental coronary artery occlusion. *Proc. Nat. Acad. Sci.* 77:6619, 1980.
7. Endo, T., et al. Comparative effects of nicardipine, a new calcium antagonist, on size of myocardial infarction after coronary artery occlusion in dogs. *Circulation* 74:420, 1989.
8. Erbel, R., et al. Combination of calcium channel blocker and thrombolytic therapy in acute myocardial infarction. *Am. Heart J.* 115:529, 1988.
9. Geary, G. G., et al. Failure of nifedipine therapy to reduce myocardial infarct size in the baboon. *Am. J. Cardiol.* 49:331, 1982.
10. Gibson, R. S., et al. Diltiazem and reinfarction in patients with non-Q-wave myocardial infarction. *N. Engl. J. Med.* 315:423, 1986.
11. Gottleib, S. O., et al. Nifedipine in acute myocardial infarction: An assessment of left ventricular function, infarct size, and infarct expansion: a double blind, randomised, placebo controlled trial. *Br. Heart J.* 59:411, 1988.
12. Held, P., Yusuf, S., and Furberg, C. Update of effects of calcium antagonists in myocardial infarction or angina in light of the second Danish Verapamil Infarction Trial (DAVIT-II) and other recent studies. *Am. J. Cardiol.* 67:1295, 1991.
13. Henry, P. D., et al. Effects of nifedipine on myocardial perfusion and ischemic injury in dogs. *Circ. Res.* 43:372, 1978.
14. Jennings, R. B., and Reimer, K. A. Lethal myocardial cell injury. *Am. J. Pathol.* 102:241, 1981.
15. Kloner, R. A., et al. Effect of a transient period of ischemia on myocardial cells. II. Fine structure during the first few minutes of reflow. *Am. J. Pathol.* 74:399, 1974.
16. Messerli, F. Cardioprotection—not all calcium antagonists are created equal. *Am. J. Cardiol.* 66:855, 1990.
17. Muller, J. E., et al. Nifedipine therapy for patients with threatened and acute myocardial infarction: A randomized, double-blind, placebo-controlled comparison. *Circulation* 69:740, 1984.
18. Multicenter Diltiazem Postinfarction Trial Research Group. The effects of diltiazem on mortality and reinfarction after myocardial infarction. *N. Engl. J. Med.* 319:385, 1988.
19. Nayler, W. G. The role of calcium in the ischemic myocardium. *Am. J. Pathol.* 102:262, 1981.
20. Neufeld, H. N. Rationale of nifedipine administration in secondary prevention after myocardial infarction. SPRINT-secondary prevention reinfarction nifedipine trial. In M. Kaltenbach and H. N. Neufeld (eds.), *5th International Adalat Symposium*. Amsterdam: Excerpta Medica, 1983.

21. Reimer, K. A., and Jennings, R. B. Effects of calcium channel blockers on myocardial preservation during experimental acute myocardial infarction. *Am. J. Cardiol.* 55:107B, 1985.
22. Reimer, K. A., et al. Animal models for protecting ischemic myocardium: Results of the NHLBI cooperative study. *Circ. Res.* 56:651, 1985.
23. Report on the Holland Interuniversity Nifedipine/Metoprolol Trial (HINT) Research Group: early treatment of unstable angina in the coronary care unit: a randomised, double blind, placebo controlled comparison of recurrent ischaemia in patients treated with nifedipine or metoprolol or both. *Br. Heart J.* 56:400, 1986.
24. Shen, R. C., and Jennings, R. B. Myocardial calcium and magnesium in acute ischemic injury. *Am. J. Pathol.* 67:417, 1972.
25. Sirnes, P. A., et al. Evolution of infarct size during the early use of nifedipine in patients with acute myocardial infarction: The Norwegian Nifedipine Multicenter Trial. *Circulation* 70:638, 1984.
26. Walker, L., et al. Effect of nifedipine in the early phase of acute myocardial infarction on enzymatically estimated infarct size and arrhythmias. *Br. Heart J.* 57:83, 1987.
27. Wilcox, R. G., et al. Trial of early nifedipine in acute myocardial infarction: The TRENT study. *Br. Med. J.* 293:1204, 1986.
28. Yellon, D. M., et al. Sustained limitation of myocardial necrosis 24 hours after coronary artery occlusion: Verapamil infusion in dogs with small myocardial infarcts. *Am. J. Cardiol.* 51:1409, 1983.
29. Zamanis, A., Verdetti, J., and Leiris, J. Reduction of ischemia-induced myocardial necrosis in the rat with permanent coronary artery occlusion under the effect of diltiazem. *J. Mol. Cell. Cardiol.* 14:53, 1982.

CHAPTER 15

PROBLEMS WITH NITROGLYCERIN AND NITRATES, INCLUDING NITRATE TOLERANCE

JONATHAN ABRAMS

When considering the adverse or unwanted effects of nitroglycerin and the organic nitrates, it is important to keep in mind that the magnitude of response of nitrate administration (i.e., vascular smooth muscle dilation) can be affected by a number of variables. The sequelae of venous and arterial vasodilation in a given individual may vary depending on a variety of factors that can modulate the nitrate response. Almost all of the common side effects produced by nitrate administration result from cerebral arterial vasodilation or the decrease in systemic blood pressure and cardiac output induced by systemic nitrate vascular dilation with subsequent reflex increase in sympathetic nervous system activity. When vascular responsiveness to nitrate vasodilation is attenuated (e.g., nitrate tolerance or resistance) or when nitrate hemodynamic effects are of less magnitude than normal, such as in congestive heart failure, the frequency and magnitude of the common adverse reactions to nitrates will be less. Conversely, in nitrate-sensitive individuals, a large fall in blood pressure may be particularly troubling. The common complaint of headache following nitrate administration does not appear to correlate with any specific pharmacologic or hemodynamic response; as with other nitrate side effects, headache appears to be less common in patients with heart failure.

The major modulators of nitrate action are listed in Table 15-1. Each will be discussed briefly before a detailed review of the adverse nitrate reactions.

REFLEX SYMPATHETIC DISCHARGE

The body's response to nitrate-induced hypotension is baroreceptor-mediated systemic and regional bed arterial vasoconstriction, often with an increase in heart rate (Fig. 15-1). The decline in systemic blood pressure is accentuated in the upright position. Decreased arterial pressure is related to systemic venous vasodilation resulting in a reduction

TABLE 15-1. *Factors That May Modulate Hemodynamic Response to Nitrates*

Reflex sympathetic nervous system activity
Status of left ventricular function
  Normal intracardiac size and pressures vs. left ventricular dysfunction, cardiac dilation, or congestive heart failure
Size of administered dose
Individual vascular reactivity
  Inherent nitrate resistance in some patients
  Presence or absence of nitrate tolerance
    partial
    complete
    cross-tolerance to other nitrates

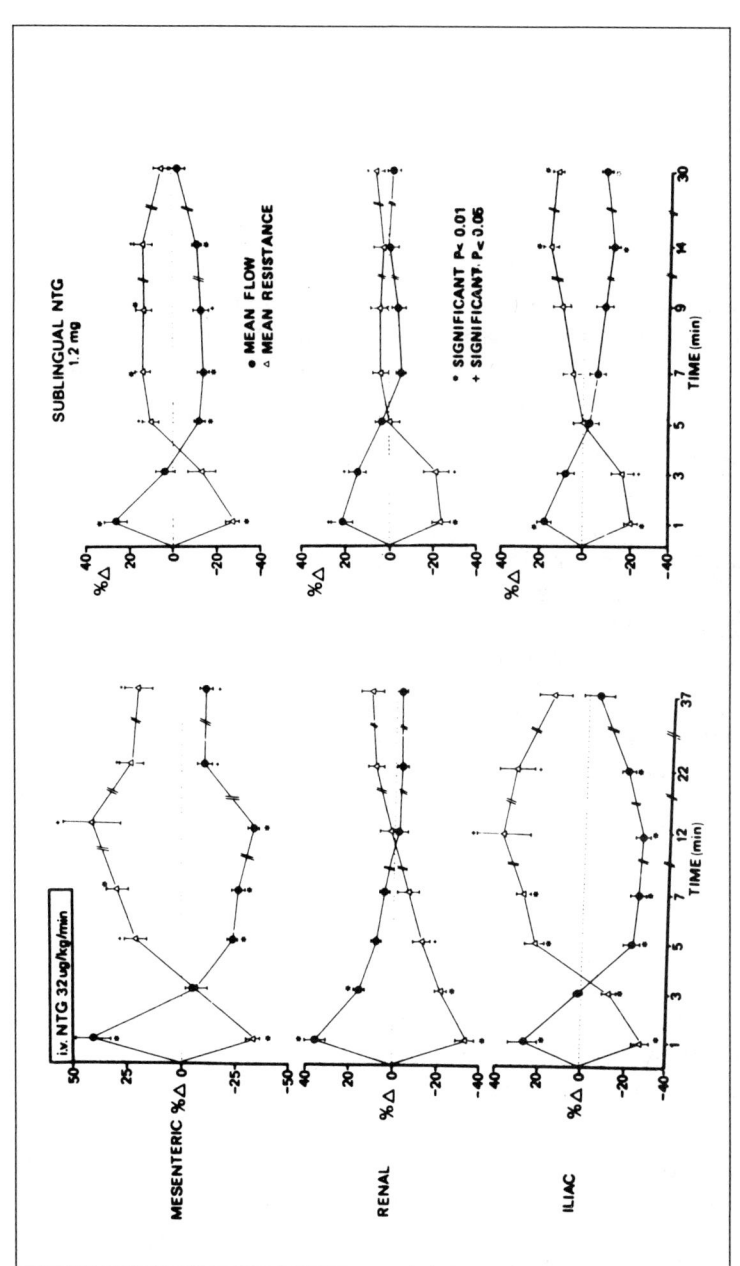

FIG. 15-1. Regional circulatory responses to intravenous and sublingual nitroglycerin in the dog. Note the initial vasodilation that occurs in the mesenteric, renal, and iliac vessels that is rapidly attenuated because of reflex sympathetic discharge, resulting in a return of vascular bed resistance toward control or even to vasoconstrictor levels. (From Ref. 69, with permission.)

TABLE 15-2. *Hemodynamic Responses and Side Effect Profile Following Nitrate Administration with Normal and Abnormal Left Ventricular Function*

	Normal LV	Abnormal LV or CHF	Symptoms If Present
Heart Rate			
Supine	↑	→	Palpitations, tachycardia
Upright	↑↑	→	Rare angina
Systolic blood pressure			
Supine	→↓	→↓	Dizziness
Upright	↓ to ↓↓	↓	Syncope (rare)

in right and left heart filling (preload) with a subsequent decrease in cardiac output and the direct arterial-arteriolar dilating effects resulting in increased arterial diameter and conductance and a decrease in systemic vascular resistance at high doses. Norepinephrine release occurs when arterial pressure is lowered [62].

The vasodilating actions of nitrates typically result in a biphasic response in many vascular beds, with early vasodilation followed by vasoconstriction (Fig. 15-1) [69]. In the presence of abnormal left ventricular function, left ventricular dilation, or overt congestive heart failure, the hypotensive response to nitrates is diminished, as cardiac output is usually maintained or even increases (see below), and reflex sympathetic discharge may not occur.

STATUS OF LEFT VENTRICULAR FUNCTION
Classic nitrate side effects are most prominent in patients with intact left ventricular function and a normal-sized heart. However, in the presence of left ventricular dysfunction, intracardiac dimensions may not measurably decrease following nitroglycerin (NTG) although intracardiac pressures predictably fall; cardiac output is not reduced after NTG in the presence of congestive heart failure, and even when peripheral vascular resistance decreases, systemic blood pressure usually is well maintained. Table 15-2 outlines the differences in hemodynamic responses to NTG and side effects in individuals with normal cardiac function compared to those with significant left ventricular dysfunction or overt congestive heart failure.

VASCULAR REACTIVITY
Individual responsiveness to nitrate administration in normal subjects and cardiac patients is highly variable. Little is known about this phenomenon. While nitrate plasma concentrations vary considerably after

15. PROBLEMS WITH NITROGLYCERIN AND NITRATES

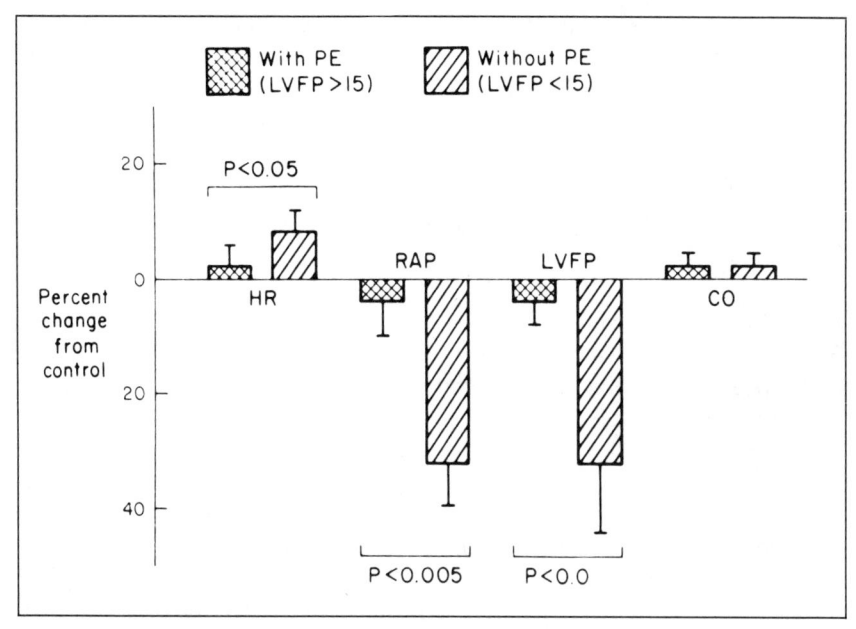

FIG. 15-2. Blunted hemodynamic response to sublingual nitroglycerin in patients with heart failure and peripheral edema. Subjects with CHF were given a sublingual nitroglycerin challenge both before and after diuresis. Note that changes in right atrial and left ventricular filling pressures were virtually nil in the presence of peripheral edema. After diuretic administration and loss of peripheral edema, the preload reduction achieved by nitroglycerin was substantial. (From Ref. 36, with permission.)

a given dose of nitrate, this alone is probably not sufficient to explain the remarkable intraindividual differences in the degree of vasodilation following NTG administration. In congestive heart failure, nitrate resistance is relatively common, and an absence of typical hemodynamic responses after nitrate administration can be seen in some patients, even when very large doses of nitroglycerin are given [7, 18, 36]. One study demonstrated restoration of vascular responses to sublingual nitroglycerin after diuretic therapy [36] (Fig. 15-2). In another investigation in severe heart failure, nitrate-resistant subjects all had an elevated right atrial pressure, but no other hemodynamic predictors were identified that separated nitrate responders from resistant subjects [18]. It is of interest that an abnormal right atrial pressure has also been correlated with decreased responsiveness to ACE inhibitors in congestive heart failure patients.

DOSAGE

With acute nitrate administration there is often a demonstrable dose-response relationship between the hemodynamic and clinical effects and the size of the nitrate dose. Blood pressure and heart rate responses in general are greater with larger doses (Fig. 15-3A.) [66]. However, following chronic administration of long-acting nitrates, the hemodynamic sequelae of a given dose are smaller, due either to some degree of the nitrate tolerance and/or counterregulatory sympathetic activity [2, 62, 69]. With repeated dosing, the dose-response relationships seen with first-dose nitrate administration may attenuate or disappear [66] (Fig. 15-3B.).

NITRATE TOLERANCE

Perhaps the most critical factor in determining the response to nitrates is the presence or absence of nitrate tolerance. The classic nitrate headache has long been known to decrease in intensity or disappear over time with repeat dosing. This is clearly a positive aspect of nitrate vascular tolerance, presumably related to a lesser dilating effect on the extra- and intracranial arteries over time. A fully reactive vascular system provides a predictable substrate for acute side effects, whereas venous and arterial circulations with attenuated vasoreactivity are less likely to result in symptomatic hypotension and/or tachycardia. The most extreme example of tolerance is a complete loss of a beneficial clinical response to nitrates demonstrable after chronic sustained action nitrate administration [50]. The phenomenon of tolerance will be discussed in more detail later in this chapter.

CONCOMITANT DRUG THERAPY

The hypotensive potential of any nitrate may be enhanced in the presence of diuretic-induced hypovolemia as well as when patients are receiving other potent vasodilators (Table 15-3). The associated use of beta blockers could blunt the compensatory reflex tachycardia following nitrate administration and might exacerbate symptoms of dizziness and near syncope after nitroglycerin. No data exist documenting this phenomenon. Use of sublingual NTG while drinking alcohol can potentiate tachycardia and hypotension in the upright posture [4] (discussed later in this chapter).

ADVERSE EFFECTS RELATING TO NITRATE PHARMACOLOGIC ACTION

Headache

The commonest side effect of acute and chronic nitrate therapy is headache. This can range from an excruciating generalized headache to a mild sensation of throbbing or fullness in the head. Some patients refuse to use sublingual NTG for angina attacks or remain extremely reluctant to do so because of this problem. Others are unable to tolerate long-

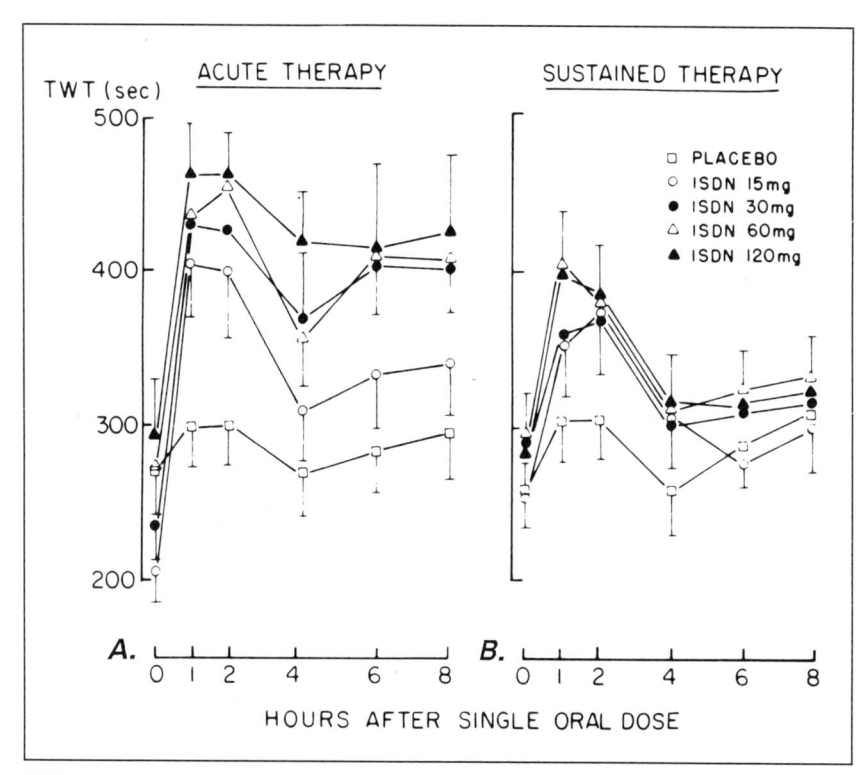

FIG. 15-3. Development of tolerance with chronic oral ISDN administration. This cohort of patients with angina were given placebo and four doses of ISDN qid, ranging from 15 to 120 mg. **A.** In the acute study without prior nitrate administration, a clear-cut dose-response relationship is seen, with improvement in exercise time to 6 to 8 hours for the highest three doses. Systolic blood pressure decreases parallel the size of the dose administered. **B.** Sustained therapy: After administration of 30 mg of oral ISDN qid for one to two weeks, the exercise protocol was repeated for each dose. Although significant antianginal effects compared to placebo were maintained at 1 and 2 hours after administration of the drug, there was no longer any significant difference from placebo 4 to 6 hours after dosing. Further, there was a relative blunting of the dose-response relationship seen with acute ISDN administration to exercise prolongation and the fall in systolic pressure. Note the attenuation of peak antianginal protection when compared to day 1. (From Ref. 66, with permission.)

TABLE 15-3. *Drug Interactions That May Result in Exaggerated Nitrate Side Effects*

Drug Classification	Mechanism
Diuretics	Hypovolemia, decreased cardiac preload
Beta blockers	Resting bradycardia, attenuation of reflex tachycardia
Calcium channel antagonists	Arterial-arteriolar vasodilation
ACE inhibitors	Arterial and venous vasodilation, decrease in cardiac filling pressures, decreased bradykinin degradation
Hydralazine, Minoxidil	Arterial-arteriolar vasodilation
Alcohol	Additive effects on blood pressure and heart rate

acting nitrates because of these headaches. The author estimates that 15 to 25 percent of individuals cannot be maintained on chronic therapy due to the headache problem.

It is presumed that headache is related to dilation of extracranial and intracerebral arteries. Intracranial pressure increases after nitrate administration. Reflex cerebral arterial vasoconstriction may play a role. No information is available regarding the precise mechanism or site of the arterial vasodilation that results in headache. Nitrate headaches usually become less severe or disappear with chronic therapy.

The disappearance of vascular tolerance to headaches is dramatically underscored by the phenomenon of nitrate dependence, demonstrated by munitions workers or those employed in nitroglycerin manufacturing factories. These individuals develop severe withdrawal headaches only after they leave the nitrate-laden work environment for several days after continuous daily nitrate exposure (Monday morning syndrome) [2, 38, 59]. Presumably, such headaches are caused by unopposed cerebral vasoconstriction. While the worker is continuously exposed to organic nitrates no symptoms are present. Employees have been known to wear NTG-impregnated headbands to avoid withdrawal symptoms. Rare cases of chest pain and acute myocardial infarction, presumably related to coronary vasospasm, have also been reported in similar circumstances [2, 33, 38].

MANAGEMENT OF NITRATE HEADACHES

Because headache is such a common problem with nitrate therapy, it is important for physicians to warn patients to anticipate this symptom before initiating nitrate therapy. Recognition that nitrate headaches usually (but not always) disappear within 1 to 2 weeks is useful so that the patient is forewarned and encouraged to continue with long-acting nitrate therapy. Patients should be alerted to the headache problem

TABLE 15-4. *Management of Nitrate Headaches*

Education
   Caution the patient that headache is common
   Counsel the patient that a decrease or disappearance of headaches typically occurs over time (3–7 days)
Short-term use of analgesics (e.g., aspirin, acetaminophen, nonsteroidals)
Begin therapy with small nitrate doses; be prepared to decrease the dose until headache tolerance occurs

through careful counseling and education. The temporary use of mild analgesics should be encouraged. If the physician is able to motivate the patient to continue nitrates until the headaches lessen or disappear, success is more likely. Reducing the nitrate dose until headache tolerance develops is another useful strategy (Table 15-4).

Dizziness and Syncope

Hypotension is often induced by acute sublingual NTG administration. Long-acting nitrates in nitrate-sensitive patients can produce alarming symptoms of dizziness, light-headedness, and even frank syncope. These are all manifestations of cerebral hypoperfusion. The timing of such symptoms depends on the formulation used and the time-course to peak hemodynamic effect. Obviously, such symptoms will immediately follow sublingual, buccal, or oral spray NTG delivery, but will occur 30 to 90 minutes after administration of most oral or topical long-acting nitrates.

If there is a concomitant vagal response with cardiac slowing, hypotensive symptoms may be more likely to occur. It is particularly worrisome if significant hypotension occurs in a patient with ischemic heart disease, particularly during acute myocardial infarction where susceptibility to vagal effects may be greater (Fig. 15-4). Bradycardia and hypotension may occasionally occur in subjects given sublingual NTG during acute attacks of anginal chest pain [11, 31, 43]. Episodes of angina can rarely be precipitated if central aortic pressure drops sufficiently in patients with symptomatic coronary atherosclerosis.

As with headaches, individuals who use NTG or long-acting nitrates should be forewarned about the possibility of severe light-headedness, particularly with initial dosing. (The author recommends having patients first try sublingual NTG tablets when they are not having chest pain so they can become familiar with nitrate side effects (if any).) The patient should be cautioned to sit or lie down promptly when dizziness first appears. For severe hypotensive episodes, patients should be put in a supine or Trendelenburg position with the legs elevated. Rarely,

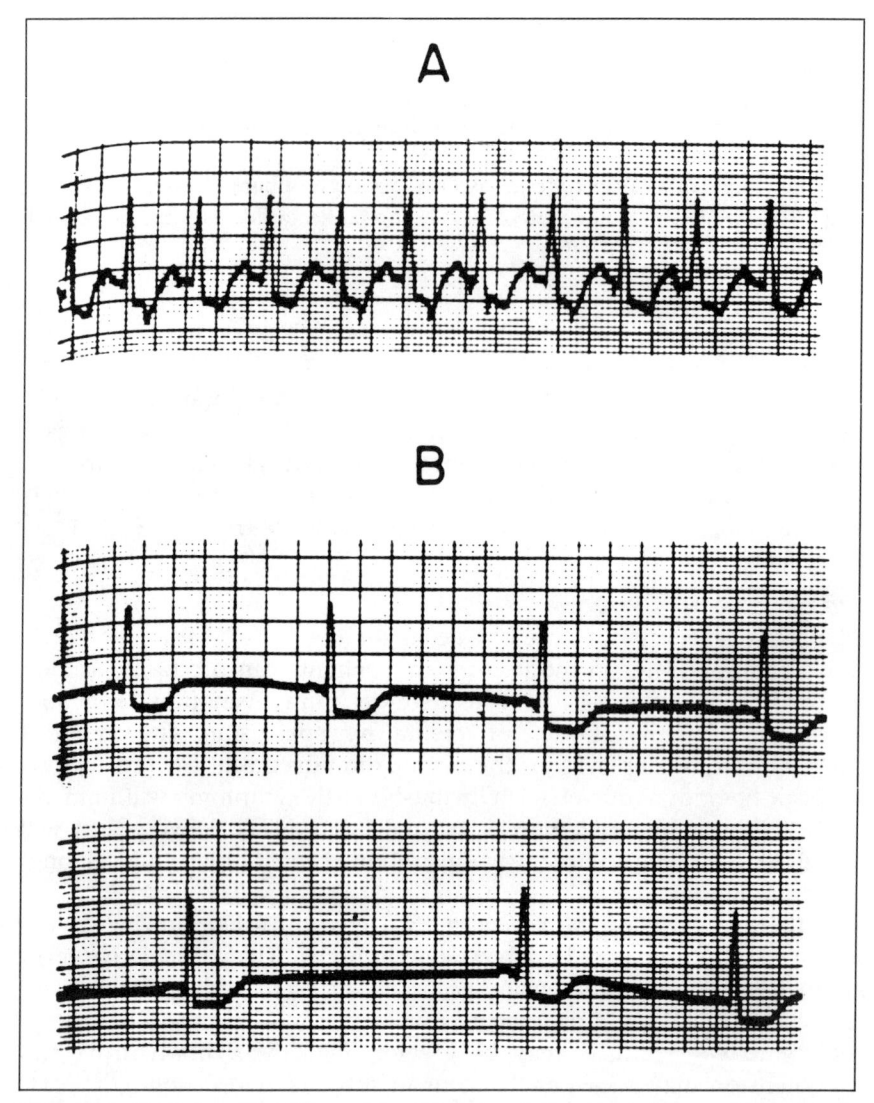

FIG. 15-4. Sinus bradycardia and hypotension following sublingual nitrate administration. These electrocardiographic strips were taken from a patient with acute myocardial infarction given sublingual nitroglycerin for chest pain; within minutes blood pressure fell and the heart rate slowed markedly. (From Ref. 11, with permission.)

intravenous fluids can be given for sustained hypotension, although this is impractical and unnecessary in the vast majority of instances.

Remember that hypovolemia, alcohol consumption, or concomitant vasoactive drug therapy are likely to potentiate the problem of dizziness and presyncope (Table 15-3).

Nausea
Occasional patients experience nausea and even vomiting following nitrate administration. If these symptoms persist, they may preclude chronic long-acting nitrate therapy.

IDIOSYNCRATIC NITRATE REACTIONS
Nitrate Bradycardia
A number of reports have documented the phenomenon of marked sinus bradycardia after sublingual NTG, particularly in the setting of acute myocardial ischemia [11, 31, 43]. This is typically compounded by arterial hypotension, resulting in symptoms of dizziness, syncope, or chest pain. This phenomenon is presumably a vasovagal-like reaction, perhaps related to sudden changes in intracardiac stretch receptors. Figure 15-4 is an example of such a reaction.

Rare reports of heart block have been documented following NTG administration. This also is likely to be a vagally-mediated phenomenon, as NTG has no depressant action on the AV node itself. In fact, the usual response to NTG administration is an acceleration of AV conduction time due to reflex sympathetic discharge [26].

The treatment of nitrate bradycardia is immediate atropine administration and/or putting the patient in the supine or Trendelenberg position.

Coronary Vasospasm
Several fascinating reports have appeared regarding workers chronically exposed to NTG in the munitions or pharmaceutical industry that implicate coronary vasospasm as a mechanism for chest pain and even acute myocardial infarction occurring after the individual is absent from the work environment for 1 to 2 days or more [2, 33, 38]. This rare manifestation of nitrate dependence appears to have little correlation in clinical medicine. The degree of nitrate exposure in these industries is pharmacologic in nature, far greater than achieved with conventional therapeutic dosing. Experienced physicians do not report nitrate withdrawal syndromes or rebound reactions that could represent reactive coronary vasospasm. Several reports, however, suggest that nitrate withdrawal could be related to serious complications in patients with coronary disease who discontinued long-acting nitrates in conjunction with a research protocol [21, 54]. Other studies are conflicting as to

whether there is rebound neurohumoral activation after nitrate administration in congestive heart failure [19, 44].

Several case reports have suggested that coronary vasospasm may represent a direct NTG effect [14], presumably idiosyncratic but conceivably related to an immediate increase in circulating catecholamines in patients given parenteral nitroglycerin.

Glaucoma

For many years it was believed that patients with glaucoma should not receive nitroglycerin. One recent report suggests that nitrates lower intraocular pressure in most patients with glaucoma, particularly in open-angle glaucoma [70]. At the present time, it appears to be safe to use nitrates in the presence of glaucoma.

Concomitant Alcohol Consumption

In the early literature on nitrate therapy there were a number of reports suggesting that there may be a particularly adverse interaction between sublingual NTG use and drinking alcohol. Over the years, it has been repeatedly stated that nitrates should be precluded in patients who actively drink. There is, however, little or no documentation of this problem. Normal volunteers who drank ethanol and then were given sublingual NTG [4] were studied. There was no synergistic reaction between ethanol and NTG. However, the blood pressure and heart rate responses to sublingual NTG were accentuated in combination with alcohol, and in the upright position, tachycardia and a significant decrease in systolic blood pressure occurred although the subjects remained asymptomatic. It is likely that in certain individuals with ischemic heart disease the combination of an excessive decrease in blood pressure and reflex sinus tachycardia could produce palpitations, dizziness, or chest pain.

ADVERSE REACTIONS DIRECTLY RELATED TO SPECIFIC NITRATE FORMULATIONS

Intravenous Nitroglycerin

METHEMOGLOBINEMIA

The potential of high concentrations of NTG to induce methemoglobinemia has long been recognized. Recent reports have documented increases in methemoglobin levels with high-dose nitrates, but the clinical significance of these observations is unclear [8, 25]. Sustained high-dose infusions of intravenous NTG or large amounts of topical NTG ointment would appear to be the likeliest formulations to result in potentially adverse plasma levels of methemoglobin. In such situations, physicians should be alert to this possibility; methemoglobin levels should be obtained in any cyanotic patient receiving large doses of nitroglycerin.

ALCOHOL INTOXICATION

The diluent used with commercial intravenous NTG preparations contains alcohol, and when high concentrations of NTG are infused for protracted periods of times, elevated blood alcohol levels could occur with resulting symptoms of excessive ethanol ingestion [26].

INTERFERENCE WITH HEPARIN THERAPY

It has recently been demonstrated that intravenous nitroglycerin may shorten the activated thromboplastin time (ATT, PTT) and thus can partially neutralize heparin action effects during systemic anticoagulation [9, 27]. This is of obvious potential importance in critical care units where intravenous nitroglycerin and heparin are often used together. Conversely, a sudden increase in PTT could occur if the nitroglycerin infusion is suddenly stopped. However, several more recent studies have been unable to confirm such an interaction between heparin and intravenous NTG, and the precise relationship between these agents remains unclear. Nevertheless, awareness of a potential effect on the PTT by intravenous NTG is appropriate for clinicians.

Topical Nitrates

Dermatitis and skin irritation is not rare following application of 2% NTG ointment or the transdermal NTG patches. Many patients note mild erythema of the skin in areas of direct contact with these formulations. Several rather unusual problems with the NTG patches have been reported, including electrical arcing with a resultant skin burn associated with D-C cardioversion and "explosion" of a nitroglycerin patch following exposure to a microwave oven!

NITRATE TOLERANCE

The most important problem in nitrate therapy is nitrate tolerance, long a controversial subject. The definition of drug tolerance includes a decreasing pharmacologic-hemodynamic effect over time, often with a need for increasing dosage to maintain a given drug effect. Nitrate tolerance has been suspected for many decades [2]. Early investigators noted the rapid attenuation of blood pressure lowering effects of organic nitrate esters used in the treatment of hypertension [58]. Subsequently, numerous other investigations have documented the decreasing effects of nitrates on systolic blood pressure with repeat dosing [66]. This is not necessarily correlated with an equivalent attenuation of other nitrate actions.

The disappearance of headache with chronic treatment is another commonly recognized aspect of nitrate tolerance. Here, of course, the appearance of apparent vascular tolerance in the cerebral circulation is welcome as a positive phenomenon.

In spite of the above observations, for many years it was believed that nitrate tolerance was not a clinically relevant issue [2]. Until very recently, most, but not all experts believed that tolerance was more of a laboratory than a patient-related phenomenon. In spite of several disturbing reports [9, 64, 66], early studies in angina and congestive heart failure were consistent with absence of tolerance [2, 20, 34]. However, since the early 1980s a large number of reports have appeared raising the specter that tolerance is a more common and serious problem than clinicians had been willing to believe. (See references 2, 3, 12, 48 for comprehensive reviews.) Studies in patients with both angina and congestive heart failure have contributed to this data base. In vivo animal [62] and human investigations in normal volunteers [37] have supported these clinical observations. Finally, the development of truly sustained acting nitrates, such as the transdermal NTG patches, have further focused attention on this issue, as these formulations appear to readily induce some degree of vascular tolerance within 24 hours after acute dosing. Limited data in long-term studies suggest that such continuous steady-state nitrate delivery may induce a total or nearly complete loss of clinical effectiveness [19, 29, 44, 50] (Fig. 15-5).

Many comparative studies, testing different formulations or different doses of the same drug, support the concept that frequent dosing regimens, high doses, or use of sustained action nitrates are more likely to induce nitrate tolerance when compared to fewer or smaller doses or administration of shorter acting nitrate compounds [3]. The concept of a nitrate-free interval has recently been emphasized and currently represents the best way to avoid nitrate tolerance.

Cellular Mechanisms of Tolerance

Recent evidence implicates a reduction in intracellular sulfhydryl or thiol groups within vascular smooth muscle cells as a putative factor in tolerance production [3, 28, 32]. Nitroglycerin and the organic nitrates exert their action through a cascade of intracellular events, as the parent nitrate ester undergoes conversion to nitric oxide (NO) and subsequently to s-nitrosothiol compounds (see Fig. 3-4) [28, 32, 41]. Both NO and nitrosothiols activate the enzyme guanylate cyclase within the cytoplasm, which in turn stimulates cyclic guanosine monophosphate (cGMP) production. This reaction is the final common pathway for smooth muscle relaxation induced by nitrates, sodium nitroprusside, and molsidomine [28, 32, 41]. It is of interest that particulate cGMP is activated by atrial natriuretic factor [41]. In addition, it appears that nitric oxide is the active component of endogenous endothelial relaxing

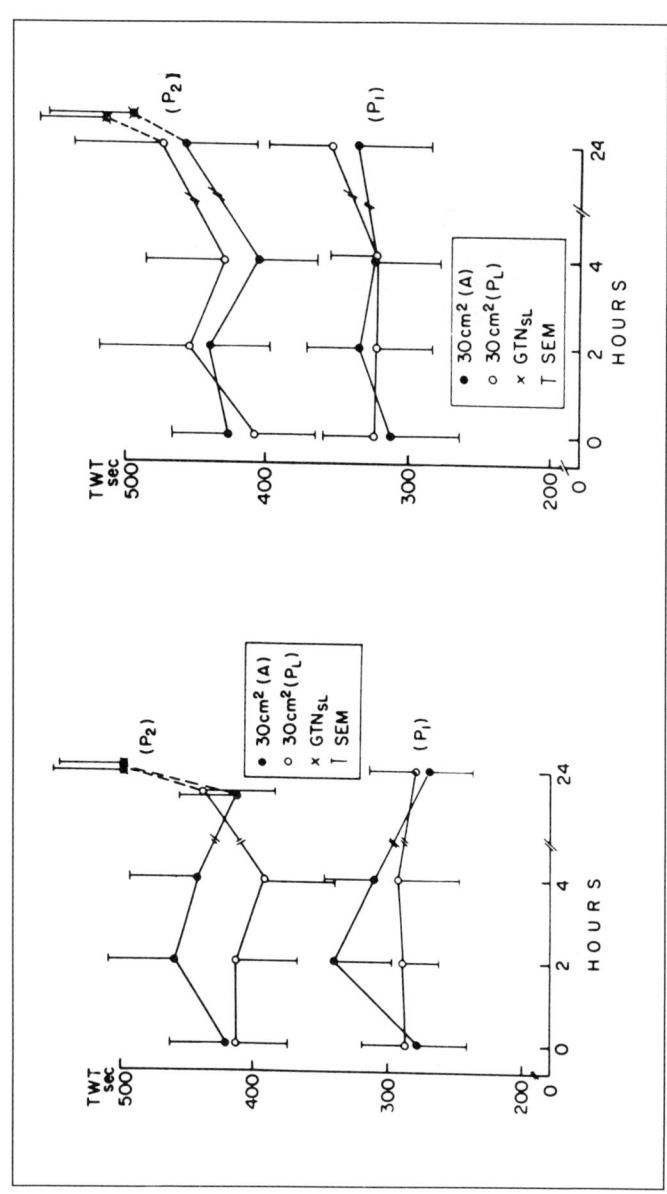

FIG. 15-5. Appearance of tolerance following continuous transdermal nitroglycerin administration. In this protocol, patients with angina were given transdermal NTG patches 15 mg/24 hours or placebo. With acute dosing (left) on the first day, treadmill walking time was prolonged over baseline at 2 and 4 hours after application of the active patch. However, by 24 hours attenuation had appeared such that there was no longer any antianginal protection compared to placebo. After 1 to 2 weeks of daily administration of the NTG patch, there was no longer any antianginal action at 2 and 4 hours; the active therapy was no different from placebo at any testing interval. (From Ref. 50, with permission.)

factor (ERDF), which also induces vascular smooth muscle relaxation and vasodilation in a flow-dependent manner and is an important regulator of arterial tone [63].

In the presence of nitrate tolerance, there appears to be a concomitant reduction in the supply of available intracellular thiols as well as a depression of guanylate cyclase activity and cGMP production. The decrease in vascular responsiveness may be partial or complete; tolerance is completely reversible if nitrate is removed from the vascular environment for sufficient time, presumably allowing for complete biochemical recovery of the cascade of nitrate conversion to nitrosothiols and restoration of maximal capability to induce cGMP [22]. Recent evidence suggests that the critical interaction of nitrate molecules with sulfhydryl donors may also involve extracellular mechanisms [23].

Other mechanisms that have been implicated in the production of nitrate tolerance include plasma volume expansion, activation of the renin-angiotensin system, and increased release of catecholamines related to counterregulatory sympathetic discharge [19, 44]. The latter phenomenon may result in pseudotolerance in the arterial circulation [62] (Fig. 15-6). In addition, a recent report suggests that neurohormonal activation might play a role in primary resistance to the beneficial effects of nitrates in patients with angina [5].

Pharmacokinetic Alterations in Tolerance

Several interesting modifications of nitrate pharmacokinetics have been documented to occur in the presence of nitrate tolerance (Table 15-5). Vascular smooth muscle nitrate metabolism is decreased; plasma levels of nitrate metabolites rise, perhaps relating to decreased nitrate clearance [22].

Venous Versus Arterial Tolerance

While it has been long believed that nitrate tolerance is an arterial phenomenon exemplified by the predictable loss of the hypotensive response to nitrates, recent evidence indicates that nitrate tolerance also affects the veins. In fact, one recent study suggested that the systemic venous bed is the major vascular circulation affected by nitrate tolerance whereas apparent arterial tolerance is actually a variant of pseudotolerance [1] (Fig. 15-6). A classic early study also documented the rapid onset of venous tolerance in the absence of arterial tolerance [71, 72]. More work needs to be done to resolve this issue.

CLINICAL STUDIES

Many recent investigations in angina as well as heart failure using varied nitrate formulations and dosing regimens have documented the ap-

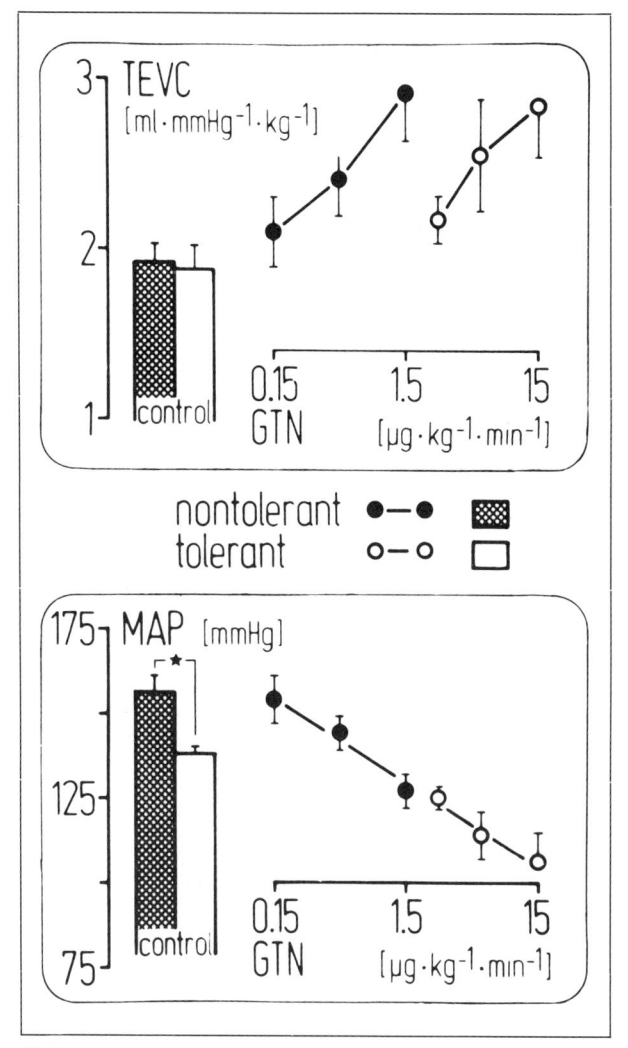

FIG. 15-6. Vascular nitrate tolerance: differential effects on veins and arteries. In this dog study, the animals were given a 4-day infusion of intravenous nitroglycerin to induce tolerance. The upper figure demonstrates a marked shift to the right of the venous dose-response curve, as assessed by measurements of TEVC (effective compliance of the total vascular bed), which reflects the capacitance of the venous circulation. Although there appeared to be arterial tolerance as well, as manifest by a failure of the mean arterial pressure (MAP) to decrease below baseline, when the animals were subjected to ganglionic blockade, there was a fall in the MAP in the tolerant dogs (open circles) without a shift in the NTG dose-response curve. These data suggest that true venous tolerance was produced, but that the arterial attenuation is in fact a pseudo-tolerance. Sympathetic activation was also demonstrated by documentation of increased catecholamine release in arterial blood. (From Ref. 62, with permission.)

TABLE 15-5. *Alterations in Nitrate Metabolism in Presence of Tolerance*

Decreased nitrate vascular clearance
Decreased arterial-venous nitrate gradient
Increased nitrate plasma levels
Decreased rate of nitrate metabolism in smooth muscle of blood vessel
Decreased activation of intracellular guanylate cyclase and formation of cyclic GMP

pearance of nitrate tolerance [9, 12, 19, 44, 48, 50, 64, 66]. Most earlier publications were not able to implicate clinically relevant tolerance in spite of attenuation of the arterial vasodilating properties of these drugs. Some of these studies employed nitrate dosing regimens that may actually have been salutary by allowing for a sufficient nitrate-free interval between the last regularly administered dose of the day and the first dose of nitrate the following morning that would maintain vascular responsiveness [16, 20, 34].

The most important work on nitrate tolerance in North America has come from the laboratory of Dr. John O. Parker in Ontario, Canada. This prolific investigator has published numerous studies indicating that tolerance is readily demonstrable in patients with angina by employing frequent nitrate dosing schedules or 24-hour sustained nitrate delivery [15, 48, 49, 50, 51, 52, 66]. Parker's work has documented a shortened duration of hemodynamic action and antianginal efficacy as well as a modest decrease in peak effect with qid dosing using oral ISDN (Figs. 9-5 and 15-3). His findings have confirmed that responsiveness to sublingual NTG is typically maintained in the tolerant state and that a nitrate-free interval restores full nitrate responsiveness [51].

In Europe, the work of Rudolph, Blasini, Silber, and Tauchert has consistently favored the presence of tolerance, while investigations of Distante et al. and Schneider et al. have not been supportive that nitrate tolerance is common. These studies, mostly in angina pectoris, have utilized a variety of nitrate formulation and dosing strategies. Many published trials support the concept that large doses, frequent administration, and sustained acting compounds are likely to produce nitrate tolerance. On the other hand, other studies from Europe have not been consistent with the appearance of significant tolerance, and this controversy is not completely resolved at this time. The interested reader is referred to several recent reviews of this subject [3, 12, 48, 61].

TRANSDERMAL NITROGLYCERIN

The popular NTG patches have focused considerable attention on the issue of nitrate tolerance because of the unexpected demonstration that

NTG effectiveness is frequently attenuated within 24 hours after patch administration. Numerous studies in angina and congestive heart failure have shown a waning efficacy of nitrate at 24 hours [29, 30, 44, 47, 50, 55, 65], although some Italian trials have demonstrated that tolerance at 24 hours is not present in all patients [39, 56]. Long-term data with transdermal nitroglycerin (TDNTG) are conflicting; Parker's early small study suggested a complete loss of effect with chronic dosing with TDNTG [50] (Fig. 15-5). However, an Italian multicenter trial demonstrated persistent nitrate effects in some subjects after 7 days of continuous treatment [39]. More recent investigations, employing intermittent transdermal nitroglycerin compared to continuous application, have also confirmed the loss of efficacy during daily 24-hour patch administration [13, 35, 42, 60].

The pharmacokinetic basis for the development of nitrate tolerance with the patches appears to be the sustained, steady-state level of NTG, without a nadir of low or near absent plasma nitrate concentrations. Studies with other long-acting formulations, including sustained release 5-ISMN [67], an ISDN ointment [53], and high-dose oral ISDN-sustained release capsules have reached similar conclusions [61]. Several recent reports have implicated continuous intravenous NTG infusion as a potential cause of nitrate tolerance [46, 68, 73]. A recent investigation by Parker demonstrated that bid and tid dosing with oral ISDN produced much less evidence for tolerance than qid dosing in the same patients [49], underscoring the problem of relatively constant nitrate delivery in enhancing the likelihood of tolerance induction (Fig. 9-5). Elkayam has provided similar data comparing qid to tid ISDN administration in heart failure [20].

Implications for Nitrate Therapy

Nitrate tolerance is clearly more common than previously thought. Some have maintained that treadmill testing is too rigorous a technique to detect relatively modest nitrate effects and argue that the widespread clinical acceptance and success of long-acting nitrates (e.g., control of patient symptoms) is often discordant with exercise test laboratory data that support the appearance of tolerance. Nevertheless, the results from many trials of disparate design are consistent with the observation that nitrate tolerance is predictably inducible by frequent nitrate administration and/or the use of sustained action or large doses of nitrates.

The deliberate institution of a nitrate-free interval of at least 8 to 10 hours is a valuable strategy to restore or maintain nitrate responsiveness. This approach has been recently documented to be important in therapy with transdermal NTG patches [13, 17, 35, 57, 60] and oral ISDN [20, 49, 61]. Table 15-6 summarizes those aspects of nitrate dosing regimens that potentiate the development of tolerance.

It is clear that successful use of nitrates requires appropriately de-

TABLE 15-6. *Dosing Factors That Promote Development of Nitrate Tolerance*

Sustained action nitrate formulations
Continuous nitrate delivery (e.g., patch, intravenous)
Large doses
Frequent doses
Failure to provide a sufficient duration of nitrate-free period

signed dosing strategies. These are not difficult to create; the regimen should vary with the nature of nitrate formulation. Table 9-3 provides suggestions as to how best to administer available nitrate formulations while avoiding the development of nitrate tolerance.

NITRATE-FREE INTERVAL

In vitro and in vivo experiments indicate that removal of vascular smooth muscle from exposure to nitrates will restore blood vessel reactivity after a period of time. It has been suggested that the failure to develop nitrate tolerance may be related in part to a phasic decline in plasma nitrate concentrations, perhaps with a minimal threshold concentration that would vary for different nitrate compounds [22, 61]. It is unlikely that the organic nitrate must disappear completely from the circulating blood, but rather that nitrate levels be allowed to decrease substantially over a protracted period of time on a daily basis.

Two important large trials have been recently completed that confirm the desirability of intermittent NTG patch administration. A major trial of continuous therapy in over 500 subjects given a wide range of doses (15 to 105 mg per 24 hours) was completely negative after 6 to 8 weeks of daily patch application [40]. No improvement in antianginal efficacy was observed in any dosing group compared to placebo, even in the very large dose groups. On day one, an anti-ischemic action was confirmed only at 4 hours after administration. A newly published trial of 200 patients given intermittent NTG patch therapy (12 hours on—12 hours off) demonstrated a continued antianginal action over a 1-month period [17]. Some attenuation of duration of NTG action was noted, and there was a suggestion of patch-off angina in a small group of patients (Fig. 15-7). These data are consistent with the concept that intermittent nitrate therapy is a viable approach to avoid significant tolerance. The safety of such a dosing strategy remains to be resolved [1].

It is possible that the veins have a different time course of nitrate tolerance development as well as reversal than the arteries; venous nitrate metabolism is more avid and complete than that of the arteries and arterioles [22, 24]. There may also be differences in the ability of

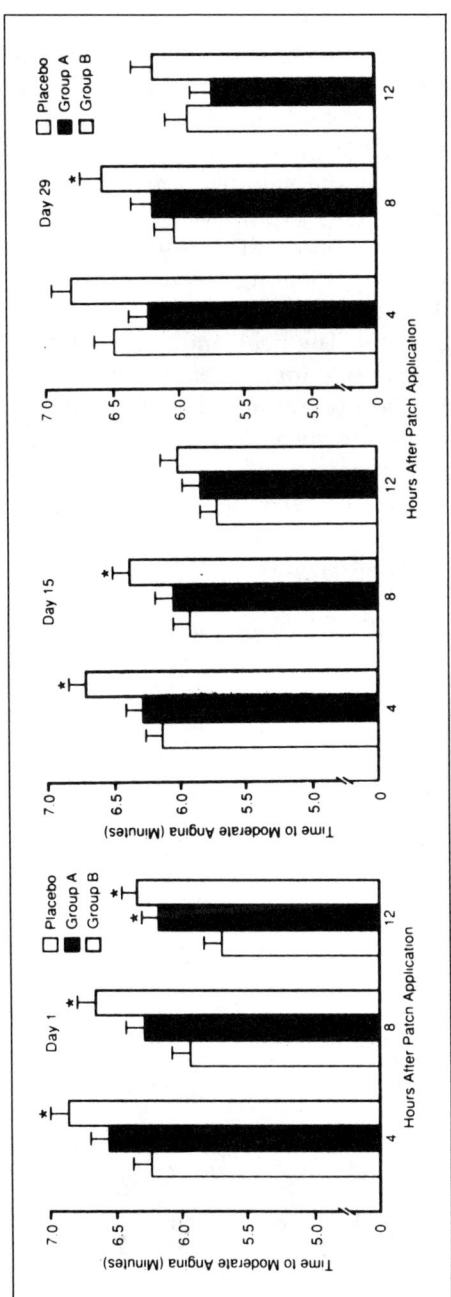

FIG. 15-7. Lack of development of significant tolerance with chronic intermittent transdermal nitroglycerin. In this large study of 206 patients, preservation of antianginal effects of transdermal NTG when compared to placebo patches was noted at 2 and 4 weeks after daily 12-hour administration of transdermal nitroglycerin with subsequent removal for 12 hours. Note that there was a significant difference from placebo on all three study days at 4 and 8 hours for the high dose group B (30 to 40 cm^2) although the 4-hour test period on day 29 did not achieve statistical significance, probably because of an increase in placebo exercise time at that testing interval. The patches failed to significantly improve angina at 12 hours after administration at all test intervals during chronic administration. This study confirms data from a number of smaller trials indicating that an intermittent dosing regimen with transdermal nitroglycerin, with patch removal for 10 to 12 hours daily, preserves nitroglycerin responsiveness in patients with effort angina. (From Ref. 17, with permission.)

various nitrate formulations, such as NTG, ISDN, and 5-ISMN, to produce tolerance.

The minimum duration of time required for a nitrate-free interval that will maintain vascular reactivity is uncertain. Parker's early data suggested that no more than 21 hours is necessary when using oral ISDN [48, 51]; this is obviously not practical for chronic dosing. His more recent study indicated that tid dosing, with the last dose of oral ISDN given at 5:00 P.M. and the first dose at 8:00 A.M., maintained antianginal activity [49] (Fig. 9-5). It is likely that the time interval necessary for disappearance of tolerance varies with the nitrate formulation employed. The longer acting the formulation, as well as the longer the vascular exposure (e.g., 24-hour application of transdermal NTG patches or infusion of intravenous NTG), the longer will be the likely requisite nitrate-free time interval. Experimental data and one recent clinical report appear to confirm this [45]. The peak and nadir levels of plasma and tissue nitrates may also be important [61], but plasma nitrate concentrations are not available to clinicians. Yet plasma nitrate concentrations are useful to help investigators resolve issues relative to the design of tolerance avoidance dosing strategies.

In conclusion, it is highly desirable for physicians deliberately to include a nitrate-free interval when devising a nitrate dosing regimen for patients. Therapeutic strategies that include the principles outlined in the above discussion should provide for predictable nitrate responsiveness and maintained clinical efficacy of these most useful agents [1].

REFERENCES

1. Abrams, J. Interval therapy to avoid nitrate tolerance: Paradise regained? *Am. J. Cardiol.* 64:931–34, 1989.
2. Abrams, J. Nitroglycerin tolerance and dependence. *Am. Heart J.* 99:113, 1980.
3. Abrams, J. Tolerance to organic nitrates. *Circulation* 74:1181, 1986.
4. Abrams, J., Schroeder, K., Raizada, V., Gibbs, D. Potentially adverse effects of sublingual nitroglycerin during consumptioin of alcohol. *J.A.C.C.* 15:226A, 1990.
5. Agabati-Rosei, E., Muiesan, M. L., Beschi, M., et al. Antianginal efficacy of transdermal nitroglycerin as related to adrenergic and renin-aldosterone systems. *Circulation* 76(Supp IV) IV:128, 1987.
6. Andrien, P., and Lemberg, L. An unusual complication of intravenous nitroglycerin. *Heart-Lung* 15:534, 1986.
7. Armstrong, P. W., Armstrong, J. A., and Marks, L. S. Pharmacokinetic-hemodynamic studies of nitroglycerin ointment in congestive heart failure. *Am. J. Cardiol.* 46:670, 1980.
8. Arsura, E., Lichstein, E., Guadagnino, V., et al. Methemoglobin levels produced by organic nitrates in patients with coronary artery disease. *J. Clin. Pharmacol.* 24:160, 1984.
9. Blasini, R., Froer, K. L., Blumel, and Rudolph. W. Wirkungverlust von

isosorbiddnitrat bei langzeitbehandlung der chronischen herzinsuffizienz. *Herz* 7:250, 1982.
10. Col, J., et al. Propylene glycol-induced heparin resistance during nitroglycerin infusion. *Am. Heart J.* 110:171, 1986.
11. Come, P. C., and Pitt, B. Nitroglycerin-induced severe hypotension and bradycardia in patients with acute myocardial infarction. *Circulation* 54:624, 1976.
12. Cowan, J. C. Nitrate tolerance. *Int. J. Cardiol.* 12:1, 1986.
13. Cowan, J. C., Bourke, J. P., Reid, D. S., and Julian, D. G. Prevention of tolerance to nitroglycerin patches by overnight removal. *Am. J. Cardiol.* 60:271, 1987.
14. Dalal, J. J., McCans, J. L., and Parker, J. O. Nitroglycerin-induced coronary vasoconstriction. *Cath. Cardiovasc. Diag.* 10:33, 1984.
15. Dalal, J. J., Yao, L., and Parker, J. O. Nitrate tolerance: Influence of isosorbide dinitrate on the hemodynamic and antianginal effects of nitroglycerin. *J.A.C.C.* 2:115, 1983.
16. Danahy, D. T., and Aronow, W. S. Hemodynamics and antianginal effects of high dose oral isosorbide dinitrate after chronic use. *Circulation* 56:205, 1977.
17. Demots, H., and Glasser, S. P. Intermittent transdermal nitroglycerin therapy in the treatment of chronic stable angina. *J.A.C.C.* 13:786–93, 1989.
18. Elkayam, U., Henriquez, B., Weber, L., et al. Lack of hemodynamic effect of high dose transdermal nitroglycerin in severe heart failure. *Circulation* 70(Suppl II):II-381, 1984.
19. Elkayam, U. Roth, A., Henriquez, B., et al. The hemodynamic and hormonal effects of high-dose transdermal nitroglycerin in patients with chronic congestive heart failure. *Am. J. Cardiol.* 56:555, 1985.
20. Elkayam, U., Jamison, M., Roth, A., et al. Oral isosorbide dinitrate in chronic heart failure: tolerance development of qid vs tid regimen. *J.A.C.C.* 13:176A, 1989.
21. Franciosa, J. A., Nordstrom, L. A., Cohn, J. N. Nitrate therapy for congestive heart failure. *J.A.M.A.* 240:443, 1978.
22. Fung, H.-L. Pharmacokinetic determinants of nitrate action. *Am. J. Med.* 76(6A):22, 1984.
23. Fung, H.-L., Chong, S., Kowaluk, K., et al. Mechanisms for the pharmacologic interaction of organic nitrates with thiols. Existence of an extracellular pathway for the reversal of nitrate vascular tolerance by N-acetylcysteine. *J. Pharmacol. Exp. Ther.* 245:524–30, 1988.
24. Fung, H.-L., Sutton, S. C., and Kamiya, A. Blood vessel uptake and metabolism of organic nitrates in the rat. *Pharmacol. Exp. Ther.* 228:334, 1984.
25. Gibson, G. R., Hunter, J. B., Raabe, D. S., et al. Methemoglobinemia produced by high-dose intravenous nitroglycerin. *Ann. Int. Med.* 96:615, 1982.
26. Gould, L., Reddy, C. V. R., Swamy, C. R. N., and Dorismond, J. C. The effect of nitroglycerin on atrioventricular conduction in man. *Am. J. Med.* 60:922, 1976.
27. Habbab, M., and Haft, J. Heparin resistance induced by intravenous nitroglycerin: A word of caution when both drugs are used concomitantly. *Arch. Int. Med.* 147:856, 1987.
28. Ignarro, L. J., Lippton, H., Edwards, J. C., et al. Mechanism of vascular smooth muscle relaxation by organic nitrates, nitrites, nitroprusside and nitric oxide: Evidence for the involvement of s-nitrosothiols as active intermediates. *J. Pharmacol. Exp. Ther.* 218:739, 1981.
29. Jordan, R. A., Seth, L., Caesbolt, P., et al. Rapidly developing tolerance to

transdermal nitroglycerin in congestive heart failure. *Ann. Int. Med.* 104:295–98, 1986.
30. Jordan, R. A., Seth, L., Henry, D. A., et al. Dose requirements and hemodynamic effects of transdermal nitroglycerin compared to placebo in patients with congestive heart failure. *Circulation* 71:980–86, 1985.
31. Khan, A. H., and Carleton, R. A. Nitroglycerin-induced hypotension and bradycardia. *Arch. Int. Med.* 141:984, 1981.
32. Kukovetz, W. R., and Holzmann, S. Mechanisms of nitrate-induced vasodilatation and tolerance on a biochemical base. *Z. Kardiol.* 74(Suppl 1):39, 1985.
33. Lange, R. L., Reid, M. S., Tresch, D. D., et al. Non-atheromatous ischemic heart disease following withdrawal from chronic industrial nitroglycerin exposure. *Circulation* 46:666, 1972.
34. Lee, G., Mason, D. T., and DeMaria, A. Effects of long-term oral administration of isosorbide dinitrate on the antianginal response to nitroglycerin. Absence of cross-tolerance and self-tolerance shown by exercise testing. *Am. J. Cardiol.* 41:82, 1978.
35. Luke, R., Sharpe, N., and Coxon, R. Transdermal nitroglycerin in angina pectoris: Efficacy of intermittent application. *J.A.C.C.* 10:642, 1987.
36. Magrini, F., and Niarchos, A. P. Ineffectiveness of sublingual nitroglycerin in congestive heart failure in the presence of massive peripheral edema. *Am. J. Cardiol.* 45:841, 1980.
37. Manyari, D. E., Smith, E. R., and Spragg, J. Isosorbide dinitrate and glyceryl trinitrate: Demonstration of cross tolerance in the capacitance vessels. *Am. J. Cardiol.* 55:927, 1985.
38. Morton, W. E. Occupational habitation to aliphatic nitrates and the withdrawal hazard of coronary disease and hypertension. *J. Occup. Med.* 19:197, 1977.
39. Muiesen, G., Asabiti-Rosen, E., Muiesen, L., et al. A multicenter trial of transdermal nitroglycerin in exercise-induced angina: Individual antianginal response after repeated administration. *Am. Heart J.* 112(1):233–38, 1986.
40. Multicenter Transdermal Nitroglycerin Trial, in press.
41. Murad, F. Cyclic guanosine monophosphase as a mediator of vasodilation. *Clin. Invest.* 78:1, 1987.
42. Nabel, E. G., Barry, J., Mead, K., et al. Effects of high dose transdermal nitrates on ambulatory ischemia and tolerance (Abstract). *Circulation* 76(Supp IV):IV-128, 1987.
43. Nemerovski, M., and Shah, P. K. Syndrome of severe bradycardia and hypotension following sublingual nitroglycerin administration. *Cardiology* 67:180, 1981.
44. Olivari, M. T., Carlyle, P. F., Levine, B., and Cohn, J. N. Hemodynamic and hormonal response to transdermal nitroglycerin in normal subjects and in patients with congestive heart failure. *J.A.C.C.* 2:872, 1983.
45. Packer, M., Gottlieb, S., Kessler, P. D., et al. Overnight withdrawal of nitroglycerin therapy does not prevent the development of nitrate tolerance in severe heart failure. *J.A.C.C.* 11:43A, 1988.
46. Packer, M., Lee, W. H., Kessler, P. D., et al. Prevention and reversal of nitrate tolerance in patients with congestive heart failure. *N. Engl. J. Med.* 317:799, 1987.
47. Packer, M., Medina, N., Yoshak, M., and Lee, W. H. Factors limiting the response to transdermal nitroglycerin in severe chronic heart failure. *Am. J. Cardiol.* 57:260, 1986.
48. Parker, J. O. Nitrate tolerance. *Am. J. Cardiol.* 60:44H, 1987.
49. Parker, J. O., Farrell, B., Lahey, K. A., and Moe, G. Effect of intervals

between doses on the development of tolerance to isosorbide dinitrate. *N. Engl. J. Med.* 316:1440, 1987.
50. Parker, J. O., and Fung, H.-L., Transdermal nitroglycerin in angina pectoris. *Am. J. Cardiol.* 54:471, 1984.
51. Parker, J. O., Fung, H.-L., Ruggirello, D., and Stone, J. A. Tolerance to isosorbide dinitrate: Rate of development and reversal. *Circulation* 68:1074, 1983.
52. Parker, J. O., VanKoughnett, K. A., and Farrell, B. Comparison of buccal nitroglycerin and oral isosorbide dinitrate for nitrate tolerance in stable angina pectoris. *Am. J. Cardiol.* 56:724, 1985.
53. Parker, J. O., Van Koughnett, K. A., and Fung, H.-L. Transdermal isosorbide dinitrate in angina pectoris: Effect of acute and sustained therapy. *Am. J. Cardiol.* 54:8, 1984.
54. Rehnqvist, N., et al. Abrupt withdrawal of long-term (≥ 1 year) prophylactic nitrate therapy in stable angina pectoris (Abstract). *Cardiovasc. Drugs Ther.* 1:279, 1987.
55. Reichek, N., Priest, C., Zimrin, D., et al. Antianginal effects of nitroglycerin. *Am. J. Cardiol.* 54:1–7, 1984.
56. Scardi, S., Pivotti, F., Fonda, F., et al. Effect of a new transdermal therapeutic system containing nitroglycerin on exercise capacity in patients with angina pectoris. *Am. Heart J.* 110:546, 1985.
57. Schaer, D. H., Buff, L. A., and Katz, R. J. Sustained antianginal efficacy of transdermal nitroglycerin patches using an overnight 10-hour nitrate-free interval. *Am. J. Cardiol.* 61:46, 1988.
58. Schelling, J., and Lasagna, L. A study of cross-tolerance to circulatory effects of organic nitrates. *Clin. Pharmacol. Ther.* 8:256, 1966.
59. Schwartz, A. M. The cause, relief and prevention of headaches arising from contact with dynamite. *N. Engl. J. Med.* 235:651, 1946.
60. Sharpe, N., Coxon, R., Webster, M., and Luke, R. Hemodynamic effects of intermittent transdermal nitroglycerin in chronic congestive heart failure. *Am. J. Cardiol.* 59:895, 1987.
61. Silber, S. Clinical relevance of nitrate tolerance. In J. N. Cohn and R. Rittinghausen (eds.), *Mononitrates*. Berlin: Springer-Verlag, 1985. P. 130.
62. Stewart, D. J., Elsner, D., Sommer, O., et al. Altered spectrum of nitroglycerin action in long-term treatment: Nitroglycerin-specific venous tolerance with maintenance of arterial vasodepressor potency. *Circulation* 75:573, 1986.
63. Stewart, D. J., Holtz, J., and Bassenge, E. Long-term nitroglycerin treatment: Effect on direct and endothelium-mediated large coronary artery dilation in conscious dogs. *Circulation* 75:847, 1987.
64. Tauchert, M., Jansen, W., Osterspey, A., et al. Dose dependence of tolerance during treatment with mononitrates. *Z. Kardiol.* 72(Suppl 3):218, 1983.
65. Thadani, U., Brady, D. C., Klutts, S. J., et al. Dose titration and duration of effects of transdermal nitroglycerin patches in angina pectoris. *Circulation* 72(Suppl III):III-431, 1985.
66. Thadani, U., Fung, H.-L., Darke, A. C., and Parker, J. O. Oral isosorbide dinitrate in angina pectoris. Comparison of duration of action and dose response relationship during acute and sustained therapy. *Am. J. Cardiol.* 49:411, 1982.
67. Thadani, U., Hamilton, S. F., Olson, E., et al. Duration of effects and tolerance of slow-release isosorbide-5-mononitrate for angina pectoris. *Am. J. Cardiol.* 59:756, 1987.
68. Thadani, U., Sharma, M., Thompson, D., et al. Intravenous nitroglycerin and tolerance in unstable angina. *Circulation* 76(Suppl IV) IV:128, 1987.

69. Vatner, S. F. Pagani, M., Rutherford, J. D., et al. Effects of nitroglycerin on cardiac performance and regional blood flow distribution in conscious dogs. *Am. J. Physiol.* 234(3):H244, 1978.
70. Wizemann, A., Wizemann, V., and Krey, H. Organic nitrates—a new principle in glaucoma therapy? In P. R. Lichtler, H.-L. Engel, A. Schrey, and H. J. C. Swan (eds.) *Nitrates III.* Berlin: Springer-Verlag, 1981. Pp. 582–86.
71. Zelis, R., and Mason, D. T. Isosorbide dinitrate. Effect on the vasodilator response to nitroglycerin. *J.A.M.A.* 234:166, 1975.
72. Zelis, R., Mason, D. T., Spahn, J. G., and Amsterdam, E. A. The mechanism of action of nitroglycerin in the relief of angina pectoris: Reduction of myocardial oxygen requirements by vasodilation and its attenuation by the chronic administration of isosorbide dinitrate. *Ann. Int. Med.* 72:779, 1970.
73. Zimrin, D., Reichek, N., Bogin, K., et al. Antianginal effects of nitroglycerin over 24 hours. *Circulation* 77:1376, 1988.

CHAPTER 16

PROBLEMS WITH BETA BLOCKER THERAPY

STEPHEN F. HAMILTON
BETH H. RESMAN-TARGOFF
EDWIN G. OLSON
UDHO THADANI

The beta-adrenergic receptor blocking drugs have widespread utility in clinical practice but the use of these agents has resulted in many adverse reactions. This chapter will review problems associated with beta blocker therapy in the hope that knowledge of potential therapeutic problems will promote judicious use and a reduction in the incidence of adverse reactions to these agents. Problems associated with beta blockers that are an extension of their pharmacologic action will receive special attention since these adverse effects should be predictable and therefore avoidable. There are times, however, when clinical judgment suggests the use of these agents in situations that are considered relative contraindications and some increased risk of toxicity is accepted. However, these situations demand increased patient monitoring.

PREDICTABLE ADVERSE REACTIONS

The predictable adverse reactions to beta blocker therapy are discussed below (Table 16-1).

Cardiovascular (Beta-1 Effects)

The cardiovascular side effects of the beta blockers are, most commonly, symptomatic bradycardia (Fig. 16-1) [22], hypotension, and ventricular dysfunction. These are beta-1 side effects and are extensions of the pharmacologic actions of these agents. Patients with little myocardial reserve are at increased risk for these adverse reactions. There is no convincing data proving that agents with intrinsic sympathomimetic activity cause fewer side effects. All these side effects have been noted with beta-1 selective and nonselective agents.

TABLE 16-1. *Predictable Adverse Reactions to Beta Blocker Therapy*

Cardiovascular manifestations (Beta-1 effects)
  Bradycardia
  Hypotension
  Ventricular dysfunction
Peripheral vascular manifestations (Beta-2 effects)
  Increased total peripheral resistance
  Decreased blood supply to extremities
  Muscle fatigue
Respiratory dysfunction (Beta-2 effects)
  Bronchospasm
  Dyspnea
Carbohydrate homeostasis (Beta-2 effects)
  Inhibition of insulin release
  Inhibition of metabolic response to hypoglycemia
  Inhibition of hemodynamic response to hypoglycemia

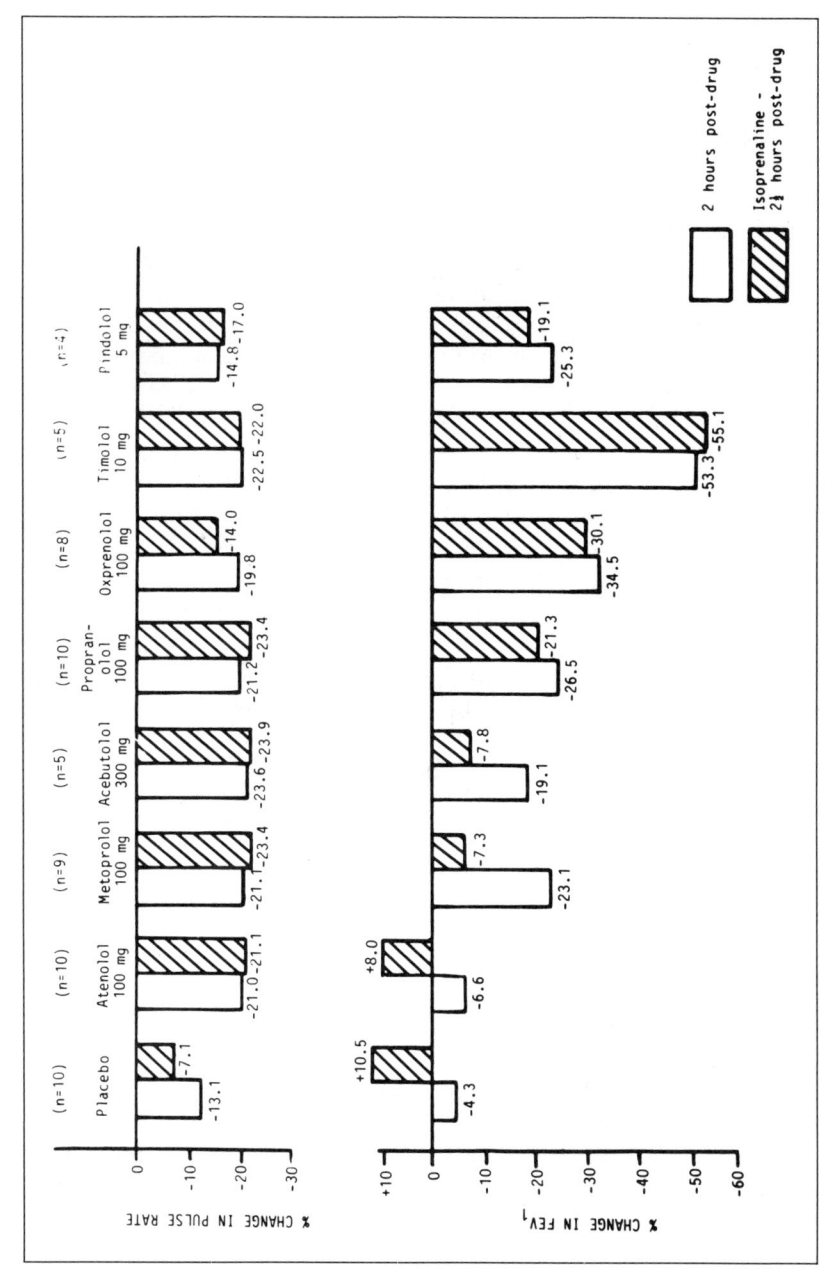

FIG. 16-1. Effect of various beta blockers (as a percentage change from baseline) and isoprenaline (isoproterenol) upon standing pulse rate (beats per minute) and FEV-1 (liters). (From Ref. 23, with permission.)

Esmolol is a cardioselective, ultra short acting (half-life = 9 minutes), intravenous beta blocker used to slow the ventricular response rate in supraventricular tachycardia. A rapid reduction in heart rate of 15 to 20 percent under baseline is usually achieved; however, significant hypotension has been reported in as many as 44 percent of patients [147]. Other serious side effects appear to occur much less often. The recovery from these side effects is rapid compared to other available intravenous beta blockers [147].

Ophthalmic application of timolol has been associated with the adverse reactions mentioned earlier. Most studies of normal volunteers or patients with glaucoma exclude patients with heart disease; when decreases in heart rate or blood pressure were noted, most subjects were asymptomatic. Doses of timolol ophthalmic drops can produce serum concentrations similar to trough levels seen with chronic oral therapy. Boger et al. [12] reported an average decrease of 9 beats per minute in heart rate after the application of ophthalmic timolol but two patients had decreases of 28 beats per minute. All subjects remained asymptomatic. Another report noted that resting and exercise pulse rates were reduced by 0.8 mg (two drops in each eye) of ophthalmic timolol [1]. A third report noted that, while resting pulse had been unaffected by ophthalmic timolol, a significant tachycardia of 10 to 15 beats per minute over baseline occurred 2 weeks after abrupt discontinuation of ophthalmic timolol [129]. Betaxolol is an agent that appears to be beneficial in glaucoma and may have fewer side effects than timolol.

The use of beta blockers is contraindicated in atrioventricular block greater than first degree since complete heart block is a risk with further suppression of nodal conduction. Further, the ventricular rate in Wolff-Parkinson-White Syndrome can be accelerated by beta blockers.

Peripheral Vascular (Beta-2 Effects)
The adverse effects of the beta blockers on the peripheral vascular system include increasing total peripheral resistance, decreased blood supply to the extremities, and muscle fatigue. The effects are caused by blockade of the beta-2 receptor. Increasing sympathetic tone stimulates the beta-2 receptors in peripheral arteries, which results in a decreased total peripheral resistance, a fall in diastolic pressure, and an increase in muscle perfusion. Blockade of the beta-2 receptor will diminish each of these effects.

INCREASED TOTAL PERIPHERAL RESISTANCE
The response to infusions of adrenaline (increased systolic (beta-1) and decreased diastolic pressure) has been altered by pretreatment with nonselective beta-receptor blockade. Two studies have shown that pretreatment with a nonselective beta blocker and subsequent adrenaline infusion results in a diminished rise in systolic pressure and unchanged

or increased diastolic pressure [70, 157]. The lack of vasodilation or actual increase in total peripheral resistance in response to adrenaline in these subjects is due to a combination of beta-2 blockade, causing a diminished ability to dilate, and unopposed alpha mediated vasoconstriction. This effect is less pronounced when selective beta-1 blockers are used in the low dosage range. Similar results have been reported in patients subjected to stress (simulated automobile driving, smoking cigarettes, or hypoglycemia). These subjects may show an increased mean arterial pressure and a fall in peripheral perfusion [27, 82, 154].

COLD HANDS AND FEET

Patients occasionally report varying degrees of symptomatic cold hands and feet, most frequently in colder climates. The mechanism may be a decrease in cardiac output and an inability to increase blood supply to the extremities. Therefore, beta blockers with beta-1 selectivity, intrinsic sympathomimetic activity, or associated alpha blockade could be beneficial in these patients. McSorley and Warren [104] reported that beta-1 selective agents are less likely to reduce skin temperature, but the data could be strengthened by further study. Also, patients with intermittent claudication reported worsening of symptoms on beta blockers and beta-1 selective agents were of no advantage. The primary mechanism in these patients is likely to be a decrease in cardiac output (beta-1) associated with widespread atheromatous disease [128]. No convincing data support the use of agents with intrinsic sympathomimetic activity or alpha blockade in these patients.

RAYNAUD'S PHENOMENON

A report by Marshall et al. [95] reported a 50 percent incidence of Raynaud's phenomenon in hypertensive patients being treated with beta blockers. The incidence with methyldopa was 5 percent in this report. There have also been reports of peripheral gangrene [48, 124, 153, 155]. The normal fall in digital arterial pressure in response to cooling has been shown to be exaggerated during propranolol treatment, but the mechanism of this reaction is unclear. It has been suggested that a possible enhancement of alpha-receptor sensitivity known to occur during beta blockade may be responsible [165].

Muscle Fatigue (Beta-2 Effect)

Muscle fatigue is a frequent complaint of patients being treated with beta blockers. The problem is complex and multiple organ systems are likely to be involved. Some authors describe muscle fatigue under peripheral vascular disturbances that may be responsible for symptoms in many patients, but metabolic and psychological factors may also be involved. The numerous possible mechanisms all seem to involve the beta-2 receptor. Muscle perfusion is reduced by a decreased cardiac output and by inhibition of vasodilation as a result of beta blocker therapy. There is a resulting decrease in delivery of oxygen, glucose, and free fatty acids along with an accumulation of lactic acid with beta blocker therapy [46]. The metabolic alterations that may be associated with beta blockade include impaired glycogenolysis in both the liver and muscle [80]. There is also modification of potassium transport across the red blood cell membrane that could be functional in the muscle [17, 130].

Psychological factors relating to fatigue will be discussed in the section titled Unpredictable Adverse Reactions: Central Nervous System. As for the other mechanisms mentioned, a beta-1 selective agent would be of theoretical advantage. Unfortunately, a number of studies have failed to show an unequivocal advantage of beta-1 selectivity. One study did indicate that comparable doses of metoprolol had an advantage over propranolol when muscle fatigue was evaluated objectively by treadmill exercise [91]. Mean treadmill walking time to exhaustion was 152 minutes on placebo, 117 minutes on metoprolol, and 88 minutes on propranolol. Propranolol caused a greater decrease in serum glucose and a more pronounced rise in free fatty acid concentrations compared to metoprolol. However, this well-documented, objective evidence may not directly relate to fatigue during normal daily life.

The complaint of lower limb fatigue has been reported during normal daily exertion in some patients on both beta-1 selective and nonselective agents [54]. Full beta blockade has been shown to decrease muscle work performance in daily life [145]. These effects have been assessed by maximal work capacity [3] or perceived exertion [122] for both selective and nonselective beta blockers.

Respiratory Dysfunction (Beta-2 Effects)

Blockade of the beta-2-adrenergic receptors in the lung has resulted in predictable respiratory dysfunction in select groups of patients (Fig. 16-1) [22]. The mechanism for this effect is not completely understood but seems to be related to unopposed parasympathetic activity following beta blockade in patients with predisposing risk factors. Bronchospasm in patients with reactive airway disease that was considered to be potentially fatal was reported early after the widespread use of propranolol [102, 103]. Asthmatic patients show an increased responsiveness to histamine or acetylcholine after beta blockade [103, 172]. This evidence suggests that patients who smoke, have bronchitis or other forms of dyspnea may be at increased risk of bronchospasm during beta blocker treatment and should be monitored carefully. Beta-1 selective agents may be of benefit in these groups. Beta-1 selective agents have been shown to cause less deterioration of respiratory function than nonselective agents in asthmatic patients [143, 151]. The response to beta-2 agonists is less likely to be diminished when selective beta-1 blockers are used [142,151]. Therefore, if these patients experience bronchospasm when being treated with a nonselective beta blocking agent, they would likely receive more benefit from beta-2 agonists if a selective beta-1 blocker were used.

Ophthalmic application of timolol (a nonselective beta blocker) for treatment of glaucoma has been associated with significant episodes of respiratory dysfunction. The Food and Drug Administration has compiled 22 reports of cases of status asthmaticus, including one death, associated with timolol ophthalmic drops [5, 42]. These effects were not noted in normal subjects but were found to be significant in patients with reactive airway disease or chronic obstructive pulmonary disease [1, 42, 137, 138]. Five patients with chronic obstructive airway disease who continued to take all oral medications had a significant fall in 1 second forced expiratory volume 15 minutes after the instillation of one drop of 0.5% timolol ophthalmic in each eye. This effect was sustained for 3 hours and dyspnea developed in four of the five subjects [138]. A similar dose and design were used to study patients with reactive airway disease. A mean 26 percent fall in the 1 second forced expiratory volume was recorded for the nine subjects. Two subjects terminated the study early due to severe dyspnea [137].

Carbohydrate Homeostasis (Beta-2 Effect)

Alterations of carbohydrate homeostasis as a result of blockade of the beta-2 receptor is the final predictable adverse effect of beta blockers discussed in this chapter. Catecholamines stimulate the release of insulin from the Islets of Langerhans; therefore, beta blockade can result in elevated serum glucose concentrations in susceptible subjects. In addition, the metabolic and hemodynamic responses to hypoglycemia mediated by catecholamines are diminished by beta blockade. Each of these effects will be discussed as well as the place for selective beta blockers in therapy.

HYPERGLYCEMIA

The concern that beta blockade could precipitate diabetes mellitus by inhibiting insulin release is unsubstantiated. However, glycemic control of diabetic patients may be disrupted or made more difficult in the presence of beta blockers. Wright et al. [170] have reported impaired glucose control in diabetic patients. However, the rise in glucose is reported to be small when beta-1 selective agents are used [161, 170].

METABOLIC RESPONSE TO HYPOGLYCEMIA

The control of glucose mobilization from the liver during periods of hypoglycemia is largely under the control of the beta-adrenergic receptors, primarily the beta-2 receptors [73]. A delayed recovery from periods of hypoglycemia during beta blocker use, especially with nonselec-

TABLE 16-2. *Unpredictable Adverse Reactions to Beta Blocker Therapy*

Central nervous system effects
  Vivid or disturbing dreams
  Lethargy
  Depression
  Acute confusion
  Hallucinations
Gastrointestinal effects
  Mild indigestion
  Nausea
  Constipation
Skin reactions (uncommon)
Sexual dysfunction
  Impotence
Neuromuscular effects
  Myasthenic syndrome
  Worsening of myasthenia gravis or myotonia

tive agents, has been reported by several authors [21, 57, 63, 78, 113, 141, 144]. Hypoglycemia as a result of beta blockade is rare but has been reported during periods of extreme exertion [64], prolonged starvation [49], and in neonates born to women treated with beta blockers [131]. Hypoglycemia has also been reported with the use of timolol ophthalmic drops [4, 158].

HEMODYNAMIC RESPONSE TO HYPOGLYCEMIA

Diminished hemodynamic response to hypoglycemia is a result of blockade of both beta-1 and beta-2 receptors. Blockade of beta-1 receptors interferes with the compensatory increase in heart rate and systolic blood pressure while blockade of beta-2 receptors interferes with the compensatory fall in diastolic pressure caused by hypoglycemia [90]. The nonselective agents may cause a marked increase in blood pressure associated with severe bradycardia [82].

UNPREDICTABLE ADVERSE REACTIONS

Beta blocker therapy may produce unpredictable adverse reactions (Table 16-2). These reactions are discussed below.

Central Nervous System (CNS)

There are beta receptors in the brain, and all beta blockers can cross the blood brain barrier and exert effects. See Chapter 7 for a discussion of beta blocker distribution to the central nervous system. The most often reported CNS effects are sleep disturbances, vivid and disturbing dreams, lethargy, depression, acute confusion and hallucinations [101, 115]. Impairment of psychomotor function has also been reported [121]. The less lipophilic beta blockers, such as atenolol and nadolol, are often substituted for the more lipophilic beta blockers, such as metoprolol, propranolol, or pindolol, when CNS side effects occur. However, as is discussed in Chapter 7, the water-soluble agents can accumulate in the cerebrospinal fluid and adverse effects are possible.

The Boston Collaborative Drug Surveillance Program [53] reported an overall incidence of CNS side effects of 3.1 to 4.3 percent while the incidence of depression was noted to be 1.6 percent. Visual hallucinations were reported in 11 of 77 patients taking a mean daily dose of 254 mg of propranolol [39]. In hospitalized patients (a group who may be more sensitive to CNS side effects) who were receiving propranolol there were reports of light-headedness (1.5 percent), tiredness and drowsiness (1.2 percent), and insomnia (0.5 percent) [52]. Other reported effects include visual and tactile disturbances of perception [38].

A review of the use of propranolol in psychiatry reported 18 cases of psychosis [2]. Waal described 27 patients with depressive symptoms, including two suicides and two other patients who required antidepressant therapy. The incidence of depression-type symptoms increased with increasing dose with 50 percent of those treated with 120 mg per day for 3 months being affected [160]. There have been many suggestions of CNS side effects from ophthalmic timolol. However, only three detailed cases of CNS side effects have been reported. These included two cases of hallucinations [168, 171] and one case of depression, weight loss, and attempted suicide [4]. The effects occurred within 3 months to 1 year of initiating treatment and symptoms stopped when the eye drops were discontinued.

More recently, objective assessment of CNS toxicity with beta blocker therapy has been attempted. Numerous studies have been reported that attempt to use psychometric testing to evaluate differences in CNS effects of various beta blocking agents. These tests are in early development and little normative data exist; the reliability and validity data are not always available. Therefore, the results of these studies should be cautiously interpreted [93]. The majority of these tests favor the hydrophilic agents (e.g., atenolol) over the lipophilic agents (e.g., metoprolol) [10, 120, 156]. However, McDevitt has reviewed the effects of beta blockers with psychometric performance studies in normal volunteers [96]. The results of the chronic dosing studies suggest that the effects of beta blockers may be sporadic and may not be more significant with lipophilic beta blocking agents [96]. These effects of either lipophilic or hydrophilic beta blocking drugs were comparable to CNS effects of diazepam [96]. Three recent studies favor atenolol over pindolol [40], propranolol [20, 164], or metoprolol [164]. Daily doses of atenolol 100 mg or pindolol slow release 20 mg were compared using a highly sensitive analog scale in a 24-week outpatient study of 107 hypertensive patients, many of whom experienced CNS complaints before beta blocker therapy. The atenolol group had significantly fewer sleep disturbances. No other differences in vivid dreams or fatigue, muscle cramps, sexual disturbances or gastrointestinal side effects reached statistical significance [40]. Before treatment, the atenolol group had a 38 percent incidence of sleep disturbances, whereas the pindolol group had a 33 percent incidence. After 12 weeks of treatment, the incidence of sleep disturbances changed to 27 percent versus 44 percent and at 24 weeks, 18 percent versus 48 percent for atenolol and pindolol, respectively. A study comparing lipophilic beta blockers (metoprolol or propranolol) to atenolol in 14 hypertensive patients who had experienced hallucinations ($N = 2$) or nightmares ($N = 12$) within the previous two years while on metoprolol ($N = 9$), propranolol ($N = 4$), or pindolol ($N = 1$) favored the hydrophilic agent atenolol. Fourteen patients experienced a total of 54 episodes of nightmares or hallucinations on the lipophilic agents compared to three patients experiencing eight episodes while on atenolol in this double-blind 4-week crossover study [164]. These subjects were not poor metabolizers of the lipophilic beta blockers. A similar study design used in patients who experienced significant side effects with lipophilic beta blockers also favored atenolol for a reduction of several CNS side effects [20].

Gastrointestinal (GI)
Gastrointestinal disturbances are common in all drug trials, often occurring as frequently with placebo as with active drug. Information on beta blocker GI disturbances is no different. The most frequent GI complaints of patients on beta blocker therapy include mild indigestion, nausea, or constipation in the minority of patients. It is not possible to explain these vague effects based on beta blockade in the GI tract. There is little evidence that these complaints are more frequent than the placebo response [96]. The evidence is similar for ophthalmic timolol [5].

Skin Reactions
Beta blockers cause comparatively few skin reactions and those that occur are not related to beta blockade [67, 96]. The cutaneous reactions associated with practolol are unique and covered later in this chapter. There have been about 44 reports of dermatologic reactions to ophthalmic timolol. Alopecia and stomatitis are the most common, but urticarial manifestations have also been reported [138].

Sexual Dysfunction
Sexual dysfunction is a common complaint of patients being treated for hypertension, and this affects quality of life for many patients. Even

without treatment, impotence is more frequent in hypertensive subjects than in nonhypertensive control groups [15]. The frequency of combination antihypertensive therapy makes identification of a specific drug as a causative factor very difficult.

In a trial of treatment of mild hypertension, impotence occurred in 14 percent of patients after 12 weeks of therapy with propranolol compared to 9 percent of the control patients [105]. This difference was not statistically significant. Impotence has been reported with other beta blockers and some of these reports are convincing [79, 106]. However, it is not clear whether this effect is specific for beta blockade or a coincidental finding. There is one case report of erectile dysfunction relieved when propranolol was replaced by atenolol [8]. Erectile dysfunction may be related to adrenergic blockade, which decreases penile blood flow. Erection is believed to be mediated predominantly through cholinergic pathways causing vasodilation. However, the vasculature of the corpora cavernosa and corpus spongiosum are supplied with adrenergic and cholinergic fibers. Therefore, sympathetic pathways acting on beta-2 receptors may be involved in erection. There has been a study that demonstrated reduced penile blood flow in impotent patients on propranolol [41]. The addition of alpha blockade to beta blockade in the treatment of hypertension could theoretically increase the incidence of sexual dysfunction.

Neuromuscular Side Effects

Interference with neuromuscular transmission has been demonstrated in rats treated with beta blockers [84]. Further, there are occasional reports of propranolol, oxprenolol [62], and practolol [66] inducing a myasthenic syndrome or unmasking myasthenia gravis. One case report described worsening of myasthenia gravis within 24 hours of starting ophthalmic timolol [139]. Propranolol has also been reported to worsen myotonia [11].

MISCELLANEOUS PROBLEMS WITH BETA BLOCKER THERAPY

The following sections describe miscellaneous problems encountered with beta blocker therapy (Table 16-3).

Long-Term Adverse Effects

CARCINOGENICITY
Early beta blockers have been associated with tumor generation in laboratory animals. Pronethalol, the first beta blocker to gain wide clinical use, was withdrawn because it was associated with thymic

TABLE 16-3. *Miscellaneous Problems with Beta Blocker Therapy*

Long-term adverse effects
  Carcinogenicity
Practolol syndrome
  Psoriasis-like lesions
  Ocular disorders
  Sclerosing peritonitis
Overdosage
  Bradycardia
  Hypotension
  Low output cardiac failure
  Cardiogenic shock
  Bronchospasm
  Grand mal seizures
Beta blocker withdrawal
  Rebound hypertension
  Rebound angina
Use in pregnancy
  Low birth weight
  Neonatal bradycardia
  Neonatal hypoglycemia
Use in the elderly
  May require dosage reduction

tumors and lymphosarcomata in mice [119]. Tolamolol and pametolol were similarly withdrawn from early trials because of an association with mammary tumors in mice and rats at higher dosages [45]. These tumors were alarming but usually occurred in one species of animal and after high dosages were administered. Fortunately, the beta blockers currently in use have not shown any tumorigenic tendencies and are considered safe by the Food and Drug Administration. Postmarketing surveillance has not identified increased cancer rates with these drugs in humans.

Practolol Syndrome

The practolol syndrome is presented here because of the infrequent but severe lesions reported and for a historical perspective on beta blocker side effects. An excellent detailed review of this syndrome has been published [74]. Some patients being treated with practolol developed one or more of three different manifestations of this syndrome: skin reactions resembling psoriasis, a series of ocular disorders, and a form of sclerosing peritonitis. Some of these reactions were mild and patients usually developed only one manifestation. However, there were reports of blindness or peritoneal adhesions, which required surgery. Some cases of death were also reported. Most nonfatal manifestations subsided when practolol was stopped and some patients later were successfully treated with other beta blockers without development of similar lesions. No similar reaction has been detected with postmarketing surveillance of any other beta blocker currently marketed.

Overdosage with Beta Blockers

The response to superpharmacologic doses of beta blockers does not lend itself to controlled clinical studies; however, rare reports of poisoning exist. It is clear that beta blockers have a large therapeutic index and are remarkably safe. Several case reports have been reviewed [29] and Frishman et al. have an excellent review of overdosage [44]. The predominant features of overdosage with beta blockers are bradycardia, hypotension, low cardiac output failure, and cardiogenic shock. Fatalities have occurred when the heart is unable to respond to pharmacologic or electrical stimulation. Bronchospasm may occur and grand mal seizures have been reported. The lipophilic agents are rapidly absorbed and probably exhibit saturable first-pass absorption. This is likely to lead to significant CNS depression, but since these agents have a short half-life, they will be eliminated hepatically if cardiac output can be maintained. The hydrophilic beta blockers are less well absorbed and may be less likely to affect the brain. However, they are longer acting and cardiac output must be maintained to insure adequate renal perfusion for elimination of these agents. Other ancillary properties may be important in overdosage. Frishman et al. [44] reported two cases of pindolol overdosage where, presumably, the intrinsic sympathomimetic activity caused an increase in blood pressure and tachycardia. Membrane stabilizing activity may result in further myocardial depression [127].

In general, the management of beta blocker overdosage involves removing the agent, if possible, by emesis or lavage and providing cardiovascular and respiratory support. Bradycardia is first treated with 0.5 to 3 mg of intravenous atropine and an isoproterenol infusion of 4mg/min if needed. Finally, transvenous pacing may be required. Bronchospasm usually responds to beta-2 stimulants and theophylline, while diazepam is used to treat seizures. Finally, glucose is given to treat hypoglycemia. As the patient recovers, evidence of beta blocker withdrawal may require treatment with alpha blockade or clonidine to decrease sympathetic outflow from the central nervous system.

Beta Blocker Withdrawal

Abrupt withdrawal of long-term beta blocker therapy has been associated with symptoms of rebound hypertension and rebound anginal episodes [58]. It is beyond the scope of this chapter to review fully rebound hypertension, but a few comments are in order since many patients have concomitant hypertension and coronary artery disease. Any treatment for hypertension should be gradually withdrawn over a period of at least 2 to 4 weeks. When abrupt withdrawal of beta blockers cannot be avoided in hypertensive patients, monitoring of blood pressure response is critical. A rise to pretreatment blood pressure is expected. When treatment is withdrawn, however, or when the rate of rise is rapid, an "overshoot phenomenon" can result in a hypertensive emergency. This may be aborted by careful (hourly) monitoring of vital signs and early treatment within the first 12 hours of withdrawal.

The occurrence of rebound anginal episodes after beta blocker withdrawal was first suggested by Wilson et al. [167] in 1969, who reported that 7 of 19 patients experienced status anginosus when placebo was substituted for oxprenolol. Further, a convincing double-blind crossover trial documented a 50 percent incidence of rebound ischemia after discontinuing propranolol [107]. There are also two reports that fail to show an increase in angina in hospitalized patients awaiting coronary catheterization [111, 140]. These patients were likely to have less exercise or other provocation for anginal episodes than the patients in the previously mentioned studies. The mechanism of this withdrawal phenomenon is complex and several possible factors may be involved. It is clear that these side effects do not occur in all subjects and do not show a strong correlation with dose.

The possible factors involved in the increase in anginal symptoms after abrupt withdrawal of beta blockade include first, a continuation of physical activity without therapy to reduce myocardial oxygen demand. A second factor may involve increased or hypersensitive response to baseline endogenous beta stimulation. This may be a result of increased numbers of post-synaptic beta receptors that developed during long-term beta blockade [169]. Elevations of circulating catecholamines after withdrawal may be a factor [112] but the supporting evidence is weak and this is not the case in many subjects [81, 92]. Increased affinity of catecholamines for the existing receptors may be involved. Finally, propranolol therapy causes a favorable shift in the oxyhemoglobin dissociation curve [86], diminishes platelet aggregation [43], and suppresses renin release [13]. Reversal of any of these effects could increase anginal symptoms in some patients. Regardless of the precise mechanism, it is clear that beta blockade should be withdrawn gradually in patients with ischemic heart disease and other therapies should be instituted to decrease myocardial oxygen demand.

Beta Blockade in Pregnancy

Beta blockers are used during pregnancy for the treatment of hypertension, arrhythmias, thyrotoxicosis, or cardiomyopathies, hypertrophic or obstructive. The majority of information deals with hypertension and pregnancy. It is not surprising that little information exists regarding pregnancy and ischemic heart disease. Therefore, only a brief review will be presented here.

When the alarming fetal mortality and morbidity of untreated hypertension is considered, the benefits of drug therapy often outweigh the risks. This is the case for beta blockers. Many studies confirm the benefit of propranolol [30, 150], oxprenolol [47], sotalol [118], atenolol [24, 152], acebutolol [24, 26], and pindolol [24] in the treatment of hypertensive pregnant subjects. Adverse effects have been reported. The most common have been low birth weight and neonatal bradycardia and hypoglycemia. These effects have been noted in many of the above studies but are usually transient. Low birth weight may be a result of diminished placental perfusion, which has been demonstrated in some animal models but not in humans.

Severe hypertension is associated with diminished placental perfusion and only one study found intrauterine growth retardation associated with propranolol therapy for any condition other than hypertension [123]. One retrospective study of severely hypertensive pregnant patients suggested that propranolol may be associated with unfavorable outcomes, but other drugs and factors could not be ruled out [87]. Since beta blockade prevents the response to hypoxia and could be associated with placental insufficiency, it is reasonable to choose other antihypertensive agents as the first choice in severe hypertension. There is no evidence that beta blockers are teratogenic and nursing infants do not seem to achieve doses capable of causing beta blockade [88]. Most studies of the use of propranolol to treat thyrotoxicosis during pregnancy failed to show an increased incidence of low birth weight infants or other ill effects on the fetus or neonate [14, 83].

Beta Blockade in Elderly Patients

It is often presumed that elderly patients have more frequent and perhaps more severe side effects of drug therapy. While it is prudent to be conscious of physiologic alterations during aging, there is little evidence that beta blockade causes an alarming rate of adverse reactions in this population. With aging, there can be a decrease in total body water, an increase in body fat, and a decrease in lean body mass. However, if these changes take place, they apparently are not dramatic enough to cause a remarkable change in the effect of beta blockade. There does not appear to be any significant increase in side effects with prudent use of beta blockers in the elderly [52]. In practice, the beta blockers are well tolerated in hypertensive elderly patients [166]. However, lower doses and the beta-1 selective agents were used more frequently [166].

DRUG INTERACTIONS WITH BETA BLOCKERS

When the treatment of a patient requires more than one drug, potential drug interactions must be considered. Given the large and growing number of potent pharmacologic agents for use in seriously ill patients, it is easily understood that no one can be aware of every potential

TABLE 16-4. *Drugs Documented to Have Significant Interactions with Beta Blocker Therapy*

Barbiturates	Methimazole
Cimetidine	Oral contraceptives
Epinephrine	Prazosin
Hydralazine	Propylthiouracil
Indomethacin	Rifampin
Insulin	Theophylline
Lidocaine	Verapamil

interaction. This topic is manageable, however, if one considers the mechanism of action or pharmacologic class of each drug in a patient's therapeutic regimen and whether those mechanisms will interact to the potential harm of the patient. The potentially harmful interactions include changes in the pharmacodynamic response by alterations in pharmacokinetic properties (absorption, distribution, metabolism, or excretion), or additive or competing changes in physiologic response. This section is presented as a guideline to understanding significant adverse drug interactions and it should not be considered an exhaustive review of this extensive topic (Table 16-4). Weak evidence exists for many drug interactions; these will not be covered [9, 50]. Where there is any doubt, specialists in drug and therapeutic information evaluation should be consulted.

Indomethacin

Indomethacin is known to elevate blood pressure and several studies suggest that it can blunt the hypotensive effects of beta blockers. In a single-blind placebo-controlled study [28], the mean diastolic blood pressures of seven patients treated with either pindolol (15 mg per day) or propranolol (80 to 160 mg per day) were recorded after 10 days of indomethacin or placebo. The mean diastolic blood pressures during two control periods (before and after the study), while on beta blocker therapy, were approximately 83 mm Hg, which was not significantly different from the placebo period. However, the diastolic blood pressure increased to a mean of 97 mm Hg after 10 days of indomethacin (100 mg per day). Similar results were found when indomethacin (100 mg per day) was added to propranolol [162], oxprenolol [132], and atenolol [133]. Sulindac did not reduce the antihypertensive effect of atenolol in the last study mentioned; therefore no conclusions can be stated for other nonsteroidal anti-inflammatory agents. Antihypotensive effects have been reported for aspirin (5 gm/24 hours) and sulfinpyrazone (400 mg twice daily), but more study is needed [37, 149].

Antiarrhythmics

LIDOCAINE
The pharmacokinetic interaction between several beta blockers and lidocaine is well established. Propranolol [11, 18, 116, 135, 148] and nadolol [135] both decreased the clearance of lidocaine by approximately 15 to 50 percent and increased the steady-state serum lidocaine concentrations by 20 to 30 percent in normal volunteers. Similar results have been reported for metoprolol [18]; however, conflicting data exist. Atenolol and pindolol have been studied and no apparent interaction exists [109]. However, caution should be used whenever any beta blocker is combined with lidocaine in patients with compromised cardiac function. This interaction could result from either decreased hepatic blood flow and/or decreased cardiac output. It is surprising that only two well-described cases of lidocaine intoxication from this interaction exist [57].

Other antiarrhythmic agents have been studied. Coadministration of disopyramide and beta blockers are possibly harmful to any patient with a low ejection fraction because both agents depress contractility. However, this interaction is not well studied in this population. Preliminary evidence of a drug interaction between procainamide and propranolol could not be confirmed in a well-controlled study [117]. Quinidine can significantly increase the total serum concentration and the concentration of the active (-) enantiomer in subjects who were extensive metabolizers of metoprolol [85]. (See Chapter 7 for a discussion of polymorphic oxidative metabolism of metoprolol.) Propranolol, which is not subject to polymorphic oxidative metabolism, is unaffected by quinidine [36]. Further, quinidine disposition is unaltered by propranolol [36, 71, 77].

Antihypertensives

CLONIDINE
The concurrent use of clonidine and beta blockers involves complex interactions. The most serious interaction may occur when clonidine is abruptly discontinued. The withdrawal symptoms, which can include agitation, headaches, and rebound hypertension, are associated with an increase in circulating catecholamines. When the beta-adrenergic receptors are blocked, there is a condition of unopposed alpha-adrenergic stimulation [7, 89, 146, 159]. This situation can become expressed as severe rebound hypertension and may also occur when a patient is switched from clonidine to beta blocker therapy. The most specific treatment is reinstitution of small doses of clonidine. Labetalol may also prevent this reaction by virtue of its combined alpha and beta blockade. This interaction is complex and would seem to be more likely with

nonselective beta blockers; however, it has been reported with atenolol [89].

HYDRALAZINE

Hydralazine and beta blockers interact in several ways. The combined use of beta blockers and hydralazine is well established in hypertension where both agents act to decrease blood pressure. Further, the beta blockers diminish the reflex tachycardia often associated with hydralazine.

Another interaction involves an increase in the oral bioavailability of the lipophilic beta blockers (propranolol, oxprenolol, and metoprolol) by hydralazine [16, 59, 68, 69, 99, 136]. Since these lipophilic beta blockers exhibit clearance that is highly correlated with hepatic blood flow, hydralazine may be responsible for a hemodynamically mediated decrease in hepatic first-pass extraction. Hydralazine shows a dose-dependent effect in increasing the bioavailability of propranolol by 50 to 110 percent. This effect is not seen when subjects are fasting or when they take sustained release formulations of propranolol. The bioavailability of beta blockers that do not undergo extensive first-pass extraction (acebutolol, atenolol, nadolol, and timolol) is not increased [68, 100]. The serum concentration of hydralazine may be increased by propranolol [134] but is not affected by oxprenolol [59].

METHYLDOPA

Two cases of a paradoxical hypertensive reaction from the combination of methyldopa and the nonselective beta blockers propranolol [114] and oxprenolol [97] have been reported. In the first, a patient already taking methyldopa experienced a cerebrovascular accident and was given an intravenous dose of propranolol, then developed a hypertensive response. The second case involved a patient taking methyldopa and oxprenolol who developed severe hypertension (200/150 mm Hg) with the addition of a nonprescription cold product containing phenylpropanolamine. The blood pressure dropped to 140/110 mm Hg with the discontinuation of the nonprescription product. Presumably both these reactions involved unopposed alpha stimulation.

PRAZOSIN

The extent and duration of the first-dose hypotensive effect of prazosin may be increased with beta blockade. The blunting of the compensatory increase in heart rate and perhaps contractility is the likely mechanism. This has been reported for both selective and nonselective beta blockers [31]. The addition of beta blockers to the regimen of patients stable on prazosin does not seem to cause acute hypotension.

Anti-Infectives

RIFAMPIN
Treatment of patients with enzyme-inducing agents such as rifampin can increase the first-pass hepatic metabolism of propranolol and metoprolol [13, 40, 78]. The effects seen with 1200 mg/day of rifampin were not greater than with 600 mg/day. This would seem to be true for other lipophilic beta blockers. The clinical consequences of this decreased bioavailability have not been determined.

Barbiturates

PENTOBARBITAL
Barbiturates, which are known enzyme-inducers, markedly decrease the bioavailability of lipophilic beta blockers. The mechanism appears to involve an increase in first-pass hepatic clearance. Pentobarbital decreased the area under the serum concentration–time curve of metoprolol by 32 percent [55], while the bioavailability of timolol (not lipophilic) was not changed [94].

Calcium Channel Antagonists

NIFEDIPINE, DILTIAZEM, AND VERAPAMIL
The combined use of beta blockers and calcium channel antagonists is beneficial in many patients with angina pectoris. However, caution must be used, especially in patients with minimal myocardial reserve. The reflex sympathetic activity resulting from vasodilation caused by nifedipine usually offsets its negative inotropic effects. However, in patients receiving beta blockers, the combined negative inotropic effects may become evident. Nifedipine has no appreciable effect on AV conduction. In contrast, verapamil and diltiazem both have additive effects to beta blockers in depressing contractility and AV conduction. Severe bradycardia and congestive heart failure can result. High-grade AV block may also occur. Beta blockers do not appear to cause alterations in the pharmacokinetics of calcium channel antagonists. However, verapamil may increase metoprolol (lipophilic) but not atenolol (not lipophilic) serum concentrations [98].

Beta-Adrenergic Blockers
There is no reason to prescribe more than one beta blocker at one time to any patient.

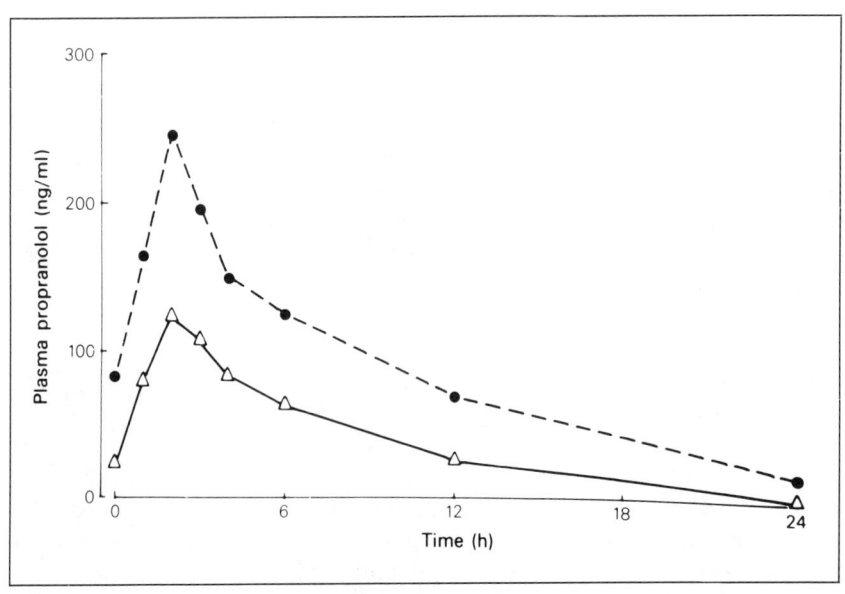

FIG. 16-2. Mean plasma concentrations of propranolol, as a function of time, following the last oral dose of propranolol 80 mg as monotherapy (▲) and after combination with cimetidine 200 mg on day 7 (●) ($N = 6$). (From Ref. 110, with permission.)

H-2 Antagonists

CIMETIDINE

Several studies have demonstrated that cimetidine can significantly increase serum concentrations of propranolol [25, 35, 61, 110, 126] (Figs. 16-2 and 16-3). The mechanism of this interaction may be a reduction in hepatic blood flow or competitive inhibition of hepatic metabolism. The clinical consequences of this interaction have been difficult to document; bradycardia was reported in one study, and one case report of bradycardia with hypotension exists [23, 35]. The data are less convincing, but this interaction may also be seen with metoprolol. Atenolol, pindolol, and nadolol, which are not lipophilic, are not involved in this interaction.

RANITIDINE

Similar data exist for an interaction between metoprolol and ranitidine as for propranolol and cimetidine. However, the extent of beta blockade of exercise-induced tachycardia was not different in the ranitidine or control group. A larger body of data exists that disputes these findings (Figs. 16-4 and 16-5) [72]. The interaction is considered unlikely since

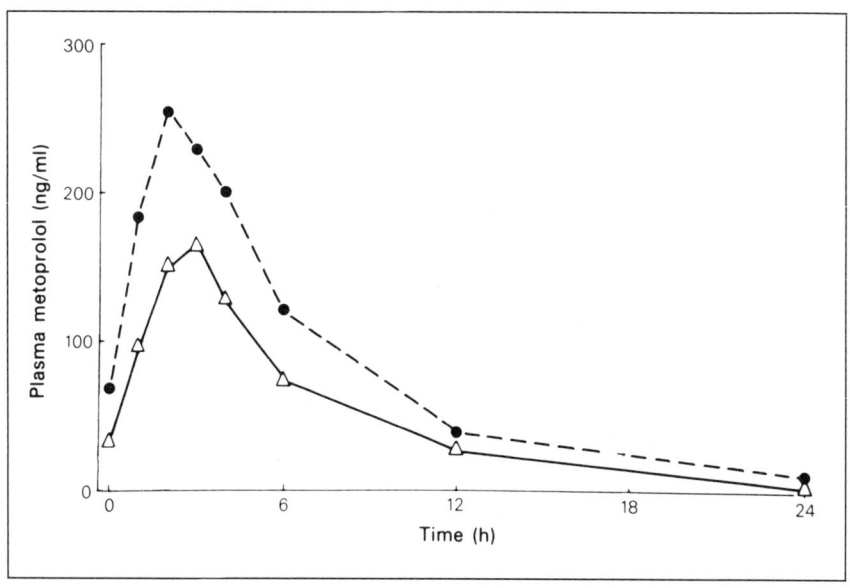

FIG. 16-3. Mean plasma concentrations of metoprolol, as a function of time, following the last oral dose of metoprolol 100 mg as monotherapy (▲) and after combination with cimetidine 200 mg on day 7 (●) ($N = 6$). (From Ref. 110, with permission.)

ranitidine does not alter the clearance of antipyrine. Further, several authors have failed to show an interaction between propranolol and ranitidine [60, 126].

Hypoglycemics

INSULIN
Beta-adrenergic blockade can alter the physiologic response to hypoglycemia. Gluconeogenesis or glycogenolysis may be blunted with nonselective beta blockade. Hemodynamically, there may be a significant increase in diastolic pressure and no increase in heart rate with hypoglycemia. The agents with intrinsic sympathomimetic activity and cardioselective agents may be safer in diabetic patients. There is conflicting evidence that propranolol can blunt tolbutamide-stimulated insulin release [109, 110].

Methylxanthines

THEOPHYLLINE
Beta blockers can cause bronchospasm in patients with reactive airway disease. The cardioselective agents in low doses may produce less

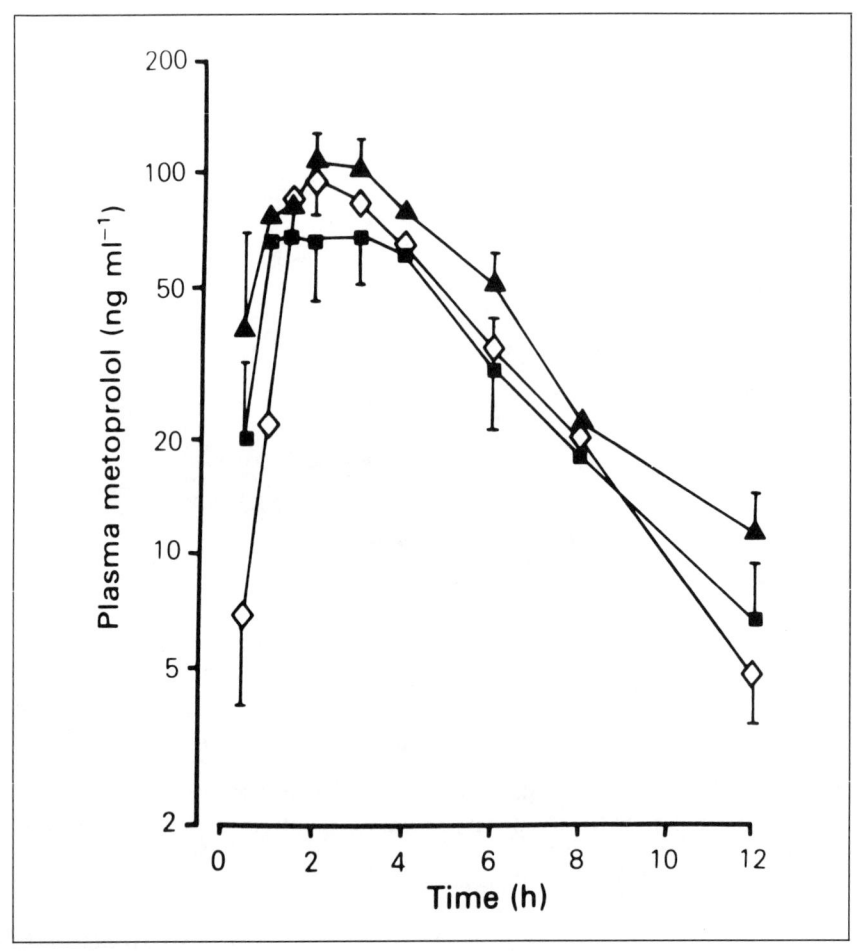

FIG. 16-4. Plasma concentrations following orally administered metoprolol 100 mg before (■), during (▲), and after (◇) ranitidine. Mean of six subjects ± s.e. mean. (From Ref. 72, with permission.)

bronchospasm in patients with obstructive airway disease. Also, propranolol has been reported to decrease theophylline clearance by 30 to 50 percent [19, 108]. This could lead to theophylline toxicity when propranolol is added to the regimens of patients with high therapeutic serum concentrations of theophylline. Metoprolol did not significantly reduce the mean theophylline clearance in a group of unselected subjects. However, in smokers (subjects with high theophylline clearance), metoprolol did appear to reduce theophylline clearance [19].

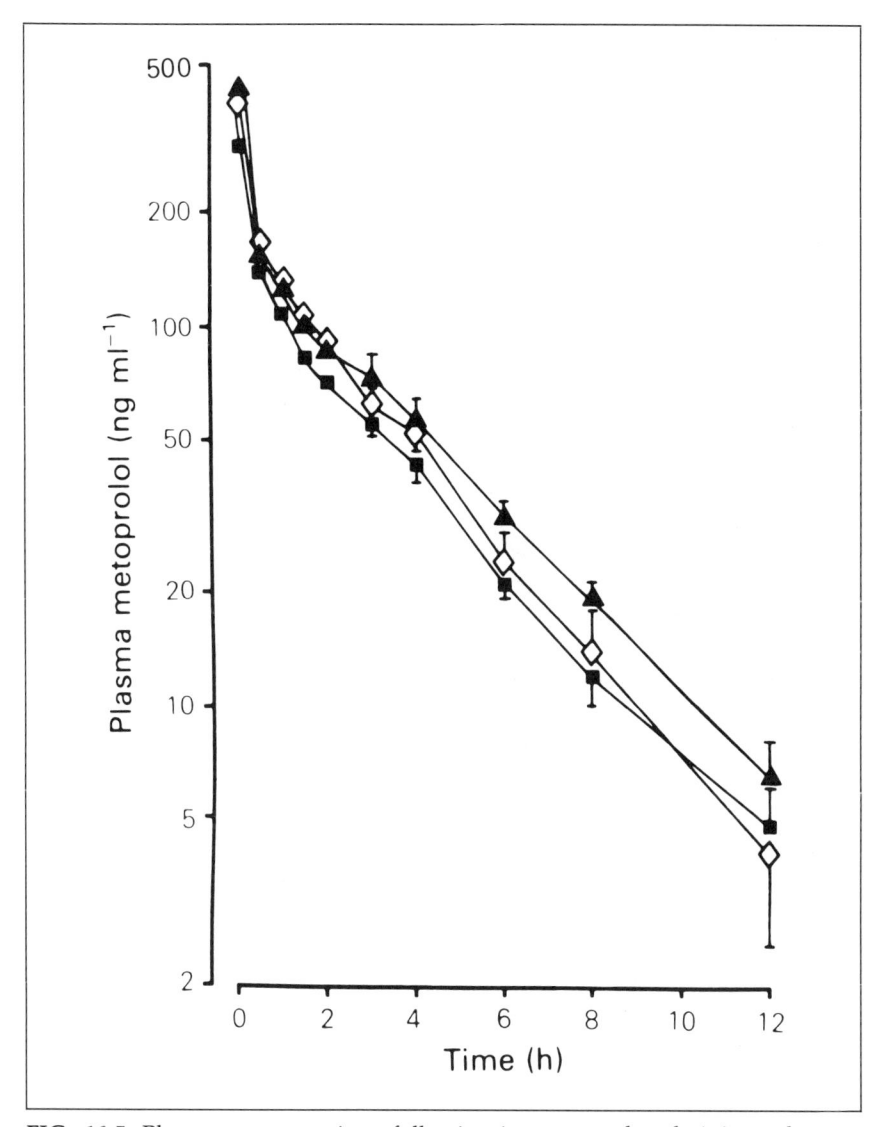

FIG. 16-5. Plasma concentrations following intravenously administered metoprolol 50 mg before (■), during (▲), and after (◇) ranitidine. Mean of six subjects ± s.e. mean. (From Ref. 72, with permission.)

Oral Contraceptives

ESTROGEN CONTRACEPTIVES

The pharmacokinetic profiles of single oral doses of several different beta blockers administered to 69 women have been compared based on whether or not the women were users of low-dose estrogen contraceptives [75, 76]. The mean area under the serum concentration–time curve for metoprolol was approximately 40 percent greater in the women who were users of the oral contraceptives. The effect of beta blockade was not measured. No changes for other beta blockers reached statistical significance.

Sympathomimetics

EPINEPHRINE

Besides the obvious interaction between beta agonists and antagonists, administration of epinephrine to patients on propranolol has resulted in dramatic rises in both systolic and diastolic blood pressure and significant bradycardia [65, 125]. This effect was not seen when epinephrine was administered to a subject receiving metoprolol [65]. Therefore, this effect may be a result of nonselective beta blockade.

Thyroid Hormones/Anti-Thyroid Agents

METHIMAZOLE AND PROPYLTHIOURACIL

There is convincing evidence that the clearance of lipophilic (flow-dependent extraction) beta blockers such as propranolol and metoprolol is significantly (greater than 80 percent) higher in hyperthyroid as compared to euthyroid patients [6, 32, 33, 34, 56, 163]. The clearance of nonlipophilic beta blockers is probably not affected [6, 56]. The result of treatment that renders a hypothyroid patient euthyroid could be associated with excessive beta blockade if the patient is on propranolol or metoprolol. Hypothyroidism has been studied and no consistent effects have been reported for alteration of beta blocker kinetics.

REFERENCES

1. Affrime, M. B., Lowenthal, D. T., Tolbert, J. A., et al. Dynamics and kinetics of ophthalmic timolol. *Clin. Pharmacol. Ther.* 27:471, 1980.
2. Ananth, J., and Lin, K. M. Propranolol in psychiatry: Therapeutic uses and side effects. *Neuropsychobiology* 15:20, 1986.
3. Anderson, S. D., Bye, P. T. P., Perry, C. P., et al. Limitation of work performance in normal adult males in the presence of beta-adrenergic blockade. *Aust. N. Z. J. Med.* 9:515, 1979.
4. Angelo-Nielsen, K. Timolol topically and diabetes mellitus. *J.A.M.A.* 244:2263, 1980.

5. Anon. Additional information on timolol adverse reactions. *FDA Drug Bull.* 10:24, 1980.
6. Aro, A., Anttila, M., Korhonen, T., and Sundquist, H. Pharmacokinetics of propranolol and sotalol in hyperthyroidism. *Eur. J. Clin. Pharmacol.* 21:373, 1982.
7. Bailey, R. R., and Neale, T. J. Rapid clonidine withdrawal with blood pressure overshoot exaggerated by beta-blockade. *Br. Med. J.* 1:942, 1976.
8. Bathen, J. Propranolol erectile dysfunction relieved. *Ann. Intern. Med.* 88:716, 1978.
9. Bax, N. D. S., Lennard, M. S., Tucker, G. T., et al. The effect of beta-adrenoceptor antagonists on the pharmacokinetics and pharmacodynamics of warfarin after a single dose. *Br. J. Clin. Pharmacol.* 17:553, 1984.
10. Betts, T. A., and Alford, C. Beta-blockers and sleep: A controlled trial. *Eur. J. Clin. Pharmacol.* 28(Suppl):65, 1985.
11. Blessing, W., and Walsh, J. C. Myotonia precipitated by propranolol therapy. *Lancet* 1:73, 1977.
12. Boger, W. P., Puliafito, C. A., Steinert, R. F., and Langston, D. P. Long-term experience with timolol ophthalmic solution in patients with open-angle glaucoma. *Ophthalmology* 85:259, 1978.
13. Buhler, F. R., Laragh, J. H., Vaughan, E. D., et al. Antihypertensive action of propranolol: Specific antirenin responses in high and normal renin forms of essential, renal, renovascular and malignant hypertension. *Am. J. Cardiol.* 32:511, 1973.
14. Bullock, J. L., Harris, R. E., and Young, R. Treatment of thyrotoxicosis during pregnancy with propranolol. *Am. J. Obstet. Gynecol.* 121:242, 1975.
15. Bulpitt, C. J., Dollery, C. T., and Carne, S. Change in symptoms of hypertensive patients after referral to hospital clinic. *Br. Heart J.* 38:121, 1976.
16. Byrne, A. J., McNeil, J. J., Harrison, P. M., et al. Stable oral availability of sustained release propranolol when co-administered with hydralazine or food: Evidence implicating substrate delivery rate as a determinant of presystemic drug interactions. *Br. J. Clin. Pharmacol.* 17(Suppl 1):45s, 1984.
17. Carlsson, E., Fellenius, E., Lundborg, P., and Svensson, L. Beta-adrenoceptor blockers, plasma-potassium, and exercise. *Lancet* 2:424, 1978.
18. Conrad, K. A., Byers, J. M., Finley, P. R., and Burnham, L. Lidocaine elimination: Effects of metoprolol and of propranolol. *Clin. Pharmacol. Ther.* 33:133, 1983.
19. Conrad, K. A., and Nyman, D. W. Effects of metoprolol and propranolol on theophylline elimination. *Clin. Pharmacol. Ther.* 28:463, 1980.
20. Cove-Smith, J. R., and Kirk, C. A. CNS-related side effects with metoprolol and atenolol. *Eur. J. Clin. Pharmacol.* 28(Suppl):69, 1985.
21. Deacon, S. P., and Barnett, D. Comparison of atenolol and propranolol during insulin-induced hypoglycaemia. *Br. Med. J.* 2:272, 1976.
22. Declamer, P. B. S., Chatterjee, S. S., Cruickshank, F. M., et al. Beta-blockers and asthma. *Br. Heart J.* 40:184, 1978.
23. Donovan, M. A., Heagerty, A. M., Patel, L., et al. Cimetidine and bioavailability of propranolol. *Lancet* 1:164, 1981.
24. Dubois, D., Petitcolas, J., Temperville, B., et al. Treatment of hypertension in pregnancy with beta-adrenoceptor antagonists. *Br. J. Clin. Pharmacol.* 13(Suppl):375s, 1982.
25. Duchin, K. L., Stern, M. A., Willard, D. A., and McKinstry, D. N. Comparison of kinetic interactions of nadolol and propranolol with cimetidine. *Am. Heart J.* 108:1084, 1984.
26. Dumez, Y., Tchobroutsky, C., Hornych, H., and Amiel-Tison, C. Neonatal effects of maternal administration of acebutolol. *Br. Med. J.* 283:1077, 1981.

27. Dunn, F. G., Lorimer, A. R., and Lawrie, T. D. V. Objective measurement of performance during acute stress in patients with essential hypertension: Assessment of the effects of propranolol and metoprolol. *Clin. Sci.* 57(Suppl):413s, 1979.
28. Durao, V., Prata, M. M., and Goncalves, L. M. P. Modification of antihypertensive effect of beta-adrenoceptor-blocking agents by inhibition of endogenous prostaglandin synthesis. *Lancet* 2:1005, 1977.
29. (Editorial) Self-poisoning with beta-blockers. *Br. Med. J.* 1:1010, 1978.
30. Eliahou, H. E., Silverberg, D. S., Reisin, E., et al. Propranolol for the treatment of hypertension in pregnancy. *Br. J. Obstet. Gynaecol.* 85:431, 1978.
31. Elliott, H. L., McLean, K., Sumner, D. J., et al. Immediate cardiovascular responses to oral prazosin—Effects of concurrent beta-blockers. *Clin. Pharmacol. Ther.* 29:303, 1981.
32. Feely, J., Crooks, J., and Stevenson, I. H. The influence of age, smoking and hyperthyroidism on plasma propranolol steady state concentration. *Br. J. Clin. Pharmacol.* 12:73, 1981.
33. Feely, J., Crooks, J., and Stevenson, I. H. Plasma propranolol steady state concentrations in thyroid disorders. *Eur. J. Clin. Pharmacol.* 19:329, 1981.
34. Feely, J., Stevenson, I. H., and Crooks, J. Increased clearance of propranolol in thyrotoxicosis. *Ann. Intern. Med.* 94:472, 1981.
35. Feely, J., Wilkinson, G. R., and Wood, A. J. J. Reduction of liver blood flow and propranolol metabolism by cimetidine. *N. Engl. J. Med.* 304:692, 1981.
36. Fenster, P., Perrier, D., Mayersohn, M., and Marcus, F. I. Kinetic evaluation of the propranolol-quinidine combination. *Clin. Pharmacol. Ther.* 27:450, 1980.
37. Ferrara, L. A., Mancini, M., Marotta, T., et al. Interference by sulfinpyrazone with the antihypertensive effects of oxprenolol. *Eur. J. Clin. Pharmacol.* 29:717, 1986.
38. Fleming, P. D., and Drachman, D. A. Propranolol, hallucinations, and sleep disturbance. *Am. J. Psychiatry* 139:540, 1982.
39. Fleminger, R. Visual hallucinations and illusions with propranolol. *Br. Med. J.* 1:1182, 1978.
40. Foerster, E. C., Greminger, P., Siegenthaler, W., et al. Atenolol versus pindolol: Side-effects in hypertension. *Eur. J. Clin. Pharmacol.* 28(Suppl):89, 1985.
41. Forsberg, L., Gustavii, B., Hojerback, T., and Olsson, A. M. Impotence, smoking, and beta-blocking drugs. *Fertil. Steril.* 31:589, 1979.
42. Fraunfelder, F. T., and Barker, A. F. Respiratory effects of timolol. *N. Engl. J. Med.* 311:1441, 1984.
43. Frishman, W. H., Christodoulou, J., Weksler, B., et al. Abrupt propranolol withdrawal in angina pectoris: Effects on platelet aggregation and exercise tolerance. *Am. Heart J.* 95:169, 1978.
44. Frishman, W., Jacob, H., Eisenberg, E., and Ribner, H. Clinical pharmacology of the new beta-adrenergic blocking drugs. Part 8. Self-poisoning with beta-adrenoceptor blocking agents: recognition and management. *Am. Heart J.* 98:798, 1979.
45. Frishman, W., Silverman, R., Strom, J., et al. Clinical pharmacology of new beta-adrenergic blocking agents. Part 4. Adverse effects. Choosing a beta-adrenoreceptor blocker. *Am. Heart J.* 98:256, 1979.
46. Frisk-Holmberg, M., Jorfeldt, L., and Juhlin-Dannfeldt, A. Influence of alprenolol on hemodynamic and metabolic responses to prolonged exercise in subjects with hypertension. *Clin. Pharmacol. Ther.* 21:675, 1977.
47. Gallery, E. D. M., Saunders, D. M., Hunyor, S. N., and Gyory, A. Z.

Randomized comparison of methyldopa and oxprenolol for treatment of hypertension in pregnancy. *Br. Med. J.* 1:1591, 1979.
48. Gokal, R., Dornan, T. L., and Ledingham, J. G. G. Peripheral skin necrosis complicating beta-blockage. *Br. Med. J.* 1:721, 1979.
49. Gold, L. A., Merimee, T. J., and Misbin, R. I. Propranolol and hypoglycemia: The effects of beta-adrenergic blockade on glucose and alanine levels during fasting. *J. Clin. Pharmacol.* 20:50, 1980.
50. Grabowski, B. S., Cady, W. J., Young, W. W., and Emery, J. F. Effects of acute alcohol administration on propranolol absorption. *Int. J. Clin. Pharmacol. Ther. Toxicol.* 18:317, 1980.
51. Graham, C. F., Turner, W. M., and Jones, J. K. Lidocaine-propranolol interactions. *N. Engl. J. Med.* 304:1301, 1981.
52. Greenblatt, D. J., and Koch-Weser, J. Adverse reactions to propranolol in hospitalized medical patients: A report from the Boston Collaborative Drug Surveillance Program. *Am. Heart J.* 86:478, 1973.
53. Greenblatt, D. J., and Koch-Weser, J. Adverse reactions to beta-adrenergic receptor blocking drugs: A report from the Boston Collaborative Drug Surveillance Program. *Drugs* 7:118, 1974.
54. Grimby, G., and Smith, U. Beta-blockade and muscle function. *Lancet* 2:1318, 1978.
55. Haglund, K., Seideman, P., Collste, P., et al. Influence of pentobarbital on metoprolol plasma levels. *Clin. Pharmacol. Ther.* 26:326, 1979.
56. Hallengren, B., Nilsson, O. R., Karlberg, B. E., et al. Influence of hyperthyroidism on the kinetics of methimazole, propranolol, metoprolol and atenolol. *Eur. J. Clin. Pharmacol.* 21:379, 1982.
57. Hansson, B. G., Dymling, J. F., Hedeland, H., and Hulthen, U. L. Long-term treatment of moderate hypertension with the beta-1-receptor blocking agent metoprolol: I. Effect of maximal working capacity, plasma catecholamines and renin, urinary aldosterone, blood pressure and pulse rate under basal conditions. *Eur. J. Clin. Pharmacol.* 11:239, 1977.
58. Harrison, D. C., and Alderman, E. L. Discontinuation of propranolol therapy: Cause of rebound angina pectoris and acute coronary events. *Chest* 69:1, 1976.
59. Hawksworth, G. M., Dart, A. M., Chiang, C. S., et al. Effect of propranolol on the pharmacokinetics and pharmacodynamics of hydralazine. *Drugs* 25(Suppl 2):136, 1983.
60. Heagerty, A. M., Castleden, C. M., and Patel, L. Failure of ranitidine to interact with propranolol. *Br. Med. J.* 284:1304, 1982.
61. Heagerty, A. M., Donovan, M. A., Castleden, C. M., et al. Influence of cimetidine on pharmacokinetics of propranolol. *Br. Med. J.* 282:1917, 1981.
62. Herishanu, Y., and Rosenberg, P. Beta-blockers and myasthenia gravis. *Ann. Intern. Med.* 83:834, 1975.
63. Hoelzer, D. R., Dalsky, G. P., Clutter, W. E., et al. Glucoregulation during exercise: Hypoglycemia is prevented by redundant glucoregulatory systems, sympathochromaffin activation, and changes in islet hormone secretion. *J. Clin. Invest.* 77:212, 1986.
64. Holm, G., Herlitz, J., and Smith, U. Severe hypoglycaemia during physical exercise and treatment with beta-blockers. *Br. Med. J.* 282:1360, 1981.
65. Houben, H., Thien, T., and van't Laar, A. Effect of low-dose epinephrine infusion on hemodynamics after selective and nonselective beta-blockade in hypertension. *Clin. Pharmacol. Ther.* 31:685, 1982.
66. Hughes, R. O., and Zacharias, F. J. Myasthenic syndrome during treatment with practolol. *Br. Med. J.* 1:460, 1976.
67. Husserl, F. E., and Messerli, F. H. Adverse effects of antihypertensive drugs. *Drugs* 22:188, 1981.

68. Jack, D. B., Kendall, M. J., Dean, S., et al. The effect of hydralazine on the pharmacokinetics of three different beta adrenoceptor antagonists: metoprolol, nadolol, and acebutolol. *Biopharm. Drug Dispos.* 3:47, 1982.
69. Jackman, G. P., McLean, A. J., Jennings, G. L., and Bobik, A. No stereoselective first-pass hepatic extraction of propranolol. *Clin. Pharmacol. Ther.* 30:291, 1981.
70. Johnsson, G. Influence of metoprolol and propranolol on hemodynamic effects induced by adrenaline and physical work. *Acta Pharmacol. Toxicol.* 36(Suppl V):59, 1975.
71. Kates, R. E., and Blanford, M. F. Disposition kinetics of oral quinidine when administered concurrently with propranolol. *J. Clin. Pharmacol.* 19:378, 1979.
72. Kelly, J. G., Salem, S. A. M., Kinney, C. D., et al. Effects of ranitidine on the disposition of metoprolol. *Br. J. Clin. Pharmacol.* 19:219, 1985.
73. Kendall, M. J. Are selective beta-adrenoceptor blocking drugs an advantage? *J. R. Coll. Physicians Lond.* 15:33, 1981.
74. Kendall, M. J., and Beeley, L. Beta-adrenoceptor blocking drugs: Adverse reactions and drug interactions. *Pharmacol. Ther.* 21:351, 1983.
75. Kendall, M. J., Jack, D. B., Quarterman, C. P., et al. Beta-adrenoceptor blocker pharmacokinetics and the oral contraceptive pill. *Br. J. Clin. Pharmacol.* 17(Suppl 1):87s, 1984.
76. Kendall, M. J., Quarterman, C. P., Jack, D. B., and Beeley, L. Metoprolol pharmacokinetics and the oral contraceptive pill. *Br. J. Clin. Pharmacol.* 14:120, 1982.
77. Kessler, K. M., Humphries, W. C., Black, M., and Spann, J. F. Quinidine pharmacokinetics in patients with cirrhosis or receiving propranolol. *Am. Heart J.* 96:627, 1978.
78. Kleinbaum, J., and Shamoon, H. Effect of propranolol on delayed glucose recovery after insulin-induced hypoglycemia in normal and diabetic subjects. *Diabetes Care* 7:155, 1984.
79. Knarr, J. W. Impotence from propranolol? *Ann. Intern. Med.* 85:259, 1976.
80. Koch, G., Franz, I. W., and Lohmann, F. W. Effects of short-term and long-term treatment with cardioselective and non-selective beta-receptor blockade on carbohydrate and lipid metabolism and on plasma catecholamines at rest and during exercise. *Clin. Sci.* 61(Suppl):433s, 1981.
81. Kristensen, B. O., Steiness, E., and Weeke, J. Propranolol withdrawal and thyroid hormones in patients with essential hypertension. *Clin. Pharmacol. Ther.* 23:624, 1978.
82. Lager, I., Blohme, G., and Smith, U. Effect of cardioselective and non-selective beta-blockade on the hypoglycaemic response in insulin-dependent diabetics. *Lancet* 1:458, 1979.
83. Langer, A., Hung, C. T., McNulty, J. A., et al. Adrenergic blockade: A new approach to hyperthyroidism during pregnancy. *Obstet. Gynecol.* 44:181, 1974.
84. Larsen, A. On the neuromuscular effects of pindolol and sotalol in the rat. *Acta Physiol. Scand.* 102:35, 1978.
85. Leemann, T., Dayer, P., and Meyer, U. A. Single-dose quinidine treatment inhibits metoprolol oxidation in extensive metabolizers. *Eur. J. Clin. Pharmacol.* 29:739, 1986.
86. Lichtman, M. A., Cohen, J., Murphy, M. S., et al. Effect of propranolol on oxygen binding to hemoglobin in vitro and in vivo. *Circulation* 49:881, 1974.
87. Lieberman, B. A., Stirrat, G. M., Cohen, S. L., et al. The possible adverse effect of propranolol on the fetus in pregnancies complicated by severe hypertension. *Br. J. Obstet. Gynaecol.* 85:678, 1978.

88. Liedholm, H., Melander, A., Bitzen, P. O., et al. Accumulation of atenolol and metoprolol in human breast milk. *Eur. J. Clin. Pharmacol.* 20:229, 1981.
89. Lilja, M., Jounela, A. J., Juustila, H. J., and Paalzow, L. Abrupt and gradual change from clonidine to beta blockers in hypertension. *Acta Med. Scand.* 211:375, 1982.
90. Lloyd-Mostyn, R. H., and Oram, S. Modification by propranolol of cardiovascular effects of induced hypoglycaemia. *Lancet* 1:1213, 1975.
91. Lundborg, P., Astrom, H., Bengtsson, C., et al. Effect of beta-adrenoceptor blockade on exercise performance and metabolism. *Clin. Sci.* 61:299, 1981.
92. Maling, T. J. B., and Dollery, C. T. Changes in blood pressure, heart rate, and plasma noradrenaline concentration after sudden withdrawal of propranolol. *Br. Med. J.* 2:366, 1979.
93. Mann, A. H. Beta-blockers and psychometric performance: The clinical relevance of psychometric testing. *Eur. J. Clin. Pharmacol.* 28(Suppl):31, 1985.
94. Mantyla, R., Mannisto, P., Nykanen, S., et al. Pharmacokinetic interactions of timolol with vasodilating drugs, food and phenobarbitone in healthy human volunteers. *Eur. J. Clin. Pharmacol.* 24:227, 1983.
95. Marshall, A. J., Roberts, C. J. C., and Barritt, D. W. Raynaud's phenomenon as side effect of beta-blockers in hypertension. *Br. Med. J.* 1:1498, 1976.
96. McDevitt, D. G. Beta-blockers and psychometric performance: Studies in normal volunteers. *Eur. J. Clin. Pharmacol.* 28(Suppl 1):35, 1985.
97. McLaren, E. H. Severe hypertension produced by interaction of phenylpropanolamine with methyldopa and oxprenolol. *Br. Med. J.* 2:283, 1976.
98. McLean, A. J., Knight, R., Harrison, P. M., and Harper, R. W. Clearance-based oral drug interaction between verapamil and metoprolol and comparison with atenolol. *Am. J. Cardiol.* 55:1628, 1985.
99. McLean, A. J., Skews, H., Bobik, A., and Dudley, F. J. Interaction between oral propranolol and hydralazine. *Clin. Pharmacol. Ther.* 27:726, 1980.
100. McLean, A. J., Wilhelm, D., and Heinzow, B. G. Stable oral availability of atenolol coadministered with hydralazine: Comparison with propranolol, metoprolol and other beta-adrenoceptor antagonists. *Drugs* 25(Suppl 2):131, 1983.
101. McNeil, J. J., and Louis, W. J. A double-blind crossover comparison of pindolol, metoprolol, atenolol and labetalol in mild to moderate hypertension. *Br. J. Clin. Pharmacol.* 8(Suppl):163s, 1979.
102. McNeill, R. S. Effect of a beta-adrenergic-blocking agent, propranolol, on asthmatics. *Lancet* 2:1101, 1964.
103. McNeill, R. S., and Ingram, C. G. Effect of propranolol on ventilatory function. *Am. J. Cardiol.* 18:473, 1966.
104. McSorley, P. D., and Warren, D. J. Effects of propranolol and metoprolol on the peripheral circulation. *Br. Med. J.* 2:1598, 1978.
105. Medical Research Council Working Party on Mild to Moderate Hypertension. Adverse reactions to bendrofluazide and propranolol for the treatment of mild hypertension. *Lancet* 2:539, 1981.
106. Miller, R. A. Propranolol and impotence. *Ann. Intern. Med.* 85:682, 1976.
107. Miller, R. R., Olson, H. G., Amsterdam, E. A., and Mason, D. T. Propranolol-withdrawal rebound phenomenon: Exacerbation of coronary events after abrupt cessation of antianginal therapy. *N. Engl. J. Med.* 293:416, 1975.
108. Miners, J. O., Wing, L. M. H., Lillywhite, K. J., and Robson, R. A. Selectivity and dose-dependency of the inhibitory effect of propranolol on theophylline metabolism in man. *Br. J. Clin. Pharmacol.* 20:219, 1985.
109. Miners, J. O., Wing, L. M. H., Lillywhite, K. J., and Smith, K. J. Failure

of 'therapeutic' doses of beta-adrenoceptor antagonists to alter the disposition of tolbutamide and lignocaine. *Br. J. Clin. Pharmacol.* 18:853, 1984.
110. Mutschler, E., Spahn, H., and Kirch, W. The interaction between H2-receptor antagonists and beta-adrenoceptor blockers. *Br. J. Clin. Pharmacol.* 17(Suppl I):51S, 1984.
111. Myers, M. G., Freeman, M. R., Juma, Z. A., and Wisenberg, G. Propranolol withdrawal in angina pectoris: A prospective study. *Am. Heart J.* 97:298, 1979.
112. Nattel, S., Rangno, R. E., and Van Loon, G. Mechanism of propranolol withdrawal phenomena. *Circulation* 59:1158, 1979.
113. Newman, R. J. Comparison of propranolol, metoprolol, and acebutolol on insulin-induced hypoglycaemia. *Br. Med. J.* 2:447, 1976.
114. Nies, A. S., and Shand, D. G. Hypertensive response to propranolol in a patient treated with methyldopa—a proposed mechanism. *Clin. Pharmacol. Ther.* 14:823, 1973.
115. Nolan, B. T. Acute suicidal depression associated with use of timolol. *J.A.M.A.* 247:1567, 1982.
116. Ochs, H. R., Carstens, G., and Greenblatt, D. J. Reduction in lidocaine clearance during continuous infusion and by coadministration of propranolol. *N. Engl. J. Med.* 303:373, 1980.
117. Ochs, H. R., Carstens, G., Roberts, G. M., and Greenblatt, D. J. Metoprolol or propranolol does not alter the kinetics of procainamide. *J. Cardiovasc. Pharmacol.* 5:392, 1983.
118. O'Hare, M. F., Murnaghan, G. A., Russell, C. J., et al. Sotalol as a hypotensive agent in pregnancy. *Br. J. Obstet. Gynaecol.* 87:814, 1980.
119. Paget, G. E. Carcinogenic action of pronethalol. *Br. Med. J.* 2:1266, 1963.
120. Panizza, D., and Lecasble, M. Effect of atenolol on car drivers in a prolonged stress situation. *Eur. J. Clin. Pharmacol.* 28(Suppl):97, 1985.
121. Patel, L., and Turner, P. Central actions of beta-adrenoceptor blocking drugs in man. *Med. Res. Rev* 1:387, 1981.
122. Pearson, S. B., Banks, D. C., and Patrick, J. M. The effect of beta-adrenoceptor blockade on factors affecting exercise tolerance in normal man. *Br. J. Clin. Pharmacol.* 8:143, 1979.
123. Pruyn, S. C., Phelan, J. P., and Buchanan, G. C. Long-term propranolol therapy in pregnancy: Maternal and fetal outcome. *Am. J. Obstet. Gynecol.* 135:485, 1979.
124. Rees, P. J. Peripheral skin necrosis complicating beta-blockade. *Br. Med. J.* 1:955, 1979.
125. Reeves, R. A., Boer, W. H., DeLeve, L., and Leenen, F. H. H. Nonselective beta-blockade enhances pressor responsiveness to epinephrine, norepinephrine, and antiotensin II in normal man. *Clin. Pharmacol. Ther.* 35:461, 1984.
126. Reimann, I. W., Klotz, U., and Frolich, J. C. Effects of cimetidine and ranitidine on steady-state propranolol kinetics and dynamics. *Clin. Pharmacol. Ther.* 32:749, 1982.
127. Richards, D. A., and Prichard, B. N. C. Self-poisoning with beta-blockers. *Br. Med. J.* 1:1623, 1978.
128. Rodger, J. C., Sheldon, C. D., Lerski, R. A., and Livingstone, W. R. Intermittent claudication complicating beta-blockade. *Br. Med. J.* 1:1125, 1976.
129. Ros, F. E., and Dake, C. L. Timolol eye drops: Bradycardia or tachycardia? *Doc. Ophthalmol.* 48:283, 1980.
130. Rosa, R. M., Silva, P., Young, J. B., et al. Adrenergic modulation of extrarenal potassium disposal. *N. Engl. J. Med.* 302:431, 1980.

131. Rubin, P. C. Beta-blockers in pregnancy. *N. Engl. J. Med.* 305:1323, 1981.
132. Salvetti, A., Arzilli, F., Pedrinelli, R., et al. Interaction between oxprenolol and indomethacin on blood pressure in essential hypertensive patients. *Eur. J. Clin. Pharmacol.* 22:197, 1982.
133. Salvetti, A., Pedrinelli, R., Alberici, P., et al. The influence of indomethacin and sulindac on some pharmacological actions of atenolol in hypertensive patients. *Br. J. Clin. Pharmacol.* 17(Suppl 1):108s, 1984.
134. Schafer-Korting, M., and Mutschler, E. Pharmacokinetics of bendroflumethiazide alone and in combination with propranolol and hydralazine. *Eur. J. Clin. Pharmacol.* 21:315, 1982.
135. Schneck, D. W., Luderer, J. R., Davis, D., and Vary, J. E. Effects of nadolol and propranolol on plasma lidocaine clearance. *Clin. Pharmacol. Ther.* 36:584, 1984.
136. Schneck, D. W., and Vary, J. E. Mechanism by which hydralazine increases propranolol bioavailability. *Clin. Pharmacol. Ther.* 35:447, 1984.
137. Schoene, R. B., Abuan, T., Ward, R. L., and Beasley, C. H. Effects of topical betaxolol, timolol, and placebo on pulmonary function in asthmatic bronchitis. *Am. J. Ophthalmol.* 97:86, 1984.
138. Schoene, R. B., Martin, T. R., Charan, N. B., and French, C. L. Timolol-induced bronchospasm in asthmatic bronchitis. *J.A.M.A.* 245:1460, 1981.
139. Shaivitz, S. A. Timolol and myasthenia gravis. *J.A.M.A.* 242:1611, 1979.
140. Shiroff, R. A., Mathis, J., Zelis, R., et al. Propranolol rebound—A retrospective study. *Am. J. Cardiol.* 41:778, 1978.
141. Simonson, D. C., Koivisto, V., Sherwin, R. S., et al. Adrenergic blockade alters glucose kinetics during exercise in insulin-dependent diabetics. *J. Clin. Invest.* 73:1648, 1984.
142. Sinclair, D. J. M. Comparison of effects of propranolol and metoprolol on airway obstruction in chronic bronchitis. *Br. Med. J.* 1:168, 1979.
143. Skinner, C., Gaddie, J., Palmer, K. N. V., and Kerridge, D. F. Comparison of effects of metoprolol and propranolol on asthmatic airway obstruction. *Br. Med. J.* 1:504, 1976.
144. Smith, U., Blohme, G., Lager, I., and Lonnroth, P. Can insulin-treated diabetics be given beta-adrenergic-blocking drugs? *Br. Med. J.* 281:1143, 1980.
145. Stone, R. Proximal myopathy during beta-blockade. *Br. Med. J.* 2:1583, 1979.
146. Strauss, F. G., Franklin, S. S., Lewin, A. J., and Maxwell, M. H. Withdrawal of antihypertensive therapy: Hypertensive crisis in renovascular hypertension. *J.A.M.A.* 238:1734, 1977.
147. Sung, R. J., Blonski, L., Kirchenbaum, J., et al. Clinical experience with esmolol, a short-acting beta-adrenergic blocker in cardiac arrhythmias and myocardial ischemia. *J. Clin. Pharmacol.* 26(Suppl A):A15, 1986.
148. Svendsen, T. L., Tango, M., Waldorff, S., et al. Effects of propranolol and pindolol on plasma lignocaine clearance in man. *Br. J. Clin. Pharmacol.* 13(Suppl 2):223s, 1982.
149. Sziegoleit, W., Rausch, J., Polák, G., et al. Influence of acetylsalicylic acid on acute circulatory effects of the beta-blocking agents pindolol and propranolol in humans. *Int. J. Clin. Pharmacol. Ther. Toxicol.* 20:423, 1982.
150. Tcherdakoff, P. H., Colliard, M., Berrard, E., et al. Propranolol in hypertension during pregnancy. *Br. Med. J.* 2:670, 1978.
151. Thiringer, G., and Svedmyr, N. Interaction of orally administered metoprolol, practolol and propranolol with isoprenaline in asthmatics. *Eur. J. Clin. Pharmacol.* 10:163, 1976.
152. Thorley, K. J., McAinsh, J., and Cruickshank, J. M. Atenolol in the treat-

ment of pregnancy-induced hypertension. *Br. J. Clin. Pharmacol.* 12:725, 1981.
153. Thulesius, O. Beta-adrenergic blockade and vasospasm. *Acta Med. Scand.* 625(Suppl):41, 1978.
154. Trap-Jensen, J., Carlsen, J. E., Svendsen, T. L., and Christensen, N. J. Cardiovascular and adrenergic effects of cigarette smoking during immediate non-selective and selective beta adrenoceptor blockade in humans. *Eur. J. Clin. Invest.* 9:181, 1979.
155. Vale, J. A., and Jefferys, D. B. Peripheral gangrene complicating beta-blockade. *Lancet* 1:1216, 1978.
156. Van Gelder, P., Alpert, M., and Tsui, W. H. A comparison of the effects of atenolol and metoprolol on attention. *Eur. J. Clin. Pharmacol.* 28(Suppl):101, 1985.
157. van Herwaarden, C. L. A., Fennis, J. F. M., Binkhorst, R. A., and van't Laar, A. Haemodynamic effects of adrenaline during treatment of hypertensive patients with propranolol and metoprolol. *Eur. J. Clin. Pharmacol.* 12:397, 1977.
158. Velde, T. M., and Kaiser, F. E. Ophthalmic timolol treatment causing altered hypoglycemic response in a diabetic patient. *Arch. Intern. Med.* 143:1627, 1983.
159. Vernon, C., and Sakula, A. Fatal rebound hypertension after abrupt withdrawal of clonidine and propranolol. *Br. J. Clin. Pract.* 33:112, 1979.
160. Waal, H. J. Propranolol-induced depression. *Br. Med. J.* 2:50, 1967.
161. Waal-Manning, H. J. Metabolic effects of beta-adrenoreceptor blockers. *Drugs* 11(Suppl 1):121, 1976.
162. Watkins, J., Abbott, E. C., Hensby, C. N., et al. Attenuation of hypotensive effect of propranolol and thiazide diuretics by indomethacin. *Br. Med. J.* 281:702, 1980.
163. Wells, P. G., Feely, J., Wilkinson, G. R., and Wood, A. J. J. Effect of thyrotoxicosis on liver blood flow and propranolol disposition after long-term dosing. *Clin. Pharmacol. Ther.* 33:603, 1983.
164. Westerlund, A. Central nervous system side-effects with hydrophilic and lipophilic beta-blockers. *Eur. J. Clin. Pharmacol.* 28(Suppl):73, 1985.
165. White, C. B., and Udwadia, B. P. Beta-adrenoceptors in the human dorsal hand vein, and the effects of propranolol and practolol on venous sensitivity to noradrenaline. *Br. J. Clin. Pharmacol.* 2:99, 1975.
166. Wikstrand, J., and Berglund, G. Antihypertensive treatment with beta-blockers in patients aged over 65. *Br. Med. J.* 285:850, 1982.
167. Wilson, D. F., Watson, O. F., Peel, J. S., and Turner, A. S. Trasicor in angina pectoris: A double-blind trial. *Br. Med. J.* 2:155, 1969.
168. Wilson, R. P., Spaeth, G. L., and Poryzees, E. The place of timolol in the practice of ophthalmology. *Ophthalmology* 87:451, 1980.
169. Wolfe, B. B., Harden, T. K., and Molinoff, P. B. In vitro study of beta-adrenergic receptors. *Ann. Rev. Pharmacol. Toxicol.* 17:575, 1977.
170. Wright, A. D., Barber, S. G., Kendall, M. J., and Poole, P. H. Beta-adrenoceptor-blocking drugs and blood sugar control in diabetes mellitus. *Br. Med. J.* 1:159, 1979.
171. Yates, D. Syncope and visual hallucinations, apparently from timolol. *J.A.M.A.* 244:768, 1980.
172. Zaid, G., and Beall, G. N. Bronchial response to beta-adrenergic blockade. *N. Engl. J. Med.* 275:580, 1966.

CHAPTER 17

PROBLEMS WITH CALCIUM ANTAGONIST THERAPY

CHARLES R. LAMBERT
CARL J. PEPINE

Although calcium channel antagonists are generally well tolerated, both minor and major adverse reactions can occur. In addition, a possible withdrawal syndrome has been reported with abrupt discontinuation of these agents. In this chapter we will review the evidence for such a withdrawal syndrome and consider the problems of left ventricular depression as well as other adverse reactions that have been reported with calcium channel antagonist therapy.

CALCIUM CHANNEL ANTAGONISTS WITHDRAWAL SYNDROME

Substance withdrawal is a recognized phenomenon occurring after abrupt discontinuation of addicting drugs. Recently, withdrawal syndromes have been described in association with clonidine, beta-adrenergic blocker, and nitrate discontinuation, and concern has arisen over the possibility of such a syndrome in patients abruptly withdrawn from calcium channel antagonists. In the sections below, we will summarize the evidence in support of and against the existence of a clinically important calcium channel antagonist withdrawal syndrome. In addition, we will briefly discuss some potential mechanisms for such a phenomenon and make some recommendations for discontinuation of calcium channel antagonists in patients with ischemic heart disease based on the available data.

Evidence Supporting a Calcium Channel Antagonist Withdrawal Syndrome

In 1982 Shick and coworkers [44] described a multicenter, randomized, double-blind withdrawal study comparing placebo to nifedipine in 38 patients with vasospastic angina. A significant increase in angina frequency was observed upon withdrawal from nifedipine therapy, and in two patients this increase was greater than 50 percent above the baseline level. These investigators felt that a withdrawal effect was probably operant in these patients although no objective indicators of recurrent myocardial ischemia were supplied. Freedman et al. [13] reported the results of both controlled and uncontrolled withdrawal of verapamil treatment in a similar group of 24 patients. Nine of these patients had recurrent angina within 48 hours of drug discontinuation, suggesting the possibility of a withdrawal syndrome. Again, no objective documentation of myocardial ischemia was collected. Moses and coworkers [33] reported an increase of angina frequency in five of seven patients with rest angina withdrawn from nifedipine therapy. One patient sustained a myocardial infarction in this period, again suggesting the existence of a calcium channel antagonist withdrawal syndrome.

Several reports have raised the possibility of coronary artery spasm in the perioperative period after coronary artery bypass surgery secondary to acute calcium channel antagonist withdrawal [8, 21]. These reports suffer from lack of angiographic documentation, and the clinical events described cannot be differentiated from the sequelae of thrombosis or embolism. Even if coronary artery spasm had been documented in these cases, etiologies other than calcium channel antagonist withdrawal that may contribute to coronary vasospasm in the perioperative period cannot be excluded on the basis of the data provided.

Perhaps the most convincing evidence supporting a calcium channel antagonist withdrawal syndrome is the report of Subramanian and coworkers [46]. Five patients were studied with continuous FM electrocardiographic monitoring during periods of self- or physician-prescribed discontinuation of verapamil or diltiazem therapy. All these patients developed recurrent angina associated with ischemic ST-T abnormalities that were not preceded by increased heart rate. Exacerbations were ameliorated with reinstitution of therapy with calcium channel antagonists and were felt to represent a substance withdrawal syndrome. This report offers the best objective evidence for such a syndrome to date.

Evidence Against a Calcium Channel Antagonist Withdrawal Syndrome

Gottlieb and Gerstenblith [17] studied 81 patients with angina at rest in a prospective, double-blind, randomized withdrawal trial of nifedipine versus placebo. Thirty-nine patients were withdrawn at the time of coronary artery bypass surgery for uncontrolled angina or left main coronary artery disease. No significant differences were noted between patients withdrawn from placebo versus nifedipine for surgery with regard to myocardial infarction, hypotension, vasodilator requirements, or arrhythmias in the perioperative period. The remaining 42 patients completed a 2-year protocol of nitrates and propranolol in addition to placebo or nifedipine. They were then hospitalized for controlled withdrawal of the study drug (placebo or nifedipine). No significant differences between groups were seen on serial exercise stress testing or in the number or duration of ischemic ST segment abnormalities on continuous electrocardiographic monitoring. Rest angina occurred during the withdrawal period in five patients, four of who were on nifedipine; however, these patients had persistent rest angina prior to the withdrawal period. Among the 34 stable patients who underwent withdrawal, none had recurrence of rest angina. Thus, in this study, no objective evidence for a clinically significant calcium channel antagonist withdrawal syndrome was seen. It should be noted, however, that the drug withdrawal period used in this study extended over 3 days and, thus, these observations are not strictly comparable to those made by Subramanian and coworkers [46] with abrupt drug discontinuation.

Just as the studies cited earlier [13, 33, 44] suggested the possibility of a calcium channel antagonist withdrawal syndrome in certain patients, similar studies by other investigators have failed to detect exacerbation of symptoms or signs of ischemia upon discontinuation of drug in placebo-controlled trials. Thus, controlled studies of diltiazem [39], and verapamil [19] in variant angina patients have failed to yield any suggestion of a withdrawal syndrome. Similarly, no evidence of withdrawal has been observed in patients with coronary artery spasm after discontinuation of treatment with nifedipine [18] or nicardipine [15]. In other studies, discontinuation of calcium channel antagonists in the setting of hypertension [1] or unstable angina [38] did not seem to provoke changes suggesting withdrawal.

From consideration of the evidence presented thus far, it appears that a calcium channel antagonist withdrawal syndrome does not occur in the majority of patients treated with these agents. There is some objective evidence, however, that withdrawal does occur in certain individuals. It is of interest in this light to consider some potential mechanisms for calcium channel antagonist withdrawal in the hope that some insight might be gained to aid in identification of patients at risk.

Possible Mechanisms for Calcium Channel Antagonist Withdrawal

Clonidine withdrawal syndrome is felt to be a dose-related state of sympathetic overactivity with increased blood and plasma levels of catecholamines [16]. Sympathetic overactivity has also been implicated in the beta-adrenergic blocker withdrawal syndrome [32]. Possible pathophysiologic mechanisms for overactivity include increased number of postsynaptic beta receptors [51], increased central sympathetic tone [35], and unfavorable changes in the oxyhemoglobin dissociation curve [28].

Calcium channel antagonists can suppress the release of catecholamines from both the adrenal medulla and sympathetic nerve terminals and can act as alpha-2 adrenergic-receptor blockers [3]. Sympathetic hyperactivity has also been implicated in the withdrawal syndrome associated with discontinuation of nitroprusside therapy [9]. This has led to consideration of adrenergic overactivity or rebound as a possible mechanism for calcium channel antagonist withdrawal as in the clonidine and beta blocker withdrawal syndromes. In this light, Frishman and coworkers [14] studied 20 patients with stable angina pectoris and found that, although verapamil treatment decreased catecholamine release during exercise, abrupt withdrawal did not produce evidence for a rebound effect.

Subramanian and coworkers [46] suggested that a state of altered coronary artery reactivity might be produced upon abrupt withdrawal of chronic calcium channel antagonist therapy. Recently, Nelson and coworkers offered experimental evidence supporting this concept [36].

Contractile activity of aortic smooth muscle obtained at surgery from patients who had or had not received calcium channel antagonists preoperatively was compared. Contractions of specimens from patients previously taking calcium channel antagonists showed prolonged relaxation times as well as increased peak tension and rate of change of tension development. These changes were independent of stimulation mode and reflect hyperresponsiveness associated with acute withdrawal of calcium channel antagonists.

It is also of interest in this regard that the patients reported by Freedman and coworkers [13] felt to have recurrent angina induced by calcium channel antagonist withdrawal all resumed smoking at that time. Smoking is another factor known to alter vascular reactivity and may have been a contributing mechanism in those patients. Vascular hyperresponsiveness has recently been demonstrated in an animal model for nitrate withdrawal [41]. No animal model for study of the calcium withdrawal syndrome has been described.

Recently, preliminary evidence for increased platelet alpha-2 receptor affinity for agonist has been cited as a possible mechanism for the calcium channel antagonist withdrawal syndrome. Such changes might induce platelet hyperaggregation and coronary vasoconstriction [31].

Conclusions

Taking all available information into account, it appears that the vast majority of patients with ischemic heart disease suffer no ill effects when calcium channel antagonist therapy is discontinued abruptly. However, a small number of patients will experience an exacerbation of symptoms and/or signs of myocardial ischemia in this circumstance. Subramanian and coworkers [46] estimated the incidence of this phenomenon in ischemic heart disease patients as 3.5 percent. Why certain individuals seem predisposed to calcium channel antagonist withdrawal while others are not remains unknown. Currently there is no method to distinguish between these two groups beforehand. It is possible that concurrent use of long-acting nitrates or other anti-ischemic agents masks or modifies the potential effect of calcium channel antagonist withdrawal. Possible mechanisms for withdrawal from calcium channel antagonists include induction of abnormalities in sympathetic nervous system function, alterations in vascular reactivity, and changes in platelet physiology.

We recommend a conservative approach to withdrawal of chronic calcium channel antagonist therapy in patients with ischemic heart disease. In stable patients these medications should be tapered over a 3-day period. In patients with unstable angina syndromes, a similar tapering schedule may be used; however, this is best accomplished during in-hospital observation and monitoring. When possible, other anti-ischemic agents such as long-acting nitrates should be continued.

No data are available pertaining to the possibility of a withdrawal syndrome when calcium channel antagonists are abruptly discontinued in patients with hypertrophic cardiomyopathy or tachydysrhythmias. Until such data are available, caution should also be used when discontinuing chronic calcium channel antagonist therapy in these patients.

DEPRESSION OF VENTRICULAR FUNCTION

As outlined elsewhere in this volume, all calcium channel antagonists depress myocardial contractile state. The potencies of nifedipine, verapamil, and diltiazem in this regard are similar in vitro; however, they may differ greatly in vivo. This difference between effects seen in the tissue bath and in the intact organism is due to a combination of autonomic reflex changes, loading alterations, and actual blood levels achievable in vivo with the various agents. As outlined below, these interactions lead to a general rank order for myocardial depression in vivo of verapamil greater than diltiazem greater than nifedipine, although there may be some patient to patient variability in this regard. In this section we will review some of the clinical and experimental data available regarding the importance of ventricular depression with calcium channel antagonist therapy.

Verapamil

Animal studies uniformly demonstrate depression in left ventricular contractile state by verapamil, which is potentiated by beta-adrenergic blockade [34, 49]. In an early study of the acute effects of intravenous verapamil in patients with either coronary artery disease or valvular heart disease, Singh and coworkers showed a decrease in mean arterial pressure and systemic vascular resistance that was associated with an increase in left ventricular end-diastolic pressure and a decrease in the first derivative of left ventricular pressure (dP/dt). Although there were no changes in left ventricular minute work or cardiac index, these data demonstrate a negative, albeit small, inotropic effect of the drug [45]. Ferlinz and coworkers studied 20 patients with coronary artery disease and found no evidence of myocardial dysfunction during acute administration of verapamil as a 0.1 mg/kg bolus followed by an infusion of 0.005 mg/kg/min [11]. The expected decreases in mean arterial pressure and systemic vascular resistance were seen; however, cardiac index, circumferential fiber shortening, and ejection fraction were improved, suggesting no net negative inotropic effect. Klein and coworkers studied a group of 38 patients having varied baseline ejection fractions during acute verapamil administration using serial radionuclide angiography [23]. All patients showed at least a transient period during which left ventricular ejection fraction was depressed. In patients with ejection fractions greater than 35 percent, this decrease was followed by an overshoot, presumably due to reflex mechanisms. The patients with ejection fractions less than 35 percent had no overshoot. Depression of left ventricular function in this study was also shown to be dose-dependent. Vlietstra and coinvestigators studied 25 patients during acute verapamil administration and found no gross depression of left ventricular function when indexed by end-diastolic pressure or ejection fraction [48]. Indeed, cardiac index was increased with drug administration; however, a small increase in end-diastolic volume index was observed with no change in heart rate, suggesting a compensated myocardial depressant effect. Ferlinz and Citron studied 14 patients with congestive heart failure during administration of verapamil intravenously and found acute improvements in ejection fraction, velocity of fiber shortening, and cardiac index [10]. In addition, no changes in heart rate or pulmonary capillary wedge pressure were observed.

Thus, although not observed in all studies, verapamil appears to have a definite negative inotropic effect demonstrable in humans during acute administration if looked for closely enough. This effect is not, however, profound enough to appear clinically important with reasonable baseline left ventricular function and may be masked entirely by reflex mechanisms. It has become apparent that the myocardial depressant effects of verapamil may be additive with beta-adrenergic blockade and that this combination of agents may indeed produce clinically important cardiac dysfunction. Although many case reports have documented individual instances of such problems, several clinical studies have also been done to better define its importance.

Packer and coworkers administered varying doses of oral verapamil to patients receiving propranolol or metoprolol and documented a dose-dependent depression of cardiac index and stroke volume index and increase in left ventricular filling pressure [37]. This depression was not seen with verapamil rechallenge after withdrawal of beta-adrenergic blockade. Kieval and coworkers also studied the effects of verapamil administration on left ventricular function in patients taking propranolol, although verapamil was given intravenously [22]. Verapamil administration was associated with the expected decrease in arterial pressure and systemic vascular resistance; however, no increase in cardiac index or velocity of circumferential fiber shortening was observed. Thus, although no overt left ventricular failure was produced, cardiac function was depressed to a degree that might be of concern in patients with minimal contractile reserve.

Diltiazem
Several animal investigations have shown that diltiazem has little effect on left ventricular function in normal hearts [34, 49]. It is interesting,

however, to consider the effects of diltiazem described by Porter and coworkers [40] in an experimental model of congestive heart failure produced by aortocaval fistula and subsequent volume overload. Although diltiazem had no effect on left ventricular function before creation of the fistula, significant depression was observed when baseline left ventricular dysfunction was produced by volume overload.

Recently Walsh and coworkers studied the effects of diltiazem administration to patients with New York Heart Association class III–IV congestive heart failure [50]. The mean left ventricular ejection fraction for this patient group was 26 percent. Diltiazem was administered initially as an intravenous infusion (100 to 200 mg/kg/min) for 40 minutes followed by 90 to 120 mg orally every 8 hours for 24 hours. Drug administration was associated with a fall in mean arterial pressure (18 percent), decreased heart rate (23 percent), increased cardiac index (20 percent), increased stroke volume index (50 percent), decreased pulmonary wedge pressure (34 percent), and no change in dP/dt. Thus, in this patient population, no deleterious effects were seen with diltiazem administration with regard to myocardial depression, although several patients were observed to have transient junctional rhythms during the intravenous infusion.

Nifedipine

As noted earlier, available calcium channel antagonists have similar potency in vitro with regard to myocardial depression. This equivalence is lost in vivo secondary to reflex mechanisms and loading changes. These factors are most prevalent for nifedipine since, relative to clinically tolerable doses, this agent provokes the most marked vasodilation of the three available calcium channel antagonists. Associated with this decrease in arterial tone is a reflex tachycardia, which is additive (via the Bowditch effect) in masking any myocardial depressant effects of the drug. If the reflex alterations are prevented in animal studies, a negative inotropic effect can be unmasked, which is easily demonstrated with intracoronary administration of the drug [49]. Similar findings have been reported with intracoronary administration of nifedipine in humans [43]. Since nifedipine is relatively more potent as a vasodilator in clinically tolerable doses than the other available calcium channel antagonists, a great deal of attention has been paid to its possible role in improving ventricular function in the setting of heart failure.

In 1980, Klugman and coworkers reported the effects of administration of nifedipine, 20 mg sublingually, to 11 patients with congestive heart failure [24]. Acute decreases in mean arterial pressure, pulmonary capillary wedge pressure, left ventricular end-diastolic pressure, systemic vascular resistance, and left ventricular end-diastolic volume were associated with no change in heart rate and increases in cardiac index, ejection fraction, and stroke volume index. Thus, in these patients, acute administration of nifedipine was associated with a favorable hemodynamic response and no evidence suggesting left ventricular depression was observed. In a similar study, Matsumoto and coworkers observed similar effects on cardiac index and systemic vascular resistance in a group of eight patients with mild to moderate congestive heart failure, although an increase in heart rate was also seen [30].

Fioretti and coworkers studied the effects of nifedipine, 20 mg sublingually, on hemodynamics in 12 patients with severe aortic insufficiency [12]. Although decreases in left ventricular end-diastolic pressure, mean arterial pressure, and systemic vascular resistance were associated with a 24 percent increase in forward cardiac index, no change was observed in end-diastolic volume, ejection fraction, or stroke work index. The regurgitant fraction changed in a parallel fashion with systemic vascular resistance. Thus, the overall hemodynamic effect in these patients was favorable and no evidence for myocardial depression was seen. Ludbrook et al. studied the acute hemodynamic effects of nifedipine in 32 patients with varying degrees of baseline left ventricular dysfunction [29]. Overall, nifedipine decreased blood pressure, improved systolic left ventricular function, and did not change diastolic functional parameters. When examined with respect to left ventricular function, the most favorable effects were seen in patients with elevated end-diastolic pressures and volumes. In these patients, improvements were documented in systolic and diastolic function, and myocardial energetic state was also affected favorably.

Elkayam and coworkers utilized afterload reduction with either nifedipine or hydralazine in patients with congestive heart failure in order to look more carefully for a possible myocardial depressant effect of the former [7]. When similar decreases in arterial pressure were induced, nifedipine treatment was associated with smaller increases in stroke volume index, cardiac index, and stroke work index, suggesting a slight negative inotropic effect only partially offset by its afterload reduction properties. A similar study was reported using nitroprusside instead of hydralazine versus nifedipine in 11 patients with congestive heart failure, again suggesting a slight negative inotropic effect of nifedipine [6]. Elkayam and coworkers also studied 20 congestive heart failure patients with acute nifedipine administration in a manner similar to the studies noted above and found some improvement in cardiac index but no change in pulmonary capillary wedge pressure, right atrial pressure, pulmonary vascular resistance, or left ventricular stroke work index [5].

Nicardipine

Recently, nicardipine became the third calcium channel antagonist available for use in patients with ischemic heart disease in the United States. Nicardipine is a dihidropyridine with relative coronary vascular selectivity [25–27]. Although a negative inotropic effect can be demonstrated with direct injection of nicardipine into the left main coronary artery in patients, the magnitude of the effect is much less than that seen with nifedipine [47]. Similarly, when nicardipine is administered in relatively high intravenous doses to patients with severe left ventricular dysfunction, a downward shift of the end-systolic pressure-volume relation can be seen; however, this is associated with an improvement in cardiac output [2]. No depression of left ventricular function has been seen when nicardipine has been given in conjunction with beta-adrenergic blocking agents [42]. Nicardipine may actually augment ventricular function in some experimental models probably via the coronary turgor effect [26]. Thus, most experimental and clinical evidence suggests that, of the calcium channel antagonists currently available, nicardipine has the least myocardial depressant activity.

Conclusions

None of the currently available calcium channel antagonists appears to exert clinically significant negative inotropic effects in patients with normal ventricular function, although with sophisticated techniques myocardial depression can be demonstrated with verapamil and possibly diltiazem [20]. In the setting of ischemia or dysrhythmia, all three agents may improve ventricular function by addressing the cause. In patients with depressed ventricular function, verapamil may depress it further and should be avoided especially in the setting of concomitant beta-adrenergic blockade. Nifedipine appears to have little myocardial depression in most studies due to potent vasodilatory actions of the drug at therapeutic doses. Its myocardial depression is masked by reflex sympathetic responses and afterload reduction. Diltiazem appears to be intermediate between verapamil and nifedipine in terms of clinically important myocardial depression; however, studies with this agent are limited. Nicardipine has the least myocardial depression of available agents. Overall, currently available data do not support use of calcium channel antagonists as primary agents for afterload reduction in patients with heart failure. Newer investigational agents with phosphodiesterase inhibitory and partial calcium agonistic properties may prove more useful in this regard.

MISCELLANEOUS PROBLEMS WITH CALCIUM CHANNEL ANTAGONIST THERAPY

Side effects and adverse reactions with calcium channel antagonist therapy are all secondary to the primary action of these compounds on cellular calcium flux and general inhibition of muscle contraction and/or stimulus secretion coupling. All available agents have been reported to cause severe hypotension and circulatory collapse. Treatment in this situation consists of fluid administration, calcium gluconate (10 gm over 10 minutes) and, if needed, vasopressor and inotropic support. Similarly, severe bradycardia, advanced AV block, or asystole may occur and are best treated with calcium, atropine, isoproterenol, and pacing if needed. In the unusual instance of a rapid ventricular response to a supraventricular dysrhythmia caused by conduction down an accessory pathway, which is precipitated by calcium channel antagonist therapy, cardioversion or therapy with lidocaine or procainamide may be needed. Problems with antidysrhythmia therapy and calcium channel antagonists are outlined elsewhere in this volume.

Minor side effects associated with nifedipine therapy include hypotension, headache, and peripheral edema. Recently a comparative clinical trial was completed assessing the side effects with nifedipine versus nicardipine [4]. Although all side effects tended to be less in the nicardipine treatment phase, the incidence of dizziness was significantly reduced. Verapamil more frequently causes constipation, conduction disturbances, and may also cause peripheral edema; however, caution must be used to exclude exacerbation of underlying congestive heart failure as the cause of the latter. Diltiazem is relatively free of adverse effects but has also been noted to cause edema. All the calcium channel antagonists have been noted to interact with the pharmacokinetics of other drugs. This will be covered elsewhere in this volume.

REFERENCES

1. Anavekar, S. N., et al. Verapamil in the treatment of hypertension. *J. Cardiovasc. Pharmacol.* 3:287, 1981.
2. Aroney, C., et al. Inotropic effect of nicardipine in patients with heart failure: Assessment by left ventricular end-systolic pressure-volume analysis. *J. Am. Coll. Cardiol.* 14:1331, 1989.
3. Arqueros, L., and Daniesi, A. J. Analysis of the inhibitory effect of verapamil on adrenal medullary secretion. *Life Sci.* 23:2415, 1978.
4. DeWood, M. A., and Wolbach, R. A. Randomized double-blind comparison of side effects of nicardipine and nifedipine in angina pectoris. *Am. Heart J.* 119:468, 1990.
5. Elkayam, U., et al. Acute hemodynamic effect of oral nifedipine in severe chronic congestive heart failure. *Am. J. Cardiol.* 52:1041, 1983.
6. Elkayam, U., et al. Comparison of hemodynamic responses to nifedipine and nitroprusside in severe chronic congestive heart failure. *Am. J. Cardiol.* 53:1321, 1984.
7. Elkayam, U., et al. Differences in hemodynamic response to vasodilation due to calcium channel antagonism with nifedipine and direct acting agonism with hydralazine in chronic refractory heart failure. *Am. J. Cardiol.* 54:126, 1984.
8. Engelman, R. M., et al. Rebound vasospasm after coronary revascularization in association with calcium antagonist withdrawal. *Ann. Thorac. Surg.* 37:469, 1984.

9. Fahmy, N. R., et al. Propranolol prevents hemodynamic and humoral events after abrupt withdrawal of nitroprusside. *Clin. Pharmacol. Ther.* 36:470, 1984.
10. Ferlinz, J., and Citron, P. D. Hemodynamic and myocardial performance characteristics after verapamil use in congestive heart failure. *Am. J. Cardiol.* 51:1339, 1983.
11. Ferlinz, J., Easthope, J. L., and Aronow, W. S. Effects of verapamil on myocardial performance in coronary disease. *Circulation* 59:313, 1979.
12. Fioretti, P., et al. Afterload reduction with nifedipine in aortic insufficiency. *Am. J. Cardiol.* 49:1728, 1982.
13. Freedman, S. B., Richmond, D. R., and Kelly, D. T. Long term follow up of verapamil and nitrate treatment for coronary artery spasm. *Am. J. Cardiol.* 50:711, 1982.
14. Frishman, W. H., et al. Comparative effects of abrupt withdrawal of propranolol and verapamil in angina pectoris. *Am. J. Cardiol.* 50:1191, 1982.
15. Gelman, J., et al. Nicardipine for angina pectoris at rest and coronary artery spasm. *Am. J. Cardiol.* 56:232, 1985.
16. Goldberg, A. D., Raftery, E. B., and Wilkinson, P. Blood pressure and heart rate and withdrawal of antihypertensive drugs. *Br. Med. J.* 1:1243, 1977.
17. Gottlieb, S. O., and Gerstenblith, G. Safety of acute calcium antagonist withdrawal: Studies in patients with unstable angina withdrawn from nifedipine. *Am. J. Cardiol.* 55:27E, 1985.
18. Hill, J., et al. Long-term responses to nifedipine in patients with coronary spasm who have an initial favorable response. *Am. J. Cardiol.* 52:26, 1983.
19. Johnson, S. M., et al. A controlled trial of verapamil for Prinzmetal's variant angina. *N. Engl. J. Med.* 304:862, 1981.
20. Josephson, M. A., and Singh, B. N. Use of calcium antagonists in ventricular dysfunction. *Am. J. Cardiol.* 55:81B, 1985.
21. Kay, R., Blake, J., and Rubin, J. Possible coronary spasm rebound to abrupt nifedipine withdrawal. *Am. Heart J.* 103:308, 1982.
22. Kieval, J., et al. The effects of intravenous verapamil on hemodynamic status of patients with coronary artery disease receiving propranolol. *Circulation* 65:653, 1982.
23. Klein, H. O., et al. The acute hemodynamic effects of intravenous verapamil in coronary artery disease: Assessment by equilibrium gated radionuclide ventriculography. *Circulation* 67:101, 1983.
24. Klugmann, S., Salvi, A., and Camerini, F. Haemodynamic effect of nifedipine in heart failure. *Br. Heart J.* 43:440, 1980.
25. Lambert, C. R., et al. Effects of nicardipine on exercise and pacing induced myocardial ischemia in angina pectoris. *Am. J. Cardiol.* 60:471, 1987.
26. Lambert, C. R., et al. Effects of nicardipine on myocardial function in vitro and in vivo. *Circulation* 81:III-39, 1990.
27. Lambert, C. R., and Pepine, C. J. Acute antianginal hemodynamic effects of nicardipine in coronary artery disease. *Am. Heart J.* 119:457, 1990.
28. Lichtman, M. A., et al. Effect of propranolol on oxygen binding to hemoglobin in vitro and in vivo. *Circulation* 49:881, 1974.
29. Ludbrook, P. A., et al. Acute hemodynamic responses to sublingual nifedipine: Dependence on left ventricular function. *Circulation* 65:489, 1982.
30. Matsumoto, S., et al. Hemodynamic effects of nifedipine in congestive heart failure. *Am. J. Cardiol.* 46:476, 1980.
31. Mehta, J., and Lopez, L. Calcium blocker withdrawal phenomenon: Increase in affinity of alpha 2 adrenoceptors for agonist as a potential mechanism. *Am. J. Cardiol.* 58:242, 1986.
32. Miller, R. R., et al. Propranolol withdrawal rebound phenomenon. *N. Engl. J. Med.* 293:416, 1975.

33. Moses, J. W., et al. Efficacy of nifedipine in rest angina refractory to propranolol and nitrates in patients with obstructive coronary artery disease. *Ann. Int. Med.* 94:425, 1981.
34. Nakaya, H., Schwartz, A., and Millard, R. W. Reflex chronotropic and inotropic effects of calcium channel blocking agents in conscious dogs: Diltiazem, verapamil, and nifedipine compared. *Circ. Res.* 52:302, 1983.
35. Nattel, S., Rangno, R. E., and Van Loon, G. Mechanism of propranolol withdrawal phenomenon. *Circulation* 59:1158, 1979.
36. Nelson, D. O., et al. Altered human vascular activity following withdrawal from calcium channel blockers. *J. Cardiovasc. Pharmacol.* 6:1249, 1984.
37. Packer, M., et al. Hemodynamic consequences of combined beta adrenergic and slow calcium channel blockade in man. *Circulation* 65:660, 1982.
38. Parodi, O., Maseri, A., and Simonetti, I. Management of unstable angina at rest by verapamil. *Br. Heart J.* 41:161, 1979.
39. Pepine, C. J., et al. Effect of diltiazem in patients with variant angina: A randomized double blind trial. *Am. Heart J.* 101:719, 1981.
40. Porter, C. B., et al. Differential effects of diltiazem and nitroprusside on left ventricular function in experimental chronic volume overload. *Circulation* 68:685, 1983.
41. Reeves, W. C., et al. Coronary artery spasm after abrupt withdrawal of nitroglycerin in rabbits. *Am. J. Cardiol.* 55:1066, 1985.
42. Rousseau, M. F., et al. Hemodynamic and cardiac effects of nicardipine in patients with coronary artery disease. *J. Cardiovasc. Pharmacol.* 6:833, 1984.
43. Serruys, P. W., et al. Regional wall motion from radiopaque markers after intravenous and intracoronary injections of nifedipine. *Circulation* 63:584, 1981.
44. Shick, E. C., et al. Randomized withdrawal from nifedipine: Placebo-controlled study in patients with coronary artery spasm. *Am. Heart J.* 104:690, 1982.
45. Singh, B. N., Phil, D., and Roche, A. Effects of intravenous verapamil on hemodynamics in patients with heart disease. *Am. Heart J.* 94:593, 1977.
46. Subramanian, V. B., et al. Calcium antagonist withdrawal syndrome: Objective demonstration with frequency modulated ambulatory ST segment monitoring. *Br. Med. J.* 286:520, 1983.
47. Terris, S., et al. Direct cardiac and peripheral vascular effects of intracoronary and intravenous nifedipine. *Am. J. Cardiol.* 58:25, 1986.
48. Vlietstra, R. E., et al. Effect of verapamil on left ventricular function: A randomized placebo controlled study. *Am. J. Cardiol.* 51:1213, 1983.
49. Walsh, R. A., Badke, F. R., and O'Rourke, R. A. Differential effects on systemic and intracoronary calcium channel blocking agents on global and regional left ventricular function in conscious dogs. *Am. Heart J.* 102:341, 1981.
50. Walsh, R. A., et al. Beneficial hemodynamic effects of intravenous and oral diltiazem in severe congestive heart failure. *J. Am. Coll. Cardiol.* 3:1044, 1984.
51. Wolfe, B. B., Harden, T. K., and Milinoff, P. B. In vitro study of beta adrenergic receptors. *Ann. Rev. Pharmacol. Toxicol.* 17:575, 1977.

CHAPTER 18

AN APPROACH TO ANTIANGINAL DRUG THERAPY

DAVID HOEKENGA
JONATHAN ABRAMS

INITIATING TREATMENT

A variety of approaches can be taken during the initiation of drug therapy in patients with angina pectoris. The equivalent efficacy of each of the three available classes of agents provides a rationale to begin therapy with any of the drugs, according to physician experience and bias. However, many patients have individual coexisting conditions that should be taken into account before initiation of medical therapy for angina. Selecting a proper antianginal agent is important because patients are usually on these drugs for many years. Several factors should be taken into consideration in choosing an antianginal drug appropriate for a particular patient, including (1) the presumed mechanism of the patient's ischemia, (2) the method of action of the particular drug, (3) convenience and cost of drug administration, (4) possible side effects of the drug, (5) the usefulness of the drug in treating other concomitant conditions, (6) significant contraindications to a particular antianginal agent, and (7) patient ability to comply with a drug regimen (see Table 18-1).

The available antianginal drugs are thoroughly discussed elsewhere in this book briefly. Each class of agents will be reviewed with the side effect profile and dosing guidelines being emphasized.

Nitrates

Nitrates are effective antianginal agents that are safe, relatively inexpensive, and available in a wide variety of delivery forms. Rare patients have severe hypotension on nitrate therapy. This important adverse side effect can often be detected by administering 0.4 mg of sublingual nitroglycerin to the patient before initiation of long-term therapy. Nitrate-induced headaches are a relatively common side effect of therapy but can often be avoided or reduced in intensity by using a low initial dose (for example, 10 mg of isosorbide dinitrate), then titrating the dose upward over several days or longer. In most patients without a history of migraine or vascular headaches, nitrate-induced headaches are mild

TABLE 18-1. *Factors to be Considered in Selecting Antianginal Drugs*

Mechanism of the patient's ischemia (spasm, fixed or mixed angina)
Method of action of the drug
Convenience and cost of drug administration
Side effects of the drug
Usefulness of the drug in treating other medical conditions
Contraindications to a particular antianginal agent
Patient ability to comply with a drug regimen

TABLE 18-2. *An Approach to Antianginal Therapy*

Try sublingual nitroglycerin. If successful add a long-acting nitrate (oral, buccal, or cutaneous).
If angina is not controlled, add:
  A beta blocker (see Table 18-3)
  A calcium channel antagonist (see Table 18-4)
If angina is not controlled:
  Consider cardiac catheterization for possible bypass surgery or coronary angioplasty
  Consider triple therapy if there is no clinical heart failure

---

and transient (subsiding in a 5 to 10 day period). A mild analgesic, such as acetaminophen, taken during the early days of therapy, is often beneficial.

Long-term nitrate therapy can be effectively delivered by use of oral isosorbide dinitrate, buccal nitroglycerin, or 2% nitroglycerin ointment. While nitroglycerin transdermal patches have been a popular form of therapy, the antianginal effect of these preparations does not predictably last the full 24 hours; daily application may induce a complete state of tolerance. Many believe that nitrate tolerance is more of a problem with these preparations than with other formulations. Recent reports suggest that patches should be used during the day, when patients are likely to experience angina, and removed during sleeping hours, when angina is usually rare or absent (see Chapter 16).

Recommended initial doses of nitrate therapy include 10 to 20 mg of isosorbide dinitrate PO tid-qid; 1/2 inch of nitroglycerin ointment to the skin qid; 1 mg of buccal nitroglycerin; or 10 mg of transdermal nitroglycerin (see Table 18-2). The final dose should be carefully determined after efficacy in angina relief and the side effects (if any) have been evaluated.

In any case, when a nitroglycerin preparation is chosen as the therapy of choice, the starting dose should be increased until angina is under control or side effects intervene. One of the advantages of initiating nitroglycerin therapy for patients with angina pectoris is the relatively limited number of side effects and their generally innocuous nature. Nevertheless, approximately 20 to 30 percent of patients cannot tolerate these drugs for long-term therapy because of headaches.

Beta Blockers

As with nitrates, the initiation of beta blocker therapy should begin with relatively low doses, such as 20 mg of propranolol PO qid, 80 mg of long-acting propranolol, or 50 mg of atenolol once each day. Adverse effects, which are more debilitating and numerous with beta blockers than with nitrates, are usually evident during the first few days of

TABLE 18-3. *When to Use a Beta Blocker for the Treatment of Angina*

If the patient also has:
 Postmyocardial infarction (within the past 2 years)
 Hypertension
 A history of supraventricular tachycardia
 A prominent exertional component to angina
 Documented ventricular arrhythmias

treatment but may be subtle and manifest only after weeks or even months of therapy.

Effective daily doses of propranolol range from a minimum of 40 mg to a maximum of 480 mg per day; most patients respond to daily doses in the range of 160 mg to 320 mg. Introduction of once daily, longer acting beta blockers such as atenolol and nadolol or other beta blockers that can be taken only twice a day such as metoprolol can also improve patient compliance.

Optimal beta blocker therapy exists when a patient has substantially diminished anginal symptoms, no major side effects, and moderate bradycardia (resting heart rate of 50 beats per minute). The resting heart rate alone may not reflect adequate beta blockade. Blunting of the heart rate and blood pressure response during exercise has been shown to be a simple measure of adequate beta blocker therapy [30]. A poor clinical response to treatment with beta blockers with no decrease or an increase in symptoms may indicate worsening of congestive heart failure, inadequate dosage, misdiagnosis of angina, or provocation of coronary artery spasm.

Cardioselective beta blockers, which have a dominant effect on beta-1 receptors located largely in the heart (see Chapter 7), may be useful in patients with chronic obstructive pulmonary disease, asthma, or diabetes mellitus (see Table 18-3). Unfortunately, at the relatively high dose levels often needed for treatment of angina, all currently available agents become much less cardioselective. The clinical benefits of intrinsic sympathomimetic activity in a beta blocker remain to be proven, although agents with this property (such as pindolol and acebutolol) would be logical choices in patients with resting bradycardia, postural hypotension, or severe peripheral vascular disease.

Unlike the nitroglycerin compounds and calcium channel antagonists, beta blocker therapy should not be terminated abruptly. In patients with angina pectoris, sudden beta blocker withdrawal can precipitate rebound hypertension and tachycardia, causing a marked increase in myocardial oxygen requirements (see Chapter 17). Rarely these rebound effects may aggravate ischemia or even precipitate acute myocardial infarction [26]. Beta blocking agents can usually be safely tapered over a 5 to 10 day period.

Calcium Channel Antagonists

The currently available calcium channel antagonists are each different in their physiologic actions and also differ in their adverse effect profile, unlike the nitrates and beta blockers. Verapamil causes moderate vasodilation, a mild decrease in contractility, and some decrease in atrioventricular (AV) conduction. Nifedipine causes marked vasodilation, no decrease in contractility or atrioventricular conduction, and the most prominent reflex sympathetic response. Diltiazem is intermediate in effect with moderate vasodilation, a mild decrease in left ventricular contractility, and a mild depression of AV conduction; diltiazem can significantly decrease S-A node function. The calcium channel antagonist selected for an individual patient should be individually chosen on the basis of these varying physiologic effects.

The effective dose of nifedipine varies from 30 mg to 120 mg per day, with rare patients benefiting from up to 180 mg per day. Side effects are frequent, including skin flushing, headaches, palpitations, and dizziness with initiation of nifedipine therapy. Ankle edema unrelated to heart failure may develop with chronic dosing. The starting dose of 10 mg three times a day can be rapidly increased to 20 mg three times a day within 48 to 72 hours if side effects are not severe and angina is still not well controlled. Higher doses may be necessary in some subjects. The new long-acting nifedipine (GTS) compound appears to be better tolerated than standard nifedipine.

Dose ranges for verapamil and diltiazem are narrower, with most patients responding best to 360 mg per day of each agent. Side effects of verapamil include slowing of the heart rate, constipation, and occasional peripheral edema. Plasma half-life of verapamil increases with long-term therapy, and the frequency of administration may be decreased in some cases after 1 to 2 weeks of treatment. In patients on digoxin, verapamil causes a 70 percent increase in free digoxin (a 45 percent increase is noted with nifedipine) [23].

Diltiazem has proved effective in daily doses of 120 to 360 mg. Because of its short elimination half-time, diltiazem is often given four times a day. However, some studies have shown it to be effective when given three times a day. The usual initial dose is 30 mg three to four times per day. In many patients the dose can then be titrated up relatively quickly. While many patients are controlled on 240 mg per day, some will need 360 to 480 mg daily in divided doses for optimal antianginal effect. In general, diltiazem is well tolerated and has a low incidence of associated side effects. In fact, when compared to the other calcium channel antagonists, beta blockers, and nitrates, diltiazem appears to have the lowest incidence of side effects of any of these agents. Side

TABLE 18-4. *When to Use a Calcium Channel Antagonist for the Treatment of Angina*

If the patient also has:
  Suspected coronary artery spasm or vasoconstriction
  Congestive heart failure (not verapamil)—use with caution
  Hypertension
  Insulin-dependent diabetes mellitus
  Peripheral vascular disease
  Bronchospasm
  Raynaud's phenomenon

effects of diltiazem include transient elevation of liver enzymes, peripheral edema, and asymptomatic sinus bradycardia. A change in therapy is usually not required because of these adverse effects, although rarely a drug rash is noted that does necessitate cessation of therapy.

Calcium channel antagonists are often useful in patients who have angina with concomitant hypertension, suspected coronary spasm, hypertension, or insulin-dependent diabetes mellitus (see Table 18-4).

Both diltiazem and verapamil have recently become available in sustained-release formulation, which is recommended for stabile angina patients. Several new dihydropyridine calcium channel antagonists are now available (isradapine, nicardipine), but not in sustained-release form. They offer no obvious advantage to the initial three blockers. Bepridil, a drug that also prolongs the QT interval, has been released, but only as a drug for refractory angina (due to serious side effects, including precipitation of ventricular arrythmias).

COMBINATION THERAPY

As little as 12 years ago, only two agents—sublingual nitroglycerin and oral propranolol—were available and widely believed to be effective for the treatment of angina. Now a wide variety of drugs in each of three different groups—nitrates, beta blockers, and calcium channel antagonists—are used in patients with angina pectoris. One of the most frequent conditions for which a cardiologist prescribes multiple drug therapy is the treatment of moderate to severe angina pectoris. The advantages of combination therapy include the ability to combine agents of different classes to utilize a variety of pharmacologic mechanisms to decrease myocardial oxygen demand. In addition, the nitrates and calcium channel antagonists have the ability to increase myocardial oxygen supply in some patients. When combination therapy is utilized, lower dosages of each drug may often be employed, with a diminution of specific drug-related side effects.

The disadvantages of combination therapy include the fact that patients must take many pills each day, often on differing time schedules, with a resulting increase in noncompliance. The cost of therapy rises, particularly with use of the more recently developed agents (diltiazem, nifedipine, newer beta blockers, nitroglycerin patches). In addition, patients are exposed to more side effects by using drugs of a variety of different classes. It is also possible that interactions can occur between various drugs that would limit their effectiveness.

In picking a drug regimen for an individual patient when combination therapy is indicated, two general approaches can be taken. One is a plan as to how to increase drug therapy by adding various agents in a predetermined fashion with a structured dosing schedule. The second approach is to tailor the selection of drugs according to the individual anginal syndrome, taking into account other cardiologic or medical conditions that might be harmed or helped by the combination therapy.

In reviewing combination drug therapy for angina pectoris, we should consider various double therapies that are commonly used (i.e., the combination of beta blockers and nitrates, beta blockers and calcium channel antagonists, and, least common, calcium channel antagonists and nitrates).

Many severely symptomatic patients will require triple therapy, utilizing a nitrate, beta blocker, and calcium channel antagonist.

Double Therapy

While some patients with mild to moderate angina are controlled with a single drug, most patients with moderate or severe angina require double or triple agent therapy to obtain adequate control of their angina pectoris. For instance, in our clinic population, we follow over 1,000 referred patients with angina pectoris. Approximately 20 percent of these patients are on monotherapy, 30 percent are on triple therapy, with a remaining 50 percent on two antianginal agents.

Experience with the three possible drug combinations used in double therapy is discussed below.

NITRATE AND BETA BLOCKERS

The combination of beta blockers and nitrates has several theoretical advantages and has been proven to be a useful strategy for the treatment of moderate to severe angina pectoris. As these were the first two agents clinically available in the United States, much more experience has accrued with these two classes of angianginal agents than with any other combination. The major physiologic effects of beta blockers and nitrates are complementary. Beta blockers reduce oxygen demand by decreasing heart rate, blood pressure, and contractility, particularly with physical activity. At the same time they may increase left ventricular size, an unwanted effect, and most increase peripheral vascular resis-

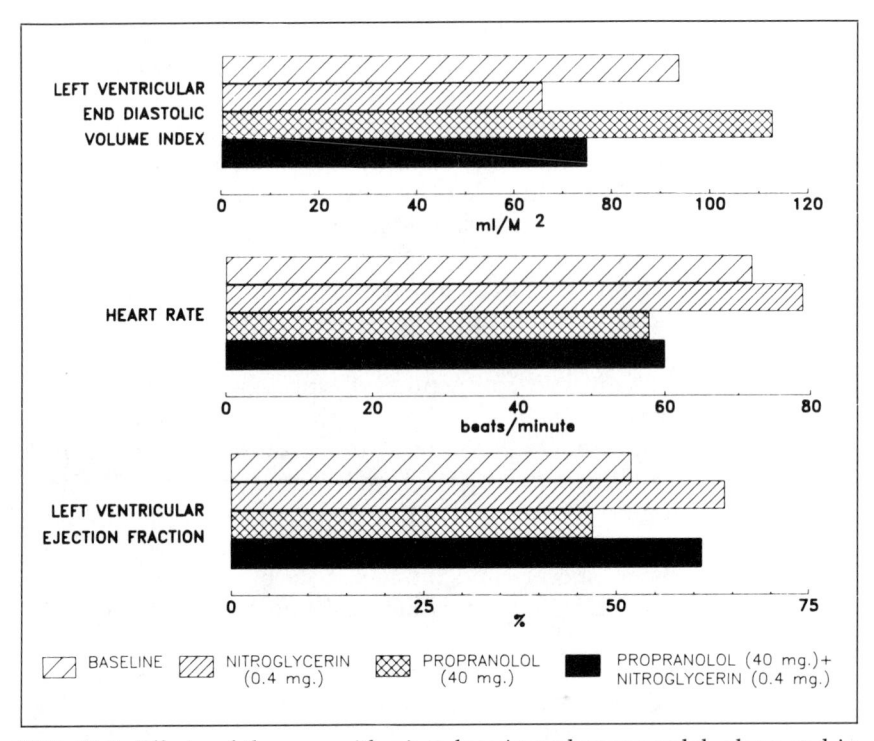

FIG. 18-1. Effects of therapy with nitroglycerin and propranolol, alone and in combination, on selected hemodynamics in patients with coronary artery disease ($N = 12$). Nitroglycerin blocked the increase in left ventricular end-diastolic volume seen with propranolol ($p < .001$). Propranolol blocked the increase in heart rate seen with nitroglycerin ($p < .001$). Nitroglycerin also largely reversed the fall in ejection fraction seen with propranolol. (Modified from Ref. 29.)

tance. Nitrates also reduce myocardial oxygen consumption, but these drugs produce reflex increases in cardiac contractility and heart rate. Nitrates decrease left ventricular volumes as well as end-diastolic pressure while increasing coronary blood flow. Thus, the undesirable effect of each class (tachycardia with nitrates, increased heart size and systemic resistance with beta blockers) is offset by concomitant utilization of the other drug. The combination of nitrates and beta blockers may be particularly desirable when coronary vasoconstriction is believed to play a role in the anginal syndrome (mixed angina) or when there is concern that a beta blocker might induce cardiac failure.

A number of investigations have confirmed the theoretical advantages of the nitrate/beta blocker combination in acute trials. In one study by Steele et al., therapy with propranolol prevented the reflex increase in heart rate seen with nitroglycerin [29]. Nitroglycerin induced a decrease in left ventricular end-diastolic volume and an increase in ejection fraction (Fig. 18-1).

Several long-term studies have examined the combination of nitrates and beta blockers in patients with angina pectoris. Schaumann showed benefit after the addition of isosorbide dinitrate to metoprolol [25] and another study showed that the addition of isosorbide dinitrate to pindolol diminished the symptoms of angina at four and eight weeks [6]. In contrast, Jensen et al. failed to find an improvement in exercise tolerance in 12 patients when isosorbide dinitrate was added to metoprolol over a three-week period [13]. Likewise, Müller et al., in a crossover study involving placebo, methopranolol, and isosorbide-5-mononitrate given over a two-week period, was unable to show that the combination of the drugs was superior to either drug given alone [19].

Overall the evidence that chronic therapy with both a nitrate and a beta blocker is superior to either drug given individually is mixed at this time. A large amount of anecdotal experience would suggest that this is an effective combination. Further trials with long-term usage of beta blockers and nitrates are indicated.

CALCIUM CHANNEL ANTAGONISTS AND NITRATES

The combination of nitrates and one of the available calcium channel antagonists has become common in clinical practice. Complementary physiologic effects of these two classes of agents should be beneficial. However, the additive effects of peripheral vasodilation, if excessive, could cause a sufficient decrease in both venous and arterial tone and lead to a significant fall in blood pressure.

Few controlled studies have compared the clinical effectiveness of a nitrate and calcium channel antagonist combination in stable angina pectoris. Some of the studies using this drug regimen have been done in patients with coronary artery spasm or variant angina. Freedman et al. used verapamil and nitrates in the treatment of 37 patients with coronary artery spasm [9]. Twenty-one months after initiation of therapy, 31 patients remained on calcium channel antagonists while 16 patients were also taking isosorbide dinitrate. Twenty-one patients were asymptomatic, and nine were improved with only one to four attacks per month. In another study Winniford et al. compared the combination of verapamil or nifedipine and isosorbide dinitrate to isosorbide alone in patients with active variant angina [35]. Patients treated with isosorbide dinitrate averaged 24 chest pain attacks per week; double therapy reduced the frequency of angina dramatically to one to four episodes of pain per week.

As both of these studies were in patients with dominant coronary artery spasm, the conclusions may not be applicable to patients with advanced atherosclerosis and effort angina pectoris who are not felt to have spasm as a prominent factor.

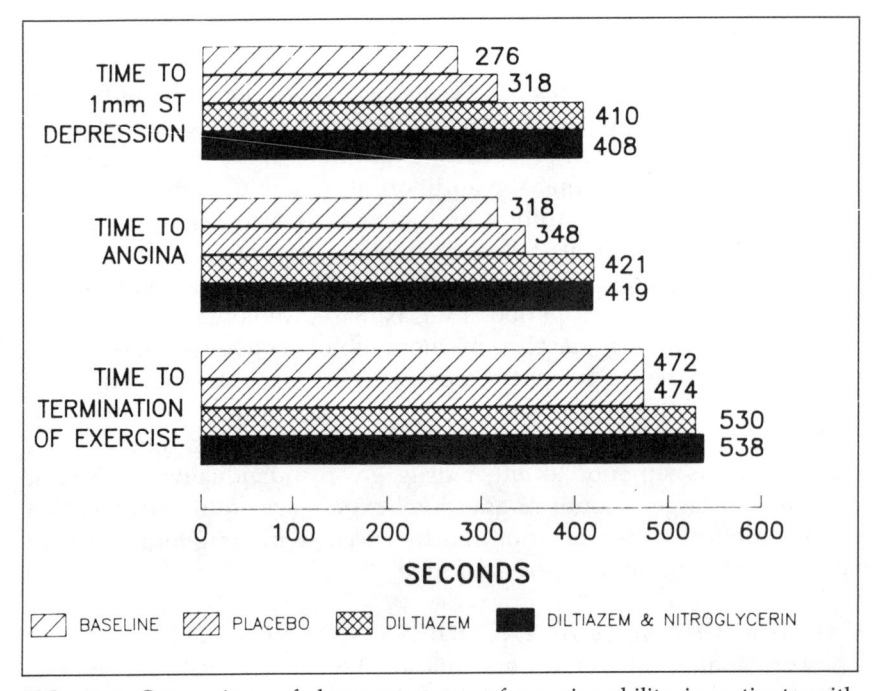

TIME TO 1mm ST DEPRESSION
- BASELINE: 276
- PLACEBO: 318
- DILTIAZEM: 410
- DILTIAZEM & NITROGLYCERIN: 408

TIME TO ANGINA
- BASELINE: 318
- PLACEBO: 348
- DILTIAZEM: 421
- DILTIAZEM & NITROGLYCERIN: 419

TIME TO TERMINATION OF EXERCISE
- BASELINE: 472
- PLACEBO: 474
- DILTIAZEM: 530
- DILTIAZEM & NITROGLYCERIN: 538

(SECONDS: 0–600)

FIG. 18-2. Comparison of three measures of exercise ability in patients with stable angina pectoris ($N = 12$). Exercise ability increased from baseline to placebo periods with a larger increase ($p < .05$) after diltiazem therapy (240 mg/day). However, addition of nitroglycerin (maximum dose 78 mg/day) did not further increase time to angina, time to 1 mm of ST depression, or time to termination of exercise.

Two studies have compared a nitrate (isosorbide dinitrate) with a calcium channel antagonist in angina pectoris without spasm and have concluded that both agents were effective in most patients [5, 10]. We recently completed a study of the combination of diltiazem and high-dose oral nitroglycerin in patients with atherosclerosis and stable angina pectoris [10]. We studied 12 patients treated with three different regimens in a double-blind crossover protocol: (1) placebo, (2) diltiazem, (3) diltiazem plus nitroglycerin. Total exercise duration was improved by addition of diltiazem when compared to placebo but was not increased further by the addition of nitroglycerin. Exercise duration to the onset of chest pain increased 18 percent with diltiazem when compared to placebo and increased only 22 percent with diltiazem plus nitroglycerin. Diltiazem also improved exercise duration time to onset of angina and time to 1 mm of ST depression (Fig. 18-2). No further improvement was noted with the addition of nitroglycerin. We concluded that combination therapy with two vasodilators such as diltiazem and nitroglycerin did not improve control of angina pectoris in patients who were responsive to monotherapy with diltiazem. In a similar study of 18 patients, Deedwania et al. titrated subjects to stable doses of oral nitroglycerin and then added diltiazem or placebo therapy for a two-week period [5]. In this investigation, oral nitroglycerin alone improved exercise time. However, the addition of diltiazem to oral nitroglycerin therapy did not result in significant improvement in exercise parameters.

While the combination of nitrates with diltiazem, nifedipine, or verapamil is widely used in the treatment of stable angina pectoris, no controlled trials at this time demonstrate the effectiveness of these two agents over therapy with a calcium channel antagonist alone.

BETA BLOCKERS AND CALCIUM CHANNEL ANTAGONISTS

Unlike combined therapy with nitrates and calcium channel antagonists, the combination of beta blockade and calcium channel blockade has been widely studied. Interest in this combination has been spurred by the possibility of treating angina with two very different types of drugs and also because of concern about potential adverse interactions of these two groups of agents.

Several studies have been performed comparing the effects of diltiazem and a beta blocker in patients with stable angina pectoris. In one study of 24 patients, Humen et al. compared propranolol monotherapy with diltiazem monotherapy to the combination of propranolol and diltiazem [11]. In this trial, combination therapy with propranolol and diltiazem (particularly at a dose of 360 mg per day) resulted in a significant improvement in exercise capacity and a reduction in symptoms without an increase in adverse effects or deterioration of left ventricular function compared to single therapy with either drug (Fig. 18-3). In a similar group of 24 patients, Strauss and Parisi found that the angina rate diminished with the addition of diltiazem to propranolol when compared to propranolol alone or propranolol plus placebo [30]. Kenny et al. also found diltiazem and propranolol combined to be superior in effort-related angina when compared to either drug alone [14].

Other studies of the diltiazem and propranolol combination have shown different results. In a study of 12 patients with stable angina pectoris, Hung et al. combined 360 mg of diltiazem with 240 mg of propranolol. In this study diltiazem alone appeared to be as effective or more effective than the combination of diltiazem and propranolol in improving exercise tolerance and left ventricular function [12].

The combination of nifedipine and a beta blocker has been studied in a number of trials. Compared to diltiazem, nifedipine has more pronounced vasodilatory properties, resulting in marked decreases in afterload. Reflex sympathetic activation often results in tachycardia and an increase in myocardial contractility. Therefore the combination of

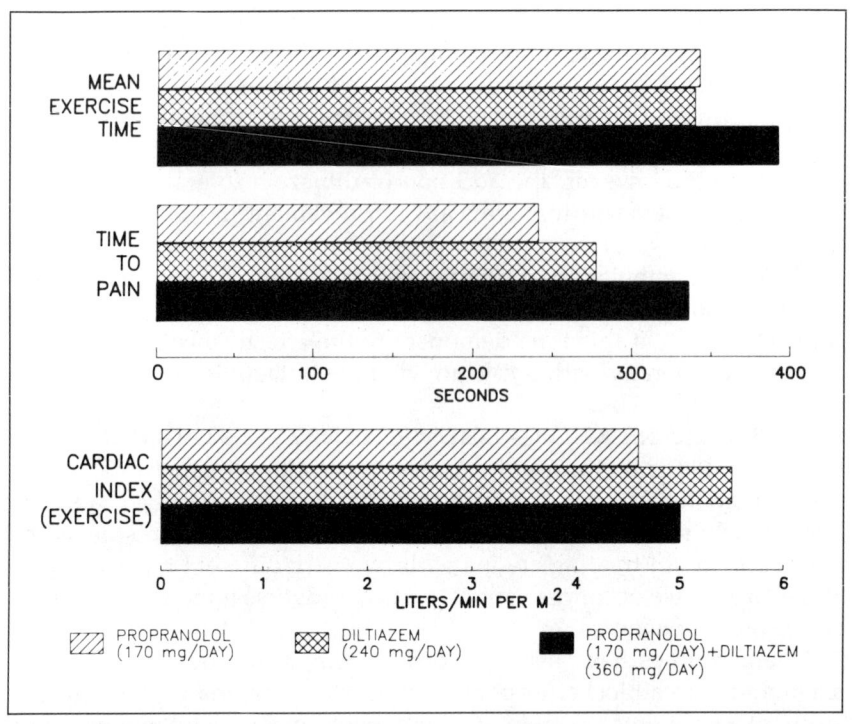

FIG. 18-3. Effects of therapy with propranolol and diltiazem, alone and in combination, in patients with stable exertional angina ($N = 24$). Total exercise time and time to onset of chest pain were similar for both forms of monotherapy but increased significantly for combination therapy ($p < .05$). Exercise cardiac index was lowest with propranolol therapy, highest with diltiazem therapy, and intermediate with combination therapy ($p < .05$ versus diltiazem). (Modified from Ref. 11.)

nifedipine and a beta blocker could be useful, particularly in patients with mild to moderate left ventricular dysfunction. In one trial reported by Braun et al., this combination was evaluated in 20 patients with stable angina pectoris [3]. Patients were studied before treatment, after four weeks of propranolol therapy, and after four weeks of combined treatment. Exercise tolerance increased on propranolol and increased further with combination therapy. Without active drug and on propranolol, exercise ejection fraction decreased significantly as measured by equilibrium radionuclide ventriculography. However, with combination therapy, there was a significant improvement in exercise ejection fraction. These authors concluded that combined propranolol and nifedipine in patients with stable angina was hemodynamically superior to therapy with propranolol alone and safe even in patients with moderately depressed LV function. In a similar study of 16 patients with stable angina, Dargie et al. showed that 30 to 60 mg per day of nifedipine combined with 240 to 280 mg per day of propranolol was effective in reducing the incidence of chest pain [4]. While each drug was significantly more effective than placebo, the combination provided even greater improvement. Additional studies with the combination of nifedipine and atenolol [8], metoprolol and nifedipine [33], and another employing the combination again of nifedipine and propranolol [18]. All concluded that combined treatment with a beta blocker and nifedipine increased antianginal efficacy compared with monotherapy with either agent without increasing adverse effects.

Case reports of patients developing symptoms of congestive failure on the combination of beta blockers and nifedipine have appeared [1]. However, in the other studies mentioned above, nearly 100 patients were given combined nifedipine and beta blockers without any instance of heart failure.

Thus, without exception, it has been found that the addition of nifedipine to beta blockade improves antianginal efficacy, often permitting a reduction in the dosage of the beta blocker. In most of these studies the calcium channel antagonist was added to previously administered beta blockers. Aggravation of angina with combination therapy seems virtually unknown. Nevertheless, the patient may experience side effects from both drugs. For example, beta blockade does not protect from the headache, flushing, hypotensive effects, or edema encountered with nifedipine. While nifedipine may counteract the cold extremities induced by beta blockade, it has little effect on such adverse effects as bronchospasm, fatigue, nightmares, and the potential precipitation of cardiac failure.

The combined administration of verapamil and a beta blocker has also been studied in patients with chronic stable angina. Early concern with this combination focused on the negative inotropic effect of verapamil (see Chapter 8), which is more pronounced when compared to the other calcium channel antagonists. The depressive effect on left ventricular contractility, along with the known decrease in LV contractile function induced by beta blockade, raised genuine concerns about this combination in the routine treatment of patients with chronic stable angina. Four chronic studies have examined this combination in patients with angina pectoris. Subramanian et al. compared treatment with verapamil 360 mg per day and propranolol 120 mg per day in a group of 14 patients who had persistent angina despite previous therapy with single drug therapy [31]. The combination of 360 mg of verapamil and 120 mg of propranolol was then initiated. Mean exercise time was 4.8 minutes for placebo, 6.8 minutes for propranolol, 8.0 minutes for verapamil, and 10.1 minutes with the combination verapamil and propranolol therapy. Seven of the 14 patients became symptom free on double therapy. Left ventricular function indices were not significantly different on both

MEAN EXERCISE TIME

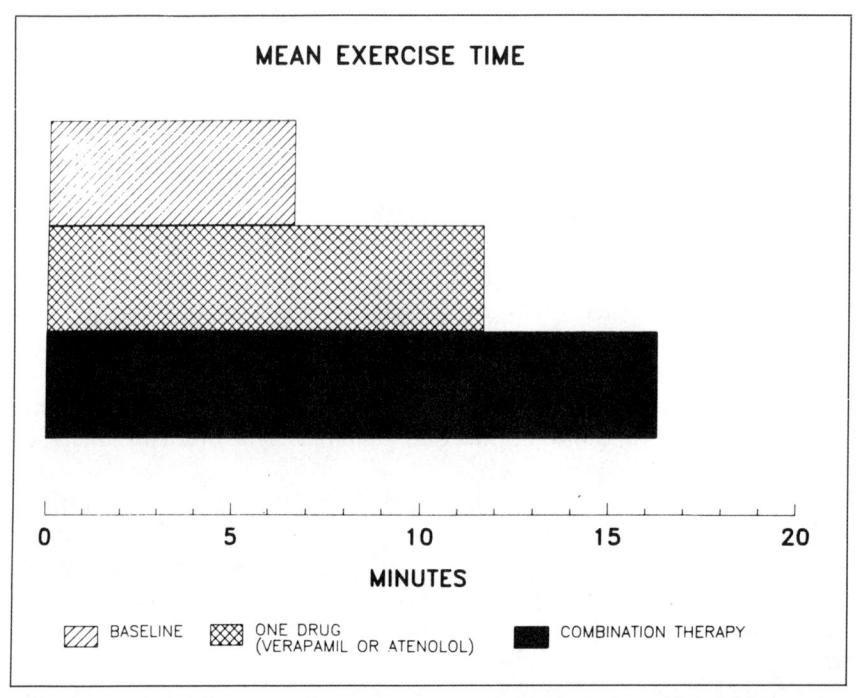

FIG. 18-4. The change in mean exercise time in patients with stable angina (N = 18) after chronic therapy with atenolol (200 mg/day), verapamil (360 mg/day) (*middle bar*) compared to baseline (*top bar*). The bottom bar represents chronic combination therapy with atenolol (100 mg/day) plus verapamil (360 mg/day). A large improvement in exercise time is apparent from baseline (6.7 min) to one drug (11.7 min) to combination therapy (16.3 min). (Modified from Ref. 15.)

drugs from those obtained with propranolol alone. Raferty treated 14 patients with the combination propranolol and verapamil using the same dosage as Subramanian [24]. In this trial, mean exercise time was increased significantly on combination therapy, and 10 of 13 patients showed an improvement in symptomatology. Lessem studied 18 patients treated with 360 mg of verapamil per day and 100 mg of atenolol per day for a period of 6 weeks [15]. Maximum exercise time increased more with the combination than with single drug therapy with either agent (Fig. 18-4). No serious adverse hemodynamic effects were recorded. Left ventricular ejection fraction with exercise actually increased 4.6 percent with the combination therapy. These authors concluded that combination beta blocker and verapamil therapy is safe and effective in chronic stable angina pectoris. In a large study involving 42 consecutive patients with angina resistant to therapy with verapamil or beta blockers alone, McGourty et al. used combination therapy and followed subjects for a period of 6.5 months [16]. Patients with heart failure, heart block, or uncontrolled hypertension were excluded from the trial. Eighty-one percent of the patients reported an improvement in the number of anginal attacks with a mean reduction from 17 attacks to five attacks per week. Side effects necessitated withdrawal of one or both drugs in six patients. The most common complication was mild left ventricular failure. These authors suggest that the combination of beta blockers and verapamil may be used in a relatively unselected group of patients with difficult-to-control angina.

Several investigators have examined the hemodynamic consequences of the combination of verapamil and a beta blocker. Packer et al. showed that 120 mg of verapamil given to patients receiving high doses of propranolol or metoprolol showed a decrease in cardiac index of .38 L/min/M^2, a 6 beat per minute decrease in heart rate and a 2.2 mm Hg rise in pulmonary capillary wedge pressure [22]. Two patients in this study developed asymptomatic but marked hypotension. In a similar intravenous study performed by Silke et al., combination therapy reduced systemic arterial pressure and heart rate without a change in cardiac output or systemic vascular resistance [27]. The authors concluded that in patients with stable coronary artery disease the cardiac depressant actions of verapamil were countered by its arterial vasodilatory properties.

In summary, the combined use of a beta blocker and a calcium channel antagonist has been shown to be more effective than monotherapy with either drug alone in many patients with stable angina. The data are particularly convincing for a nifedipine–beta blocker combination. The potential hazards of a negative chronotropic (verapamil or diltiazem and a beta blocker) or a negative inotropic (verapamil and beta blocker) have not been shown to be a major problem. Nevertheless, marked cardiac slowing, AV conduction disturbances, or the precipitation of congestive heart failure are potentially limiting in susceptible subjects. Patients with intrinsic bradycardia or depressed LV function should be started on combination therapy with great caution; nifedipine is the safest calcium channel antagonist for bradycardic individuals, while diltiazem or nifedipine should be carefully administered to subjects with major left ventricular dysfunction.

The use of a nitrate with a calcium channel antagonist has not been documented to be an effective antianginal combination. Nitrate–beta blocker therapy has theoretical advantages, but little data to demonstrate clear-cut efficacy despite widespread clinical use.

Triple Therapy

Patients with severe angina unresponsive to double therapy frequently undergo coronary angiography with the hope that an intervention will allow a reduction in medical therapy. However, a subgroup of patients, in our experience as high as 30 percent, may be unsuitable for percutaneous transluminal coronary angioplasty and/or coronary artery bypass grafting. In this group with persistent angina on double therapy, three antianginal agents may be used. Traditionally, the combination has consisted of a nitrate, beta blocker, and calcium channel antagonist for the control of severe angina rather than using two drugs from within a class of agents plus a second type of antianginal agent.

Several studies have looked at the usefulness of triple therapy in obtaining additional control of angina pectoris. In a study by Nesto et al., 16 patients with three or more episodes of angina pectoris per week, despite therapy with long-acting nitrates and beta blockers, were studied [20]. Patients were either on nadolol, metoprolol, or propranolol as a beta blocker. Sixty-two percent of the patients were on propranolol with a mean dose of 168 mg/day. Nitrate therapy consisted of nitroglycerin ointment or isosorbide dinitrate, with the majority being on oral isosorbide at a mean dose of 120 mg/day. Nifedipine at a mean dose of 95 mg/day was added to the nitrate and beta blocker therapy. On two agents, all exercise tests were limited by angina. With the addition of a calcium channel antagonist, only eight patients stopped their exercise test because of angina. Mean duration of exercise increased with the addition of calcium channel antagonist from 431 to 532 sec ($p < 0.001$). An improvement in global left ventricular function at comparable workloads was also noted. These authors conclude that exercise-induced ischemia in these patients, who were receiving maximum doses of beta blockers and nitrates, was significantly reduced when nifedipine was added. In a similar study, White et al. studied the effects of oral nifedipine in patients who were symptomatic despite therapy with beta adrenoreceptor blocking drugs and nitrates [34]. Patients were treated with 80 to 120 mg/day of nifedipine in addition to baseline medication. On this therapy the duration of exercise increased by a mean of 21 percent with nifedipine ($p < 0.005$). While 14 patients were limited by angina pectoris at baseline, only 5 patients were limited by angina pectoris after nifedipine treatment.

A similar study with another calcium channel antagonist was performed by Boden et al. in 12 patients on beta blockers and nitrates [2]. Diltiazem in a dose of 90 mg qid was combined with maximally tolerated propranolol and isosorbide dinitrate. In this study, angina pectoris was abolished during peak exercise in 8 of the 12 patients with the addition of diltiazem. Diltiazem increased the exercise duration from 276 to 310 seconds. Reduction of rate pressure product at submaximal and peak workload indicated that patients could perform a high level of external work before the onset of ischemia.

Negative results with maximal (triple) drug therapy were reported in a study by Tolins et al. [32]. In this study, patients on propranolol therapy were given nifedipine of 20 mg or isosorbide dinitrate, or both drugs, 1½ hours before exercise. Exercise duration was 467 seconds with propranolol and increased to 556 seconds with isosorbide dinitrate and to 636 seconds with nifedipine. However, exercise duration with all three drugs was only 597 seconds. Improvement with the nifedipine combination was greater than that with isosorbide dinitrate plus propranolol. In this study, the exercise duration was actually worse in nine of 16 patients when all three drugs were given than when the two-drug combination of propranolol and nifedipine was used. However, this was an acute study with only one dose of nitrate and/or calcium channel antagonist being given before the exercise test.

In general the studies performed using triple therapy in patients with severe angina pectoris are encouraging. Most report a decrease in angina and increases in exercise ability with therapy using nitrates, beta blockers, and calcium channel antagonists. Caution is raised by the Tolins study, even though it was an acute trial, suggesting that in some patients two-drug combinations were even more efficacious than triple-drug therapy. Several experts have commented that triple therapy has little objective support in the research literature. We believe, however, that in *symptomatic* anginal subjects on double therapy, a careful institution of a third compound will usually result in clinical benefit.

STRATIFICATION OF PATIENTS INTO SUBSETS FOR THERAPY WITH A SPECIFIC DRUG

Other Cardiovascular Diseases

HYPERTENSION
Either beta blockers or calcium channel antagonists should be used as first-line treatment for recent-onset angina in hypertensive subjects. Although more clinical experience has accumulated for the beta blockers, calcium channel antagonists are effective in the treatment of hypertension.

IMPAIRED LEFT VENTRICULAR FUNCTION OR CONGESTIVE HEART FAILURE
Use of nitrates or calcium channel antagonists is indicated when cardiac mechanical function is significantly impaired. Nitrates are also effective in patients with mitral regurgitation. Gross cardiomegaly in a patient with angina is a relative contraindication for the initial use of beta-adrenergic blocking therapy. Beta blockers should probably not be given when there is a history of definite congestive heart failure; verapamil should be employed with great caution in such patients. Nifedipine

may improve the performance of the compromised left ventricle because of its marked afterload-reducing action. All calcium channel antagonists have the potential to further reduce left ventricular function that is impaired. Caution should be used in any patient with an ejection fraction less than 30 percent when beginning a calcium channel antagonist.

POSTMYOCARDIAL INFARCTION
Recently reported trials of beta blocker administration after acute myocardial infarction demonstrate that recurrent infarction, sudden death, and overall cardiovascular mortality are decreased in treated subjects compared with control subjects. The presumption is that these drugs may decrease the incidence of recurrent myocardial ischemia and/or malignant ventricular dysrhythmias. We believe that a history of prior infarction is a relative indication for use of beta blocking therapy in angina. Similar data for nitrates (positive) and calcium channel antagonists (conflicting) are not strong enough to make recommendations for these agents in the routine post-MI patient with angina.

ARRHYTHMIAS
For the unusual angina patient with recurrent supraventricular tachycardia or paroxysmal atrial fibrillation, verapamil or a beta blocker are clearly the first-line choices. Although there have been many efforts to demonstrate a decrease in ventricular ectopic activity with beta-adrenergic blocking therapy, the efficacy of these drugs in suppressing ventricular dysrhythmias is controversial. Antiarrhythmic activity may be the mechanism for the decrease in sudden death found in the postmyocardial infarction trials with beta blockers, and data from the BHAT study [17] and a postinfarction metoprolol trial [21] are consistent with this hypothesis.

Beta blockers, verapamil, and possibly diltiazem are contraindicated in patients with angina who have significant atrioventricular block or sinus node dysfunction.

Noncardiac Diseases

CHRONIC OBSTRUCTIVE PULMONARY DISEASE AND ASTHMA
Calcium channel antagonists or nitrates are preferred in patients with bronchospasm who have angina. Beta blockers should be avoided. All beta blockers can potentially aggravate bronchospasm or may even provoke an acute attack. Cardioselective beta blockers, such as metoprolol and atenolol, in low dose can be used in some patients with pulmonary disease. However, cardioselectivity is lost as beta blocker

dosage is increased. Drugs with partial antagonist activity, such as acebutolol, may be less likely to provoke bronchospasm.

DIABETES MELLITUS

In patients with diabetes, beta blockers may mask the symptoms associated with hypoglycemia, except sweating. By inhibiting glycogenolysis, the agents may prolong hypoglycemia after excessive insulin administration. These problems generally do not arise in patients who are not taking insulin. If beta blockers are used, beta-1 selective agents in low dose are preferable. However, calcium channel antagonists, especially verapamil or diltiazem, are generally preferred in patients with diabetes mellitus. Since diabetics are vulnerable to autonomic insufficiency and postural hypotension, the systemic vasodilation caused by calcium channel antagonists, particularly nifedipine, may be troublesome. Remember that diabetic patients are more likely to have silent ischemia, so additional testing with Holter monitoring may be necessary even if anginal attacks are reduced.

RAYNAUD'S PHENOMENON

Since nifedipine has proved effective as therapy for Raynaud's phenomenon [28], the combination of angina and Raynaud's could be effectively treated with this agent. Diltiazem is also beneficial for Raynaud's phenomenon but verapamil is less effective.

MIGRAINE

In migraine headaches, a beta blocker is usually preferable as initial therapy for angina pectoris. Calcium channel antagonists such as verapamil or diltiazem may also be used.

HYPERTHYROIDISM

In hyperthyroidism, beta blockers are effective in controlling the tachycardia, anxiety, palpitations, excess sweating, and tremors associated with this condition [7]. Therefore, they would be an excellent choice in the rare patient with coexisting angina pectoris.

CONCLUSIONS

A wide variety of drugs is available to the physician for the therapy of angina, and it is hoped that some of these agents may positively alter the natural history of ischemic heart disease. This fortunate situation demands a choice among the three major classes of antianginal drugs when treatment is initiated, as well as a determination of the most appropriate maintenance therapy for a patient already being treated for angina. It is possible to tailor therapy to the underlying pathophysiology of angina in many cases, and an intelligent analysis of the clinical picture usually provides a rationale for selecting one of the three groups of antianginal drugs. Although some empiricism is still necessary, particularly in the use of double or triple therapy, our therapeutic armamentarium has been enriched with effective agents that can improve and possibly prolong the life of patients with angina pectoris.

REFERENCES

1. Anastassiades, C. J. Nifedipine and beta-blocker drugs. *Br. Med. J.* 281:1251–52, 1980.
2. Boden, W. E., Bough, E. W., Reichman, M. J., et al. Beneficial effects of high-dose diltiazem in patients with persistent effort angina and β-blockers and nitrates: A randomized, double-blind, placebo-controlled cross-over study. *Circulation* 71:1197–1205, 1985.
3. Braun, S., Terdiman, R., Berenfeld, D., and Laniado, S. Clinical and hemodynamic effects of combined propranolol and nifedipine therapy versus propranolol alone in patients with angina pectoris. *Am. Heart J.* 108:478–85, 1985.
4. Dargie, H. J., Lynch, P. G., Krikler, D. M., et al. Nifedipine and propranolol: A beneficial drug interaction. *Amer. J. Med.* 71:676–82, 1981.
5. Deedwania, P. C., Andrew, H. T., Thao, T. P., and White, K. L. Diltiazem fails to augment the anti-anginal efficacy of nitroglycerin. *Circulation* 70:II-190, 1984.
6. Delmare, J. Double-blind comparative study of pindolol alone and its association with a nitrate derivative. *Nouv. Presse Med.* 7:2733–34, 1978.
7. Feely, J., and Peden, N. Uses of β-adrenoreceptor blocking drugs in hyperthyroidism. *Drugs* 27:425, 1984.
8. Findlay, I. N., MacLeod, K., Ford, M., et al. Treatment of angina pectoris with nifedipine and atenolol: Efficacy and effect on cardiac function. *Br. Heart J.* 55: 240–45, 1986.
9. Freedman, S. B., Richmond, D. R., and Kelly, D. T. Long-term follow-up of verapamil and nitrate treatment for coronary artery spasm. *Amer. J. Cardiol.* 50:711–15, 1982.
10. Hoekenga, D. E., Moss, J., and Abrams, J. A comparison of diltiazem monotherapy to the combination of diltiazem and oral nitroglycerin in stable angina pectoris. *Amer. Heart J.* (submitted).
11. Humen, D. P., O'Brien, P., Purves, P., et al. Effort angina with adequate beta-receptor blockade: Comparison with diltiazem alone and in combination. *J. Amer. Coll. Cardiol.* 7:329–35, 1986.
12. Hung, J., Lamb, I. H., Connolly, S. J., et al. The effect of diltiazem and propranolol, alone and in combination, on exercise performance and left ventricular function in patients with stable effort angina: A double-blind, randomized, and placebo-controlled study. *Circulation* 68:560–67, 1983.
13. Jensen, G., Trautner, F., Rasmussen, S., and Hesse, B. Isosorbide dinitrate (ISDN) in effort-induced angina pectoris despite beta-blocking treatment. Clinical and hematological effects assessed by isotope angiocardiography. *Ugeskr. Laeger* 133:3247–50, 1982.
14. Kenny, J., Kiff, P., Holmes, J., and Jewitt, D. E. Beneficial effects of diltiazem

and propranolol, alone and in combination, in patients with stable angina pectoris. *Br. Heart J.* 53:43–46, 1985.
15. Lessem, J. Combined therapy with Ca-antagonists and beta-adrenergic receptor blocking agents in chronic stable angina. *Acta Med. Scand.* 681(Suppl):83–90, 1984.
16. McGourty, J. C., Silas, J. H., and Solomon, S. A. Tolerability of combined treatment with verapamil and beta blockers in angina resistant to monotherapy. *Postgrad. Med. J.* 61:229–32, 1985.
17. Morganroth, J., Lichstein, E., Hubble, E., and Harrist, R. Effect of propranolol on ventricular arrhythmias in the β-blocker heart attack (BHAT). *Circulation* 66:II-328, 1982.
18. Morse, J. R., and Nesto, R. W. Double-blind crossover comparison of the anti-anginal effects of nifedipine and isosorbide dinitrate in patients with exertional angina receiving propranolol. *J. Amer. Coll. Cardiol.* 6:1395–1401, 1985.
19. Müller, G., Uberbacher, H. J., and Glocke, M. Coronary therapeutic effects of low dose IS-5-MN compared to the combination of IS-5-MN + methopranolol and placebo. *Med. Welt.* 34:321–27, 1983.
20. Nesto, R. W., White, H. D., Ganz, P., et al. Addition of nifedipine to maximal beta-blocker nitrate therapy: Effects on exercise capacity and global left ventricular performance at rest and during exercise. *Amer. J. Cardiol.* 55:3E–5E, 1985.
21. Olsson, G., and Rehnqvist, N. Antiarrhythmic effects of chronic post-infarction metoprolol therapy. *Circulation* 66:II-144, 1982.
22. Packer, M., Meller, J., Medina, N., et al. Hemodynamic consequences of combined beta-adrenergic and slow calcium channel blockade in man. *Circulation* 65:660–68, 1982.
23. Pepine, C. J., Feldman, R. L., and Conti, C. R. Comprehensive drug management of angina pectoris. *Cardiovasc. Clin.* 14:139–51, 1984.
24. Raferty, E. B. Calcium blockers and beta blockers: Alone and in combination. *Acta Med. Scand.* 694(Suppl):188–96, 1984.
25. Schaumann, H.-J. Additional treatment of angina pectoris with a betablocker. *Therapiewoche* 33:2333–42, 1983.
26. Shiroff, R. A., Mathis, J., and Zelis, M. D. Propranolol rebound—a retrospective study. *Amer. J. Cardiol.* 41:778–80, 1978.
27. Silke, B., Verma, S. P., Nelson, G. I. C., et al. The effects on left ventricular performance of verapamil and metoprolol singly and together in exercise-induced angina pectoris. *Amer. Heart J.* 109:1286–93, 1985.
28. Smith, C. D., and McKendry, R. J. P. Controlled trial of nifedipine in the treatment of Raynaud's phenomenon. *Lancet* 2:1299, 1982.
29. Steele, P. P., Maddoux, G., Kirch, D. L., and Vogel, R. A. Effects of propranolol and nitroglycerin on left ventricular performance in patients with coronary arterial disease. *Chest* 73:19–23, 1978.
30. Strauss, W. E., and Parisi, A. F. Superiority of combined diltiazem and propranolol therapy for angina pectoris. *Circulation* 71:951–57, 1985.
31. Subramanian, B., Bowles, M. J., Davies, A., and Raferty, E. B. Combined therapy with verapamil and propranolol and chronic stable angina. *Amer. J. Cardiol.* 49:126–32, 1983.
32. Tolins, M., Weir, E. K., Chesler, E., and Pierpont, G. L. "Maximal" drug therapy is not necessarily optimal in chronic angina pectoris. *J. Amer. Coll. Cardiol.* 3:1051–57, 1984.
33. Uusitalo, A., Arstila, M., Bae, E. A., et al. Metoprolol, nifedipine, and the combination in stable effort angina pectoris. *Amer. J. Cardiol.* 57:733–37, 1986.

34. White, H. D., Polak, J. F., Wynne, J., et al. Addition of nifedipine to maximal nitrate and beta-adrenoreceptor blocker therapy in coronary artery disease. *Amer. J. Cardiol.* 55:1303–07, 1985.
35. Winniford, M. D., Gabliani, G., Johnson, S. M., et al. Concomitant calcium antagonist plus isosorbide dinitrate therapy for markedly active variant angina. *Amer. Heart J.* 108:1269–73, 1984.

CHAPTER 19

WHEN TO USE ANGIOPLASTY OR BYPASS SURGERY

BARRY F. ROSE
CARL J. PEPINE

Despite advances in pharmacologic therapy of patients with coronary artery disease, coronary revascularization procedures are often necessary either to relieve symptoms because of failure of drug therapy alone or to attempt to improve long-term prognosis in certain patient subsets. Revascularization procedures currently available for general clinical use include percutaneous transluminal coronary angioplasty (PTCA) and coronary artery bypass graft (CABG) surgery, in addition to thrombotic drug therapy for acute myocardial infarction. Newer alternative revascularization procedures such as laser angioplasty directional atherectomy and vascular endoprosthesis are considered new or experimental and will not be discussed.

Traditionally, CABG surgery was done with saphenous vein but now increasingly also includes one or both internal mammary arteries. It is acknowledged that both CABG surgery and PTCA may provide effective revascularization, that is, improved blood flow to potentially ischemic myocardium and thereby provide both subjective (i.e., relief of symptoms) and objective improvement in myocardial ischemia through increases in coronary flow [51, 54, 59, 60, 64, 75, 83, 117, 120]. The relative value of these two procedures, however, in the various coronary disease syndromes remains to be determined by controlled clinical trials.

Patients with coronary artery disease have varied clinical presentations including any of the following alone or in combination: (1) chronic stable effort angina, (2) unstable rest angina, (3) acute myocardial infarction, and (4) silent ischemia. When a patient presents with one of the above, the physician must decide if revascularization therapy is appropriate as an addition to drug therapy and which revascularization therapy is most appropriate. To this end, the following discussion will compare the effectiveness of PTCA and CABG procedures with each other and with drug therapy alone. Regarding long-term efficacy of revascularization procedures, we shall consider problems of graft occlusion with CABG surgery and problems of restenosis with PTCA. The role of repeat revascularization in patients who present with angina after previous PTCA or CABG surgery will also be addressed. These considerations are particularly important in determining the relative value of each of these therapies when used either alone or in combination in any given patient.

CHRONIC STABLE ANGINA PECTORIS

General Considerations

FACTORS PREDICTING PROGNOSIS
Before examining results of revascularization treatment in chronic stable angina, it is important to review factors that predict prognosis in these patients. Years ago, Burggraf and Parker, among others, recognized the

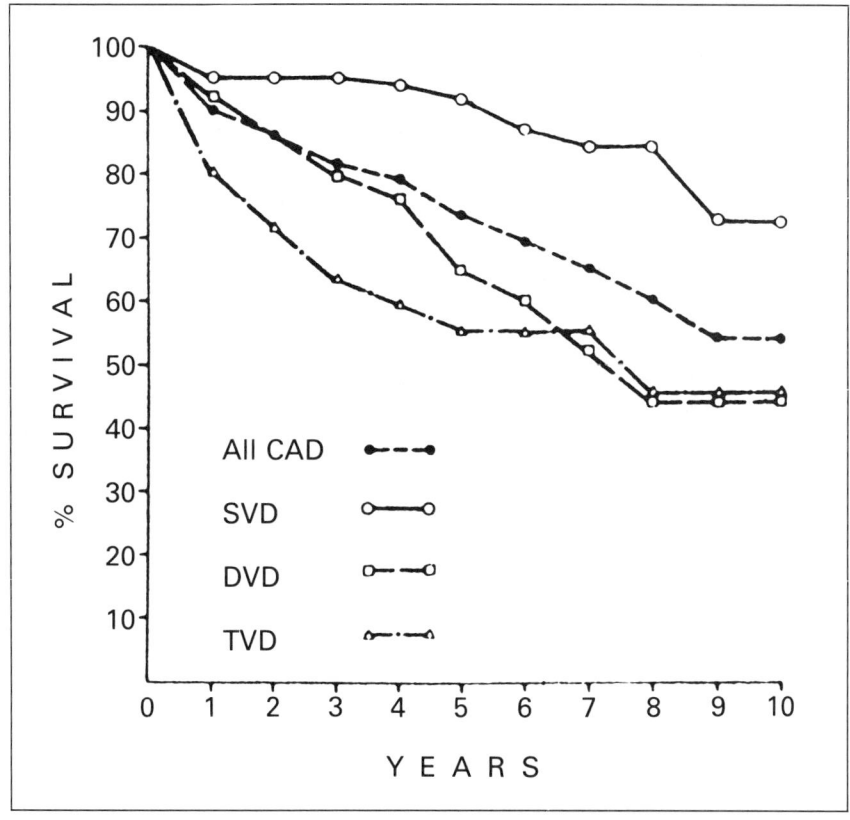

FIG. 19-1. Survival related to extent of coronary artery involvement. CAD = coronary artery disease; SVD = single vessel disease; DVD = double-vessel disease; TVD = triple-vessel disease. (From Ref. 16, with permission of the American Heart Association, Inc.)

importance of the extent and severity of coronary artery disease on long-term survival (Figs. 19-1 and 19-2) [16]. The extent of coronary artery disease and severity of left ventricular dysfunction are clearly two important predictors of mortality in patients with chronic stable angina pectoris (Fig. 19-3) [106]. It is also well established that there is an increased risk of cardiac events, including death, in patients with objective evidence for transient myocardial ischemia. Treadmill exercise with electrocardiographic and blood pressure monitoring, thallium-201 perfusion scans, and noninvasive left ventricular imaging have received the most attention in this regard. Patients with ischemia occurring at low workloads (less than or equal to 6.5 METS) or heart rates (less than or equal to 120 beats per minute), those with 2.0 mm or greater ST segment depression, prolonged recovery period ST segment depression (greater than 6.0 min), ST shifts in multiple leads, exercise-induced

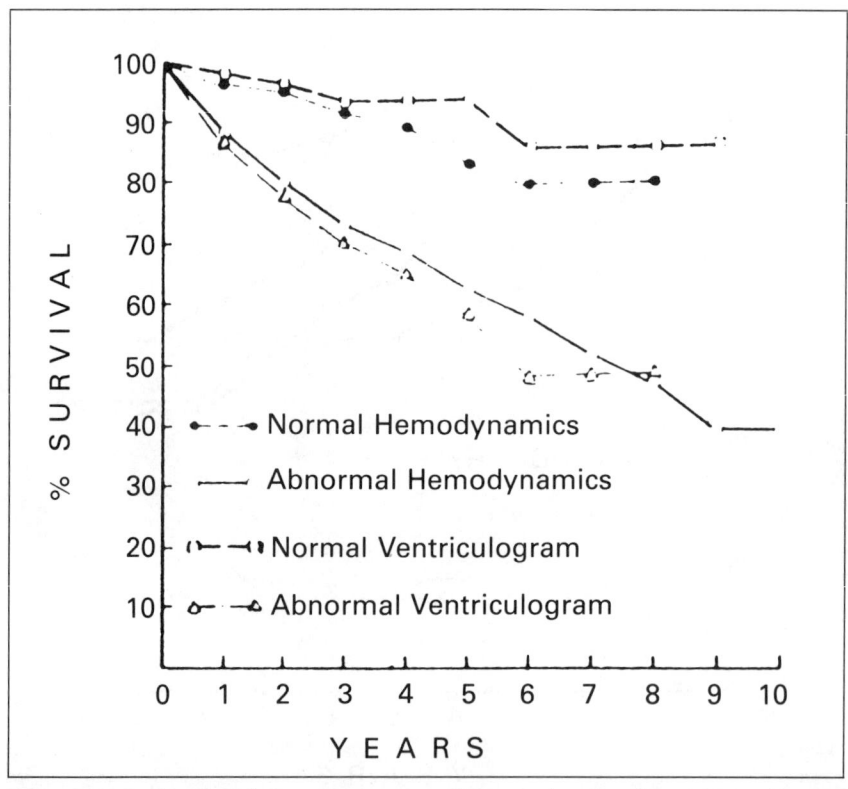

FIG. 19-2. Survival with coronary artery disease related to hemodynamics and ventriculography. (From Ref. 16, with permission of the American Heart Association, Inc.)

ventricular tachycardia, or those failing to increase their blood pressure with exercise are at highest risk [6, 38, 74]. Similarly, patients with increased lung uptake or an enlarged cardiac pool of thallium-201, new perfusion defects at low workloads, and multiple new defects are at high risk. Likewise, patients with an ejection fraction of less than or equal to 35 percent and those with greater than or equal to 5 percent decrease in exercise ejection fraction are at high risk. Other demographic factors such as age, sex, and diabetes are also important determinants of morbidity and mortality.

PATIENTS WITH DISABLING SYMPTOMS AND OPTIMAL THERAPY

There is general agreement that revascularization is of proven value in patients with disabling chest pain due to transient myocardial ischemia that continues to recur with optimal medical therapy. Optimal medical therapy is expected to vary from patient to patient and is meant to be

19. WHEN TO USE ANGIOPLASTY OR BYPASS SURGERY

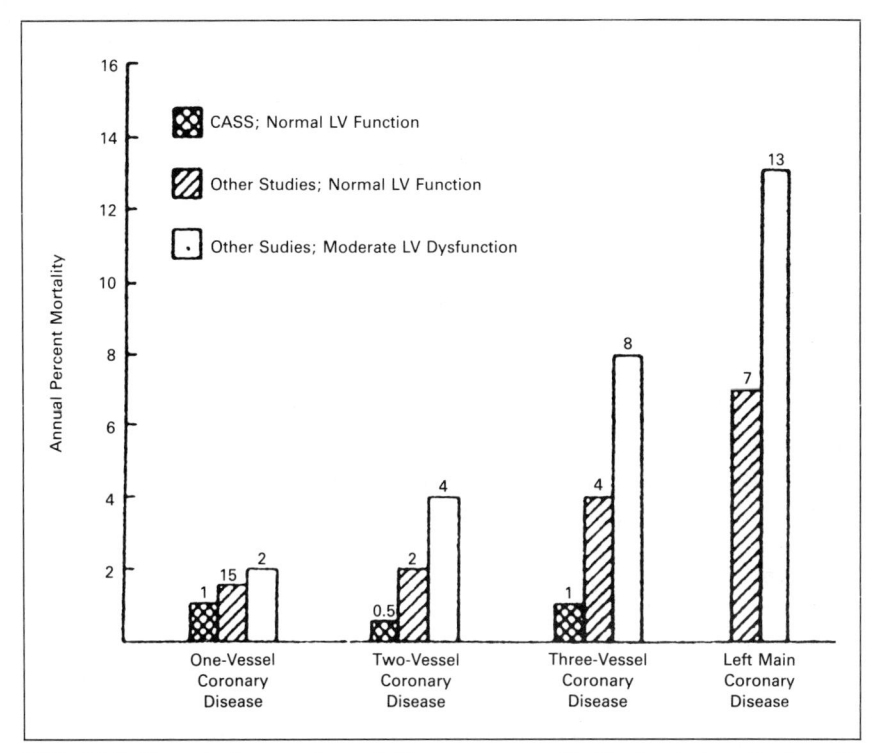

FIG. 19-3. Expected annual mortality among medically treated patients with coronary artery disease and chronic angina pectoris. Values (rounded off) are from the recent Coronary Artery Surgery Study (CASS) trial or are estimates based on a number of other studies and are presented according to the number of disease vessels and the extent of left ventricular (LV) dysfunction. Patients with left main coronary disease were excluded from the CASS trial. (From Ref. 106, with permission.)

individualized. Optimal medical therapy should include modification of aggravating factors, for example, obesity, hypertension, and smoking, in addition to drugs such as nitrates, calcium channel antagonists, and beta-adrenergic blockers. Failure of optimal therapy then implies that symptoms due to ischemia or side effects of medications result in an unacceptable life-style. In patients meeting this definition the decision for revascularization therapy is usually not difficult. The more difficult decision is when to recommend revascularization in those who are less symptomatic or have no symptoms in an attempt to improve long-term prognosis as opposed to medical therapy alone.

RESULTS IN SPECIFIC PRACTICE ENVIRONMENTS

Before addressing results of revascularization procedures, it is important to point out that the actual results of these highly technical procedures (e.g., CABG and PTCA) vary widely from one practice setting to another even in similar patients. For example, while the overall surgical mortality in the Coronary Artery Surgery Study (CASS) report was approximately 3 percent, the actual mortality rate at individual sites, all of which were selected because of excellence in CABG surgery, ranged from less than 1 percent to greater than 12 percent [57]. Similar findings of a wide range of surgical mortality rates were also noted in the Veterans Administration (VA) Cooperative Trial [84]. Although some of this variability can be accounted for by the varied patient mix at the different centers, most probably relates directly to technical factors. For example, in CASS mortality for patients over 60 years of age was greater than 6 percent, and females of all ages had approximately twice the mortality of males. Similar variability is present in results of PTCA. Thus, it is imperative for clinicians to interpret results discussed below in light of their own practice settings when attempting to make decisions relative to revascularization in any given patient.

Coronary Artery Bypass Graft Surgery

LEFT MAIN AND SINGLE-VESSEL CORONARY OBSTRUCTION

Three major multicenter randomized trials addressed results of surgery in chronic effort angina. The VA cooperative study randomized 596 patients to either surgical (286 patients) or medical (310 patients) treatment groups [84]. Despite criticism regarding high surgical mortality and graft occlusion rates, this study clearly demonstrated improved survival in the subgroup of patients with left main obstruction randomized to initial surgery (Fig. 19-4). These results were confirmed by the European Coronary Surgery Study Group (ECSSG) [40, 41]. As a result, the CASS excluded patients with left main disease from randomization [20]. Data from several observational-type studies supported the beneficial effect of surgery on survival in patients with left main obstruction [23]. Because it was evident from nonrandomized trials that as a group patients with single-vessel disease had relatively low mortality, the ECSSG excluded patients with single-vessel obstruction. The other two randomized trials confirmed that similar 5- to 7-year survival rates were obtained in patients with single-vessel obstruction when comparing initial medical and surgical treatment.

Thus, initial surgery is considered the treatment of choice, regardless of symptom status, in patients with left main coronary obstruction greater than 50 percent diameter narrowing. There is no clear advantage with single-vessel obstruction, in terms of improved mortality over 5 to 7 years, in using initial surgery compared with medical treatment alone. Therefore, treatment choice for patients with single-vessel obstruction should be based on other considerations (i.e., symptoms and indicators of high risk). It should be emphasized that all of the randomized trials

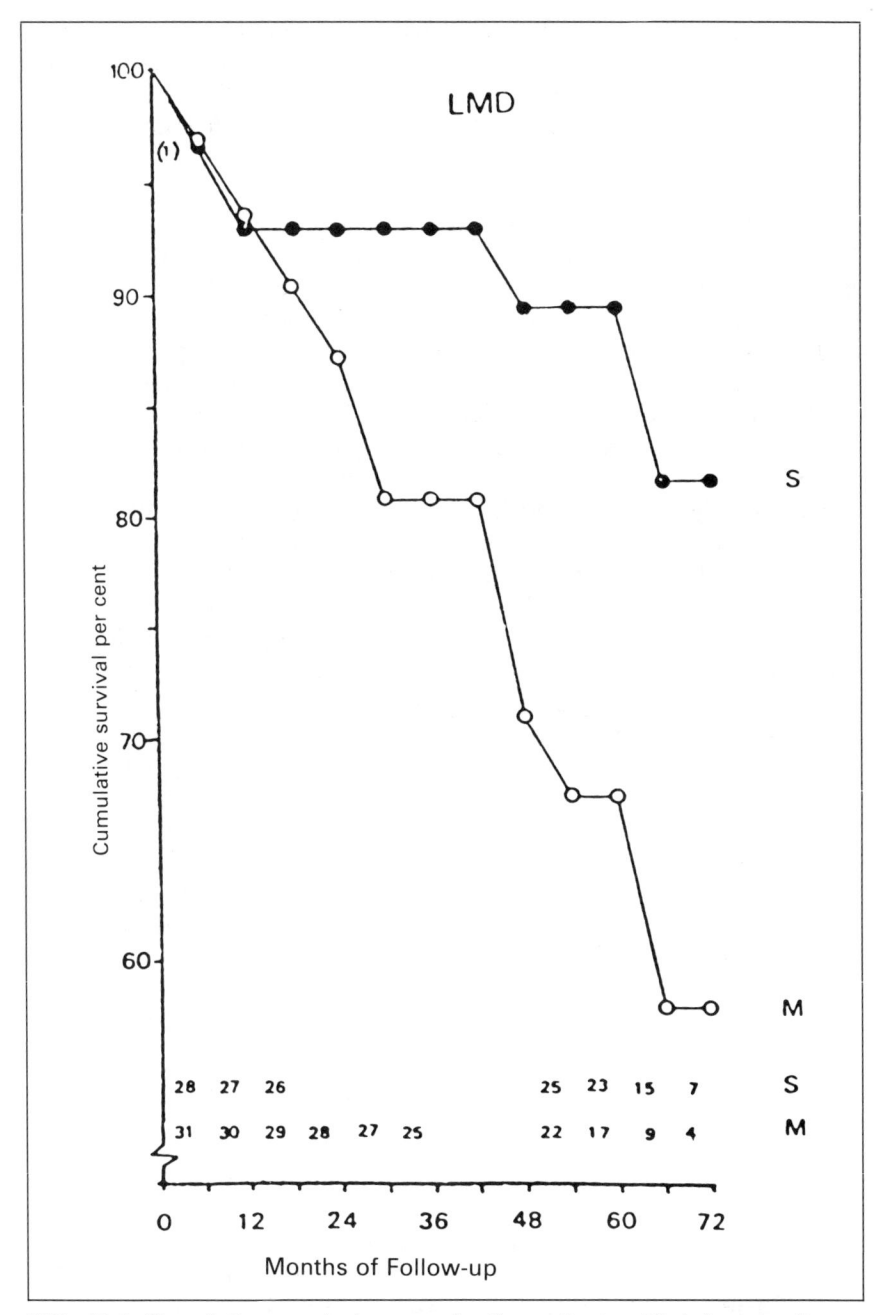

FIG. 19-4. Cumulative survival curves for the patients with left main disease (LMD). M = medical group; S = surgical group. (From Ref. 41, with permission of the American Heart Association, Inc.)

compare initially assigned treatment groups. Hence, those assigned initial medical therapy who undergo CABG surgery for whatever reason several months later continue to remain in the medically assigned group for the purposes of the study. Thus, these results refer only to initial treatment choice.

MULTIVESSEL CORONARY ARTERY OBSTRUCTION

Despite general agreement in the groups discussed earlier, disagreement occurs when comparing patients with multivessel coronary disease. In patients with multivessel disease and good ventricular function both the CASS and VA studies demonstrated similar survival rates for those assigned initial medical and surgical treatment. However, the ECSSG found significantly increased survival in patients with triple-vessel disease when treated surgically compared to those assigned medical treatment (94 percent versus 80.4 percent, 6-year survival rate). The explanation for different results in the ECSSG compared with the two U.S. studies is probably related to different patient populations.

Recently, Bonow and Epstein critically reviewed these studies and noted that 42 percent of ECSSG patients had either class III or IV angina whereas CASS excluded patients with severe angina from randomization [14]. An observational study of patients with severe angina from the nonrandomized population of the CASS registry demonstrated improved survival in surgically treated patients who had multivessel disease [56]. It seems reasonable to conclude that patients with multivessel disease and severe symptoms may have improved survival with CABG surgery. Since the 5-year survival rates in surgically treated patients are similar in both CASS and ECSSG, Bonow and colleagues also attributed some of the disparity to higher mortality in medically assigned patients. In a group of 117 patients with either mild angina or who were asymptomatic and prospectively followed for 4 years after referral, it has been suggested that a subgroup of patients with triple-vessel coronary artery disease and preserved left ventricular function who are at high risk for death when treated medically may be identified by treadmill testing [13]. Forty-three patients with triple vessel coronary artery disease had a 4-year survival of 88 percent. No deaths occurred in 12 patients without exercise-induced ST shifts whereas 31 patients with a positive ST segment response during exercise had a 4-year survival of 82 percent (annual mortality 4.5 percent). Data from the CASS Registry on 5303 patients who underwent treadmill testing at the time of catheterization showed surgical treatment to be more beneficial in patients exhibiting at least 1 mm of ST segment depression and in those who could only exercise to stage I Bruce protocol or less [115]. Seven-year survival in patients in this subgroup was 58 percent when treated medically and 81 percent when treated surgically.

The ECSSG patients with two-vessel disease with one stenosis involving the proximal left anterior descending artery also had improved survival with surgery (Fig. 19-5). Several nonrandomized, observational-type studies provide further support for the prognostic importance of proximal left anterior descending artery stenosis [63]. An initial report from the CASS registry data suggested that patients with proximal stenosis in any vessel had a poorer prognosis than patients with the same number of diseased vessels but with distal stenosis [80]. A subsequent review of data in 903 patients with combined proximal left anterior descending and left circumflex stenosis (the majority not meeting randomization criteria) demonstrated improved 5-year survival in those treated surgically versus medically (85 percent versus 55 percent) [21].

When comparing patients who had both multivessel disease and poor left ventricular function, defined as an ejection fraction less than 50 percent, long-term follow-up from both the VA and CASS studies suggests that surgery offers improved survival [33, 61, 89, 114]. Patients with an ejection fraction of less than 50 percent were excluded from the ECSSG.

RECOMMENDATIONS

Based on review of major trials in patients with chronic stable angina and our knowledge of predictors of high risk based on results of non-invasive testing studies, it would appear that the following subgroups should have improved survival with surgery: (1) left main disease; (2) triple-vessel disease with depressed left ventricular function; (3) triple-vessel disease with normal left ventricular function in patients with moderate to severe angina; (4) double-vessel disease with normal left ventricular function when one of the occluded vessels is the proximal left anterior descending artery; and (5) some patients who appear to be at high risk based on risk stratification by noninvasive tests, that is, those with ischemia provokable at low workloads or of severe magnitude.

Percutaneous Transluminal Coronary Angioplasty

Initially, PTCA was introduced for use only in a highly select group of patients with single-vessel disease and good ventricular function. Appropriate candidates were described as having proximal, discrete, noncalcific, concentric stenosis with recent onset angina. Since patients with mild angina and single-vessel disease usually do well with medical therapy in terms of 5-year survival and surgery has not been shown to reduce mortality infarction rates, PTCA was often reserved for those with unsatisfactory symptom responses to medical therapy. The question remains as to whether an alternative form of revascularization,

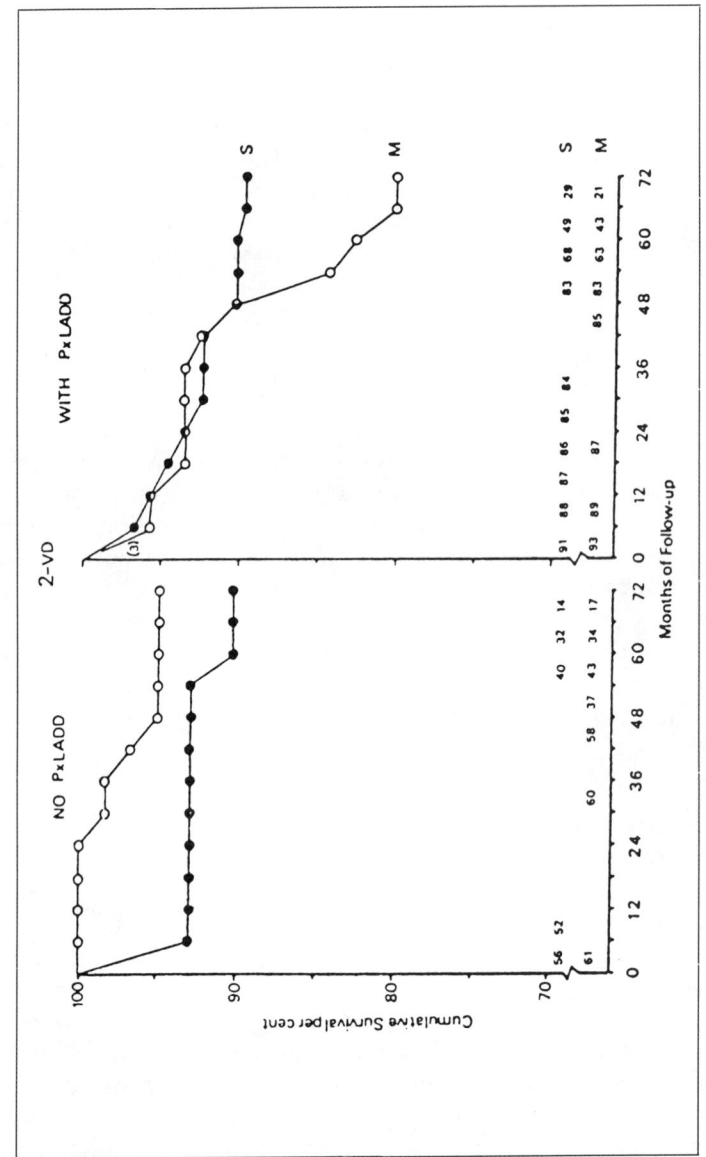

FIG. 19-5. Cumulative survival curves for patients with two-vessel disease (2-VD) subdivided into two subsets according to absence and presence of proximal left anterior descending disease (PxLADD). M = medical group; S = surgical group. (From Ref. 41, with permission of the American Heart Association, Inc.)

such as PTCA, will offer results different from CABG surgery. Also, results of PTCA compared to medical therapy alone are unknown. These issues are currently being addressed by NHLBI and VA cooperative studies. More recently, PTCA has been applied to increasing numbers of patients with multivessel disease and another NHLBI sponsored controlled trial is addressing this issue. At this time, PTCA seems to have some favorable cost and logistical advantages over CABG surgery. However, until results of controlled trials are available, clinical judgment must be used to select candidates. Some arbitrary guidelines are in order.

LEFT MAIN AND SINGLE-VESSEL DISEASE
Presently, in patients with single-vessel disease, PTCA appears more clearly indicated for those whose life-styles are limited by symptoms, drug therapy itself, or stress tests suggesting high risk ischemia based on recent guidelines [6]. With respect to left main disease, it would appear that surgery is the currently preferred revascularization approach because of unacceptable long-term results in a few patients who were treated with PTCA when the procedure was introduced [51]. However, patients with protected left main disease, where at least one patent graft supplies a left coronary branch, are acceptable PTCA candidates.

MULTIVESSEL DISEASE
Frequently, the question arises as to whether patients with multiple-vessel disease, who would be expected to benefit from CABG revascularization, should be given the option for revascularization by PTCA. This question is important because of concerns about PTCA efficacy in multivessel disease related to primary success rate, completeness of revascularization, and possible increased rates of complication and restenosis. Dorros et al. reported results of multiple-vessel PTCA in a series of 309 patients [35]. Initial angiographic success was achieved in 87 percent of lesions and in 285 of 309 (92 percent) patients. The complication rate was similar to that of PTCA performed in patients with single-vessel disease. Follow-up studies showed that only 20 percent had clinical evidence of lesion recurrence, including those who underwent repeat PTCA. On long-term follow-up 85 percent of patients had sustained clinical improvement.

Cowley et al. reported results of PTCA on 84 patients with two-vessel disease, 14 with triple-vessel disease, and two with four-vessel disease [26]. Two hundred and seventy-three lesions were attempted in these 100 patients with an angiographic success rate of 90 percent and clinical improvement in 95 percent. These investigators reported the clinical success rate to be higher than their total PTCA population (including patients with single-vessel disease) for the same time period. It should be noted that case selection may have affected results as revascularization by PTCA was recommended when lesions were felt amenable to such therapy. Most importantly, in this report the incidence of complications was not appreciably different from that of PTCA in patients with single-vessel disease. Sustained improvement was noted in many patients as 64 percent were event free and 50 percent were asymptomatic after a mean follow-up of approximately 2 years. There was no statistically significant difference in recurrence rate comparing patients with multiple-vessel PTCA (34 percent) and patients with single-vessel PTCA (28 percent) who had PTCA performed during the same time period at that institution.

The importance of complete revascularization for relief of angina with CABG surgery has been discussed in detail elsewhere [27]. One CABG study followed consecutive patients undergoing CABG surgery with repeat angiography 1 year after operation [26]. Complete revascularization was defined as all major vessels greater than or equal to 1.5 mm in diameter with stenosis of greater than or equal to 50 percent being bypassed. When correlating symptoms with both graft patency and completeness of revascularization, asymptomatic patients had 91 percent graft patency as compared to only 27 percent graft patency in unimproved patients. Likewise, 87 percent of patients completely revascularized with all grafts patent were asymptomatic. Only 42 percent of those patients incompletely revascularized were asymptomatic. From these findings after CABG surgery, one would also expect that complete revascularization should be important after PTCA in patients with multivessel disease.

Mabin et al. addressed completeness of revascularization in an experience with 229 patients undergoing PTCA, 86 of whom had multivessel disease [72]. Overall success rate was 67 percent (153 patients) for the series, 61 percent for patients with single-vessel disease, and 77 percent for those with multivessel disease. Of the 153 patients in whom PTCA was initially successful, revascularization was considered complete, that is, no residual diameter stenosis greater than 70 percent in 87 of 143 patients with single-vessel disease and 31 of 86 patients with multivessel disease. The chance of event-free survival (e.g., no angina recurrence, myocardial infarction, death, repeat PTCA or CABG surgery) was directly influenced by completeness of revascularization. All patients with multivessel disease obtaining complete revascularization had no angina on follow-up whereas only 57 percent of those patients with partial revascularization were asymptomatic. At 6 months 79 percent of patients with complete revascularization had event-free survival compared with only 43 percent of those who had a residual stenosis (Fig. 19-6).

A subsequent study suggested that despite high primary success rates, defined as dilation of the critical lesion, complete revascularization

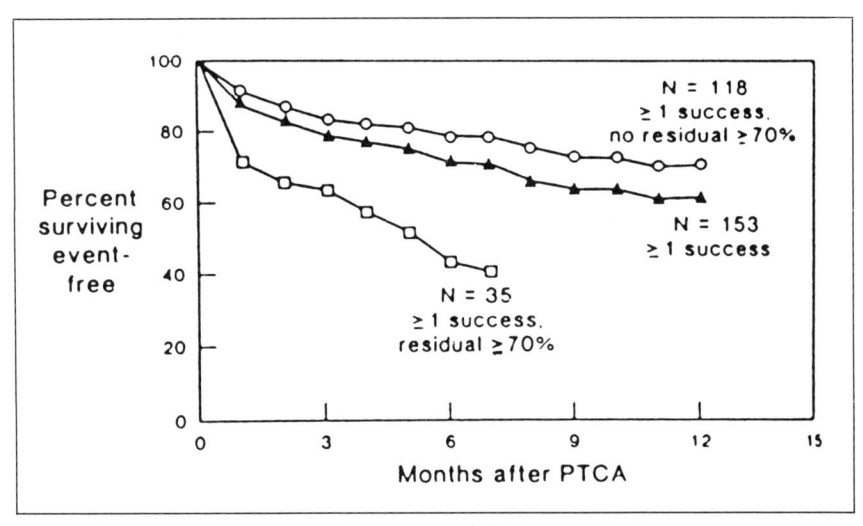

FIG. 19-6. Event-free survival after successful dilation of at least one vessel ($N = 153$) and in subgroups: with complete revascularization (no residual stenosis, $N = 118$) and with incomplete revascularization (one or more residual stenoses $\geq 70\%$, $N = 35$). The difference between results in the two subgroups is significant ($p < 0.001$). (From Ref. 72, with permission of the American Heart Association, Inc.)

was obtained in only 46 percent of patients with multivessel disease who had obtained primary success [112]. As with the Mabin et al. study [72], cardiac events, need for second revascularization procedure, and evidence for residual myocardial ischemia by exercise testing were more frequent in the incompletely revascularized group despite initial clinical improvement.

RECOMMENDATIONS

It is apparent that with optimal case selection initial success rates with PTCA may be similar for patients with single- and multivessel disease. It is also evident that on long-term follow-up patients with single-vessel disease are more likely to sustain improvement than patients with multivessel disease. However, many patients with multivessel disease also may have sustained long-term benefit after PTCA. In patients who have restenosis or recurrence of symptoms either repeat PTCA or CABG surgery may be readily performed with a very high success rate.

It is our opinion that PTCA and CABG surgery are complementary to each other and may be used at different stages in the course of a given patient's generally progressive obstructive disease. Even when PTCA results in acute occlusion, surgical treatment may be performed with the same relatively low operative mortality/morbidity rates that are enjoyed without the attempted PTCA. For those in whom PTCA is unsuccessful and without complication, CABG surgery may be performed electively [1, 75, 90]. The results of Mabin and colleagues suggest that event-free survival in patients treated with unsuccessful PTCA and prompt CABG surgery is as good as or better than that in patients who had successful PTCA of at least one vessel.

In summary, based on results of several controlled trials, it is possible to identify subgroups of patients with chronic stable angina in whom CABG surgery improves prognosis. At this time similar controlled trials have not been done with PTCA but should evolve in the near future. Until that time use of PTCA must be based on clinical judgment in situations where PTCA appears to offer a reasonable alternative to CABG surgery. This judgment is influenced largely by coronary anatomic features of the lesions under consideration.

Special Considerations

REPEAT REVASCULARIZATION

It must be recognized that any revascularization therapy directed toward coronary artery disease is often temporary because of the progressive course of the atherosclerotic process. With regard to CABG surgery, Bourassa and colleagues demonstrated through follow-up studies that 15 to 20 percent of saphenous vein CABGs are occluded by 1 year and that only 60 percent remain patent at 11 years [15]. Those grafts remaining patent often have evidence of important atherosclerotic stenosis. Others have suggested that there may be increased progression of native coronary artery disease in vessels that have been bypassed. Thus, as a consequence of graft occlusion, stenosis, and/or progression of native coronary artery disease, disabling angina recurs at a rate of up to 5 percent a year following initially successful CABG surgery. Thus, many patients become candidates for reoperation with increased risk of complications and possibly increased mortality [44]. Long-term relief of angina is not as effective with repeat surgery [70, 102]. Loop et al. reported a series of 1000 patients undergoing reoperation from 1969 to 1982 [70]. Although angina was completely relieved in 65 percent to 75 percent of patients 5 years after initial CABG surgery, only 52 percent were angina-free 5 years after reoperation. Internal mammary arteries are increasingly used as conduits since patency rates in uncontrolled trials appear higher, averaging about 90 percent at 10 years [7, 8, 69]. Nonrandomized studies suggest that survival may be increased in patients with internal mammary artery as compared to saphenous vein CABGs [18, 71].

Although reoperation can be performed successfully with slight increase in mortality and complications, PTCA is an attractive alternative form of therapy for patients with signs or symptoms of ischemia due to bypass graft occlusion. PTCA can be performed on either grafted native vessels or bypass grafts [12, 24, 36, 37]. In reports that evaluate the occurrence of restenosis with respect to site of PTCA, distal graft-native artery anastomosis seems to behave similarly to native coronary arteries whereas, the aortosaphenous vein graft anastomosis and vein graft body are associated with high rates of restenosis that approximate 50 percent. Also, the risk of infarction is higher with PTCA of lesions in the body of saphenous vein grafts, presumably due to embolic debris.

Graft occlusion after CABG surgery is not the same as restenosis after PTCA. Restenosis occurs in 20 to 45 percent of cases undergoing successful PTCA and usually occurs within 4 to 6 months of dilation. Factors associated with increased risk of restenosis may include diabetes, unstable angina, proximal left anterior descending lesion, high-grade residual postangioplasty diameter reduction or increased residual transstenotic gradients, and also lower balloon-artery diameter ratios (see Table 19-1) [55, 65, 67]. Even though there are limitations to the studies, no drug intervention has convincingly altered restenosis rates including trials using coumadin, aspirin, sulfinpyrizone, methyl predvisolone, nifedipine, or diltiazem. The etiology of restenosis remains unclear. This process probably is related to a form of accelerated atherosclerosis and includes platelet activation, thrombosis, noncellular components, smooth muscle cell injury, and proliferation. As opposed to reoperation following CABG surgery, repeat PTCA for restenosis can be done with a high success rate and few complications [76, 118].

HIGH-RISK GROUPS

Although some report that elderly patients undergoing CABG surgery have similar perioperative mortality when compared with younger individuals [98], the CASS demonstrated a significantly increased risk [47]. Part of the reason for this disparity may relate to chronologic versus physiologic age. Reports on the role of PTCA in the elderly vary. One suggests similar initial success rates, complications, and long-term clinical improvement as compared to younger individuals [100]. Another suggests a slightly lower primary success rate and higher complication rate [81]. However, in this latter study the magnitude of difference, though statistically significant, was small and may not be clinically important. Thus, both PTCA and CABG surgery are feasible in the elderly. Others considered at high risk for CABG surgery include those with depressed left ventricular function and those with poor general medical condition. In select patients PTCA may be considered palliative for those at high risk for CABG surgery [110].

UNSTABLE REST ANGINA

General Considerations
The definition of unstable angina varies and this fact continues to hamper management of patients with this ischemic syndrome. Most con-

TABLE 19-1. *Factors Associated with Increased Restenosis Risk from Currently Available Studies*

	Often Associated	Occasionally Associated	Not Associated
Patient	Angina: CCS class, variant or spasm, new onset/short duration	Male sex Diabetic Unstable angina Hypertension No MI Hypercholesteremia Smoking post PTCA	Age Calcium channel antagonists Aspirin
Angiographic	Stenoses: high grade, LAD, aorto SVBG anastomosis, SVBG body, branch point, chronic total, ostial and proximity Small artery	Eccentric stenosis	Stenosis: length, distal SVBG anastomosis Multivessel LV function
Procedural	High prestenosis gradient High final stenosis gradient High-grade residual stenosis Absence of tear	Balloon/artery diameter < 1 Brief inflation	Number of inflation Inflation pressure

Abbreviations: CCS = Canadian Cardiovascular Society; MI = myocardial infarction; LAD = left anterior descending; PTCA = percutaneous transluminal angioplasty; SVBG = sayphen vein bypass graft; LV = left ventricular function.
Source: Modified from B. Rose, and C. J. Pepine, Restenosis Following PTCA: Patterns, Recognition and Results of Repeat Angioplasty. In S. Goldberg (ed.), *Cardiovascular Clinics.* Philadelphia: F. A. Davis, 1988. P. 238. Reproduced with permission.

sider patients with angina of increasing severity and frequency occurring with ordinary activities of daily living or at rest as qualifying for this definition [91]. Management, in addition to hospitalization, includes intensive drug therapy, usually consisting of nitrates, calcium channel antagonists, and beta blockers. Attempts to identify and correct possible aggravating factors such as hypertension or anemia must be made.

Currently, there is general agreement that most unstable angina patients have a recent change in coronary artery obstruction and an increased risk of serious events. For this reason, all patients with unstable angina are candidates for coronary angiography at some point in order to delineate the extent and severity of underlying coronary artery disease. Patients with continued or recurrent symptoms despite medical therapy should undergo urgent coronary angiography in preparation for possible PTCA or CABG surgery. These patients appear to be at highest risk for early events [46]. Waiting even 48 hours will mean that some patients will proceed to events. Others may argue that patients whose symptoms stabilize quickly with medical therapy need not be subjected to catheterization because studies such as the NHLBI Cooperative Study in which patients were randomized to either initial medical or surgical therapy showed no significant differences in in-hospital or late nonfatal myocardial infarction or mortality [85]. However, it is important to note that the window for surgical therapy in this study was 7 days during which myocardial infarction or death might have occurred. Further, randomization was done only after coronary angiography; those with left main coronary stenosis (approximately 10 percent) were sent promptly to surgery, and those without important stenosis (presumable spasm) were excluded. Even with these exclusions totaling approximately 20 percent of the remaining patients randomized to initial medical therapy, 35 percent had class III or IV angina at 1 year and would have required coronary angiography during that period to assess anatomy. Subsequently, a very high percentage of patients initially assigned medical treatment eventually required CABG surgery for relief of symptoms. It should also be recognized that other high-risk patients, that is, those with poor left ventricular function and myocardial infarction within the previous 3 months, were excluded from randomization. Finally, it is important to emphasize that waiting for recurrent chest pain in patients receiving medical therapy may not be appropriate because a substantial number will have recurrent ischemia in the absence of angina. For example, Gottlieb et al. studied 70 patients with unstable rest angina after instituting therapy with calcium channel antagonists, beta blockers, and nitrates [50]. Although only eight (11 percent) had recurrent angina, 37 (53 percent) had recurrent ischemia documented by transient electrocardiographic changes. This group of patients with recurrent silent ischemia experienced 16 of 20 events (myocardial infarction or revascularization for recurrent angina) occurring over the first 30 days after presentation for unstable angina. The results have been extended to 2 years when a significant difference between the two groups was noted in terms of death and myocardial infarction. These results have been confirmed by others.

Based on the above considerations, there is general agreement that patients presenting with unstable angina warrant early coronary angiography and ambulatory ECG monitoring for recurrent silent ischemia after drug therapy is initiated.

Because underlying coronary anatomy is of uppermost importance in considering potential revascularization, we will digress briefly to consider some of the many angiographic studies performed in patients with unstable angina. Despite various postulated mechanisms, for example, vasomotion, microthrombus, or both, it is apparent that severe underlying coronary artery disease is present in the majority of patients with unstable angina [3, 97, 99]. Patients with unstable angina have a greater progression in both extent and severity of coronary diseases than patients with stable angina [62, 82]. Angiographic studies have identified intraluminal thrombi at increased frequency in patients with unstable angina [17, 19]. The shorter the interval between a rest pain episode and angiographic study, the higher the frequency of intracoronary thrombus [19]. Prognostic importance of thrombosis is suggested by studies demonstrating decreased mortality and infarction rate in patients treated with either antiplatelet agents or anticoagulants [17, 68, 111]. Potential concern relative to feasibility of PTCA in unstable angina was noted after Mabin and colleagues reported an extraordinarily high rate of acute occlusion in patients with thrombi at the dilation site prior to PTCA [73]. These data were collected, however, before use of steerable wire, balloon catheter guiding systems. These workers also reversed heparinization with protamine shortly after PTCA. A follow-up study in patients whose heparinization was not reversed and in whom steerable, low-profile dilation systems were used showed patients with intraluminal thrombi to be at a slightly greater but not statistically significant risk of acute occlusion compared with patients without thrombi [109].

Coronary Artery Bypass Graft Surgery

Clearly, CABG surgery has been demonstrated to be efficacious for relief of pain due to myocardial ischemia in patients with unstable angina. In the NHLBI Cooperative Trial only 11 percent of patients randomized to CABG surgery had class III or IV symptoms after 1 year compared with 36 percent of those randomized to medical therapy [85]. This statistically significant difference was present even though high-risk patients with left main stenosis or poor left ventricular function were eliminated. This controlled trial supported results from large numbers of nonrandomized trials confirming that CABG surgery is effective for relief of pain in patients with unstable angina. Relative to improved survival, however, no significant difference was found between patients randomized to CABG surgery and those randomized to initial medical therapy alone. The surgical mortality and postoperative infarction rate were considerably higher than we would expect today. Likewise, medical therapy has improved with the addition of calcium channel antagonists, intravenous nitrates, and aspirin, and with improved detection of myocardial infarction by MB isoenzyme of creatine kinase (MB-CK). Whether the results of the NHLBI Trial are still applicable is unknown.

Percutaneous Transluminal Coronary Angioplasty

PTCA was suggested effective for unstable angina by Williams and colleagues [119]. Seventeen unstable angina patients underwent PTCA and had a beneficial clinical response, objective evidence for relief of ischemia, and a low incidence of complications. De Feyter and colleagues reported an initial success rate of 93 percent with a low complication rate in 60 patients presenting with unstable angina refractory to maximum medical therapy [31]. Interestingly, PTCA was the most frequently used procedure in those patients who required revascularization because of continued symptoms. Observational data from the NHLBI PTCA Registry compared acute and long-term effects of PTCA in patients with unstable angina with similar patients with stable angina and patients with unstable angina from the CASS Registry who underwent CABG surgery [143]. Success rates were comparable in both PTCA groups. There were no differences in mortality or myocardial infarction rates between the unstable angina groups treated with either type of revascularization procedure. Interestingly, there was a statistically higher percentage of patients within the PTCA group who had long-term symptom improvement than within the CABG group. Although it has been suggested that PTCA performed in the unstable angina setting may be associated with higher restenosis rates compared with PTCA performed in stable angina, the studies noted above and those by Meyer et al. and Quigley et al. have demonstrated similar initial success, restenosis, and complication rates [77, 79, 96].

The importance of completeness of revascularization for continued long-term alleviation of ischemia has been reviewed in patients with chronic stable angina. Presumably, this principle also applies to unstable angina. Some have performed qualitative analysis attempting to delineate the reason why patients become unstable. This has given rise to the concept of the "culprit lesion." Ambrose et al., in two separate studies, suggest that eccentric lesions can be identified much more frequently in patients with unstable angina than stable angina. Further, these lesions are presumed to be ischemia-producing stenoses as they occur in myocardial areas predicted to become ischemic based on the leads showing ECG changes or myocardial segments showing reversible thallium-201 perfusion defects [4, 5]. Wohlgelernter et al. were able to identify the "culprit lesion" in a high percentage of patients. They suggested that PTCA of such lesions can be an effective alternative revascularization procedure to CABG surgery in unstable angina patients with multivessel disease [121]. In a group of 27 patients with medically refractory unstable angina and multivessel disease, a culprit lesion was identified and successful PTCA performed in 89 percent with resolution of symptoms. Long-term follow-up confirmed continued clinical improvement in most, as only 17 percent of patients had recurrent angina. This group suggested that unique morphologic features of the culprit lesion provide a greater opportunity to treat the ischemia-producing lesion by PTCA. Thus, potential for long-term, functional improvement may be greater in unstable angina than in chronic stable angina with multivessel disease.

RECOMMENDATIONS

Until additional studies are available, current preference for revascularization in unstable angina patients is CABG surgery for patients with left main disease and the majority of patients with multivessel disease. PTCA is reserved for those patients with single-vessel disease and selected cases of multivessel disease where all major coronary branches supplying the three left anatomic ventricular regions with important stenosis can be approached. Patients with an obviously identifiable culprit lesion with surgical contraindications or those at high risk for surgery are likely to be considered for PTCA. PTCA is an effective alternative to CABG surgery in many patients and initial concerns regarding acute occlusion or reocclusion in the presence of intraluminal thrombus, high restenosis rates, decreased effectiveness, and higher complication rates as compared with stable angina have not been confirmed.

ANGINA DUE TO CORONARY ARTERY SPASM

General Considerations

There is a consensus that myocardial ischemia is a result of variable contributions of processes acting to limit or reduce coronary blood supply and/or increase myocardial oxygen demand. Atherosclerosis, dynamic coronary artery narrowing, and thrombosis act to influence coronary blood flow, as discussed elsewhere in this volume. Within the general spectrum of patients with myocardial ischemia, coronary artery spasm is responsible in a minority subgroup termed *variant angina*. This term refers to individuals who have chest pain primarily at rest associated with ST segment elevation. A larger group of patients also have coronary artery spasm during chest pain associated with a wide variety of ST or T wave changes. A smaller number of both groups have little atherosclerotic obstruction. This small group of patients responds well to nitrates and calcium channel antagonists. However, the majority of patients with coronary artery spasm are more likely to have dynamic obstruction superimposed on atherosclerotic stenosis, and some will have intracoronary thrombus. Currently, there are no published controlled studies comparing medical and revascularization therapy in the patients with coronary spasm.

Several reports have examined the role of revascularization in this latter subgroup. David et al. first reported results of PTCA in 11 patients with variant angina who had underlying coexisting coronary stenosis [28]. Despite initial success, persistence of symptoms requiring calcium channel antagonists and a high restenosis rate was noted. Corcos and colleagues also demonstrated in a series of 21 patients a high restenosis rate, but after repeat angioplasty 75 percent of patients were asymptomatic requiring no medical therapy, suggesting that PTCA did play a role in management of spasm superimposed on organic stenosis [25]. More recently, Bertrand et al. suggested a high incidence of restenosis when PTCA was performed on dynamic narrowing when compared to that observed in patients with fixed stenosis [10]. Leisch et al. have confirmed that although PTCA is initially highly effective in patients with variant angina, there is a higher restenosis rate than in patients with fixed stenosis [66].

The results of surgical treatment of patients with proven or suspected coronary spasm are summarized in (Table 19-2) [22]. It is apparent that CABG surgery can be done on patients with spasm superimposed on atherosclerotic lesions but results are not as favorable as those found when CABG surgery is done in patients without spasm. Perioperative death, myocardial infarction, and recurrent angina or myocardial infarction are not infrequent. Likewise, isolated case reports suggest that CABG surgery is not useful in patients with coronary spasm who do not have important atherosclerotic obstruction. Plexectomy combined with CABG surgery has been suggested, but these results are not encouraging.

Recommendations

It would appear that vigorous medical therapy (nitrates plus calcium channel antagonists) should be utilized in all patients with coronary spasm. If patients have recurrent symptoms or signs of ischemia that can be documented as due to spasm, PTCA may be an appropriate consideration for select patients. CABG surgery may be a consideration in very few patients, particularly those with multivessel disease when spasm is not diffuse because of the reported higher restenosis rate.

Because of the possibility of recurrent spasm, patients undergoing either PTCA or CABG surgery should continue to receive intravenous nitroglycerin and calcium channel antagonists during surgery and in

TABLE 19-2. *Medical and Surgical Treatment of Patients with Coronary Stenosis and Evidence of Coronary Artery Spasm*

Report	Patients (N)	Early or Perioperative Death	Early or Perioperative Myocardial Infarction	Average Follow-Up	Late Death	Late Myocardial Infarction	Angina	Decreased or no Angina
University of Florida								
Surgical	21	1	1	3.5 years	1	2	9	10
Medical	27	2	0	3.5 years	2	2	17	6
"Surgical" Reports	89	12	13	12.2 months	2	0	24	51
Pasternak et al.								
Surgical	38	3	3	32.3 months	2	2	5	28
Medical	16	0	1	32.3 months	1	0	7	8
Schick et al.								
Surgery								
Preinfarction	40	0	7	30 months	0	0	10	30
Recent infarction	12	3	—	30 months	0	2	2	7
NHLBI[a] Trial								
Surgical	37	6	—	42 months	0	10	5	26
Medical	42	3	—	42 months	0	6	29	10
Bertrand et al.								
CABG[b]	13	2	1	36 months	—	—	2	10
CABG plus plexectomy	22	2	0	20 months	—	—	1	19

[a]NHLBI = National Heart, Lung and Blood Institute.
[b]CABG = coronary artery bypass graft.
Source: From Ref. 22, with permission.

the postoperative period. After discharge, they should also be maintained on oral nitrates and calcium channel antagonists for some time (at least 6 months or longer). Only after an appropriate asymptomatic interval when it is proven that recurrent ischemia does not occur in either a painful or silent form should judicious withdrawal of antispasm therapy be contemplated.

EVOLVING MYOCARDIAL INFARCTION

General Considerations

It has been demonstrated that in survivors of myocardial infarction, left ventricular ejection fraction is probably the single best predictor of prognosis. Accordingly, recent emphasis has been directed toward myocardial salvage in an attempt to limit extent of myocardial necrosis during the evolving phase of acute myocardial infarction. This includes medical therapy aimed at reducing myocardial oxygen demand and improving supply. This consists of bed rest, alleviation of anxiety, oxygen, pain relief, beta blockers, and nitrates.

The importance of acute thrombotic coronary occlusion in acute myocardial infarction has been documented by DeWood and colleagues and confirmed by subsequent acute interventional studies [34]. Several trials have documented improved left ventricular function with reperfusion and subsequent reduction in mortality in early treatment groups. However, controversy persists regarding: (1) subsets of patients who are candidates for thrombolytic therapy, (2) timing of infusion, (3) percentage of patients actually obtaining reperfusion, (4) presence of residual stenosis, (5) potential for continued decrease in flow reserve and ischemia, and (6) propensity for reocclusion and reinfarction.

Evidence from several studies suggests early intervention is of the utmost importance. In the GISSI Trial [48], 11,806 patients with acute myocardial infarction were randomized on presentation to treatment with either 1.5 million units of intravenous streptokinase over 1 hour or conventional therapy. To be eligible patients had to present within 12 hours of the onset of symptoms. Analysis showed that only patients receiving streptokinase within 3 hours of presentation had statistically significant reduction in 21-day mortality, whereas those treated at 3 to 6 hours had important trends toward reduced mortality. Thus, extent of beneficial effect is directly rated to the time between onset and initiation of reperfusion therapy. There is evidence to suggest that some patients with collateral or partially patent infarct-related arteries show improvement in left ventricular function when treated with streptokinase at a later time after onset of symptoms [101]. Also, it is difficult to determine the precise onset of infarction in some patients who present with recurrent, prolonged painful episodes.

Another factor contributing to efficacy of thrombolytic therapy is initial patency rate. Logically one would expect that patients who obtain reperfusion should have limited necrosis and, therefore, improved left ventricular function that may translate to improved survival. Although results vary, approximately 50 percent of patients treated with intravenous streptokinase and 80 percent of patients treated with intracoronary streptokinase have successful reperfusion. Recent reports suggest that rTPA may result in higher initial reperfusion rates. The Western Washington Randomized Trial suggested that after 1 year of follow-up the early difference in mortality observed at 30 days between patients given intracoronary streptokinase and control patients was no longer statistically significant. However, when results are analyzed according to whether actual reperfusion was established, a significant difference in 1-year mortality emerged favoring those in whom reperfusion was achieved. Patients obtaining reperfusion had a 1-year mortality of only 2.5 percent compared with 23.1 percent in those with partial and 14.6 percent in those who did not obtain reperfusion. The latter two groups did not differ significantly [58].

Coronary Artery Bypass Graft Surgery

It has been recognized for some time that CABG surgery may be performed shortly after onset of acute myocardial infarction with relatively low mortality. Some argue that a potential advantage of CABG surgery is that, in addition to reperfusing the infarct-related artery, revascularization of noninfarct, but potentially ischemic, myocardium may occur. In an observational-type study, Phillips and colleagues performed CABG surgery in 75 patients, 6.5 hours (mean) after onset of infarction with an operative mortality of only 1.3 percent [94]. There were only two late deaths in the series with a follow-up of 18 months (mean). Both deaths occurred in patients who presented with hypotension requiring vasoactive medications. Selinger et al. reported a series of 101 patients with anterior wall myocardial infarction who underwent emergency CABG surgery with an operative mortality of only 2 percent [105]. Long-term mortality was only 5 percent compared with 28 percent in patients treated without CABG surgery in the same hospitals over the same time period. More recently, another nonrandomized study suggested that early reperfusion by CABG surgery may limit infarction size and improve left ventricular function [113]. Patients with early CABG surgery had significantly higher ejection fractions determined at late follow-up (more than 2 months) compared with nonoperated patients or those patients reperfused late (more than 4 hours) after onset of symptoms.

Percutaneous Transluminal Coronary Angioplasty

Alternative forms of reperfusion other than thrombolysis or CABG surgery have been used in the early hours of infarction in an attempt to improve initial patency rates, thereby possibly improving long-term mortality rates.

Several uncontrolled trials have demonstrated the efficacy of PTCA either alone or in combination with streptokinase in acute myocardial infarction [52, 53, 78]. In the largest of these, Hartzler and colleagues reported results on PTCA performed in 78 consecutive patients who presented with acute infarction. Sixty-three (81 percent) patients were successfully managed by PTCA with or without streptokinase. Only four of those initially successfully reperfused had acute reocclusions. Repeat catheterization in the majority demonstrated improved regional wall motion and increase in ejection fraction. At 6.6 months of follow-up, 97 percent were asymptomatic and 15 percent required repeat PTCA for restenosis [53]. Experience with PTCA and acute infarction at the University of Florida was also favorable (Fig. 19-7) [93, 95]. Angioplasty was initially successful in 25 (86 percent) of 29 patients. Four patients developed acute reocclusion within 12 hours and four had a late reocclusion. Once again, left ventricular function was better preserved in patients with patent arteries. Of 21 patients obtaining initial success 17 (81 percent) remained patent at follow-up. Thus, initial patency rates with PTCA alone or in combination with streptokinase are comparable to those of intracoronary streptokinase. Although associated with a slightly higher acute reocclusion rate, frequency of restenosis is similar to that in patients undergoing angioplasty for chronic stable angina.

In addition to time to reperfusion after presentation and actual recanalization, the presence of a residual lesion with potential for continued ischemia, reocclusion, and risk of reinfarction must also be considered. For example, in the GISSI study there were 238 reinfarctions in the streptokinase treatment group compared to 124 reinfarctions in the control group [48]. Gold et al. suggested that improved overall reflow rate in patients with both streptokinase followed by PTCA versus streptokinase alone resulted in lower recurrent in-hospital ischemic events and reocclusions or reinfarction [49]. Others documented that there were increased rates of reperfusion with combined chemical and mechanical recanalization [39]. In those patients who received thrombolytic therapy alone, reocclusion was more frequent in those with a higher degree of residual coronary artery luminal narrowing. Those patients treated with PTCA had less residual stenosis and lower reocclusion rates with improvement in regional wall motion.

A recent prospective randomized trial assigned patients to either streptokinase or PTCA and, although both groups had similar primary reflow success rates, residual stenosis decreased more significantly with greater ejection fraction and improved regional wall motion was noted in the PTCA group. These results suggested more effective preservation of left ventricular function when PTCA was used [88]. Similarly, Fung et al. randomized a small group of patients to either PTCA or streptokinase, and despite similar initial reperfusion rates, residual stenosis

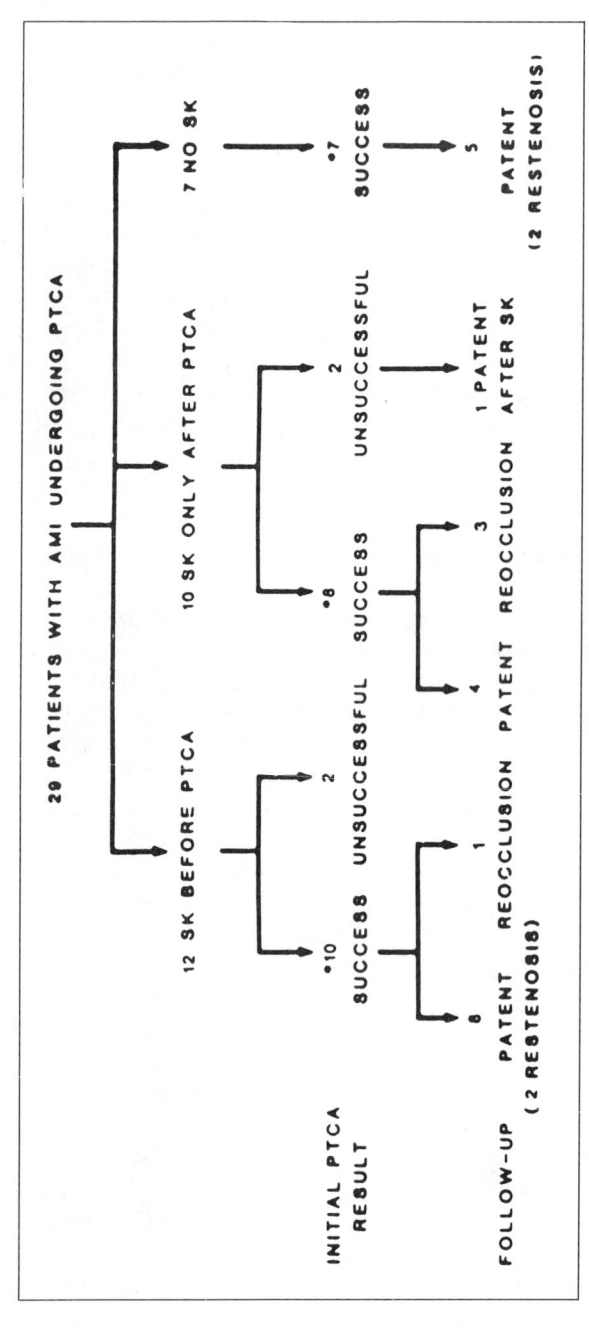

FIG. 19-7. Summary of the influence of adjunctive streptokinase (SK) administration on the result of percutaneous transluminal coronary angioplasty (PTCA) in acute myocardial infarction (AMI). No effect of adjunctive SK administration was apparent on PTCA result at follow-up evaluation. Asterisks indicate that one patient in the group receiving SK before PTCA, one patient in the group receiving SK after PTCA, and two in the group taking no SK have not been restudied. (From Ref. 95, with permission.)

was significantly higher in the streptokinase group [45]. The PTCA group had a markedly reduced frequency of exercise-induced ischemia as detected by thallium-201 tomography after recovery.

Thus, because of logistical reasons and the presence of residual stenosis following thrombolytic therapy, the current preferred approach to management of acute myocardial infarction would appear to be early PTCA if a team is readily available. Patients who present at other times would be given thrombolytic therapy followed by PTCA for those with high-degree residual stenosis causing recurrent ischemia. All patients treated with thrombolysis should be considered for cardiac catheterization in order to detect residual stenosis or other coronary artery stenosis.

Recommendations
It is generally agreed that either CABG surgery or PTCA may be performed in patients with evolving myocardial infarction. In controlled trials, because reperfusion therapy with streptokinase or rTPA is beneficial, reperfusion therapy is recommended over conservative medical management for patients presenting within 6 hours of onset of the event. For those presenting between 6 and 12 hours, some benefit has been suggested, but this remains controversial. Revascularization by PTCA or CABG surgery is also likely to be of benefit, though it must be emphasized that this has not yet been proven by controlled trials. Although both PTCA and CABG surgery can safely be performed within the first hours of evolving myocardial infarction case selection, logistics and costs of maintaining standby surgical and/or catheterization teams present major difficulties. These difficulties represent major limitations for treating the majority of patients with either of these approaches. Neither procedure is likely to become commonplace, although PTCA may be preferred in this setting because of longer delays associated with initiation of surgical reperfusion since coronary angiography must be done first.

POSTMYOCARDIAL INFARCTION
General Considerations
The postmyocardial infarction period is known to be associated with substantial morbidity and mortality. Accordingly, attempts to identify those at risk are now part of standard medical care in the postinfarction period. Many studies have identified factors in addition to left ventricular function as being important in predicting prognosis during this period [9, 29]. Of these, the presence of postinfarction angina or ischemia detected by predischarge stress testing appears to alter significantly prognosis in patients with similar degrees of left ventricular

function. Schuster et al. followed 70 patients with early postinfarction angina with either ischemia at a distance or ischemia in the infarct zone and noted a 56 percent mortality at 6 months [104]. Ischemia at a distance was associated with a particularly high mortality rate of 72 percent. De Feyter et al. noted increased mortality in patients with either ejection fractions less than 30 percent or triple-vessel disease as compared to patients with either ejection fractions greater than 30 percent or single- or double-vessel disease [30]. In this study, patients who were able to complete 10 minutes of exercise had a much lower reinfarction rate as compared with those who did not complete 10 minutes. Thus, in patients with continued postinfarction angina, those with preserved left ventricular dysfunction and detectable ischemia and those with triple-vessel coronary artery disease might be expected to have improved prognosis if revascularization were to be performed.

Coronary Artery Bypass Graft Surgery

Intuitively, one would expect that relief of ischemia by CABG surgery in the postinfarction period would be associated with improved survival. In an observational study, Akhras et al. followed 119 patients with relatively uncomplicated myocardial infarction and performed exercise treadmill testing 2 weeks postinfarction [2]. Those patients who had positive treadmill tests underwent coronary angiography at 6 weeks. Patients with significant triple-vessel disease, critical proximal left anterior descending stenosis as a component of double- or triple-vessel disease, and who had refractory angina despite optimal medical therapy underwent CABG surgery within 3 months of infarction. The majority of these patients had triple-vessel disease and their exercise time averaged only 5.5 minutes. In these patients identified as possibly being high risk, CABG surgery resulted in a 1-year mortality of only 2 percent. Singh et al., in a study of 108 consecutive patients undergoing CABG surgery with angina within 30 days of infarction, demonstrated 5-year actuarial survival to be 87 percent [107]. This suggests that CABG surgery may be associated with reduced mortality when done in patients with postinfarction angina.

However, three randomized controlled trials of CABG surgery versus medical therapy showed no distinct benefit in favor of surgery for patients without severe postinfarction angina. Norris et al. were the first to address this issue in 100 consecutive patients who had second or third infarctions [86]. The majority had triple-vessel disease, and most had depressed left ventricular function (ejection fractions less than 50 percent). They were all either asymptomatic or only minimally symptomatic and were randomized to receive either CABG or medical therapy. No difference in mortality was found in follow-up to 4.5 years (mean). This same group terminated a similar randomized trial in the patients following a first infarction when no trends were observed in favor of surgery [87]. Likewise, group C of CASS randomized an even larger group of postmyocardial infarction patients to CABG or medical therapy. Again, no improvement was seen in the CABG surgery group [20].

In the postmyocardial infarction period, revascularization by CABG surgery is clearly indicated in patients who have signs or symptoms of recurrent myocardial ischemia. Recurrence of ischemia in this setting is in itself indicative of high risk, and successful CABG surgery will prevent recurrent ischemia and has the potential to improve survival. The latter has not been proven in controlled trials and is unlikely to be tested on ethical grounds. For postinfarction patients who are not symptomatic, risk stratification is in order. For those with clinical or noninvasively detected indicators of high risk, coronary angiography is in order. If high-risk anatomy is found, for example, left main or three-vessel disease, or high-risk ventricular dysfunction (i.e., ejection fractions less than or equal to 40 percent), strong consideration may be given to a recommendation for CABG surgery. It should be emphasized that this recommendation relates to potential for modifying risk and has not been tested in controlled trials.

Percutaneous Transluminal Coronary Angioplasty

Recently, De Feyter performed PTCA in 53 patients with unstable angina between 48 hours and 30 days after acute myocardial infarction [32]. PTCA was initially successful in 47 of the 53 patients with 4 of the 6 patients with unsuccessful PTCA having reinfarctions. The procedure-related myocardial infarction rate was somewhat higher than that expected for elective PTCA done for chronic stable angina. The majority of patients in this study had single-vessel disease, as patients with multivessel disease were often offered CABG surgery. Angina recurred more frequently in patients with multivessel disease who had undergone PTCA of only the ischemia-related vessel (8 of 17, 47 percent) than in patients with single-vessel disease (6 of 30, 20 percent). This difference, however, apparently was not statistically significant. During 6 months of follow-up, there were no late cardiac deaths, but recurrent myocardial infarction developed in two patients.

It would appear that patients who are postmyocardial infarction, have abnormal left ventricular function, recurrent signs or symptoms of ischemia, or multivessel disease are at increased risk for adverse events. Revascularization with PTCA may be offered in settings where CABG surgery is considered as discussed above. It would appear at present that patients with single-vessel coronary disease, excluding the left main, may be better PTCA candidates, whereas the majority of those with multivessel disease may be better CABG surgery candidates.

SILENT ISCHEMIA

Silent or asymptomatic myocardial ischemia, present in the majority of patients with stable effort angina, has been reported to account for approximately 75 percent of all ischemic episodes [103]. Gottlieb et al. reported a high proportion of silent ischemic events in patients presenting with unstable angina [50]. Additionally, patients who have survived ventricular fibrillation and those who have never previously had recognizable symptoms of coronary artery disease may also have objective evidence of myocardial ischemia [92]. In these patients with coronary artery disease confirmed by angiography, silent ischemia may be detected by exercise treadmill testing and/or ambulatory ECG monitoring.

General Considerations

Recognizing that some patients with coronary artery disease present with silent ischemia, two questions of importance are: What are the prognostic implications of silent ischemia? Is there a subgroup that could benefit from revascularization in terms of improving long-term prognosis (i.e., survival)? It has been suggested that in patients with unstable angina silent ischemia detected by ambulatory ECG monitoring is indicative of a poor prognosis when compared to patients without transient silent ischemia [50]. Stern and Tzivoni first suggested a similar association in patients with other chest pain syndromes [108]. In a group of 80 patients, 37 were found to have transient ST-T wave changes and 43 had negative monitoring. Of the 37 patients with positive testing, 16 (43 percent) had deterioration in symptomatology over the next 6 to 12 months compared with only 3 (7 percent) of the 43 patients with negative testing. Thus, in patients with stable or unstable angina ST-T wave changes detected by ambulatory ECG monitoring are indicative of a worsened long-term prognosis. However, it is uncertain as to whether patients with silent ischemia and no symptoms demonstrating similar changes on ambulatory ECG monitoring will have a worsened prognosis. Based on results of exercise treadmill testing, one might hypothesize that such a relationship exists.

Ellestad et al. previously suggested that exercise treadmill testing demonstrating ischemia appears to have the same significance regardless of whether the ST-T changes are accompanied by symptoms [38]. Falcone et al. also examined the clinical significance of exercise-induced silent myocardial ischemia in patients with coronary artery disease [42]. These investigators compared 269 patients with chest pain and ECG changes with 204 patients who had exercise-induced ST-T wave changes but no chest pain. The two groups had similar degrees of left ventricular function and coronary artery disease. CABG surgery was performed on 113 of the patients with symptoms (45 percent) and 48 of the patients without symptoms (24 percent). After a mean follow-up of 36 months, survival in the medically treated patients in both groups was not statistically different even when patients were classified according to the number of diseased vessels. Recently, Weiner et al. reported on 2982 patients from the CASS Registry who underwent coronary angiography and exercise treadmill testing at approximately the same time and were followed for 7 years [116]. One group of 424 patients had exercise-induced ST segment depression without angina and a second group of 456 patients had exercise-induced ischemic ST segment depression and angina. The 7-year survival rates were similar in the two groups, again suggesting that patients with silent myocardial ischemia detected by treadmill testing have a long-term prognosis that is not different from patients who experience angina. Most likely, these patients can be treated similarly to patients who have angina.

Revascularization
At the time of writing there are no controlled studies of asymptomatic patients with definite ischemia comparing revascularization with medical therapy in order to determine the effect on future events or life expectancy. The postinfarction studies of Norris and the CASS group [86] are outlined above.

Recommendations
Presently, no studies are available randomizing patients with silent ischemia and mild or no symptoms to either PTCA versus CABG surgery or PTCA versus medical therapy. It is uncertain as to which patients with silent ischemia should be referred for revascularization. Based on the results of exercise testing, demonstrating that patients have similar prognoses regardless of whether symptoms are present, patients with silent ischemia and stress tests suggesting high risk should undergo coronary angiography. If high-risk anatomy (left main stenosis or three-vessel disease with poor left ventricular function) is present, either CABG surgery or PTCA, dependent on anatomy, should be considered. Patients with frequent ST-T wave changes on ambulatory ECG monitoring despite medical therapy may also be considered for revascularization.

CONCLUSIONS

This review outlines current use of revascularization options in the management of patients with various forms of coronary artery disease. A summary of preferred therapies is shown in Table 19-3.

There are several controlled clinical trials currently underway in the United States and Europe that should provide information helpful for

TABLE 19-3. *Preferred Therapy*

Syndrome	Preferred Initial Therapy				
	Medical		PTCA[a]		CABG[b]
Chronic Stable Angina					
Left main stenosis					x
3-vessel, N LV[c] function, No high-risk ischemia	x	=	?x		
3-vessel, ↓ LV function or high-risk ischemia*			x	<	x
2-vessel, one involving proximal LAD[e]			x	=	x
2-vessel, neither involving proximal LAD	x	=	x		
Single vessel	x	=	x		
Unstable Angina					
Early	x	=	?x		
Late			x	=	x
Coronary Artery Spasm					
With normal CAS	x				
Superimposed on fixed stenosis	x	≠	?x	≠	?x
Acute Myocardial Infarction ± Thrombolysis					
Early (<6 hr)			thrombolytic		
Early with high-grade residual stenosis			x		
Late with high-grade residual stenosis			x	=	x
Silent Ischemia	Same as chronic stable angina				

[a] PTCA = percutaneous transluminal coronary angioplasty.
[b] CABG = coronary artery bypass graft.
[c] LV = left ventricular.
[d] AHH/ACC task force JACC, 1986.
[e] LAD = left anterior descending.

making these choices. The pertinent features of these anxiously awaited trials are summarized in Table 19-4.

TABLE 19-4. *Summary of Clinical Trials Comparing PTCA with Other Anti-ischemic Therapy*

Study Sample Size	Coronary Angio Entry Criteria*	Registry	Planned Follow-Up Duration (Yr)	Major End Points
PTCA vs Medical Therapy				
ACME 328	1,2V >70%	yes	4	AP, ETT, D, MI, TL^{201} ANGIO, LV FUNC, REVASC, QofL
PTCA vs CABG				
BARI 2400	2,3V >50%	yes	5	D/MI, REVASC, ISCH, AP, ETT, CHF, ANGIO, LV FUNC, QofL
CABRI 2000	2,3V >50%	yes	2	AP, ETT, TL^{201}, D, MI, CHF, ANGIO
EAST 600	2,3V >50%	yes	3	ANGIO REVASC, TL^{201}, QofL
GABI 400	2,3V >70%	—	1	AP, ETT, MI, D
RITA 1000	1,2,3V >50%	yes	5	D, MI, AP, ETT, EMP, LV FUNC, REVASC

Abbreviations: ACME = angioplasty compared to medicine; BARI = bypass angioplasty revascularization investigation; CABRI = coronary angioplasty bypass revascularization investigation; EAST = Emory angioplasty surgery trial; GABI = German angioplasty bypass trial; RITA = randomized interventional treatment of angina; D = death; MI = myocardial infarction; AP = angina pectoris; ETT = exercise tolerance testing; EMP = employment status; LV FUNC = left ventricular function; REVASC = revascularization = need for additional revascularizaton; CHF = congestive heart failure; TL^{201} = stress thallium scintography; QofL: = quality of life.
*1,2,3V = single-, double-, and triple-vessel coronary artery disease >50% = 50% diameter narrowing.

REFERENCES

1. Akins, C. W., and Block, P. C. Surgical intervention for failed percutaneous transluminal coronary angioplasty. *Am. J. Cardiol.* 53:108C, 1984.
2. Akhras, F., et al. Early exercise testing and elective coronary artery bypass surgery after complicated myocardial infarction: Effect on morbidity and mortality. *Br. Heart J.* 52:413, 1984.
3. Alison, H. W., et al. Coronary anatomy and arteriography in patients with unstable angina pectoris. *Am. J. Cardiol.* 41:204, 1978.
4. Ambrose, J. A., et al. Angiographic morphology and the pathogenesis of unstable angina pectoris. *J. Am. Coll. Cardiol.* 5:609, 1985.
5. Ambrose, J. A., et al. Angiographic evolution of coronary artery morphology in unstable angina. *J. Am. Coll. Cardiol.* 7:472, 1986.

6. American College of Cardiology/American Heart Association Task Force on Assessment of Cardiovascular Procedures (Subcommittee on Exercise Testing). Guidelines for exercise testing. *J. Am. Coll. Cardiol.* 8:725, 1986.
7. Barner, H. B., Standeven, J. W., and Reese, J. Twelve-year experience with internal mammary artery for coronary artery bypass. *J. Thorac. Cardiovasc. Surg.* 90:668, 1985.
8. Bashour, T. T., Hanna, E. S., and Mason, D. T. Myocardial revascularization with internal mammary artery bypass: An emerging treatment of choice. *Am. Heart J.* 111:143, 1986.
9. Beller, G. A., and Gibson, R. S. Risk stratification after myocardial infarction. *Mod. Concepts Cardiovasc. Dis.* 55:5, 1986.
10. Bertrand, M. E., et al. Comparative results of percutaneous transluminal coronary angioplasty in patients with dynamic versus fixed coronary stenosis. *J. Am. Coll. Cardiol.* 8:504, 1986.
11. Bresnahan, D. R., et al. Angiographic occurrence and clinical correlates of intraluminal coronary artery thrombus: Role of unstable angina. *J. Am. Coll. Cardiol.* 6:285, 1985.
12. Block, P. C., et al. Percutaneous angioplasty of stenoses of bypass grafts or of bypass graft anastomotic sites. *Am. J. Cardiol.* 53:666, 1984.
13. Bonow, R. O., et al. Exercise-induced ischemia in mildly symptomatic patients with coronary-artery disease and preserved left ventricular function. *N. Engl. J. Med.* 311:1339, 1984.
14. Bonow, R. O., and Epstein, S. E. Indications for coronary artery bypass surgery in patients with chronic angina pectoris: Implications of the multicenter randomized trials. *Circulation* 72:V-23, 1985.
15. Bourassa, M. G., et al. Long-term fate of bypass grafts: The Coronary Artery Surgery Study (CASS) and Montreal Heart Institute experiences. *Circulation* 72:V-71, 1985.
16. Burggraf, G. W., and Parker, J. O. Prognosis in coronary artery disease: Angiographic, hemodynamic and clinical factors. *Circulation* 51:146, 1975.
17. Cairns, J. A., et al. Aspirin, sulfinpyrazone, or both in unstable angina: Results of a Canadian Multicenter Trial. *N. Engl. J. Med.* 313:1369, 1985.
18. Cameron, A., Kemp, H. G., and Green, G. E. Bypass surgery with the internal mammary artery graft: 15 year follow-up. *Circulation* 74:III-30, 1986.
19. Capone, G., et al. Frequency of intracoronary filling defects by angiography in angina pectoris at rest. *Am. J. Cardiol.* 56:403, 1985.
20. CASS Principal Investigators and their Associates. Coronary Artery Surgery Study (CASS): A randomized trial of coronary artery bypass surgery (Survival Data). *Circulation* 68:939, 1983.
21. Chaitman, B. R., et al. Participating CASS Hospitals. The role of coronary bypass surgery for "left main equivalent" coronary disease: The Coronary Artery Surgery Study Registry. *Circulation* 74:III-17, 1986.
22. Conti, C. R. Large vessel coronary vasospasm: Diagnosis, natural history and treatment. *Am. J. Cardiol.* 55:41B, 1985.
23. Conti, R. C., et al. Left main coronary artery stenosis: Clinical spectrum, pathophysiology and management. *Prog. Cardiovasc. Dis.* 22:73, 1979.
24. Corbelli, J., et al. Percutaneous transluminal coronary angioplasty after previous coronary artery bypass surgery. *Am. J. Cardiol.* 56:398, 1985.
25. Corcos, T., et al. Percutaneous transluminal coronary angioplasty for the treatment of variant angina. *J. Am. Coll. Cardiol.* 5:1046, 1985.
26. Cowley, M. J., et al. Coronary angioplasty of multiple vessels: Short-term outcome and long-term results. *Circulation* 72:1314, 1985.
27. Cukingnan, R. A., et al. Influence of complete coronary revascularization on relief of angina. *J. Thorac. Cardiovasc. Surg.* 79:188, 1980.

28. David, P. R., et al. Percutaneous transluminal coronary angioplasty in patients with variant angina. *Circulation* 66:695, 1982.
29. DeBusk, R. F., et al. Identification and treatment of low-risk patients after acute myocardial infarction and coronary-artery bypass graft surgery. *N. Engl. J. Med.* 314:161, 1986.
30. De Feyter, P. J., et al. Prognostic value of exercise testing, coronary angiography and left ventriculography 6–9 weeks after myocardial infarction. *Circulation* 66:527, 1982.
31. De Feyter, P. J., et al. Emergency coronary angioplasty in refractory unstable angina. *N. Engl. J. Med.* 313:342, 1985.
32. De Feyter, P. J., et al. Coronary angioplasty for early postinfarction unstable angina. *Circulation* 74:1365, 1986.
33. Detre, K. M., et al. Long-term mortality and morbidity results of the Veterans Administration randomized trial of coronary artery bypass surgery. *Circulation* 72:V-84, 1985.
34. DeWood, M. A., et al. Prevalence of total coronary occlusion during the early hours of transmural myocardial infarction. *N. Engl. J. Med.* 303:897, 1980.
35. Dorros, G., et al. Complex coronary angioplasty: Multiple coronary dilatations. *Am. J. Cardiol.* 53:126C, 1984.
36. Douglas, J. S., et al. Percutaneous transluminal coronary angioplasty in patients with prior coronary bypass surgery. *J. Am. Coll. Cardiol.* 2:745, 1983.
37. El Gamal, M., et al. Percutaneous transluminal angioplasty of stenosed aortocoronary bypass grafts. *Br. Heart J.* 52:617, 1984.
38. Ellestad, M. H., and Wan, M. K. Predictive implications of stress testing: Follow-up of 2700 subjects after maximum treadmill stress testing. *Circulation* 51:363, 1975.
39. Erbel, R., et al. Percutaneous transluminal coronary angioplasty after thrombolytic therapy: A prospective controlled randomized trial. *J. Am. Coll. Cardiol.* 8:485, 1986.
40. European Coronary Surgery Study Group. Long-term results of prospective randomised study of coronary artery bypass surgery in stable angina pectoris. *Lancet* ii:1174, 1982.
41. European Coronary Surgery Study Group. Prospective randomized study of coronary artery bypass surgery in stable angina pectoris: A progress report on survival. *Circulation* 65:II-67, 1982.
42. Falcone, C., et al. Clinical significance of exercise-induced silent myocardial ischemia in patients with coronary artery disease. *J. Am. Coll. Cardiol.* 9:295, 1987.
43. Faxon, D. P., et al. Role of percutaneous transluminal coronary angioplasty in the treatment of unstable angina. Report from the National Heart, Lung and Blood Institute Percutaneous Transluminal Coronary Angioplasty and Coronary Artery Surgery Study Registry. *Am. J. Cardiol.* 53:131C, 1983.
44. Foster, E. D. Reoperation for coronary artery disease. *Circulation* 72:V-59, 1985.
45. Fung, A. Y., et al. Prevention of subsequent exercise-induced periinfarct ischemia by emergency coronary angioplasty in acute myocardial infarction: Comparison with intracoronary streptokinase. *J. Am. Coll. Cardiol.* 8:496, 1986.
46. Gazes, P. C., et al. Preinfarctional (unstable) angina—a prospective study—ten year follow-up: Prognostic significance of electrocardiographic changes. *Circulation* 43:331, 1973.
47. Gersh, B. J., et al. Coronary arteriography and coronary artery bypass

surgery: Morbidity and mortality in patients ages 65 years or older. A report from the Coronary Artery Surgery Study. *Circulation* 67:483, 1983.
48. GISSI. Effectiveness of intravenous thrombolytic treatment in acute myocardial infarction. *Lancet* i:397, 1986.
49. Gold, H. K., et al. Combined intracoronary streptokinase infusion and coronary angioplasty during acute myocardial infarction. *Am. J. Cardiol.* 53:122C, 1984.
50. Gottlieb, S. O., et al. Silent ischemia as a marker for early unfavorable outcomes in patients with unstable angina. *N. Engl. J. Med.* 314:1214, 1986.
51. Grüntzig, A., Senning, A., and Siegenthaler, W. E. Nonoperative dilation of coronary-artery stenosis: Percutaneous transluminal coronary angioplasty. *N. Engl. J. Med.* 301:61, 1979.
52. Hartzler, G. O., et al. Percutaneous transluminal coronary angioplasty without thrombolytic therapy for treatment of acute myocardial infarction. *Am. Heart. J.* 106:965, 1983.
53. Hartzler, G. O., Rutherford, B. D., and McConahay, D. R. Percutaneous transluminal coronary angioplasty: Application for acute myocardial infarction. *Am. J. Cardiol.* 53:117C, 1984.
54. Hirzel, H. O., et al. Short- and long-term changes in myocardial perfusion after percutaneous transluminal coronary angioplasty assessed by Thallium-201 exercise scintigraphy. *Circulation* 63:1001, 1981.
55. Holmes, D. R., et al. Restenosis after percutaneous coronary angioplasty (PTCA): A report from the PTCA Registry of the National Heart, Lung and Blood Institute. *Am. J. Cardiol.* 53:77C, 1984.
56. Kaiser, G. C., et al. Survival following coronary artery bypass grafting in patients with severe angina pectoris (CASS). *J. Thorac. Cardiovasc. Surg.* 89:513, 1985.
57. Kennedy, J. W., et al. Multivariate discriminant analysis of clinical and angiographic predictors of operative mortality from the Collaborative Study in Coronary Artery Surgery (CASS). *J. Thorac. Cardiovasc. Surg.* 80:876, 1980.
58. Kennedy, W. J., et al. The Western Washington Randomized Trial of intracoronary streptokinase in acute myocardial infarction: A 12-month follow-up report. *N. Engl. J. Med.* 312:1073, 1985.
59. Kent, K. M., et al. Effects of coronary-artery bypass on global and regional left ventricular function during exercise. *N. Engl. J. Med.* 298:1434, 1978.
60. Kent, K. M., et al. Improved myocardial function during exercise after successful percutaneous transluminal coronary angioplasty. *N. Engl. J. Med.* 306:441, 1982.
61. Killip, T., Passamani, E., and Davis, K. B. Coronary artery surgery study (CASS): A randomized trial of coronary bypass surgery. Eight years follow-up and survival in patients with reduced ejection fraction. *Circulation* 72:V-102, 1985.
62. Kimbiris, D., et al. Rapid progression of coronary stenosis in patients with unstable angina pectoris selected for coronary angioplasty. *Cathet. Cardiovasc. Diagn.* 10:101, 1984.
63. Klein, L. W., et al. Prognostic significance of severe narrowing of the proximal portion of the left anterior descending coronary artery. *Am. J. Cardiol.* 58:42, 1986.
64. Lawrie, G. M., et al. Results of coronary bypass more than 5 years after operation in 434 patients: Clinical, treadmill exercise and angiographic correlations. *Am. J. Cardiol.* 40:665, 1977.
65. Leimgruber, P. P., et al. Restenosis after successful coronary angioplasty in patients with single-vessel disease. *Circulation* 73:710, 1986.

66. Leisch, F., et al. Influence of variant angina on the results of percutaneous transluminal coronary angioplasty. *Br. Heart J.* 56:341, 1986.
67. Levine, S., et al. Coronary angioplasty: Clinical and angiographic follow-up. *Am. J. Cardiol.* 55:673, 1985.
68. Lewis, H. D., et al. Protective effects of aspirin against acute myocardial infarction and death in men with unstable angina: Results of a Veterans Administration Cooperative Study. *N. Engl. J. Med.* 309:396, 1983.
69. Lewis, M. R., and Dehmer, G. J. Coronary bypass using the internal mammary artery. *Am. J. Cardiol.* 56:480, 1985.
70. Loop, F. D., et al. Trends in selection and results of coronary artery reoperations. *Ann. Thor. Surg.* 36:380, 1983.
71. Loop, F. D., et al. Influence of the internal-mammary-artery graft on 10-year survival and other cardiac events. *N. Engl. J. Med.* 314:1, 1986.
72. Mabin, T. A., et al. Follow-up clinical results in patients undergoing percutaneous transluminal coronary angioplasty. *Circulation* 71:754, 1985.
73. Mabin, T. A., et al. Intracoronary thrombus: Role in coronary occlusion complicating percutaneous transluminal coronary angioplasty. *J. Am. Coll. Cardiol.* 5:198, 1985.
74. McNeer, J. F., et al. The role of the exercise test in the evaluation of patients for ischemic heart disease. *Circulation* 57:64, 1978.
75. Meier, B., et al. Long-term exercise performance after percutaneous transluminal coronary angioplasty and coronary artery bypass grafting. *Circulation* 68:796, 1983.
76. Meier, B., et al. Repeat coronary angioplasty. *J. Am. Coll. Cardiol.* 4:463, 1984.
77. Meyer, J., et al. Treatment of unstable angina pectoris with percutaneous transluminal coronary angioplasty (PTCA). *Cathet. Cardiovasc. Diagn.* 7:361, 1981.
78. Meyer, J., et al. Percutaneous transluminal coronary angioplasty immediately after intracoronary streptolysis of transmural myocardial infarction. *Circulation* 66:905, 1982.
79. Meyer, J., et al. Percutaneous transluminal coronary angioplasty in patients with stable and unstable angina pectoris: Analysis of early and late results. *Am. Heart J.* 106:973, 1983.
80. Mock, M. B., et al. The survival of nonoperated patients with ischemic heart disease: The CASS experience (Abstract). *Am. J. Cardiol.* 49:1007, 1982.
81. Mock, M. B., et al. Percutaneous transluminal coronary angioplasty (PTCA) in the elderly patient: Experience in the National Heart, Lung and Blood Institute PTCA Registry. *Am. J. Cardiol.* 53:89C, 1984.
82. Moise, A., et al. Unstable angina and progression of coronary atherosclerosis. *N. Engl. J. Med.* 309:685, 1983.
83. Mundth, E. D., and Austen, W. G., Surgical measures for coronary heart disease (second of three parts). *N. Engl. J. Med.* 293:75, 1975.
84. Murphy, M. L., et al. Treatment of chronic stable angina: A preliminary report of survival data of the Randomized Veterans Administration Cooperative Study. *N. Engl. J. Med.* 297:621, 1977.
85. National Cooperative Study Group to Compare Surgical and Medical Therapy. II. In-hospital experience and initial follow-up results in patients with one, two and three vessel disease. *Am. J. Cardiol.* 42:839, 1978.
86. Norris, R. M., et al. Coronary surgery after recurrent myocardial infarction: Progress of a trial comparing surgical with nonsurgical management for asymptomatic patients with advanced coronary disease. *Circulation* 63:785, 1981.

87. Norris, R. M. Prognosis after recovery from first acute myocardial infarction: Determinants of reinfarction and sudden death. *Am. J. Cardiol.* 53:408, 1984.
88. O'Neill, W., et al. A prospective randomized clinical trial of intracoronary streptokinase versus coronary angioplasty for acute myocardial infarction. *N. Engl. J. Med.* 314:812, 1986.
89. Passamani, E., et al. A randomized trial of coronary artery bypass surgery: Survival of patients with a low ejection fraction. *N. Engl. J. Med.* 312:1665, 1985.
90. Pelletier, L. C., et al. Myocardial revascularization after failure of percutaneous transluminal coronary angioplasty. *J. Thorac. Cardiovasc. Surg.* 90:265, 1985.
91. Pepine, C. J. Acute and chronic heart disease: Unstable angina. In W. W. Parmley, K Chatterjee, (eds.), *Cardiology, Vol. 2, Cardiovascular Disease.* Philadelphia: Lippincott, 1989. Ch. 5.
92. Pepine, C. J. Ambulant myocardial ischemia and its prognostic implications (Editorial). *Circulation* 81:1136, 1990.
93. Pepine, C. J., et al. Percutaneous transluminal coronary angioplasty in acute myocardial infarction. *Am. Heart J.* 107:820, 1984.
94. Phillips, S. J., et al. Emergency coronary artery revascularization: A possible therapy for acute myocardial infarction. *Circulation* 60:241, 1979.
95. Prida, S. E., et al. Percutaneous transluminal coronary angioplasty in evolving acute myocardial infarction. *Am. J. Cardiol.* 57:1069, 1986.
96. Quigley, P. J., et al. Percutaneous transluminal coronary angioplasty in unstable angina: Comparison with stable angina. *Br. Heart J.* 55:227, 1986.
97. Rahimtoola, S. H., et al. Ten-year survival after coronary bypass surgery for unstable angina. *N. Engl. J. Med.* 308:676, 1983.
98. Rahimtoola, S. H., Grunkemeier, G. L., and Starr, A. Ten year survival after coronary artery bypass surgery for angina in patients aged 65 years and older. *Circulation* 74:509, 1986.
99. Rahimtoola, S. H. Coronary bypass surgery for unstable angina. *Circulation* 69:842, 1984.
100. Raizner, A. E., et al. Transluminal coronary angioplasty in the elderly. *Am. J. Cardiol.* 57:29, 1986.
101. Rogers, W. J., et al. Return of left ventricular function after reperfusion in patients with myocardial infarction: Importance of subtotal stenoses on intact collaterals. *Circulation* 69:338, 1984.
102. Schaff, H. V., et al. The morbidity and mortality of reoperation for coronary artery disease and analysis of late results with use of actuarial estimate of event-free interval. *J. Thorac. Cardiovasc. Surg.* 85:508, 1983.
103. Schang, S. J., and, Pepine, C. J. Transient asymptomatic S-T segment depression during daily activity. *Am. J. Cardiol.* 39:396, 1977.
104. Schuster, E. H., and Bulkley, B. H. Early post-infarction angina: Ischemia at a distance and ischemia in the infarct zone. *N. Engl. J. Med.* 305:1101, 1981.
105. Selinger, S. L., et al. Surgical treatment of acute evolving anterior myocardial infarction. *Circulation* 64:II-28, 1981.
106. Silverman, K. J., and Grossman, W. Current Concepts. Angina Pectoris: Natural history and strategies for evaluation and management. *N. Engl. J. Med.* 310:1712, 1984.
107. Singh, A. K., et al. Early myocardial revascularization for postinfarction angina: Results and long-term follow-up. *J. Am. Coll. Cardiol.* 6:1121, 1985.

108. Stern, S., and Tzivoni, D. Early detection of silent ischaemic heart disease by 24-hour electrocardiographic monitoring of active subjects. *Br. Heart J.* 36:481, 1974.
109. Sugrue, D. D., et al. Coronary artery thrombus as a risk factor for acute vessel occlusion during percutaneous transluminal coronary angioplasty: Improving results. *Br. Heart J.* 56:62, 1986.
110. Taylor, G. J., et al. Percutaneous transluminal coronary angioplasty as palliation for patients considered poor surgical candidates. *Am. Heart J.* 111:840, 1986.
111. Telford, A. M., and Wilson, C. Trial of heparin versus atenolol in prevention of myocardial infarction in intermediate coronary syndrome. *Lancet* i:1225, 1981.
112. Vandormael, M. G., et al. Immediate and short-term benefit of multilesion coronary angioplasty: Influence of degree of revascularization. *J. Am. Coll. Cardiol.* 6:983, 1985.
113. Vanhaecke, J., et al. Emergency bypass surgery: Late effects on size of infarction and ventricular function. *Circulation* 72:II-179, 1985.
114. The Veterans Administration Coronary Artery Bypass Surgery Cooperative Study Group. Eleven-year survival in the Veterans Administration Randomized Trial of Coronary Bypass Surgery for Stable Angina. *N. Engl. J. Med.* 311:1333, 1984.
115. Weiner, D. A., et al. The role of exercise testing in identifying patients with improved survival after coronary artery bypass surgery. *J. Am. Coll. Cardiol.* 8:741, 1986.
116. Weiner, D. A., et al. Significance of silent myocardial ischemia during exercise testing in patients with coronary artery disease. *Am. J. Cardiol.* 59:725, 1987.
117. Williams, D. O., et al. Restoration of normal coronary hemodynamics and myocardial metabolism after percutaneous transluminal coronary angioplasty. *Circulation* 62:653, 1980.
118. Williams, D. O., et al. Efficacy of repeat percutaneous transluminal coronary angioplasty for coronary restenosis. *Am. J. Cardiol.* 53:32C, 1984.
119. Williams, D. O., et al. Evaluation of the role of coronary angioplasty in patients with unstable angina pectoris. *Am. Heart J.* 102:1, 1981.
120. Williams, D. O., et al. Coronary circulatory dynamics before and after successful coronary angioplasty. *J. Am. Coll. Cardiol.* 1:1268, 1983.
121. Wohlgelernter, D., et al. Percutaneous coronary angioplasty of the "culprit lesion" for management of unstable angina pectoris in patients with multivessel coronary artery disease. *Am. J. Cardiol.* 58:460, 1986.

INDEX

Abnormal coronary circulation, and nitrates, 91
Absorption
 of beta blockers, 178, 182
 vs. bioavailability, 178
 of calcium channel antagonists, 208–211
Acebutolol, 100, 263, 268, 271
 absorption characteristics of, 182
 ancillary properties of, 180
  cardioselectivity, 119, 180, 187
  intrinsic sympathomimetic activity, 180, 188, 189, 190
  membrane stabilizing activity, 130, 180, 187
 for angina, 444
 and bronchospasm, 458
 dosage of (angina), 263, 274
 hydralazine interaction with, 412
 and hypertension in pregnancy, 409
 indications for, 179
 metabolism of, 183, 192
 molecular structure of, 117
 nifedipine compared with, 272
ACE inhibitors, 373, 376
Acetaminophen, 443
Acute myocardial infarction. *See* Myocardial infarction, acute
Adenosine diphosphate (ADP), and propranolol, 126
Adenylate cyclase, 98, 99, 106–107
Adenylate cyclase system, 142, 99–108
 and ischemia, 115
Adenosine, 5–6
Adenosine nucleolide (ADP), 15
Adrenergic activity, and acute myocardial infarction, 330
Adrenergic nervous system, 98–99
Adrenocortical extract (ACE) inhibitors, 326
Adverse effects
 of beta blockers, 194, 260–261, 277, 299, 349, 351, 396–409, 443–444, 447. *See also under* Beta blockers
 of calcium channel antagonists, 436–437
  of nicardipine, 295, 437
  ventricular depression, 432–436
  withdrawal syndrome, 428–431
 and combination therapies (angina), 453
 of nitrates, 370, 380–381, 442, 447
  dizziness or syncope, 377–379
  headache, 374, 376–377
  nausea, 379
Aging. *See* Geriatrics
Airway disease
 and beta blockers, 187, 273, 274
  propranolol, 400
  timolol, 401
 and cardioselective beta blockers, 119
Airway obstruction, reversible, calcium channel antagonists for, 208
Alcohol
 and nitrates, 376, 379, 380
 as NTG diluent, 381
 and sublingual nitroglycerin, 374
Alcohol withdrawal, beta blockers for, 98
Alpha-adrenergic receptors, 6, 98–99, 100
 and labetalol, 191
Alpha blockade
 and beta blockers, 120, 191
 and cold hands or feet, 399
 and sexual dysfunction, 405
Alprenolol, 263, 271, 346
 ancillary properties of, 180
 and angina, 270
 and myocardial infarction, 332, 338, 339, 346
Andolol, and CNS reactions, 403
Aneurysmal resection, 27

503

Aneurysms, 26
Anginal equivalents, 41
Angina pectoris, 16, 38, 39–40
  and beta blockers, 38, 98, 193, 195, 443–445, 447–449, 451–457. *See also under* Beta blockers
  beta with alpha blockers for, 191
  and beta blockers plus calcium channel antagonists, 413
  calcium channel antagonists for, 38, 301, 449–457, 483
  coronary artery/atherosclerotic stenosis caliber changes in, 83
  from coronary artery spasm, 482–485, 494
  description of feeling of, 41
  emotion- or stress-related, 235–236
  exertional, 253, 291–293, 295, 389
  and heart-rate goal, 195
  mixed, 22, 234, 252–253, 278, 447–448
  and nitrates, 38, 81, 85, 442–443, 447–451, 456–457
    nitroglycerin, 83, 86, 161, 235, 443, 446
    nitroglycerin (combination), 448, 456
  nocturnal, 248
  spontaneous improvement in, 235
  stable, 16–19, 47. *See also* Stable angina pectoris
  unstable, 19–21, 38–39, 53–58, 249–252, 479. *See also* Unstable angina pectoris
  variant (vasospastic), 22, 483. *See also* Variant angina pectoris
Angina pectoris drug therapy, approach to, 38, 442
  beta blockers, 443–445
  calcium channel antagonists, 445–446
  nitrates, 442–443
  stratification of patients for, 457–459
  therapies in combination, 446–447
    beta blockers/calcium channel antagonists, 451–456
    beta blockers/nitrates, 447–449
    calcium channel antagonists/nitrates, 449–451
    triple (beta blockers/calcium channel antagonists/nitrates), 455–457
Angina at rest, 19, 53–54

calcium channel antagonists for, 288–290
and myocardial oxygen supply, 20
and nicardipine, 295
Angiography, coronary, 45
indication of, 48
and revascularization, 489, 491, 493
and thrombosis, 46
and unstable angina, 56, 479, 480
Angioplasty. *See also* Percutaneous transluminal coronary angioplasty
  for acute myocardial infarction, 27
  laser, 53
  and unstable angina, 21
  for variant angina, 22
Angioplasty balloons, 53
Anisoylated plasminogen streptokinase activator complex (APSAC), 62, 63
Antianginal drug therapy approach. *See* Angina pectoris drug therapy, approach to
Antiarrhythmic agents, and beta blockers, 411
Antiarrhythmic effects. *See also* Arrhythmias and bepridil, 296
  of beta blockers, 194, 333–334
    atenolol, 334
    metoprolol, 334
    propranolol, 188, 334
Anticoagulants, for unstable angina pectoris, 21
Antihypertensives, beta blockers in interaction with, 411–412
Anti-infectives, beta blockers in interaction with, 413
Antiplatelet antibodies, with tPA, 63
Anti-thyroid agents, beta blockers in interaction with, 418
Aortic regurgitation, 18–19
Aortic stenosis
  and angina, 40
  and diminished vascular flow reserve, 15–16
  and heart work, 3
Approach to antianginal drug therapy. *See* Angina pectoris drug therapy, approach to
Arcus senilis, 42
Arrhythmias. *See also* Antiarrhythmic effects
  and angina therapy, 458
  beta blockers for, 98

INDEX 505

propranolol, 179, 196
and sotalol, 131
and postinfarction period, 337
Arrhythmias, ventricular. *See* Ventricular arrhythmias
Arterial stenosis. *See* Stenosis, coronary arterial
Arterial vasodilation, and nitrates, 86–87, 89
Arteriolar vasodilation, and nitrates, 87
Aspirin
　for beta blockers, 410
　for mixed angina, 23
　for myocardial infarction (acute), 61, 67
　for unstable angina, 21, 54, 251
Asthma. *See also* Airway disease; Bronchospasm
　and angina therapy, 458
　beta blockers for, 400, 444
Atenolol (tenormin), 100, 263, 268, 271, 345
　absorption characteristics of, 182
　ancillary properties of, 180, 189, 191
　as cardioselective, 119, 121, 180, 187
　for angina, 196, 444
　for angina (combination), 452, 453, 454
　antiarrhythmic effects of, 194
　and CNS reactions, 403, 403–404
　distribution of, 182
　dosing of, 196–197, 263, 274
　and hypertension, 194
　in pregnancy, 409
　indications for, 179
　interactions with
　　cimetidine, 414
　　clonidine, 412
　　hydralazine, 412
　　indomethacin, 410
　　lidocaine, 411
　　verapamil, 413
　metabolism of, 184–185
　molecular structure of, 117
　and myocardial infarction, 332, 333, 334, 338, 345–346
　and myocardial ischemia, 331
　nifedipine with, 273
　and platelet aggregation, 126
　and serum concentration, 193

and serum lipids, 127
and sexual functioning, 405
Atherectomy, 53
Atherogenic risk factor, and calcium channel antagonists, 299–300
Atherosclerosis, 2, 12, 14
　and calcium channel antagonists, 297
　and variant angina pectoris, 22
Atherosclerotic coronary artery disease, 17
Atherosclerotic lesion, and acute myocardial infarction, 24–25
Atherosclerotic stenoses
　caliber of changes of, 83
　dilation of, 82
ATP, 15
Atrioventricular node, and beta blockers, 128
Australian-Swedish Pindolol Study, 338
Autoregulation of coronary arteries, 6, 7

Balloons, 53, 56, 58–59
Barbiturates, beta blockers in interaction with, 413
Bayes theorem of conditional probability, 43
Bay *8644*, 140, 141
Bepredil, 138, 295–296, 446
Beta blockade, 98, 192–193, 260, 261
　alpha blockade with, 120
　and calcium channel antagonists, 143, 144
　chronic, 113, 123
　degree of, 261–262, 264
　and regulation of beta receptors, 112
　and silent ischemia, 279
　and unstable angina, 275
Beta Blocker Heart Attack Trial, 339, 342, 343, 344, 347, 348, 349
Beta blockers (beta-adrenergic blocking agents), 46, 98, 178, 260
　absorption of, 178, 182
　adverse effects of, 194, 260–261, 277, 299, 349, 351, 396–409, 443–444, 447
　　esmolol, 398
　　nitrates combined with, 447–449
　　oxprenolol, 405, 408
　　practolol, 349, 404, 405, 406–407

Beta blockers, adverse effects of, *(continued)*
  propranolol, 277, 399, 400, 403, 403–404, 405, 408
  timolol, 188, 398, 401, 402, 403, 404, 405
and alpha blockade, 191
ancillary properties of, 98, 130–131, 180–181, 260, 260–261, 274, 332
  cardiac selectivity, 119–120, 121, 180–181, 187, 273, 274, 444, 458
  instrinsic sympathomimetic activity, 118–119, 120, 121, 122, 180–181, 188–190, 349, 407, 444
  membrane stabilizing activity, 130–131, 180–181, 187–188, 407
  protein binding and lipophilicity, 180–181, 190–191
for angina, 38, 98, 193, 195, 443–445, 447–449, 451–457
  with alpha blockers, 191
  atenolol, 196, 444
  atenolol (combination), 452, 453, 454
  metoprolol, 196, 444
  metoprolol (combination), 448, 452, 455, 456
  nadolol, 197, 444
  nadolol (combination), 456
  propranolol, 193, 195–196
  propranolol (combination), 448, 451, 452, 453, 455, 456, 457
  timolol, 197
for angina (mixed), 278
for angina (stable), 18, 47–48, 260–274
  acute studies on, 265–266
  in comparison to other antianginal drugs, 271–273
  and concomitant disease, 273
  medium- to long-term studies on, 266–267
  and optimal dose, 261–262, 264–265, 270
  and study design, 265
for angina (unstable), 20, 54, 56, 274–277, 331, 480
for angina (variant), 277–278
antiarrhythmic effects of, 194, 458
and beta receptors, 113
selectivity among, 119–120
binding of, 190
and calcium channel antagonists combined with, 277, 300–301, 413, 451–457
  combined with (as single agents), 433, 435–436
  compared with, 272, 299, 300, 301
  in interaction with, 223–224, 413
contraindications for, 187, 350, 398, 457, 458
and diabetes mellitus, 459
vs. calcium channel antagonists, 300
distribution of, 182–183
dosing guidelines and schedules for, 194–198, 277, 349
electrophysiologic effects of, 127–131
hemodynamic effects of, 120
  blood pressure, 122–123
  cardiac output, 122
  heart rate, 120–122, 128
  metabolic effects, 127
  myocardial oxygen demand, 123–124
  myocardial oxygen supply, 124–126
  platelet effects, 126–127
  ventricular diastolic function, 123
and hypertension, 194, 457
and hyperthyroidism, 459
indications for, 179
interactions of, 374, 376, 409–418
  with calcium channel antagonists, 223–224, 413
  with nitrates, 166, 374, 376
metabolism (biotransformation) and elimination of, 183–187
and migraine, 459
for myocardial infarction (acute), 27, 58, 330–344, 347–351
  alprenolol, 346
  atenolol, 345
  metoprolol, 345
  oxprenolol, 346
  pindolol, 346
  propranolol, 344–345
  sotalol, 346
  timolol, 345
and nitrates
  combined with, 242, 251, 272, 277, 447–449, 456–457
  compared with, 242, 271–272
  in interaction with, 374, 376
and nitroglycerin (transdermal), 248
plasma concentrations or dose-response relationships for, 191–192

and postmyocardial infarction, 458
  for silent myocardial ischemia, 278–279
  structure activity relationships of, 116–118
  and venodilation, 80
Beta blocker withdrawal, 407–408, 428, 430
Beta (beta-adrenergic) receptors, 6, 98, 98–99, 100, 102–106, 178
  activation of, 116
  beta-blocker affinity to, 119–120
  and congestive heart failure, 112
  and coronary blood flow, 124
  distribution of, 125
  and ischemia, 115
  regulation of, 108–114
  spare, 111–112
Betaxolol, 268
  ancillary properties of, 180, 187, 188
  dosing schedule for, 198
  and glaucoma, 398
  indications of, 179
Bevantolol
  ancillary properties of, 180
  and angina, 270
Bioavailability
  vs. absorption, 178
  of beta blockers, 178, 182
  of calcium channel antagonists, 210
    diltiazem, 212
    verapamil, 212
Bisoprolol, ancillary properties of, 180
Black hypertensive patients, and diltiazem, 301
Blood pressure
  and beta blockers, 122–123
  and calcium channel antagonists, 301
  and nitrate administration, 370, 374
Blood pressure, systolic, 85
Bopindolol, ancillary properties of, 180
Boston Collaborative Drug Surveillance Program, 403
Bowditch staircase phenomenon, 3
Bradycardia
  from beta blockers, 396–398, 407, 409, 444
  and calcium channel antagonist therapy, 436
  and combination therapy, 455
  from nitrates, 377, 378, 379

Bronchospasm. *See also* Airway disease
  and angina therapy, 458
  and beta blockers, 119, 187, 400–401, 407
    cardioselective, 273, 274
    propanolol, 189
Bufentolol, ancillary properties of, 180
Bupranolol, ancillary properties of, 180

Calcium, intracellular ionized, and nitrate action, 85
Calcium channel(s), 138–139
Calcium channel activation, through neurohumoral influences, 142
Calcium channel antagonists (blockers), 15, 46, 138–140, 146, 208
  and acute myocardial infarction, 27, 356–367
  adverse reactions to, 428–437
    of nicardipine, 295, 437
  for angina, 38, 301, 445–446, 449–457, 483
    due to coronary spasm, 483
    for angina (exertional), 291
      diltiazem, 291–292
      nifedipine, 291
      verapamil, 293
    for angina (mixed), 253
    for angina (rest), 288
      comparison studies on, 290
      diltiazem, 288–289
      nifedipine, 289
      verapamil, 289–290
    for angina (stable), 18, 47–48
    for angina (unstable), 21, 54, 56, 480
    for angina (variant), 22, 277
  and beta blockers
    combined with, 277, 300–301, 413, 451–457
    combined with (as single agents), 433, 435–436
    compared with, 272, 299, 300, 301
    in interaction with, 223–224, 413
  and bronchospasm, 458
  contraindication for, 458
  dihydropyridines, 138, 139–140, 141, 142, 295
  and diabetes mellitus, 459

Calcium channel antagonists
(continued)
dosing guidelines for, 445
individualized, 214–218
effects on diastolic ventricular function of, 144–145
electrophysiologic effects of, 145–146
experimental
bepridil, 295–296
inmoldipine, 295
insoldipine, 295
nicardipine, 294–295
general cardiovascular effects of, 142–143
for hypertension, 296–301, 457
for hypertension plus angina pectoris, 301
indications for, 457
interactions of, 218, 437
with beta blockers, 223–224, 413
with cimetidine, 219, 220–222
with digoxin, 219–220
with nitrates, 376
potential, 223–224
with quinidine, 219, 222–223
and migraine, 459
for myocardial infarction, 58
and nitrates
combined with, 125, 242
compared with, 242
in interaction with, 376
and nitroglycerin (transdermal), 248
pharmacokinetics of (classic)
absorption, 208–211
distribution, 211–212
metabolism and elimination, 212
pharmacokinetics of (clinical), 213–214
and PTCA or CABG surgery, 485
for silent myocardial ischemia, 278, 293–294
sites of action for, 139
use dependency of inhibition for, 140–141
and venodilation, 80
and ventricular function, 432, 436
diltiazem, 433–434, 436
nicardipine, 435–436
nifedipine, 434–435, 436
verapamil, 432–433, 436
Calcium channel antagonist withdrawal syndrome, 428–431

Capillaries in heart, recruitment of, 7
Captopril, 324–325, 326
Carbohydrate homeostasis, from beta blockers, 401
Carcinogenicity, of beta blockers, 405–406
Cardiac catheterization, 41, 45
Cardiac death, sudden, 27–28
Cardiac output, and beta blockers, 122
Cardiac selectivity, of beta blockers, 119–120, 180–181, 187
and heart rate, 121
and pulmonary disease, 458
usefulness of, 444
Cardiomyopathy, hypertrophic. See Hypertrophic cardiomyopathy
Cardiomyopathy, ischemic, 28–29
Cardiovascular effects, from beta blockers, 396–398
Cartenolol, 268
ancillary properties of, 180
indications for, 179
Carvedilol, and angina, 270
CASS. See Coronary Artery Surgery Study
Catecholamines, 98, 99, 401
and beta blockade, 194, 331
and beta blocker withdrawal, 408
and calcium channel antagonists, 430
and clonidine withdrawal, 411
and congestive heart failure, 112
and myocardial infarction, 114, 330
and nitrate tolerance, 384
Catheterization, cardiac, 45
Celiprolol, 271
ancillary properties of, 180
and angina, 270
Cell death, ischemic
and calcium channel antagonists, 356
progression of, 13
Central nervous system (CNS), and beta blockers, 402–404, 407
Cerebrovascular spasm, calcium channel antagonists for, 208
Chest pain
beta blockers for, 332–333
evaluation of patient with, 41
from nitrate dependence, 376
Chronic beta blockade, 113
Chronic congestive heart failure, 39

Chronic stable angina pectoris. *See* Stable angina pectoris, chronic
Cigarettes. *See* Smoking
Cimetidine, drug interactions of
  beta blockers, 414, 415
  calcium channel antagonists, 220–222
Classic pharmacokinetics, 208
  of calcium channel antagonists, 208–212
Clinical pharmacokinetics, 208
  of calcium channel antagonists, 213–214
Clonidine
  beta blockers in interaction with, 411
  withdrawal syndrome for, 411, 428, 430
Cold cardioplegia, 55
Cold hands and feet, from beta blockers, 399
Competitive inhibition, of beta receptors, 98, 103, 105, 106, 107, 108
Concomitant drug therapy, and nitrates, 374
Congenital long Q-T syndrome, 129, 130
Congestive heart failure
  and angina therapy, 457–458
  and beta-adrenergic stimulation, 112
  and beta blockers, 188–189, 457
  and calcium channel antagonists, 218
  and cardioselective beta blockers, 119
  chronic, 39
  and digoxin combinations, 219
  and ISA beta blockers, 118
  as ischemic-heart-disease syndrome, 40
  and labetalol, 120
  and nifedipine, 434, 435
  and nitrate action, 85
  and nitrate amount, 242
  nitrate resistance in, 373
  and nitrate withdrawal, 380
  and nitroglycerin, 165
    intravenous, 327
    transdermal, 161
  symptoms of, 41
  verapamil for, 433

Contraceptives, oral, beta blockers in interaction with, 418
Coronary angiography. *See* Angiography, coronary
Coronary arteries, 6
  blood flow in, 6–7
  caliber changes in, 83
Coronary artery bypass graft surgery (CABG), 21, 27, 38, 39, 46, 48–51, 464
  for angina due to coronary spasm, 483–485, 494
  and complete revascularization, 474
  high-risk groups for, 477–479
  for myocardial infarction, 59, 486–487, 489, 494
  patients unsuitable for, 456
  and postmyocardial infarction, 490–491
  and PTCA, 52, 473, 476
  and silent ischemia, 493, 494
  for stable angina pectoris, 468–471, 472, 494
  for unstable angina pectoris, 56, 480–481, 482, 494
Coronary artery disease, 330
  and by-passed vessels, 476
  and calcium channel antagonists, 290
  clinical presentations of, 464
  diagnosis of, 45
  as mortality indicator, 464–465, 467
  and unstable angina, 480
Coronary artery spasm. *See* Spasm, coronary artery
Coronary artery stenosis, 5
Coronary Artery Surgery Study (CASS), 48, 467, 468, 470, 471, 477, 481, 491, 493
Coronary atherosclerosis, 9
  and nitrates, 91
Coronary blood flow (oxygen supply), 5–7, 21
  and nicardipine, 295
  and nifedipine, 292
  and stenosis, 9
Coronary circulation, abnormal, and nitrates, 91
Coronary circulation, normal, and nitroglycerin, 89, 90
Coronary Prevention Research Study, 338, 347

Coronary revascularization procedures. *See* Coronary artery bypass graft (CABG) surgery; Percutaneous transluminal coronary angioplasty (PTCA); Revascularization
Coronary stenosis. *See* Stenosis, coronary
Coronary thrombosis, 15. *See also* Thrombosis
 and sudden cardiac death, 27–28
 and unstable angina, 251
Coronary vascular flow reserve, diminished, 15–16
Coronary vasoconstriction, *See* Vasoconstriction, coronary
Coronary vasospasm. *See* Vasospasm, coronary
Corticosteroids
 and beta-adrenergic receptor regulation, 114
 for myocardial infarction, 58
Crescendo angina, 19, 53
"Culprit lesion," 481–482
Cyclic AMP, 99
Cyclic GMP, 142, 153–154, 155–156, 157, 382, 384
Cyclo-oxygenase inhibitors, 15
Cytochrome P-450 system, 186

D600, 139
Danish Verapamil Infarction Trial (DAVIT I), 361
Danish Verapamil Infarction Trial II (DAVIT II), 361, 363
Debrisoquine, metabolism of, 183, 184
Delivery sets, and nitroglycerin absorption, 159
Depression (psychological), from beta blockers, 402–403
Dextropropranolol, and ventricular arrhythmias, 130
Diabetes, revascularization risk in, 478
Diabetes mellitus
 and angina therapy, 459
 and beta blockers, 119–120, 273, 274, 300, 401–402, 444
 and calcium channel antagonists, 446
 vs. beta blockers, 300

Diacetolol, 183
 cardiac selectivity of, 187
 and dose-response curve, 192
Diastolic filling, and beta blockers, 123
Diastolic pressure time index (DPTI), 3–4, 7
Diazepam, 403, 407
Dichloisoproterenol, 117
Digital radiography, 45
Digoxin, interactions of (calcium channel antagonists), 219–220
Dihydropyridines, 138, 139–40, 141, 142, 295
Diltiazem, 138, 139, 141, 208
 absorption of, 210–211
 active metabolites of, 214
 adverse effects of, 437
 for angina, 291–292, 445–446
 for angina (combination), 449–450, 451, 452, 456–457
 beta blockers in interaction with, 413
 binding of, 211
 and blood flow, 143
 and cimetidine, 221
 clinical effects of, 213–214
 contraindications for, 458
 and coronary artery disease, 290
 and diabetes mellitus, 459
 with digoxin, 219, 220
 dose alterations of, 215
 and geriatrics, 216
 and heart rate, 145, 301
 and hypertension, 297, 299, 300–301
 inotropic influence of, 142
 and liver disease, 216
 metabolism of, 212
 and myocardial infarction (acute), 357, 361–362
 pharmacokinetic parameters of, 209
 potential interactions of, 223
 propranolol with, 273
 propranolol compared with, 275–276
 and quinidine, 222
 and Raynaud's phenomenon, 459
 and renal disease, 217, 217–218
 for rest angina, 288–289
 and silent ischemia, 293, 294
 in sustained-release formulation, 446
 and ventricular relaxation, 144

with verapamil, 272–273
withdrawal from, 430
Dimensions, intracardiac, and nitroglycerin, 87
Diminished coronary vascular flow reserve, 15–16
Disopyramide, 411
Dissection, coronary artery, 14
Distribution
  of beta blockers, 182–183
  of calcium channel antagonists, 211–212
Diuretics
  and hypokalemia, 119
  and nitrates, 376
Dizziness
  from nifedipine vs. nicardipine, 437
  from nitrates, 377–379
Doppler tipped catheter, 45
Dose-response relationship
  for beta blockers, 192
  and hypertension, 194
  for ISDN, 375
  and spare receptors, 111
Dosing guidelines and schedules
  for beta blockers, 194–198, 263, 274, 277, 444
  for calcium channel antagonists, 214, 218, 445
    and geriatrics, 215, 216–217
    and liver disease, 214–216
    and renal disease, 215, 217–218
  for nitrates, 241, 249, 250, 373–374, 387–388
    ISDN, 390
    and nitrate tolerance, 168
Dreams, from beta blockers, 402–403
Drug interactions
  of beta blockers, 374, 376, 409–410
    with antiarrhythmics, 411
    with anti-infectives, 413
    with barbiturates, 413
    with beta blockers (combination), 413
    with calcium channel antagonists, 223–224, 413
    with H-2 antagonists, 414–415
    with hypoglycemics, 415
    with indomethacin, 410
    with methylxanthines, 415–416
    with nitrates, 166, 374, 376
    with oral contraceptives, 418
    with sympathomimetics, 418
    with thyroid hormones/antithyroid agents, 418
  of calcium channel antagonists, 218–224, 437
    with beta blockers, 223–224, 413
    with nitrates, 376
  of nitrates
    with beta blockers, 166, 374, 376
    with calcium channel antagonists, 376
Dynamic coronary obstruction, 253

ECSSG (European Coronary Surgery Study Group), 50, 468, 469, 470, 471
Effort angina. See Exertional angina
Elderly patients
  beta blockade in, 409
  and revascularization risk, 477, 479
Electrocardiogram, 42–43
Electrophysiologic effects, of beta blockers, 127–131
Elimination
  of beta blockers, 183–187
  of calcium channel antagonists, 212
Embolism, coronary artery, 14
Endocardial viability ratio, 4
Endorphine levels, and silent ischemia, 23
Endothelium-dependent relaxing factor (EDRF), 156–157, 382–383
Endothelium-dependent vasodilators, 57, 155, 157
Epinephrine, 98, 99
  beta blockers in interaction with, 418
  and cardioselective agents, 119
  and competitive binding, 105
  and myocardial ischemia, 114–115
  and propranolol, 126
Equilibrium radionuclide angiocardiography, 43
Esmolol (brevibloc), 100, 398
  adverse effects of, 398
  ancillary properties of, 180, 187
  dosing schedule for, 197–198
  indications for, 179
  metabolism of, 185
  molecular structure of, 117
Esophageal motor dysfunction, calcium channel antagonists for, 208

Estrogen contraceptives, beta blockers in interaction with, 418
European Coronary Surgery Study Group (ECSSG), 50, 468, 469, 470, 471
European Infarction Study, 338, 346
European Multicenter Trial, 344
Evaluation of patient with ischemic heart disease, 39–45
Exercise, stenosis constriction from, 82
Exercise testing, 43–44
Exertional angina
  calcium channel antagonists for, 291–293
  and mixed angina, 253
  nicardipine for, 295
  and transdermal nitroglycerin responsiveness, 389

Factor VII, 15
Fatigue, muscle, from beta blockers, 399–400
Fats, saturated, and ischemic heart disease mortality, 38
Fatty acids
  and beta blockers, 127, 400
  and myocardial oxygen consumption, 5
Fatty streaks, 12
Fendiline, 139
Fibrinogen, 15
First-pass effect, 210
5-ISMN. *See* Isosorbide-5 mononitrate
Flunarizine, 138
Food and Drug Administration (FDA), and beta blockers, 178, 179

Gastrointestinal (GI) effects, of beta blockers, 404
Geriatrics, and calcium channel antagonists, 216–217
GISSI study, 61, 485, 487
Glaucoma
  and nitrates, 380
  timolol for, 182, 188, 398, 401
Glucose-insulin-potassium infusion, for myocardial infarction, 58
Goteborg Intravenous Metoprolol Trial, 334, 342, 345, 347
Guanine nucleotide regulatory protein, 99, 102, 106

Guanylate cyclase, 84, 153–154, 155, 156, 167–168, 382, 384

H-2 antagonists, beta blockers in interaction with, 414
Hallucinations, from beta blockers, 402–403
Headache
  migraine, 98, 208
  and nitrate administration, 370, 374, 376–377, 442
  nitroglycerin, 443
  and nitrate tolerance, 382
Health awareness education, and ischemic heart disease mortality, 38
Heart rate
  and beta blockers, 120–122, 128, 195, 262, 264, 277
  and calcium channel antagonists, 301
  diltiazem, 297
  verapamil, 297
  and nitrates, 251, 374
  and silent myocardial ischemia, 279
Heart work, 2–3
  variation in, 5
Heberden, Dr. William, 17, 40, 41
Heparin
  and intravenous nitroglycerin, 381
  with tissue plasminogen activator, 62
  for unstable angina, 21, 54
High-risk groups
  detection of, 21
  with ischemic heart disease, 40
  for revascularization, 477–479
His-Purkinje system, 129, 130
History, and ischemic heart disease, 41–42
Holland Interuniversity Nifedipine/Metoprolol Trial Research Group (HINT), 276, 362
Hyaluronidase, for myocardial infarction, 58
Hydralazine
  and beta blockers, 412
  and nitrates, 376
  and ventricular function, 435
Hydrochlorthiazide, diltiazem compared with, 300
Hypercholesterolemia, 42
Hyperglycemia, from beta blockers, 401–402

INDEX 513

Hypertension
    and angina therapy, 457
    and atenolol, 196–197
    and beta blockers, 98, 179, 194, 457
        with hydralazine, 412
        with ISA, 118
    calcium channel antagonists for, 208, 296–301, 446, 457
    and coronary artery disease, 42
    and diminished vascular flow reserve, 15–16
    and ischemic heart disease mortality, 38
    labetalol for, 120
    metoprolol for, 196
    nadolol for, 197
    nitroglycerin (intravenous) for, 327
    and nitroprusside treatment, 324
    oxprenolol for, 198
    and peripheral resistance, 190
    and pregnancy, 408–409
    propranolol for, 195–196
    rebound
        and beta blockers, 411
        from beta blocker withdrawal, 407–408, 444
    and sexual dysfunction, 404–405
    timolol for, 197
Hypertension, pulmonary
    calcium channel antagonists for, 208
    and diastolic blood flow in right coronary artery, 7
    and nitrate action, 85
Hyperthyroidism
    and angina therapy, 459
    beta blockers for, 98
    and beta receptors, 114
Hypertrophic cardiomyopathy
    and angina, 40
    and beta blockers, 123
    and calcium channel antagonist withdrawal, 431
    and diminished vascular flow reserve, 15–16
    obstructive, 3
Hypoglycemia, and beta blockers, 127, 401–402, 409, 459
Hypoglycemics, beta blockers in interaction with, 415
Hypokalemia, 119
Hypotension
    from beta blockers, 396, 407, 444
    from beta blocker/verapamil combination, 455
    from nitrate therapy, 54, 377, 378, 379, 442
    and nitroglycerin for acute myocardial infarction, 67
    and streptokinase, 61

Idocyanopindolol, and competitive binding, 105
Imaging, myocardial, 41, 44–45
Incipient heart failure, and beta blockers, 273, 274
Indomethacin, 157, 410
Infarct expansion, and nitroglycerin (intravenous), 325–326
Infarct size
    and beta blockers, 332
    and calcium channel antagonists, 356–357, 358, 359, 360, 361, 363
Infusion bags, and nitroglycerin absorption, 159
Inmoldipine, 295
Insoldipine, 295
Insulin, and beta blockers, 127, 415
Interactions. See Drug interactions
Intermediate syndrome, 19
Intermittent claudication, calcium channel antagonists for, 208
Intracardiac dimension, and nitroglycerin, 87
Intracellular ionized calcium, and nitrate action, 85
Intravenous nitroglycerine, 310
    and acute myocardial infarction in canine model, 319
    clinical trial of longer-term infusion, 314–316
    vs. nitroprusside, 324
    other clinical trials, 316–319
    recommendations for use, 326–327
    short-term hemodynamic responses, 310–313
    adverse effects of, 380–381
    for congestive heart failure, 327
    for hypertension, 327
    indications for, 310
    and infarct expansion/left ventricular modeling, 325–326
    for ischemic rest chest pain, 251
    and nitrate tolerance, 252, 387

Intravenous nitroglycerine, *(continued)*
  and nitroprusside
    and blood pressure lowering, 321
    and regional myocardial blood flow, 319–32
  pharmacokinetics of, 158, 159–160
  for postinfarction unstable angina, 327
  and PTCA or CABG surgery, 485
Intravenous thrombolytic therapy, in emergency room treatment, 326
Intrinsic sympathomimetic activity (ISA), 118
  of beta blockers, 118–119, 120, 180–181, 188–190, 444
    and cardiac output, 122
    and cold hands or feet, 399
    and heart rate, 121
Irreversible myocardial ischemia, 24
ISA. *See* Instrinsic sympathomimetic activity
Ischemic but still viable myocardium, detection of, 44–45
Ischemic cardiomyopathy, 28–29, 40
Ischemic heart disease. *See* Myocardial ischemia
Ischemic rest chest pain, intravenous NTG for, 251
Isoprenaline, 397
Isoproterenol
  and beta blockers, 99, 192–193
  and cardioselective agents, 119
  and competitive binding, 105
  structure-activity of, 116, 117
Isosorbide dinitrate (ISDN), 152, 242, 243
  for angina (combination), 448–449, 449, 456, 457
  chewable, 236
  develoment of tolerance with, 375
  intravenous, 162, 251
  nifedipine compared with, 289
  and nitrate tolerance, 387
  oral, 163–164, 239, 241, 243, 244, 245, 443
  as oral spray, 236
  pharmacokinetics of, 158, 162–164, 165
  with propranolol, 272
  and stenosis enlargement, 91
  structure of, 153

sublingual, 163, 236, 237–238, 241, 272
  sustained release or retard forms of, 242–43, 387
  transdermal, 66, 162–163
Isosorbide-5 mononitrate (5-ISMN), 152
  pharmacokinetics of, 158, 164–165
  structure of, 153
  sustained release, 387
Isradipine, 208
  absorption of, 210
  for angina (combination), 449
  and cimetidine, 221
  with digoxin, 219, 220
  and geriatrics, 217
  and liver disease, 216
  metabolism of, 212
  pharmacokinetic parameters of, 209
  and renal disease, 217
Italian Group for the Study of Streptokinase in Myocardial Infarction, 61

Johns Hopkins Hospital, studies at, 310, 325, 360

Katenserin, 15
Kinetic work, 2–3

Labetalol, 120, 263, 268, 271
  absorption characteristics of, 182
  and alpha blockade, 191
  ancillary properties of, 180, 187
  clonidine in interaction with, 411
  dosage of (angina), 263, 274
  and hypertension, 194
  indications for, 179
  molecular structure of, 117
  and myocardial ischemia, 279
  and serum lipids, 127
Laboratory investigation, for ischemic heart disease, 41
Lactate, 6, 16
Laplace's law, 3
Laser angioplasty, 53
Left main coronary artery stenosis, 40
Left main coronary obstruction or disease, 468, 469, 471, 473
Left ventricular (dys)function
  and angina therapy, 457–458
  for unstable angina, 56
  and beta blocker (plus nifedipine), 451

INDEX 515

and calcium channel antagonists, 458
  diltiazem, 433–434
  nicardipine, 435–436
  nifedipine, 434–435
  nifedipine (plus beta blocker), 451
and combination therapy, 455
as mortality indicator, 350, 464–465, 467
and myocardial-infarction necrosis, 58
and nitrates, 243, 372, 373
  nitroglycerin, 311–312, 313, 314
  nitroprusside, 323
and phenylephrine, 312–313
and postinfarction period, 337
and revascularization, 490
and surgery (with triple-vessel disease), 470, 471
and verapamil, 432
Left ventricular remodeling, and intravenous nitroglycerin, 324–326
Left ventriculography, 45
Levobunolol
  ancillary properties of, 180, 188
  indications for, 179
Lidocaine
  beta blockers in interaction with, 411
  and calcium channel antagonist therapy, 436–437
Lidoflazine, 138
Life-style alterations, 330
Ligand binding, 103, 104
Lipid-lowering agents, 330
Lipid solubility, and beta blockers, 182–183
Liver disease or dysfunction
  and calcium channel antagonists, 214–216
  and pharmacokinetics of nitrates, 165–166
  and propranolol, 191
Lung disease, obstructive, 119–120. *See also* Pulmonary disease, chronic obstructive

Membrane stabilizing activity, of beta blockers, 130–131, 180–181, 187–188, 407
Mepindolol, ancillary properties of, 180

Metabolic effects, of beta blockers, 127
Metabolism (biotransformation)
  anaerobic, 16
  of beta blockers, 183–187
  of calcium channel antagonists, 212
Methemoglobinemia, and NTG/nitrates, 380–381
Methimazole, beta blockers in interaction with, 418
Methopranolol, for angina (combination), 449
Methyldopa
  beta blockers in interaction with, 412
  and Raynaud's phenomenon, 399
Methylxanthines, beta blockers in interaction with, 415
Metoprolol (Lopressor), 100, 263, 268, 269, 345
  absorption characteristics of, 182
  acute studies with, 266, 267, 268
  adverse effects of, 400, 403, 403–404
  ancillary properties of, 181, 187, 190, 191
  for angina, 196, 444
  for angina (combination), 448, 452, 455, 456
  antiarrhythmic effects of, 194
  bioavailability of, 178
  and blood glucose recovery, 273
  as cardioselective, 119
  distribution of, 182
  dosing of, 196, 263, 274
  and hypertension, 300
  indicators for, 179
  interactions with
    antiarrhythmics, 411
    calcium channel antagonists, 413
    cimetidine, 414, 415
    epinephrine, 418
    estrogen contraceptives, 418
    hydralazine, 412
    methimazole or propylthiouracil, 418
    pentobarbital, 413
    ranitidine, 414–415, 416, 417
    rifampin, 413
    theophylline, 416
  metabolism of, 186–187
  molecular structure of, 117

Metoprolol (Lopressor),
  (continued)
  and myocardial infarction, 332, 333, 334, 335–336, 339, 342, 349, 362
  and myocardial ischemia, 279, 331
  nifedipine compared with, 276
  and platelet aggregation, 126
  and post-myocardial infarction, 345
  and propranolol, 271, 400
  and serum concentration, 193
  and serum lipids, 127
  and verapamil, 223, 433
MIAMI Trial, 336
Migraine headaches
  beta blockers for, 98
  calcium channel antagonists for, 208
Minoxidil, and nitrates, 376
Mitral regurgitation
  acute, 27
  nitrates for, 457
  in physical examination, 42
  and propranolol, 331
Mixed angina pectoris, 22, 234, 252–253
  beta blockers for, 278
  nitrates for, 234
  nitrates and beta blockers for, 447–448
  and therapy approach, 38
Molsidomine, 152
  structure of, 153
Monday morning syndrome, 376
Morbidity, for ischemic heart disease, 2
Mortality rates, 48
  for acute myocardial infarction, 25–26, 39
  from ischemic heart disease, 2, 38
  from myocardial infarction, 38
  for PTCA, 51
Multicenter Diltiazem Postinfarction Trial Research Group, 361–362
Multicenter International Study, 343, 347
Muscle fatigue, from beta blockers, 399–400
Myocardial blood flow, nitroglycerine vs. nitroprusside effects on, 320–321
Myocardial disease, hypertrophic
  calcium channel antagonists for, 208
Myocardial hypoxia, 2

Myocardial imaging, 41, 44–45
Myocardial infarction, 38, 58–67, 330
  and beta blockers, 98, 195
  and electrocardiogram, 42
  as ischemic-heart-disease syndrome, 40
  metoprolol for, 196
  pathophysiology of, 20–21
  periods of, 347
  propranolol for, 195–196
  secondary intervention for, 330
  silent, 23. *See also* Silent ischemia
  timolol for, 197
  and unstable angina, 19–20
Myocardial infarction, acute, 24–28, 39, 464
  and adrenergic activity, 330
  beta blockers for, 458
    atenolol, 197, 333
    effects on mortality, 338–344
    effects on short-term mortality, 334–338
    and post-infarction period, 331–334, 347–350
    and prevention, 331
    rationale in, 330–331
    studies on individual agents, 344–346
  calcium channel antagonists in, 356–367
  as ischemic-heart-disease syndrome, 47
  from nitrate dependence, 376
  nitroglycerin (intravenous) for, 310–319, 326–327
  nitroprusside in, 322–324
  treatment strategy for, 27
Myocardial infarction, evolving, 485–486
  coronary artery bypass graft surgery for, 486–487, 489, 494
  percutaneous transluminal coronary angioplasty for, 487–489, 494
Myocardial ischemia (ischemic heart disease), 2, 9–11, 482–483
  and beta blockers, 127, 331, 334, 458
  calcium channel antagonists for, 208, 288
    bepridil, 295–296
    nicardipine (Japan), 294
  clinical syndromes of, 40. *See also specific syndromes*
  deaths from, 38

INDEX

evaluation of patient with, 39–45
irreversible, 24
and nicardipine, 295
nitrates for, 81, 91. *See also*
  Nitrates; Nitroglycerin
pathogenesis of, 12–16
prognosis of, 40
results of, 11
reversible, 15–23
silent, 22–23, 42, 252, 278–279,
  293–294. *See also* Silent
  ischemia
transient, 465, 466–467
Myocardial ischemia, therapy for, 45–47
  chronic stable angina, 47–53
  myocardial infarction, 58–67
  unstable angina, 53–58
Myocardial oxygen consumption
  (uptake), 2–5
  and blood flow, 89
  and catecholamines, 330
  and nitroglycerin, 88
  in resting (basal) state, 3
Myocardial oxygen demand
  (requirement), 9, 47
  and beta blockers, 123–124, 127, 330
  and beta blocker withdrawal, 408, 444
  and diltiazem, 292
  and myocardial-infarction treatment, 67
  and nitrates, 87–89
  and unstable angina, 19–20
Myocardial oxygen supply, 5–8, 10, 47. *See also* Coronary blood flow
  and angina, 19
  and beta blockers, 124–126
  and myocardial ischemia, 9, 10
  silent, 278
  and unstable-angina therapy, 53
Myocardium, working, 129

Nadolol (corgard), 100, 263, 268
  absorption characteristics of, 182
  ancillary properties of, 181
  for angina, 197, 444
  for angina (combination), 456
  distribution of, 182
  dosing for, 197, 263, 274
  indications for, 179
  interactions with
    cimetidine, 414
    hydralazine, 412
  metabolism of, 185
  molecular structure of, 117
  and propranolol, 271
National Heart, Lung and Blood
  Institute (NHLBI)
  Cooperative Study of, 479, 480–481
  and PTCA, 51, 473, 481
  trial sponsored by, 55
Nausea, from nitrates, 379
Neonates, weight of, and beta
  blockers, 190
Nervous system, adrenergic. *See*
  Adrenergic nervous system
Neurohormonal compensation, and
  nitrate tolerance, 168
Neurohormonal influences, 142
  and nitrate tolerance, 384
Neuromuscular side effects, from
  beta blockers, 405
NHLBI. *See* National Heart, Lung
  and Blood Institute
Nicardipine dihydropyrine, 138, 141,
  208, 294
  absorption of, 210
  adverse effects of, 295, 437
  and cimetidine, 221–222
  with digoxin, 219, 220
  and geriatrics, 217
  and liver disease, 216
  metabolism of, 212
  and myocardial infarction (acute), 358
  pharmacokinetic parameters of, 209
  and renal disease, 217
  and silent ischemia, 293
  and vasodilation, 143
  and ventricular function, 435–436
  withdrawal from, 430
Nicorandil, 152
  structure of, 153
Nifedipine, 19, 138, 139, 140, 141, 208
  absorption of, 210–211
  adverse effects of, 437
  for angina, 445
    exertional, 292
    rest, 289
  for angina (combination), 449, 451–453, 455, 456, 457
  atenolol with, 273
  and beta blockers, 272, 413
  and blood flow, 143
  and cimetidine, 221

Nifedipine, *(continued)*
  clinical effects of, 213
  comparisons of, 272, 276–277, 294
  and coronary artery disease, 290
  and diabetes mellitus, 459
  with digoxin, 219, 220
  dose alterations of, 215
  and geriatrics, 216
  and heart rate, 145
  and hypertension, 296, 297, 298, 299, 300, 301
  and infarct expansion, 326
  inotropic influence of, 142, 143
  and liver disease, 216
  metabolism of, 212
  and myocardial infarction (acute), 357, 358, 359–360, 363, 365
  and nitroglycerin, 166
  pharmacokinetic parameters of, 209
  potential interactions of, 223
  with propranolol, 273
  protein binding for, 211
  and quinidine, 222
  and Raynaud's phenomenon, 459
  and renal disease, 217
  and silent ischemia, 293–294, 294
  in tablet, 211
  and ventricular function, 434–435, 436, 458
  and ventricular relaxation, 144
  withdrawal from, 428, 429
NIH Cooperative Study in Animal Models for Protecting Ischemic Myocardium, 358
Nimodipine, 138, 208
  and cimetidine, 221–222
  and geriatrics, 217
  and liver disease, 216
  metabolism of, 212
  pharmacokinetic parameters of, 209
  and renal disease, 217
Nisoldipine, 141
Nitrate concentration, plasma, and antianginal effects, 66
Nitrate dependence, 376, 379
Nitrates, 81–82, 152, 234
  and acute myocardial infarction, 27
  adverse effects of, 370, 374–379, 380–381, 442, 447
  for angina, 38, 81, 85, 442–443, 447–451, 456–457
    stable, 18, 234–249
    unstable, 21, 56, 250–252, 480
    variant, 22, 277

  antiplatelet activity of, 92
  and beta blockers
    combined with, 242, 251, 272, 277, 447–449, 456–457
    compared with, 242, 271–272
    in interaction with, 374, 376
  biochemical mechanisms of, 152–157
  and bronchospasm, 458
  and calcium channel antagonists
    combined with, 125, 242
    compared with, 242
    in interaction with, 376
  chemical structures of, 49
  cellular mechanisms of action of, 82–85
  central or coronary arterial effects of, 89–92
  dose-response actions of, 80
  idiosyncratic reactions from, 379–380
  indications for, 457
  interactions with, 374, 376
    beta blockers, 166, 374, 376
    calcium channel antagonists, 376
  for mixed angina, 253
  modulators for, 370
    concomitant drug therapy, 374
    dosage, 373–374
    left ventricular function status, 372
    nitrate tolerance, 374
    reflex sympathetic discharge, 370, 372
    vascular reactivity, 372–373
  nitroglycerin, 152. *See also* Nitroglycerin
  oral, 243
  and PTCA or CABG surgery, 485
  for silent myocardial ischemia, 252, 278
  specific mechanisms of action of, 84, 85–92
  topical (adverse effects), 381
  as transdermal discs, 241
  use of (short-acting), 236
  withdrawal syndrome for, 379–380, 428, 431
Nitrate tolerance, 249, 381–384
  avoidance of, 249, 250, 387–390
    through dosage, 168, 387–388
    through nitrate-free interval, 388–390
  biochemical mechanism of, 166–168

INDEX 519

cellular mechanisms of, 382, 384
clinical studies on, 384, 386
and ISDN, 375
as modulator, 374
and nitroglycerin
  for infarct expansion, 326
  intravenous, 252
  patches, 246, 443
pharmacokinetic alterations with, 384
and transdermal NTG patches, 382, 383, 386–387, 388, 389
venous vs. arterial, 384, 385, 388
Nitrendipine, 141
Nitric oxide, 154, 155, 156, 157
Nitrogen oxide-containing vasodilators (nitrovasodilators), 154, 155
Nitroglycerin, 46, 80–82, 152
adverse effects of, 374, 377, 379, 380–381, 443
for angina, 83, 86, 161, 443, 446
  stable, 16, 47–48, 235, 236–237, 238, 239, 240, 241, 242, 243, 246–248
  unstable, 54, 56, 251–252
  for angina (combination), 448, 456
buccal or transmucosal, 161, 236, 238, 239, 241, 242, 248, 251, 443
cellular mechanisms of action of, 82–84
central or coronary arterial effects of, 89–92
fear of, 241–242
intravenous, 158, 159–160, 310–319. See also Intravenous nitroglycerin
and liver blood flow, 166
loss in potency of, 236–237
for myocardial infarction, 58
and nitric oxide formation, 156
as ointment, 87, 161, 241, 243, 246, 314, 443, 456
oral, 162, 241, 243, 449–450
as oral spray, 161, 236, 237, 238, 240, 241
peripheral effects of, 85–89
pharmacokinetics of, 158, 159–162, 165
for silent myocardial ischemia, 252
structure of, 153

sublingual, 235, 236, 236–237, 241. See also Sublingual nitroglycerin
transdermal (patches or disks), 160–161, 246–248
  for angina, 86, 443
  and nitrate tolerance, 382, 383, 386–387, 388, 389
  problems with, 381
use of (short-acting), 236
Nitroprusside
  and guanylate cyclase, 154
  for myocardial infarction, 58, 322–324
  blood pressure lowering, 321
  hemodynamic effects, 312
  and ventricular function, 435
  withdrawal syndrome associated with, 430
Nitrovasodilators, mechanisms of, 57
Nonatherosclerotic ischemic heart disease, 14–15
Noncompliance, and combination therapy, 446
Norepinephrine, 98, 99
  and arterial pressure, 372
  and competitive binding, 105
  and myocardial ischemia, 114–115
Normal coronary circulation, and nitroglycerin, 89, 90
Norwegian Multicenter Timolol Study, 340, 343, 345, 347, 348
Norwegian Nifedipine Multicenter Trial, 360
Norwegian Propranolol Trials, 348
NTG. See Nitroglycerin

Obstructive lung disease, reversible, and cardioselective beta blockers, 119–120
Optimal medical therapy, 467
Oral contraceptives, beta blockers in interaction with, 418
Oral nitrates, 243. See also under specific medications
Overdosage, with beta blockers, 407
Oxprenolol, 263, 271, 346
  absorption characteristics of, 182
  acute studies with, 265–266, 267
  adverse effects of, 405, 408
  ancillary properties of, 181, 187, 188, 189, 190–191
  and angina, 270
  dosing schedule for, 198

Oxprenolol, *(continued)*
  and hypertension in pregnancy, 409
  indications for, 179
  interactions with
    hydralazine, 412
    indomethacin, 410
    methyldopa, 412
  membrane stabilizing of, 130
  molecular structure of, 117
  and myocardial infarction, 338, 346, 348, 349
Oxygen consumption of heart. *See* Myocardial oxygen consumption
Oxygen demand of heart. *See* Myocardial oxygen demand
Oxygen supply, myocardial. *See* Myocardial oxygen supply
Oxygen wastage, 5

Pacemaker tissue, and beta blockers, 128
Pametolol, 406
Paroxysmal supraventricular tachycardia (PSVT), and beta blockers, 128
Pathogenesis, of ischemic heart disease, 12–16
Patient history, and ischemic heart disease, 41–42
Penbutolol, 268
  ancillary properties of, 181
  indications for, 179
Pentobarbital, beta blockers in interaction with, 413
Peptic ulcer disease, and calcium channel antagonist therapy, 222
Percutaneous transluminal coronary angioplasty (PTCA), 38, 39, 46, 327, 464
  for angina
    due to coronary spasm, 483, 485, 494
    stable, 471, 473–476, 494
    stable (chronic), 51–53
    unstable, 55–56, 56, 57, 481–482, 494
  high-risk groups in, 477–479
  for myocardial infarction, 59, 63–65, 67, 487–489, 494
  vs. other therapies, 495
  patients unsuitable for, 456

  and postmyocardial infarction, 491–492
  and repeat revascularization, 477
  and silent ischemia, 493, 494
Perfusion pressure, 6, 8, 47
Perioperative infarction, 48, 49
Peripheral vascular disease, 42
  and beta blockers, 444
    cardioselective, 119–120
    labetalol, 120
  and beta blockers with ISA, 118
Peripheral vascular effects, from beta blockers, 398–399
Pharmacodynamics, of beta blockers
  adverse effects, 194
  antianginal effects, 193
  antiarrhythmic effects, 194
  and beta blockade, 192–193
  dosing guidelines, 194–195
  dosing schedules, 195–198
  and hypertension, 194
  plasma concentrations or dose-response relationships, 191–192
Pharmacokinetics, 157–158, 191–192, 208
  of beta blockers
    absorption, 178, 182
    distribution, 182–183
    metabolism (biotransformation) and elimination, 183–187
  of calcium channel antagonists
    classic, 208–212
    clinical, 213–214
  classic, 208
  clinical, 208
  and drug interactions, 410
  of nitrates, 157–158
    and disease states, 165–166
    in interaction with other drugs, 166
    isosorbide dinitrate, 162–164
    isosorbide-5 mononitrate, 164–165
    nitroglycerin, 159–162
Pharmacologic stress testing, 43
Phenylephrine, and nitroglycerin anti-ischemic study, 312–313
Phosphorylation, of beta receptor, 110
Physical examination, 42
Pindolol, 100, 263, 268, 270, 271, 346
  absorption characteristics of, 182
  adverse effects of, 403, 403–404

ancillary properties of, 181, 187, 188, 189, 190
for angina, 444
for angina (combination), 448
and beta receptor density, 113
comparison of, 272
and congestive heart failure, 189
elimination of, 183
and hypertension in pregnancy, 409
indications for, 179
interactions with
  cimetidine, 414
  indomethacin, 410
  lidocaine, 411
ISA of, 118
membrane stabilizing of, 130
and myocardial infarction, 346, 349
nifedipine compared with, 293–294
and platelet aggregation, 126
and serum concentration, 193
and serum lipids, 127
Plaques, 12, 14
fissuring or rupture of, 15
  and sudden cardiac death, 27, 28
  and thrombus, 24
  and unstable angina, 19–20, 53
Plasma nitrate concentration, and antianginal effects, 66
Plastics, and nitroglycerin absorption, 159
Platelet activating factor, 14
Platelet aggregation, 23
  and beta blockers, 126–127
  and calcium channel antagonists, 293
  and coronary artery spasm, 14
  intermittent, 15, 22
  and myocardial infarction (acute), 58
  and nitrates, 92
  and propranolol, 408
  and sudden cardiac death, 27, 28
  and unstable angina, 19, 39, 53, 250
Platelet occlusion, intermittent, in silent myocardial ischemia, 278, 279
Poiseuillie's law, 9
Positron-emission tomography (PET), 44
Postinfarction angina, 19
  intervention required in, 27

unstable (nitroglycerin for), 327
and verapamil, 361
Postmyocardial infarction, 489–490
and angina therapy, 458
and coronary artery bypass graft surgery, 490–491
and percutaneous transluminal coronary angioplasty, 491–492
Potassium, 6
Practolol, 263, 269, 270–271
  acute studies with, 265–266, 267
  adverse effects of, 349, 404, 405, 406–407
  ancillary properties of, 181
  and myocardial infarction, 338, 348, 349
Practolol Multicenter Trial, 348
Practolol Syndrome, 406–407
Prazosin, 100
  beta blockers in interaction with, 412
Pregnancy, beta blockade in, 408–409
Preinfarction angina, 19
Prenylamine, 138
Pressure work, 2–3
Prinzmetal's angina, 22. *See also* Variant angina pectoris
  and beta blockade, 125
  and nitrates, 91–92
Procainamide, and calcium channel antagonist therapy, 436–437
Pronethalol, 405–406
Propranolol, 100, 263, 268, 269, 270–271, 275–276, 344
  absorption characteristics of, 182
  acute studies with, 265–266, 267
  adverse effects of, 277, 399, 400, 403, 403–404, 405, 408
  ancillary properties of, 181, 187, 188, 189, 190, 190–191
  for angina, 193
  for angina (combination), 448, 451, 452, 453, 455, 456, 457
  antiarrhythmic effects of, 188, 194
  and binding, 103
  bioavailability of, 178
  and blood glucose recovery, 273
  cardiac selectivity of, 121
  comparisons with, 271, 272, 275–276, 277, 293, 400
  and competitive binding, 105
  and coronary artery size, 125
  and diltiazem/verapamil, 223, 273, 275–276

Propranolol, *(continued)*
  distribution of, 182
  and dose-response curve, 192
  dosing of, 195–196, 263, 274, 444
  and hypertension, 194, 300
    in pregnancy, 409
  and hypertension plus angina, 301
  indications for, 179
  interactions with
    antiarrhythmics, 411
    cimetidine, 414
    epinephrine, 418
    hydralazine, 412
    indomethacin, 410
    insulin, 415
    methimazole or propylthiouracil, 418
    methyldopa, 412
    procainamide, 411
    rifampin, 413
    theophylline, 416
  and ISA, 118
  and isosorbide dinitrate, 272
  membrane stabilizing activity of, 130
  metabolism of, 185–186
  and myocardial infarction, 332, 334, 338, 339–340, 341, 343, 348, 349
  and myocardial ischemia, 279, 331
  nifedipine combined with, 273, 294
  and nitroglycerin anti-ischemic study, 312–313
  nonspecific effects of, 127
  oral, 446
  and pindolol, 270
  and platelet aggregation, 126–127
  for postmyocardial infarction, 344–345
  and serum concentration, 193
  structure-activity of, 116, 117
  verapamil combined with, 294, 433
  withdrawal of (abrupt), 113
Propylthiouracil, beta blockers in interaction with, 418
Prostaglandins, 6
  and antiplatelet action, 92
  and nitrates, 85, 157
Protons, 6
Pro-urokinase, 63
PTCA. *See* Percutaneous transluminal coronary angioplasty
Pulmonary disease, chronic obstructive
  and angina therapy, 458
  and timolol adverse effects, 401

Quinidine, drug interactions of
  and beta blockers, 411
  calcium channel antagonists, 222–223
Q wave infarct, 24
Q waves, 25, 42, 58, 332

Ranitidine, beta blockers in interaction with, 414–415, 416, 417
Rauwolseine, 100
Raynaud's phenomenon
  and angina therapy, 459
  and beta blockers, 399
  and beta blockers with ISA, 118
  calcium channel antagonists for, 208
  and intrinsic sympathomimetic activity, 190
  and labetalol, 120
Receptor adenylate cyclase system, 99–108
Recombinant tissue-type plasminogen activator (rtPA), for acute myocardial infarction, 27
Reflex sympathetic discharge, and nitrates, 370, 372
Regional circulations, and nitrates, 86
Regulatory protein, 106
Reinfarction
  and beta blockers, 340, 342
  verapamil for, 361
Renal actions, of calcium channel antagonists, 297
Renal disease or failure
  and acebutolol or diacetolol, 184
  and atenolol, 185, 197
  and calcium channel antagonists, 217
  and metoprolol, 186
  and nadolol, 185, 197
  and pharmacokinetics of nitrates, 166
  and propranolol, 186, 191
  and timolol, 185
Renin-angiotension-aldosterone
  effects of calcium channel antagonists, 297, 299

INDEX 523

Reperfusion therapy, 39, 59, 67, 489
  coronary artery bypass graft surgery as, 39, 59. *See also* Coronary artery bypass graft surgery
  percutaneous transluminal coronary angioplasty as, 39, 63–65, 67. *See also* Percutaneous transluminal coronary angioplasty
  thrombolytic therapy as, 39, 59–63, 65. *See also* Thrombolytic therapy
Respiratory dysfunction, from beta blockers, 400–401
Rest angina. *See* Angina at rest
Restenosis, 477
Revascularization, 464. *See also* Coronary artery bypass graft (CABG) surgery; Percutaneous transluminal coronary angioplasty (PTCA)
  complete, 474
  decision regarding, 48, 56–57, 464, 464–467, 493
  repeat, 476–477
  and silent ischemia, 493
Reversible myocardial ischemia, 16–23
Rifampin
  beta blockers in interaction with, 413
  and verapamil, 223

Saturated fats, and ischemic heart disease mortality, 38
Scleroderma heart disease, spasm in, 14–15
Second International Study of Infarct Survival (ISIS-2), 61, 62
Serotonin, 15
Serum lipoproteins, and calcium channel antagonists, 293
Sexual dysfunction, from antihypertensive therapy, 404–405
Side effects. *See* Adverse effects
Silent myocardial infarction, 25
Silent (silent myocardial) ischemia, 23, 42, 235, 293, 492–493
  angina absent from, 40
  beta blockers for, 278–279
  calcium channel antagonists for, 293–294

as coronary-artery-disease syndrome, 464
diurnal variation of, 278–279
frequency of, 262
nitrates for, 234, 252
therapy for, 494
and transdermal nitroglycerin, 248
understanding of growing, 39
Single chain urokinase-type plasminogen activator (pro-urokinase), 63
Single photon-emission computed tomography (SPECT), 44
Skin reactions, and beta blockers, 404
Smoking (cigarettes)
  and angina, 431
  and ischemic heart disease mortality, 38
  and metoprolol, 416
  and propranolol, 186
S-nitrosothiols, 155–156, 167
Sodium nitroprusside. *See* Nitroprusside
Sotalol, 117, 263, 271, 346
  acute studies with, 265–266
  ancillary properties of, 181
  and angina, 270
  and hypertension in pregnancy, 409
  electrophysiologic activity of, 131
  and myocardial infarction, 332, 340, 346
Soterenol, and competitive binding, 103, 108
Spare receptors, 111–112
Spasm, coronary
  and acute myocardial infarction, 58
  and calcium channel antagonists, 290, 446
  and labetalol, 120
Spasm, coronary artery, 9, 14–15, 19, 20–21, 22
  angina due to, 482–485
  mixed, 22
  variant, 22, 38
  calcium channel antagonists for, 54, 288, 294
  calcium channel antagonists plus nitrates for, 449
  diltiazem for, 288
  and electrocardiogram, 43
  and nicardipine, 295

SPRINT Trial (Secondary Prevention Reinfarction Nifedipine Trial), 362
Stable angina pectoris, 17–19
  beta blockers in, 260–274
  calcium channel antagonists for, 272, 272–273
    nitrates for, 234–236, 272
      nitroglycerin, 17, 235, 236
    nitrates for (short-acting), 241
      isosorbide dinitrate (sublingual), 236, 237–238
      nitroglycerin, 235
      nitroglycerine (buccal), 236, 238, 239, 242
      nitroglycerin (fear of), 241–242
      nitroglycerin (oral spray), 236, 238, 240
      nitroglycerin (sublingual), 236, 236–237, 239
      utilization of, 236, 241
    treatment strategy for, 18–19, 235–236
Stable angina pectoris, chronic, 47–53
  beta blockers for, 47–48
    oxprenolol, 198
  calcium channel antagonists for, 47–48
  as ischemic-heart-disease syndrome, 40, 47
  nitrates for (long-acting), 242–243
    buccal nitroglycerin, 248
    dosing guidelines for, 241, 249, 250
    and nitrate tolerance, 249
    nitroglycerin, 47–48, 242, 243, 246–248
    oral, 243, 244, 245
    topical, 243, 246–248
  nitrates for (short-acting), as prophylaxis, 239, 241
  and revascularization, 464–468, 494
    coronary artery bypass graft surgery, 468–471, 472, 473, 474, 494
    high-risk groups, 477–479
    percutaneous transluminal coronary angioplasty, 471, 473–476, 494
    repeat revascularization, 476–477
Stage fright, beta blockers for, 98
Stenosis, aortic. See Aortic stenosis
Stenosis, coronary
  and angina, 40
  aortic, 15, 40
  and coronary blood flow, 7
  dilation of, 85
Stenosis, coronary arterial
  high risk from (left), 40
  nitroglycerin effects on, 90
Stenosis vasodilation, nitrates for, 91
Stereoisomers, 116, 126
Streptokinase
  for acute myocardial infarction, 27, 47, 60–61, 63, 64, 485–486, 487, 488
  and thrombolytic therapy, 46
  for unstable angina, 54
Stress, physical or mental, and myocardial contractility, 5
Stress testing, exercise, 43
Study design
  in evaluation of beta blockers in angina pectoris, 265
  and limitations of myocardial-infarction trials, 337–338
  and placebo effects (HINT), 276
Sublingual nitroglycerin, 235, 236, 236–237, 241
  adverse effects of, 378
  and alcohol, 374, 380
  for angina, 83, 443, 446
    stable, 16, 236–237
    stable (chronic), 242
    unstable, 56
  and beta blockers, 272
  and cavity size reduction, 87
  dosage for, 241
  effects of, 81, 83
  and headaches, 374, 376
  hemodynamic response to, 320, 372, 373
  lowering of content in, 159
  for myocardial infarction, 67
  and myocardial oxygen consumption, 87, 88
  and nitrate tolerance, 239, 386
  and oral spray, 238, 240
  plasma concentration rise from, 161
  regional circulatory responses to (dog), 371
  restoration of vascular responses to, 373
  and silent ischemia, 252
Sudden cardiac death, 27–28, 39
  and beta blockers for myocardial infarction, 342–344
Sulfhydryl (SH) groups, 84, 152–153, 155–156, 167, 384
Sulfinpyrazone, 410

INDEX

Sulindac, 410
Sympathomimetic activity, intrinsic.
    See Intrinsic sympathomimetic
    activity
Sympathomimetics, beta blockers in
    interaction with, 418
Syncope, from nitrates, 377–379
Syndrome X, 16

Tachycardia, 7
  and beta blockers, 412, 444
  from nifedipine, 434
  and nitrates, 447
  supraventricular
    and angina therapy, 458
    calcium channel antagonists for,
      208
    esmolol for, 197
    paroxysmal supraventicular
      (PSVT), 128
    propranolol for, 189
    verapamil for, 218
  and timolol, 398
  ventricular, 28, 130
Tachydysrhythmias, and calcium
    channel antagonist
    withdrawal, 431
Tension, 3
Tension time index (TTI), 3–5
TEVC (effective compliance of total
    vascular bed), 385
Thallium-201 scintigraphy, 41, 43, 44
Theophylline, beta blockers in
    interaction with, 415
Therapeutic drug monitoring, 192
Therapy for angina pectoris. See
    Angina pectoris drug therapy,
    approach to
Therapy for ischemic heart disease.
    See Myocardial ischemia,
    therapy for
Thrombolytic agents, for acute
    myocardial infarction, 27
Thrombolytic therapy, 39, 46
  for myocardial infarction, 59, 59–
    63, 65, 67
  nifedipine in concert with, 360
  for unstable angina, 21, 54–55, 56
Thrombosis. See also Coronary
    thrombosis
  and plaque fissuring, 24
  and unstable angina, 39, 480
Thromboxane A$_2$, 14
Thyroid hormones, beta blockers in
    interaction with, 418

Tiapamil, 138, 139
TIMI II Trial, 334, 342, 348
Timolol (blocadren), 263, 268, 345
  absorption characteristics of, 182
  adverse effects of, 188, 398, 401,
    402, 403, 404, 405,
  ancillary properties of, 181, 188
  dosing schedule for, 197
  indications for, 179
  interactions of
    hydralazine, 412
    pentobarbital, 413
  metabolism of, 185
  molecular structure of, 117
  and myocardial infarction, 332,
    339, 340, 342, 343, 345, 347,
    348, 349
  and platelet aggregation, 126
  and serum concentration, 193
Tissue plasminogen activator (tPA)
  in emergency room treatment, 326
  for myocardial infarction, 61–62,
    63
  for unstable angina (intravenous),
    54–55
Tolamolol, 263, 270–271, 406
  acute studies with, 266, 267
  ancillary properties of, 181
Topical nitrates, 243, 246–248
Transdermal nitroglycerin. See under
    Nitroglycerin
Transient myocardial ischemia
  and revascularization, 466–467
  risk from, 465
Tremor, beta blockers for, 98
Treppe phenomenon, 3

Unstable angina pectoris, 19–21, 38–
    39, 53–58, 249–250, 464, 479
  beta blockers in, 21, 54, 56, 274–
    277, 331, 480
    propranolol, 331, 275–276
  calcium channel antagonists for,
    363–365
    verapamil, 294
  as ischemic-heart-disease
    syndrome, 40, 47
  and myocardial ischemia, 235
  nitrates for, 21, 56, 250–252, 480
    nitroglycerin, 54, 56, 251–252
    postinfarction (intravenous
      nitroglycerin for), 327
  prognosis of, 53
  resting ECG with, 43

Unstable angina pectoris, *(continued)*
   revascularization for, 479–480
     coronary artery bypass surgery, 480–481, 482, 494
     percutaneous transluminal coronary angioplasty, 481–482, 494
   and silent ischemic events, 492
   and stable angina, 17
   therapy for, 54–56
   treatment strategy in, 21, 56–58
Uptake. *See* Myocardial oxygen consumption
Urokinase, for myocardial infarction, 62, 63

Valve replacement, aortic, 19
Variant (vasospastic) angina pectoris, 22, 483
   beta blockers in, 277–278
   and electrocardiogram, 43
   as ischemic-heart-disease syndrome, 40
   nifedipine in, 289, 294
   and nitrates, 91–92
   and stable angina, 18
   and therapy approach, 38
   treatment strategy for, 22
   verapamil in, 294
Vascular disease, peripheral. *See* Peripheral vascular disease
Vascular reactivity, and nitrates, 372–373
Vasoactive compounds, 6
Vasoconstriction, coronary
   and beta blockers, 54
   and emotional stress, 236
   and nitrates, 82, 91–92, 234, 235
     nitroglycerin, 89
   and nitrates-beta blocker combination, 447–448
   in silent myocardial ischemia, 278
Vasodilation, 6
   mechanisms of, 57, 155
   and nitrates, 85, 152
     nitroglycerin, 82
Vasodilation, arterial, and nitrates, 86–87
Vasodilation, arteriolar, and nitrates, 87, 89
Vasospasm, coronary
   and coronary blood tone, 47
   and nitrates, 82, 91–92, 379–380
   and unstable angina, 39, 53

Venodilation, from nitrates, 85–86
Ventricular arrhythmias, 40
   and beta blockers, 129–130
   in long Q-T syndrome, 129
   and sotalol, 131
   and spasm release, 22
Ventricular dysrhythmias, 458
Ventricular fibrillation, 28
   and epinephrine/norepinephrine, 114–115
   and postinfarction period, 336
Ventricular function
   and beta blockers, 123
   and calcium channel antagonists, 432–436
Ventricular function, left. *See* Left ventricular (dys)function
Ventricular remodeling, left, and intravenous nitroglycerin, 324–326
Ventricular tachycardia, 28, 130
Verapamil, 138, 139, 140, 141, 208
   absorption of, 210–211
   active metabolites of, 214
   adverse reactions to, 437
   for angina, 445
   for angina (combination), 449, 451, 453–455
   and arrhythmias, 458
   and beta blockers
     combined with, 223, 433
     compared with, 300
     in interaction with, 413
   binding of, 211
   and blood flow, 143
   and cimetidine, 221
   clinical effects of, 213
   contraindication for, 457–458, 458
   and coronary artery disease, 290
   and diabetes mellitus, 459
   with digoxin, 219–220, 223
   with diltiazem, 272–273
   dose alterations of, 215
   for exertional angina, 293
   and geriatrics, 217
   and heart rate, 145, 297, 301
   and hypertension, 296, 297, 299, 300
   and hypertension plus angina, 301
   inotropic influence of, 142
   and liver disease, 215–216
   metabolism of, 212
   and myocardial infarction (acute), 357, 358, 360–361, 362–363, 363

nifedipine compared with, 296
pharmacokinetic parameters of, 209
potential interactions of, 223
propranolol compared with, 272, 276
and quinidine, 222–223
and Raynaud's phenomenon, 459
and renal disease, 217
for rest angina, 289–290
and silent ischemia, 293, 294
in sustained-release formulation, 446
for tachycardia, 218
and ventricular function, 432–433, 436
and ventricular relaxation, 144, 145
withdrawal from, 428, 430
Veterans Administration Cooperative Study, 55, 322, 468, 470
Veterans Administration multicenter trial, 48

Wall stress, 3
Western Washington Randomized Trial, 486
Western Washington trial of intracoronary streptokinase, 60
Windkessel capacity, and nitroglycerine, 86
Withdrawal, 428
 of alcohol, 98
 of beta blockers, 113, 407–408, 428, 430, 444
  propranolol, 113
 of calcium channel antagonists, 428–431
 of clonidine, 411, 428, 430
 of nitrates, 379–380, 428, 431
  nitroprusside, 430
Working myocardium, and beta blockers, 129

Xantholasmas, 42
Xanthomas, 42

Yohimbine, 100